Advances in Imaging

Sikandar Shaikh

Advances in Imaging

Step Towards Precision Medicine

Springer

Sikandar Shaikh
Department of Radiodiagnosis
Shadan Institute of Medical Sciences
Hyderabad, India

ISBN 978-981-16-9534-6 ISBN 978-981-16-9535-3 (eBook)
https://doi.org/10.1007/978-981-16-9535-3

This Springer imprint is published by the registered company Springer Nature Singapore Pte Ltd.
The registered company address is: 152 Beach Road, #21-01/04 Gateway East, Singapore 189721, Singapore

ALMIGHTY GOD WHOSE BLESSINGS ARE ALWAYS THERE

MY PARENTS

MY WIFE

MY DAUGHTERS

MY MENTORS

MY TEACHERS

MY ANONYMOUS FRIEND AND WELL WISHER

MY ALL WELLWISHERS

ALL MY DEPARTMENT COLLEAGUES AND STAFF

ALL FRIENDS

MY PATIENTS BECAUSE OF WHOM I LEARNT THE ART OF MEDICINE AND STILL LEARNING EVERYDAY

Foreword

It gives me great pleasure to write a foreword for this second book by Dr Sikandar Shaikh on the ***Advances in Imaging—Step Towards Precision Medicine***. Medical Imaging has revolutionized in recent years due to the development of the technology, development of newer protocols and techniques, development of the biomarkers, molecular probes, and radiotracers. These advances are seen in all the modalities more so in relation to the Molecular Imaging. Ultrasound and Magnetic Resonance Imaging are the best examples of the transition from the anatomical to functional imaging having both the concepts of imaging. Hybrid Imaging is also playing an important role for the development of the newer technology, radiotracers, molecules, and biomarkers. These innovations have led to enhancing the concept of personalized medicine which allows for effective medical care and focussed applications for patients in preclinical stages, as well as clinical and serious diseases and disorders. The applications of these are seen in all the aspects of Oncology, Neurology, Cardiology, Infection and Inflammation, and many more. This book covers the basics of the Molecular Imaging Instrumentation, Molecular Imaging Biomarkers, Molecular Imaging in Oncology, Molecular Imaging in the Infection and Inflammation, Functional Imaging, Molecular Imaging in Precision medicine, PET-CT, PET-MR, Nanoimaging, Hypoxia Imaging, Amyloid Imaging, Translational Imaging, Multiparametric Imaging, Immunoimaging, Optical Imaging, Genetic Imaging, Stem Cell Imaging, Theranostics, Radiobiology, Robotic Imaging, Radiomics, QIBA Imaging, and Artificial Intelligence. All the applications of these imaging modalities are covered very meticulously for all possible preclinical and clinical applications. These will lead to significantly reduced morbidity and mortality world-wide. With the advances made in all the imaging modalities, it is feasible to scan within a short period of time non-invasively and quantify the underlying process with high precision and accuracy and increased disease specificity. Dr Sikandar Shaikh had described the importance of every modality and that imaging technique which is mentioned above and their critical role in various clinical applications for various pathologies. In this book, all the possible preclinical and clinical applications, their possible advantages and disadvantages over each other, possible side effects, and futuristic changes and challenges are explained in detail. This book will be an excellent guide for the quick reference for the Imaging specialists,

Radiologists, Molecular Imaging specialists, Nuclear Physicians, Scientists, Researchers, and all those involved in the Molecular imaging practice.

I have known Dr Sikandar Shaikh as a distinguished colleague and an academician par excellence in our discipline. He has been involved as a major contributor to many International Organizations. He is the current Secretary of the Indian College of Radiology. He is a President Elect of ISMRM India Chapter, an Indian Ambassador of the European Society of Hybrid Imaging, a Committee Member in World Molecular Imaging Society, Society of Paediatric Radiology, ISMRM International, European Society of Onco-imaging, and various National Indian Societies. He is a reviewer of AJR, BJR, European Radiology, JMRI, Radiology, Radiographics, Radiology Cardiothoracic Imaging, Frontiers in Oncology, and many more. He has made many presentations in various International and National Societies and has many publications in the International and National Journals. He already had written the book on *PET-CT in Infection and Inflammation* which was released in January 2021. He is also the Adjunct Professor in the Department of Biomedical Engineering at the prestigious Indian Institute of Technology, Hyderabad, India. This book in true sense will be a basic guide for the concept of the step towards the Precision Medicine. With this introduction, I wish him all the best for publishing this book and all his future endeavors.

26 September 2021

Abas Alavi, MD, MD(Hon), PHD(Hon), DSc (Hon)
University of Pennsylvania
Philadelphia, PA, USA

Foreword

Medical imaging of the human body achieved true proficiency from the discovery of the X-rays by Wilhelm Conrad Roentgen on November 8th, 1895, at the University of Würzburg and the recognition of their potential for diagnostic medicine. Medical imaging can be structured into morphological imaging for the assessment of anatomy, functional imaging for the assessment of physiological processes such as tissue perfusion or glucose metabolism as well as molecular imaging for the non-invasive characterization of tissues on a cellular level. Morphological imaging underwent dramatic change with the advent of CT and MRI allowing for the diagnostic assessment of whole-body gross anatomy in great detail. The added value of functional imaging techniques was quickly recognized with perfusion imaging in CT and MRI for stroke or myocardial imaging as well as diffusion-weighted imaging in oncological MRI. Functional PET imaging with the glucose analog ^{18}F-FDG for the assessment of cellular metabolism in oncology and inflammation imaging gained diagnostic significance with the availability of hybrid PET/CT scanners providing complementary morphological and functional diagnostic information side by side. The potential of molecular imaging in a complementing imaging concept with the non-invasive assessment of morphological, functional, and molecular information in vivo was recognized early on for preclinical and clinical imaging in precision medicine. Mainly preclinical molecular imaging techniques include optical fluorescence and bioluminescence imaging, optoacoustic imaging, or molecular ultrasound and play an important role for the preclinical development of drugs and companion image biomarkers. However, the translational gap for most functional and molecular imaging techniques remains hard to bridge particularly for reasons of standardization and validation. The broader clinical availability of novel molecular PET tracers for neurological and oncological imaging transforms PET today to a truly molecular imaging technique.

Multiparametric concepts for PET/MRI combine various morphological, functional, and molecular imaging parameters for the multi-faceted characterization of pathophysiology in vivo for clinical decision guidance in precision medicine. Radiomic features contribute alongside with ADC values and PET parameters to increase diagnostic accuracy and confidence. Prospectively, algorithm-based automated image analysis and the AI-driven warehousing of quantitative image parameter profiles have great potential to redefine the role of medical imaging in concert with digital pathology and liquid biopsy as a driver in clinical decision guidance increasing therapeutic efficiency and providing significant benefits for the patient.

26 September 2021

Clemens Cyran
Hybrid and Molecular Imaging, and Vice Chair
at the Department of Radiology
Ludwig-Maximilian's-University
Munich, Germany

Foreword

Whenever I think of humility, down to earth, knowledgeable person, I think of Dr. Sikandar. When I think of precise PET-CT science, astute knowledge of the subject, and impeccable work and research, I think of Dr. Sikandar. I think of Dr. Sikandar as a doctor, teacher, scientist, and writer of everything PET-CT. I was a professor of medicine in a small town in Maharashtra, when I came across Dr. Sikandar. Working with him was akin to working with a brilliant doctor who was precise, direct, and clever with his diagnosis. He had the ability to explain the most complex of medical problems in the easiest way. In the years I have known him ever since he is promoted a more humanistic and creative approach to the radiology in healthcare system. He is a visionary with a rare ability to express complex theories in the most eloquent manner. I strongly believe that Dr. Sikandar exemplifies the extraordinary trait of carrying medical expertise in his life and in his work. Over the years, as I got the opportunity to follow Dr. Sikandar's work, my respect and admiration for him have only grown. His compilations of research in the field of comprehensive Radiology have only provided me and the medical fraternity with scientific evidence to make a substantial difference in helping people recover from significant medical problems. I believe that his first book has stood as one of the foundational cornerstones for PET-CT in Infection and Inflammation. Now his second but first of this kind "*Advances in Imaging—Step Towards Precision Medicine*" will become a primary support model for evidence-based medicine. I wish him all the best in his every endeavor he is contemplating. I hope you have a wonderful time reading this book!

26 September 2021 Major Milind Bhrushundi, MD General Medicine
Nagpur, India

Preface

Medicine has been revolutionized in recent years to every aspect and the imaging is also the component of this revolution. The era of the anatomical imaging is being seen as transition to the functional and molecular imaging by the virtue of the various hybrid imaging modalities available. However, the future of the imaging is purely seen on the lines of the molecular imaging. And to these, various aspects of the technological revolution along with the research in the various specialties are going hand in hand for this revolution. This will become the blend of the various aspects of the Chemistry, Biology, Biochemistry, Pharmacology, Nuclear medicine, Physics, Electronics to the newer entities which are more focussed like Nanotechnology, Stem Cell research, Genetic Engineering, Biomedical Engineering, Medical Electronics, and various aspects of the blend of the subspecialties of each components mentioned above along with the various combinations used for different aspects of imaging. The molecular imaging which today is and what future will be entirely different. However, it doesn't mean that the existing imaging modalities role will be nullified. The important aspect of this will be seen as the single-shot tool shop for the medical diagnosis, investigations, follow-up after the treatment and also for the therapeutic role that is theranostics.

The various Molecular imaging components which are included in this book and discussed thoroughly are the Molecular Instrumentation, Biomarkers and Contrast Agents, Molecular Imaging in Oncology, Molecular Imaging in Infection and Inflammation, Functional Imaging, PET-CT, PET-MR, Nanoimaging, Hypoxia Imaging, Amyloid Imaging, Translational Imaging, Multiparametric Imaging, Optical Imaging, Stem cell Imaging, Immunoimaging, Gene Imaging, Robotic Imaging, Radiomics, Radiobiology, Theranostics, Artificial Intelligence, and QIBA. All these are used in various tumors, infections, and inflammations, metabolic conditions, neurological disorders, cardiac conditions, various pediatric conditions, traumatic injuries, and many other conditions where they can be used as therapeutic as well as diagnostic options. Many papers and research articles are available for the current concepts related with these modalities and agents. These are also being developed as the targeted to the disease like use of the DOPA for the Parkinsonism.

These are all under research to a very great extent and with the use of these modalities will redefine the concept of the imaging. This will be more focussed and precise to diagnose the preclinical stage as well as the non-clinical suspicion of these entities. The use of these imaging modalities will lead to more effective results and also aligning with the existing modalities so that it will be leading to the concept of the personalized medicine and which will be the basis of the precision medicine.

This book is written to stress on the various applications which will be having for the use of the specific molecular imaging modalities which are being covered in this book.

With these advancements, this book will give the comprehensive reference of the concept of the precision medicine and leading to the concept of the personalized medicine.

Hyderabad, India Sikandar Shaikh

Acknowledgements

Dr. Abas Alavi, MD, MD(Hon), PHD(Hon), DSc (Hon)
University of Pennsylvania, USA

Prof. Clemens Cyran
Professor of Radiology, Section Chief, Hybrid and Molecular Imaging, and Vice Chair at the Department of Radiology, Ludwig-Maximilian's-University Munich, Germany. President ESHI

Late Prof. Kakarla Subbarao, M.B.B.S, MS, FACR, FRCR, DSC (Hon)
Emeritus Professor of Radiology, Nizam's Institute of Medical Sciences, Hyderabad, India

Dr. Prabhakar Reddy, MD
Past President, Asia Oceania Society of Radiology (AOSR)
Past President, National Indian Radiological and Imaging Association (IRIA)
Vice President, Asian Musculoskeletal Society (AMS)

Dr. Anand Abkari, MD(RD), DMR, FICR, FAAMS
Professor Emeritus, Department of Radiodiagnosis, Deccan College of Medical Sciences, Hyderabad, India

Prof. Rammurthi. S., MD
Dean, Professor, and Head Department of Radiology and Imaging, Nizams Institute of Medical Sciences, Hyderabad, India

Dr. Hemant Patel, MD
Immediate Past President, National IRIA
Director, Gujarat Imaging Centre, Ahmedabad, India

Prof. C Amarnath
Professor and Head Department of Radiology, Immediate Past President, National IRIA

Dr. Nidhi Goyal
Senior Consultant Radiologist, Apollo Indraprastha Hospitals, New Delhi, India

Dr. Arvind Chaturvedi
Chair, Radiology and Interventional Oncology, Rajiv Gandhi Cancer Institute, New Delhi
President, Society of Oncoimaging, India

Prof. Mandapal. T.
Director and Head Department of Radiology, Care Hospitals Group, Banjara Hills, Hyderabad

Dr. Suresh Kawathekar

Retired Professor and Head Department of Radiology, MNR Medical College, Sanga Reddy, Hyderabad, India

Dr. Amit Kharat

Professor, Department of Radiology, Bharati Vidyapeeth Medical College, Pune, India

Dr. Amit Chaudhari

Assistant Professor, Department of Radiology, Tata Memorial Hospital, Mumbai

Dr. Madhur Shrivastava

Associate Professor, Department of Nuclear Medicine and PET-CT, Nizams Institute of Medical Sciences, Hyderabad, India

Doguparthi Suresh

Assistant Manager, Yashoda Hospitals, Somajiguda, Hyderabad

Mr. Madhu Mangal

Graphic Designer, New Delhi

Contents

About the Author

Sikandar Shaikh, DMRD, DNB, EdiR, MNAMS, FICR graduated from The B R Ambedkar Marathwada University, Aurangabad, Maharashtra, India. He is the Associate Professor, Shadan Institute of Medical Sciences, consultant PET-CT and radiology at Yashoda Hospitals, Somajiguda, Hyderabad, India. He has many international publications and has delivered more than 110 oral and posters presentations at various international meetings.

Dr. Sikandar is the president elect of ISMRM India Chapter. He is also Indian ambassador of European Society of Hybrid, Molecular and Translational Imaging (ESHI), research committee member of European Society of Oncoimaging (ESOI), education committee member of World Molecular Imaging Society (WMIS), oncoimaging committee member of International Society of Paediatric Radiology (SPR), governing council member of Society of Emergency Radiology (SER), Executive committee member of the Indian Society of Neuroradiology, ethics committee member at IIT Hyderabad, associate editor of JMRI (International Journal of MRI). He is the secretary of the Indian College of Radiology 2021–2023. He is the reviewer of many international radiology journals, such as *Radiographics, Radiology Cardiothoracic Imaging, Radiology Cancer Imaging, European Radiology, American Journal of Roentgenology*. He is member of various societies ESOI, SPR, ESCR, ESNR, ESSR, ESPR, ESER, RSNA, ISMRM, AMS, ESHNR and many more societies.

Abbreviations

μm	Micrometer
1H	1 hydrogen
11C-MET	11C methionine
111In	111 indium
123i	123 iodine
123I	Iodine 123
125i	125 iodine
129 XE	129 xenon
131I	Iodine 131
13C	13 carbon
15O	15 oxygen
18F-FACBC	18 fluciclovine
18F-FDOPA	18 fluorine dopamine
19F	19 fluorine
2D	2 dimensional
23Na	23 sodium
3 He	3 helium
3D	3 dimensional
31P	31 phosphorus
68Ga	Gallium 68
68Ga EDTA	[^{68}Ga] ethylenediaminetetraacetic acid
82RB	Rubidium 82
99mTC	99 m Technetium scan
AD	Alzheimer's disease
ADC	Apparent diffusion co-efficient
AFD	Anderson–Fabry disease
AI	Artificial intelligence
ANN	Artificial neural network
APDs	Avalanche photo diodes
APT	Amide proton transfer
ASL	Arterial spin labeling
ATM	Ataxia Telangiectasia Mutated
ATP	Adenosine triphosphate
AU	Gold
AUNP	Gold nanoparticle
BBB	Blood brain barrier
BCI	Brain computer interface

BGO	Bismuth Germanate
BIRADS	Breast imaging reporting and data system
BLI	Bioluminescence imaging
BOLD	Blood oxygen level dependent
BRCA	Breast cancer gene
BRCA1	Breast cancer gene 1
BRCA2	Breast cancer gene 2
BREF	Best Available Technique Reference
BRET	Bioluminescent resonance energy transfer
BSE	Bovine spongiform encephalopathy
CA	Contrast agent
CBD	Corticobasal degeneration
CBF	Cerebral blood flow
CBV	Cerebral blood volume
CCD	Charge coupled device
Cd	Cadmium
CD4+	CD4 cells
CD8+	CD 8 cells
CDN	Cyclic dinucleotide
CECT	Contrast enhanced computed tomography
CELSE	Cherenkov excited luminescence imaging
CEST	Chemical exchange saturation transfer
CEUS	Contrast enhanced ultrasound
CHO	Choline
CHT	Choline transporter
CJD	Creutzfeldt–Jakob disease
CLIO	Cross limb iron oxide
CNN	Convolutional neural network
CNR	Contrast to noise ratio
CNS	Central nervous system
CNT	Carbon nano tube
CO_2	Carbon dioxide
COPD	Chronic obstructive pulmonary disease
CRPC	Castrate-resistant prostate cancer
CSC	Cancer stem cell
CSF	Cerebrospinal fluid
CTE	Chronic traumatic encephalopathy
Cu	Copper
CuS	Copper sulfide
CXCR	CX Chemokine Receptor
CXCR4	C-X-C-R motif chemokine receptor 4
CZT	Cadmium zinc telluride
DAT	Dopamine transporter
DC	Dendritic cell
DCE MRI	Dynamic contrast-enhanced magnetic resonance imaging
DIP	Drug induced parkinsonism
DL	Deep learning
DLB	Dementia with Lewy bodies

DNA	Deoxy nucleic acid
DOI	Diffuse optical imaging
DPC	Digital photon counter
DSE MRI	Dynamic Susceptibility Imaging
DTI	Diffusion tensor imaging
DWI	Diffusion-weighted imaging
EBRT	External beam radiotherapy
ECG	Electrocardiogram
EEG	Electroencephalogram
EGFR	Epidermal growth factor receptor
EMA	European Medicine Association
EPI	Echoplanar imaging
ERBB2	Ebr-b2
ERC	Endorectal coil
EROS	Event related optical signal
ESA	European Space Agency
ESC	Embryonic stem cell
FA	Fractional anisotropy
FDA	Food and Drug Administration
FDG	Fluorodeoxy glucose
FES	Fluoro estradiol
FFP	Field free point
FI	Fluorescence imaging
FLT	Fluoro thymidine
f-MRI	Functional magnetic resonance imaging
FRET	Fluorescence resonance energy transfer
FTD	Frontotemporal dementia
G6PD	Glucose 6 phosphate dehydrogenase
GABA	γ-aminobutyric acid A
GBM	Glioblastoma multiforme
GCP II	Glutamate carboxypeptidase II
Gd	Gadolinium
GE	General Electric
GFP	Green fluorescent protein
GHZ	Giga Hertz
GIST	Gastrointestinal stromal tumor
Gluco CEST	Gluco chemical exchange saturation transfer
GS	Gleason score
Hb	Hemoglobin
HDL	High density lipoproteins
HER2	Human epidermal growth factor receptor 2
HF	Hydrogen fluoride
HIF	Hypoxia-inducible factor
ICI therapy	Immune checkpoint inhibitor
IPSC	Induced pluripotent stem cells
IV	Intravenous
IVM	Intravital microscopy
KEV	Kilo electron voltage

KRAS	Kirsten rat sarcoma viral oncogene homolog
LED	Light-emitting diode
LMRI	Lymphotropic nanoparticle enhanced magnetic resonance imaging
LN	Lymph node
LSO	Lutetium oxyorthosilicate
LYSO	Lutetium–Yttrium oxyorthosilicate
MAA	Microaggregated albumin
MAI	Magnetic acoustic imaging
MCI	Mild cognitive impairment
mci	Millicurie
Mg/dl	Milligram per deciliter
MHZ	Mega Hertz
MI	Molecular imaging
MIBC	Muscle invasive bladder cancer
MIBG	Metaiodobenzyl guanidine
Micro CT	Micro computed tomography
MION	Mono disperse iron oxide nanoparticles
ML	Machine learning
MLH1	MutL homolog 1
mMR	Molecular magnetic resonance
Mn	Manganese
MNO	Manganese oxide
MOI	Magnetic optic imaging
mp-MRI	Multiparametric magnetic resonance imaging
MPs	Misfolded proteins
MR	Medical microrobots
MRI	Magnetic resonance imaging
MRS	Magnetic resonance spectroscopy
MRSI	Magnetic resonance spectroscopy imaging
MSC	Mesenchymal stem cell
MSH2	MutS homolog 2
MSH6	mutS homolog 6
mSV	Millisieverts
MTV	Metabolic tumor volume
NaF	Sodium fluoride
NaI	Sodium iodide
NCD	Neuro cognitive disorder
NET	Neuroendocrine tumor
NFT	Neurofibrillary tangles
NIH	National Institute of Health
NIR II	Near-infrared window II
NIRS	Near-infrared spectroscopy
NK	Natural killer
nm	Nanometer
NMIBC	Non-muscle invasive bladder cancer
NMR	Nuclear magnetic resonance
NP	Nanoparticle

NSC	Neuroprogenitor stem cell
NSCLC	Non-small cell lung cancer
OA	Osteoarthritis
OCT	Optical coherence tomography
OI	Optical imaging
PA	Photo acoustic
PAI	Photo acoustic imaging
PARACEST	Para chemical exchange saturation transfer
PAT	Photo acoustic tomography
Pb	Lead
PCa	Prostate cancer
PCI	Percutaneous coronary intervention
PCr	Phosphocreatine
PD	Parkinson's disease
PDD	Parkinson's disease dementia
PDE	Photon detection efficiency
PDT	Photo dynamic therapy
PET CT	Positron emission tomography and computed tomography
PET MRI	Positron emission tomography and magnetic resonance imaging
PET	Positron emission tomography
PFC	Per Fluoro carbon
PIRADS	Prostate imaging and reporting archiving data system
PLGA	Polylactic-co-glycolic acid
PLNP	Persistent luminescence nanoparticles
PMS2	Post meiotic segregation increased 2
PMT	Photo multiplier tubes
PPP	Pentose phosphate pathway
PRRT	Peptide receptor radionuclide therapy
PSA	Prostate specific antigen
PSC	Per fluoro carbon
PSMA	Prostate specific membrane antigen
PSP	Pseudo parkinsonism
PTT	Photo thermal therapy
Q Dots	Quantum dots
QD	Quantum dot
QE	Quantum efficiency
QI	Quality indicator
QIBA	Quantitative imaging biomarker allowance
QMA	Quantitative morphometric analysis
RA	Rheumatoid arthritis
RECIST	Response evaluation criteria in solid tumors
RNA	Ribo nucleic acid
ROI	Region of interest
SC	Stem cell
Se	Selenium
SERS	Surface enhanced Raman scattering
SiPms	Silicon photo multipliers

SNR	Signal to noise ratio
SPECT	Single photon emission computed tomography
SPECT CT	Single photon emission computed tomography and computed tomography
SPIO	Super paramagnetic iron oxide
SPION	Super paramagnetic iron oxide nanoparticle
SPN	Solitary pulmonary nodule
SSTR	Somatostatin receptors
STI	Signal transduction inhibitor
STING	Stimulator of the interferon receptor
STIR	Short tau inversion recovery
SUV max	Standardized uptake value maximum
SUV	Standardized uptake value
SWNTs	Single-walled carbon nanotubes
TAM	Tumor assistant microphages
TBI	Traumatic brain injury
TCA cycle	Tricarboxylic acid
TCR	T cell receptor
TE	Time for excitation
TKI	Tyrosine kinase inhibitors
TLG	Total lesion glycolysis
TOF	Time of flight
TOLD	Tissue oxygen level dependent
TR	Time for relaxation
TRUS	Transrectal ultrasound
TSE	Transmissible spongiform encephalopathy
TSPO	Translocator protein
TURBT	Transurethral resection of bladder tumor
US	Ultrasound
USPIO	Ultrasound super paramagnetic iron oxide
VCAM	Vascular cell adhesion molecule
VCAM-1	Vascular cell adhesion molecule-1
VEGF	Vascular endothelial growth factor
VOI	Volume of interest
VPF	Vascular permeability factor
WHO	World Health Organization
Z	Atomic number
ZN	Zinc

Introduction to Precision Medicine

1

Key Points (Abstract)

The advances in imaging are based on the important aspect leading to the concept of precision medicine. The different newer imaging modalities are important for the focussed imaging leading to the tailor-made management of the diseases. Here in this book are the various research aspects leading to the precision imaging.

Keywords

Precision medicine · Molecular imaging
Probes · Genomes · Optical imaging
Nanoimaging · Stem cell imaging
Radiomics · Radiobiology

1.1 Introduction of Precision Medicine

This book is important for the advances in imaging, which will be more precise and specific to the researchers, practising imaging specialists, biomedical engineers, and scientists who are all involved in the high-end imaging stuff. This book is also useful for radiology, imaging, and students from all the specialities who are involved in the various aspects of research and high-end applications.

This book is described in 25 chapters other than the first chapter that is the introduction of this book. These 25 chapters are covering the various aspects of the newer modalities of imaging and technologies in their respective fields for the various research applications. Each chapter is designed and described in detail the concept of the imaging modality and the various protocols used in these imaging modalities along with the biggest aspect that is the advantages and disadvantages pertaining to the various applications.

The applications are based on the different presets like in oncology, infection and inflammation, cardiology, neurology, and many more in detail pertaining to that chapter. The description and discussion is also meticulously done so that the basic concept of the imaging modality, is explained with present scenarios to the futuristic applications of these imaging modalities. Every aspect of these imaging modalities is explained in detail along with their various applications.

One important point is that these applications are being mentioned in different chapters like "Nanoparticles", which have the applications in oncology, infection, and inflammation, as well as in the "Theranostics", which means the diverse role in various applications. These chapters include the relevant diagrams, figures, and images pertaining to these respective chapters.

After reading this book, it becomes important to have the basic knowledge of these various chapters and also associate with the different aspects of their applications. The chapters included are based on the modern aspects of imaging and their futuristic applica-

S. Shaikh, *Advances in Imaging*, https://doi.org/10.1007/978-981-16-9535-3_1

tions, which have specific and focussed applications leading to the concept of the tailor-made imaging and further leading to the precision medicine imaging.

Precision medicine is now being well established for the early and tailor-made approach and the management of the various disorders, and these are being based on the various genetic and environmental factors that are impacted on them. The prevention and therapeutic options are more precise and focussed for targeted interventions for the benefit of the patients. Due to the technological advancements, this precision medicine is being used for early patient screening, diagnosis of diseases, and post-treatment evaluation of particular disease.

Molecular imaging in precision medicine is for early diagnosis and for the concept of personalized treatment options. As per the National Academy of Sciences, "precision medicine is using the concept of the tailoring of disease management based on the individual patient characteristics, who is more prone for the particular disease, and in the biology and/or for the prognosis of those diseases which will be developing, based on the response to a specific line of the treatment" [1]. By this concept, there are more advantages for the focussed management reducing the cost of the patients and also the side effects of the therapy. Here, the patients' genetic and associated environmental factors are taken into consideration [2]. Different parameters like various genetic, different biomarkers and multiple phenotypes are used for the differentiation of one patient to another patient of same disease pattern [3]. Due to this, precision medicine is becoming more important due to genomics, molecular biology advancements, tumour biology, technological developments, and newer imaging concepts where scan times are reduced shortly.

This concept will be used for the screening of the suspected patients for early diagnosis, for focussed tailor-made treatment options for the patients, and for the various therapeutic options that will be used [4].

Molecular imaging has evolved significantly to become the hallmark of precision medicine in this era [5]. The cellular-level imaging can identify the disease in early preclinical states and can also classify the patients who need the particular type of therapy and for post-treatment evaluation. Different endogenous and exogenous agents are being used like biomarkers, nanoparticles, etc.

Oncology is the one having the precision oncology concept that is more useful for the evaluation of the various aspects of the personalized medicine.

"Radiomics" is also important for imaging as the mineable data that will be extracted from the available imaging modalities with the use of various algorithms [6, 7]. Another aspect is the use of quantitative imaging concepts where various features of lesion characterization like shape, size of the lesions, tumour volume, various signal intensities, CT attenuation values, standardized uptake value, and all are being used as the molecular biomarkers in the prognosis of tumour and response to therapy evaluation [8–12].

The use of molecular imaging has become crucial in every aspect for the earliest diagnosis and the evaluation of various diseases and pathologies that are not possible to get detected in the preclinical stages. The various imaging components are genetic imaging for gene evaluation of various therapies for the target genetic material to be delivered based on gene delivery and gene expression in vivo imaging. The development of various modalities and the evaluation of the different modalities like the CT molecular imaging are not established due to the contrast aspects and less sensitivity as compared to the other imaging modalities [13–15].

MRI is an important modality for better detection and characterization of soft tissue pathologies, which shows a very higher spatial resolution and contrast. In the recent years, molecular imaging modalities are used for evaluation of cell tracking, angiogenesis, apoptosis, and tissue gene imaging [16].

Radionuclide Molecular Imaging: This imaging is widely used for personalized medicine concept. PET and SPECT are used for diagnosis as well as therapeutic, and many options are available that are focussed, reasonable, and precise [17].

Ultrasound Molecular Imaging: Ultrasound is an important evolving modality of molecular imaging with the use of various ultrasound contrast agents. This can be used as preclinical diagnosis where different aspect of advanced instrumentations is being used, such as the use of the endoscopes along with the advanced, novel US-compatible imaging agents leading to the targeted ultrasound imaging.

Optical Imaging: The use of optical imaging is important for the analysis of various pathologies that are based on optical properties. The different imaging components are fluorescence imaging, bioluminescence imaging, photoacoustic imaging, and optical tomography [18].

Multimodal molecular imaging is the use of the combination of the two or more modalities of molecular imaging for the better evaluation of the various diagnosis, treatment, and monitoring. Cardiovascular diseases evaluation, multimodal functional imaging for the neurological networks like the auditory response evaluation by the functional MRI for the metabolic activity evaluation can be easily done by this imaging [19].

The various other aspects of molecular imaging are PET-CT, PET-MR, SPECT, and SPECT-CT.

The use of nanotechnology has significant impact on the diagnostic as well as the therapeutic options of various disease pathologies. This is purely based on the molecular level with the use of various nanoparticles and the various nanotube components. Theranostics is the newer concept for diagnosis, and the tailor-made therapeutic options can be used for the evaluation of preclinical disease [20].

The various newer imaging modalities like hypoxia imaging, radiomics imaging, stem cell imaging, genetic imaging, radiobiology, robotic imaging, and QIBA are the ones that will probably replace our traditional modalities. These newer modalities are more focussed with advantages as compared to the routine imaging modalities.

Conclusion: Molecular imaging and all the newer imaging modalities will be the future of precision medicine.

References

1. National Research Council, Division on Earth and Life Studies, Board on Life Sciences, et al. Toward precision medicine: building a knowledge network for biomedical research and a new taxonomy of disease. Washington, DC: The National Academies Press; 2011.
2. Obama B. The precision medicine initiative. Available at: https://www.whitehouse.gov/precision-medicine. Accessed October 7, 2015.
3. Jameson JL, Longo DL. Precision medicine—personalized, problematic, and promising. N Engl J Med. 2015;372:2229–34.
4. Herold CJ, Lewin JS, Wibmer AG, et al. Imaging in the age of precision medicine: summary of the proceedings of the 10th biannual symposium of the International Society for Strategic Studies in radiology. Radiology. 2016;279:226–38.
5. Mankoff DA. A definition of molecular imaging. J Nucl Med. 2007;48(18N):21N.
6. Kumar V, Gu Y, Basu S, et al. Radiomics: the process and the challenges. Magn Reson Imaging. 2012;30:1234–48.
7. Lambin P, Rios-Velazquez E, Leijenaar R, et al. Radiomics: extracting more information from medical images using advanced feature analysis. Eur J Cancer. 2012;48:441–6.
8. De Cecco CN, Ciolina M, Caruso D, et al. Performance of diffusion weighted imaging, perfusion imaging, and texture analysis in predicting tumoral response to neoadjuvant chemoradiotherapy in rectal cancer patients studied with 3T MR: initial experience. Abdom Radiol (NY). 2016;41:1728–35.
9. Skogen K, Schulz A, Dormagen JB, et al. Diagnostic performance of texture analysis on MRI in grading cerebral gliomas. Eur J Radiol. 2016;85:824–9.
10. Smith AD, Gray MR, del Campo SM, et al. Predicting overall survival in patients with metastatic melanoma on antiangiogenic therapy and RECIST stable disease on initial posttherapy images using CT texture analysis. AJR Am J Roentgenol. 2015;205:W283–93.
11. Hayano K, Tian F, Kambadakone AR, et al. Texture analysis of noncontrast-enhanced computed tomography for assessing angiogenesis and survival of soft tissue sarcoma. J Comput Assist Tomogr. 2015;39:607–12.
12. De Cecco CN, Ganeshan B, Ciolina M, et al. Texture analysis as imaging biomarker of tumoral response to neoadjuvant chemoradiotherapy in rectal cancer patients studied with 3-T magnetic resonance. Investig Radiol. 2015;50:239–45.
13. He W, Ai K, Lu L. Nanoparticulate X-ray CT contrast agents. SCIENCE CHINA Chem. 2015;58(5):1–8. https://doi.org/10.1007/s11426-015-5351-8.
14. Attia MF, Anton N, Chiper M, et al. Biodistribution of X-ray iodinated contrast agent in nano-emulsions is controlled by the chemical nature of the oily core. ACS Nano. 2014;8(10):10537–50. https://doi.org/10.1021/nn503973z.
15. Attia MF, Anton N, Akasov R, Chiper M, Markvicheva E, Vandamme TF. Biodistribution and toxicity of X-ray iodinated contrast agent in nano-emulsions in function of their size. Pharm Res. 2016;33(3):1–12. https://doi.org/10.1007/s11095-015-1813-0.
16. Kim HS, Woo J, Lee JH, et al. In vivo tracking of dendritic cell using MRI reporter gene, ferritin. PLoS

One. 2015;10(5) https://doi.org/10.1371/journal.pone.0125291.e0125291.
17. Choi H. Deep learning in nuclear medicine and molecular imaging: current perspectives and future directions. Nucl Med Mol Imaging. 2017;52(2):109–18. https://doi.org/10.1007/s13139-017-0504-7.
18. Thibon A, Pierre VC. Principles of responsive lanthanide-based luminescent probes for cellular imaging. Anal Bioanal Chem. 2009;394(1):107–20. https://doi.org/10.1007/s00216-009-2683-2.
19. Chiotis K, Saint-Aubert L, Savitcheva I, et al. Imaging in-vivo tau pathology in Alzheimer's disease with THK5317 PET in a multimodal paradigm. Eur J Nucl Med Mol Imaging. 2016;43(9):1686–99. https://doi.org/10.1007/s00259-016-3363-z.
20. González-Gómez MA, Belderbos S, Yañez-Vilar S, Piñeiro Y, Cleeren F, et al. Development of superparamagnetic nanoparticles coated with polyacrylic acid and aluminum hydroxide as an efficient contrast agent for multimodal imaging. Nanomaterials (Basel). 2019;9:1626.

2 Molecular Imaging and Instrumentation

Key Points (Abstract)

The development of medical technology has warranted advanced patient care, and the better, faster, easily available, cost-effective, and, most important, non-invasive imaging is the requirement of the day. With this, the evaluation of the anatomy, function, or molecular-biological components is needed for the study of the patients. These imaging modalities can be individual or combined, providing both anatomical and molecular functional information.

For this, understanding the imaging modality is very important for proper functioning especially in cases of hybrid imaging. The physical components are needed to be understood along with the instrumentation functioning that needs to be analyzed for proper applications and also for future advancements in that modality, which qualifies the above-mentioned criteria as an ideal imaging modality that till date does not exist.

Positron emission tomography (PET) and single photon emission computed tomography (SPECT) are the imaging modalities that are based on the concept of detection of gamma rays, which leave the body when the radiotracer is being injected. The sensitivity of these modalities is important, and PET has the detection capability of the picomolar tracer amounts in vivo, and with the available technology, it is up to millimetre (PET) or submillimetre (SPECT) spatial resolution. Due to this, these modalities are being used in various clinical and preclinical applications. The basic component is that the detectors used in both positron emission tomography and single photon emission computed tomography are the combination of scintillation crystals where it is converted into incident gamma radiation to visible scintillation light. The photodetector component in this uses this scintillation light and converts it into electrical pulse.

Keywords

PET · PET-CT · PET-MR · SPECT
SPECT-CT · Gamma camera · Detectors

2.1 Introduction

The first discovery of X-rays by Wilhelm Conrad Roentgen in 1895 has revolutionized the medical imaging till date [1]. Now, the role of the newer non-invasive medical imaging modalities is becoming the most important for the diagnosis and staging of various diseases. The introduction of computed tomography (CT) and magnetic resonance (MR) was done in the early [1] and late 1970s [2, 3], respectively, and they are now the most commonly used imaging modalities for structural and morphological assessment of the human anatomy [4–6] as well as pathology. The earliest changes, which happen in the form of

S. Shaikh, *Advances in Imaging*, https://doi.org/10.1007/978-981-16-9535-3_2

molecular changes, can be depicted with the use of metabolic or functional imaging modalities, which provide the earliest information of the particular disease, and this is helpful for the diagnosis and staging of many diseases. The first single photon emission tomography (SPECT) as a functional imaging modality was introduced in the early 1960s [7], and then the first positron emission tomography (PET) system was introduced in 1972 [8] followed by the first MR system in 1977 [3].

2.2 Hybrid Imaging

The word hybrid imaging denotes the combination of the two imaging modalities, anatomical and functional, or it can be functional and functional for the significantly improved diagnostic accuracy resulting in patient comfort. This can be physical combination or software combination. But the most designed ones are the hardware physical fusion. This is possible with the greater innovation, the continuous ongoing research, and the technological advances resulting in combined modality. This hybrid imaging systems are used both clinically and subclinically like research. These modalities also focus on the various technological advances that use them as complementary anatomical and biological information for analysing the pathologies as well as using the various technical aspects beneficial like image reconstruction and data correction schemes. The basic aim of these modalities is to provide very useful, complementary, and quantitative information for patient workup. These hybrid imaging is being used as the source of multiparametric assessment of diseases, which further will be more beneficial and contribute financially.

A few of the functional imaging modalities that have functional components are functional magnetic resonance imaging (fMRI) like DWI, perfusion MR, magnetic particle imaging (MPI), near-infrared spectroscopy (NIRS), and many more. PET and SPECT are also non-invasive and have the advantage of quantitative analysis of the various physiological processes at a molecular level in the body. Thus, the functional information provided by these modalities are not correlating with the various anatomical structures. The biggest drawback is the lack of high-contrast anatomical information in both these SPECT or PET modalities, and it forms the major limitation of these imaging techniques. For the excellent use of the PET or SPECT, these modalities need to be fused with anatomical imaging modalities like CT or MRI. Thus, the PET-CT and PET-MR are being developed with the combination of functional and anatomical modalities, which will significantly increase the clinical results. The SPECT-CT was first used primarily for CT-based attenuation and for scatter correction of the SPECT data [9–11]. This use of the CT-based attenuation and scatter correction now has benefits in both SPECT and PET, and this has the very shorter transmission times post-injection [12] (Diagram 2.1).

2.3 SPECT-CT

The first combined SPECT-CT design was proposed by Mirshanov in 1987 [13], but due to technical difficulties, it took around a decade for the commercial use, after the technical modifications by Blankespoor et al. [14]. Thus, the SPECT-CT has evolved rapidly, and many commercial system designs are available today (Fig. 2.1). There are two types of the design of the integrated CT components. First one is the fully diagnostic CT systems with fast-rotation detectors for the simultaneous acquisition of 16 or 64 detector rows, and the X-ray tubes provide the sufficient tube voltages with high tube current and automatic exposure control [15]. These are also capable of doing the advanced CT imaging like cardiac gating, calcium scoring, and iterative reconstruction [16, 17]. SPECT-CT systems have the rotating SPECT components with adapted rotation times and dose-optimized acquisition modes, when the CT components have the limited acquisition flexibility, which have very low tube voltages and currents [15]. The Hungarian company Mediso has developed the triple-modality SPECT/CT/PET system (Mediso

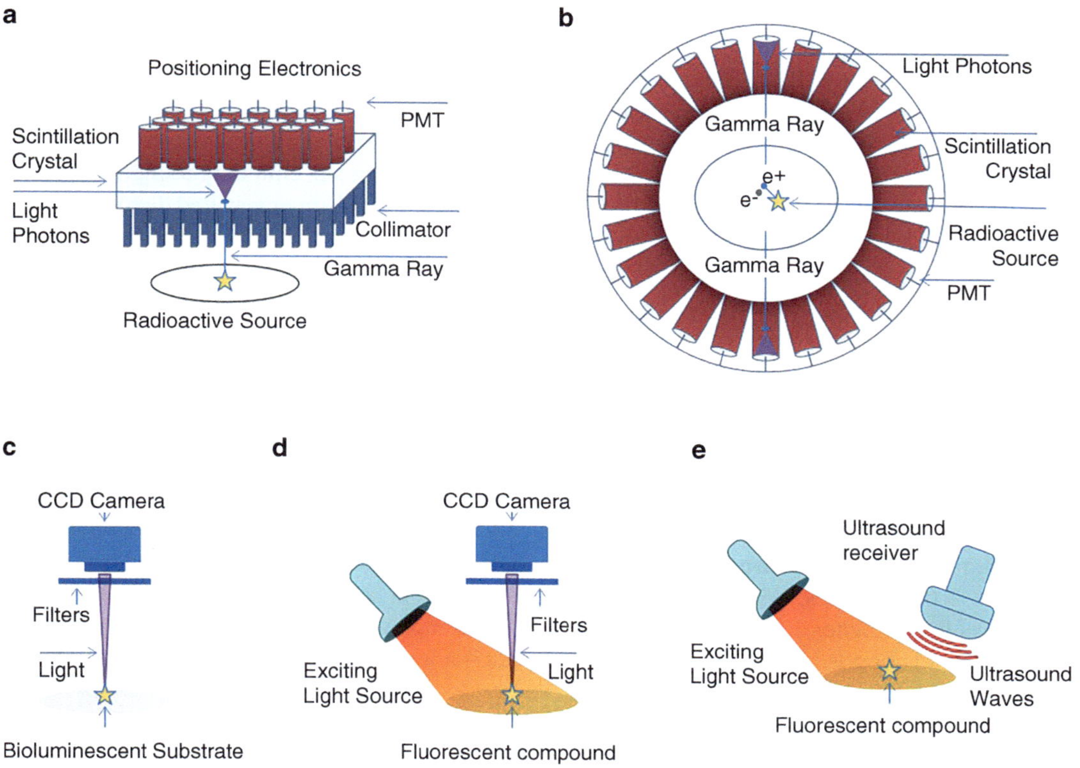

Diagram 2.1 (**a**) Composition of the nuclear medicine gamma camera, (**b**) PET scan, (**c**) optical bioluminescent imaging camera, (**d**) fluorescent imaging optical imaging camera, and (**e**) optoacoustic imaging

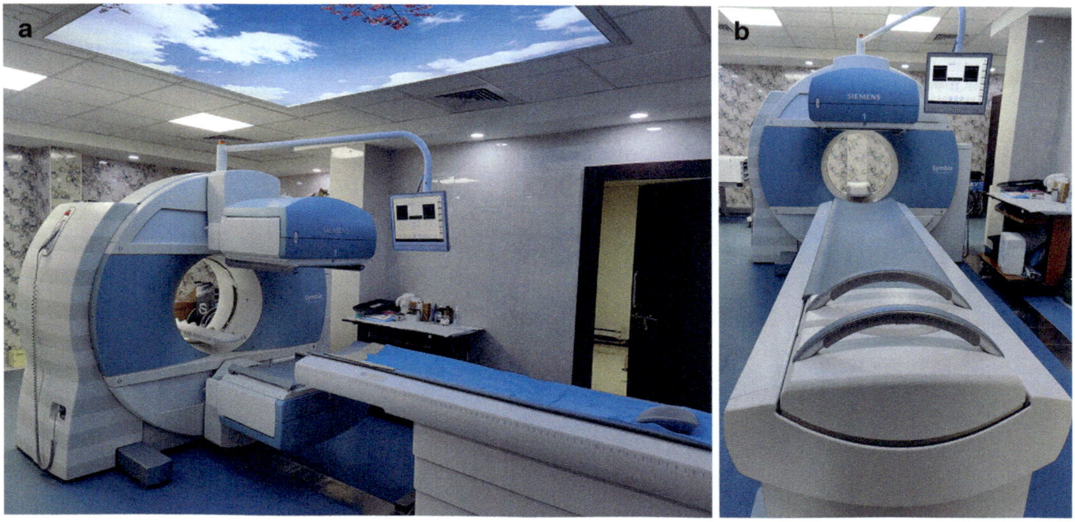

Fig. 2.1 (**a** and **b**) The SPECT-CT machine in different angles. (Courtesy Dr. Madhur Srivastava, Associate Prof. Nuclear Medicine, NIMS, Hyderabad)

AnyScan) where the combination of all these three modalities is there in a single device. Commonly, these SPECT systems are based on planar detectors having two-dimensional (2D) array of photomultiplier tubes (PMTs), which are attached to the scintillation crystal on the back with en face collimators. The photon interaction site is the center of gravity of the position-dependent energy signals from the PMTs based on the Anger logic hypothesis [18]. Due to the higher costs, the use of solid-state detectors will be restricting the adoption in smaller systems like the various application of the cardiac [19] (Fig. 2.2), brain [20], or preclinical imaging [21]. Thus, the use of SPECT-CT has a wide range of applications [22–25] (Figs. 2.3, 2.4, and 2.5). The advantages of SPECT-CT are better attenuation correction and accurate anatomical allocation of the SPECT-CT findings, which are from both modalities for the better diagnostic performance. SPECT-CT imaging is now being established in the clinical management of patients with cardiovascular disease [19].

Single photon emission computed tomography (SPECT) and PET are similar in the use of radioactive tracer and in the detection of γ-rays. SPECT radiotracers emit only a single γ-ray during decay and is being measured directly. SPECT scans are cheaper than PET scans, and one of the reasons is that the nuclides used in SPECT have longer half-life and can be relatively easily obtained as compared to PET. The various γ-emitting isotopes for SPECT are 99mTc ($t1/2$ = 6 h), 123I ($t1/2$ = 13.3 h), and 111In ($t1/2$ = 2.8 days), which are heavy radioisotopes, and all of them decay via a single photon emission. SPECT I utilized a γ camera to detect γ photons. This γ camera is rotated around the subject, and various projections are acquired during the rotation, covering all the parts to be scanned. The component used in the collimator in γ camera is a lead or tungsten that has the capability to

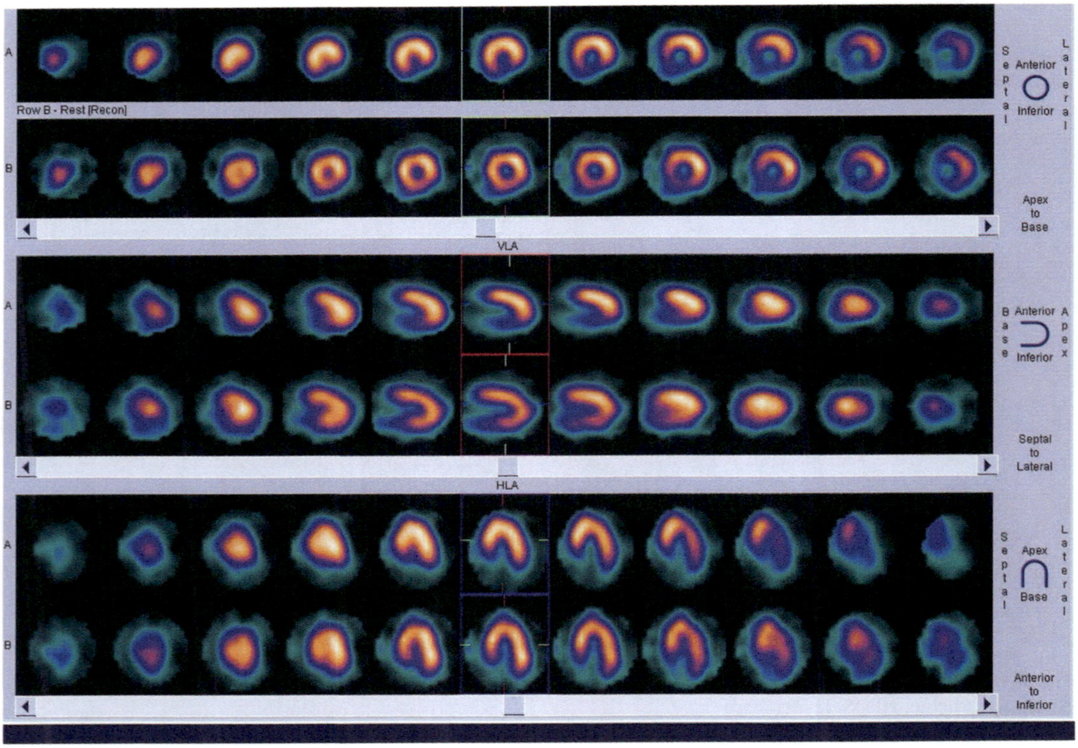

Fig. 2.2 Normal cardiac SPECT scan

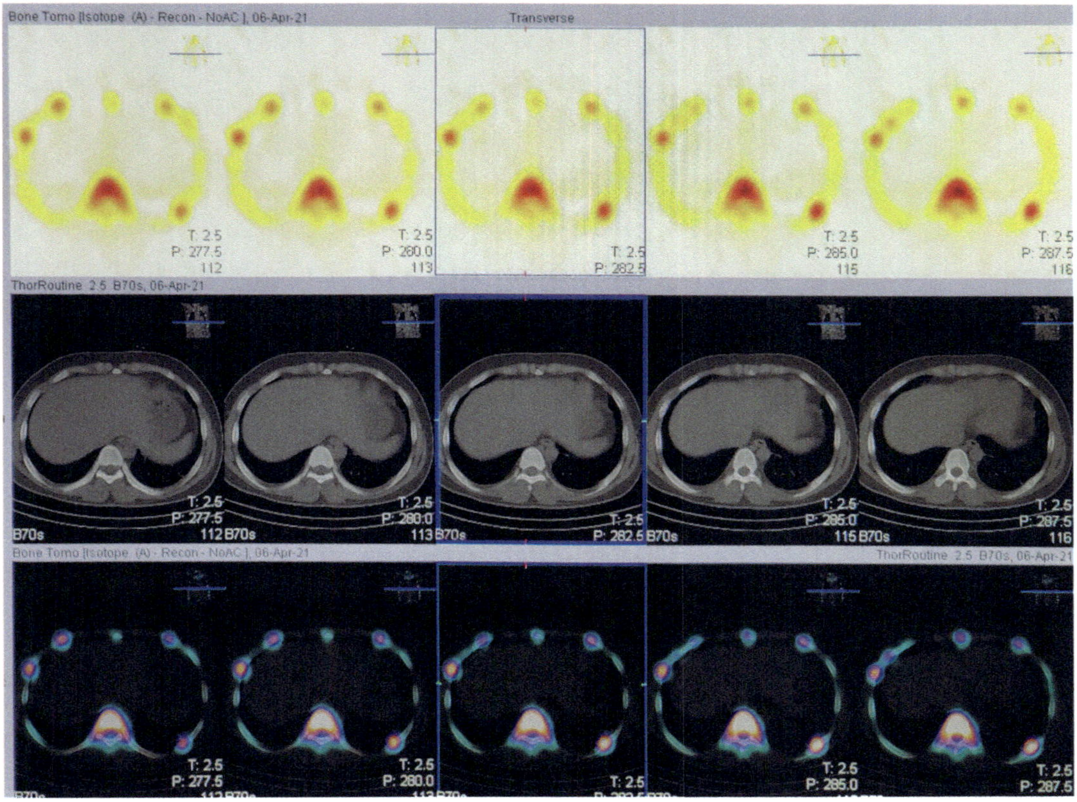

Fig. 2.3 MSK SPECT scan showing normal physiologic uptake in the vertebral bodies suggestive of physiologic uptake

reject many photos that are not travelling along the axis at right angles. The biggest disadvantage of this is that collimator absorbs most of the photons, which results in the sensitivity of SPECT in the magnitude that is far lower than PET. The spatial resolution of SPECT depended on the various collimation errors, which are usually far lower than the clinical PET. But in case of micro-SPECT, the spatial resolution has to be very high. This microSPECT, which is designed for imaging small animals, is being more widely used in preclinical studies like neurology and oncology and the drug development in small animal model. For example, Beekman et al. developed a new rodent SPECT instrument named U-SPECT-I. The spatial resolution here is of the submillimetre in 2005 [26]. Second-generation machine called U-SPECT-II is also being developed by the same group whose spatial resolution is less than half a millimetre [27]. The longer half-life radionuclides that are being used in SPECT can make it perform the longitudinal scans. The important aspect here is that the PET is not capable of distinguishing the two different radioisotopes when they are injected simultaneously as the isotopes that are positron emitters give rise to the two γ-rays of the same energy. SPECT, on the contrary, has the multiplexing capabilities of various multiple nuclides, which produce the γ-rays with different energies; thus, they enable the different image targets simultaneously [28]. For example, Hijnen et al. [29] has used the microSPECT and conducted the experiment that can quantify the biodistribution and tumour uptake of the angiogenesis tracer cyclic arginine-glycine-aspartate (cRGD) via SPECT. Recently, Hapdey et al. [30] have shown the spectral factor analysis (GSFA) method for simultaneous use and detection of the 99mTc/123I SPECT, thus proving that simultaneous 99mTc/123I imaging obtained through

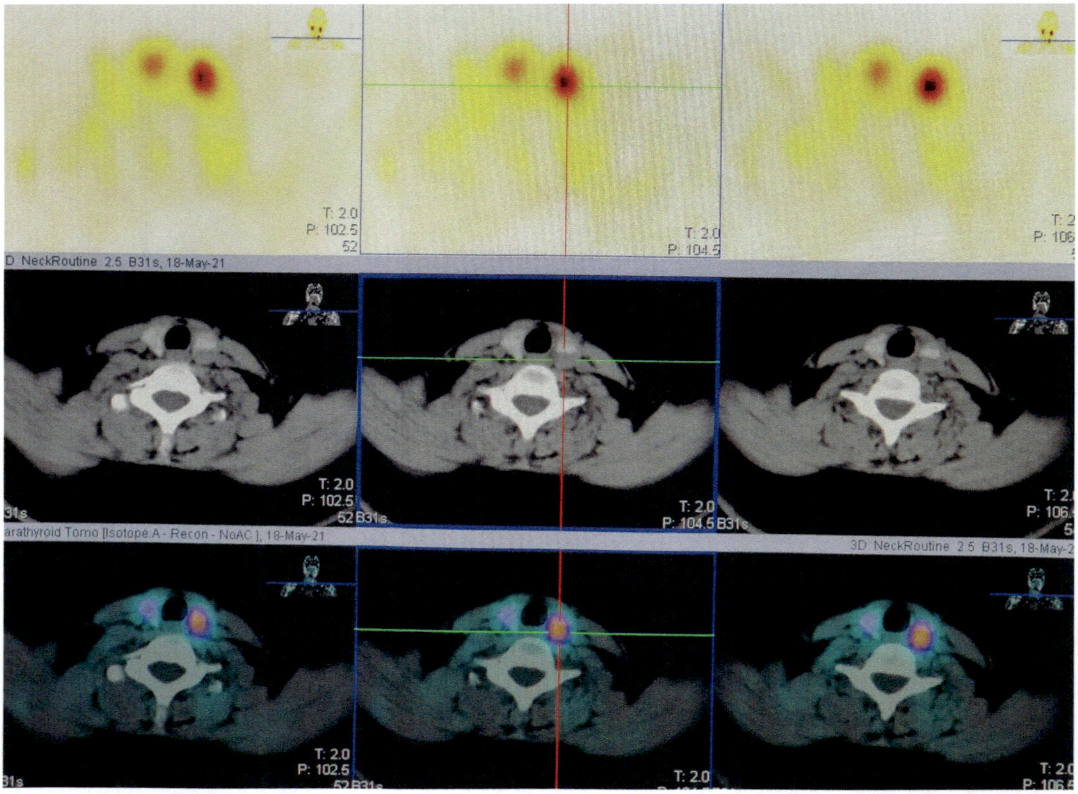

Fig. 2.4 SPECT parathyroid scan showing focal area of increased uptake in left parathyroid nodule suggestive of left parathyroid adenoma

GSFA has the same quantitative accuracy as compared to those using sequential and scatter-free 99mTc/123I imaging in the brain.

2.4 SPECT

The scintillators are divided into organic and inorganic materials and may or may not have the complementary characteristics. The organic scintillators are showing the poor light output and are very fast, while inorganic scintillators are showing high light output and a very slower decay constant [31, 32]. The atomic number of organic materials is much less as compared to the inorganic scintillators.

2.5 Properties of Photodetectors

2.5.1 Photomultiplier Tubes (PMTs)

Photomultiplier tubes (PMTs) are being used to convert scintillation light into an electrical pulse (Knoll 2000) [33–35]. The basic PMT architecture is made in the vacuum glass tube and comprised of the photocathode that emits photoelectrons when the visible light is incident to its surface, a number of dynodes that emit the secondary electrons for every incident primary photoelectron, and a single anode or an anode mesh that collects the secondary electron cloud and ultimately produces the current pulse that is proportional to the number of electrons in the

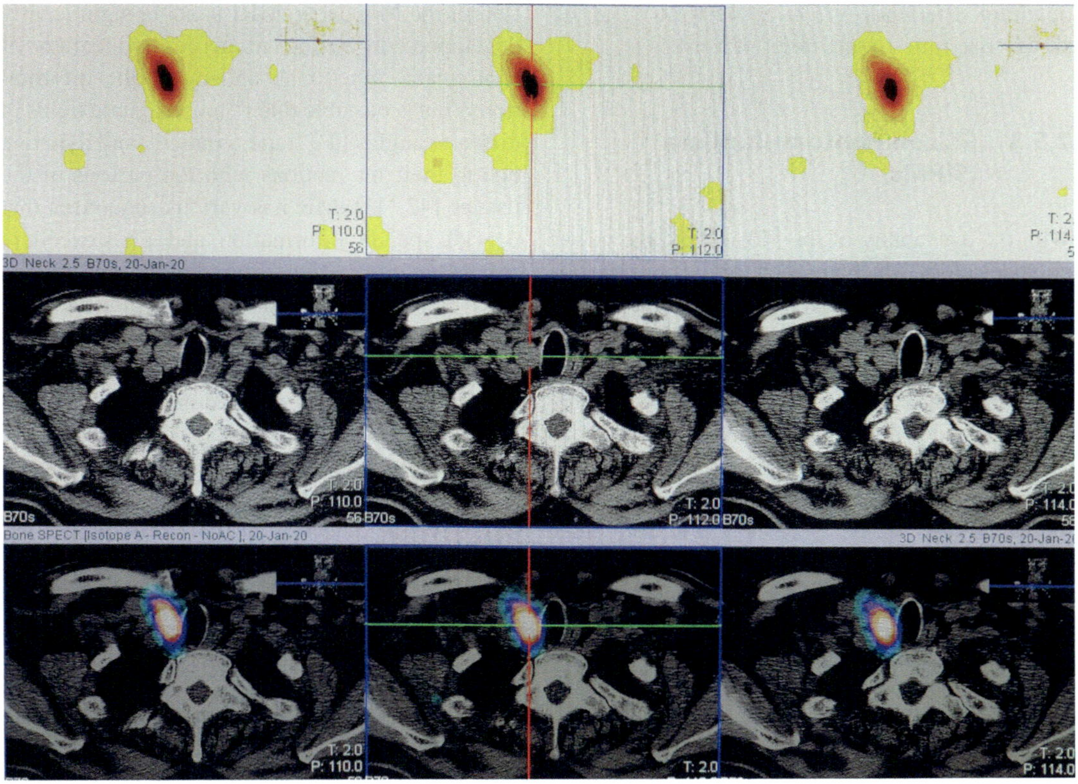

Fig. 2.5 SPECT scan again showing the nodule in the right upper paratracheal region showing diffuse uptake suggestive of adenoma

cloud. PMT performance has the low quantum efficiency (QE), which is the ratio of the number of photoelectrons produced at the photocathode to the number of incident photons at the photocathode surface (typically 25% at 420 nm). Thus, the performance of a PMT is significantly degraded inside the magnetic fields, and due to this, it will be very difficult to have the simultaneous MR/PET imaging.

2.5.2 Avalanche Photodiodes (APDs)

Avalanche photodiodes (APDs) are the semiconductor photodiodes and are significantly developed in the recent years due to the increasing demand for multimodality imaging [36–39]. The advantage of the APDs is that they are being produced in various compact sizes and their performance is not altered in the magnetic fields, thus making them more appropriate in the PET devices in the PET-MR imaging when they are being inserted in the MR. The main detector architecture of this is the p-to-n or n-to-p semiconductor junctions, which are being operated based on the voltage like the negative voltage on the p-side relative to the n-side. Within the APD, no free charge depletion region is created. When the photon is absorbed in the depletion region, the charge that will be produced is swept out towards the respective electrodes. During its process, the charge is being accelerated by the existing electric field, which will be moving towards the opposite polarity electrode and then into the avalanche region, in which many secondary electrons are produced. Here, the electron avalanche is collected by the anode and causing the current pulse. Compared with PMTs, APDs are characterized by low gain in the order of 100 by higher quantum efficiency (75% at 420 nm) and by slower rise times in the order of 5 ns.

2.5.3 Silicon Photomultipliers (SiPMs)

With the availability of the [40–42] are the newer photodetectors, which are more promising detector technology capable of multimodality imaging in nuclear medicine. Silicon photomultipliers (SiPMs) are made up of an array of individual APDs, which work in Geiger discharge mode (cells). In this mode, breakdown, every illuminated cell results in the fast (rise time ~1 ns) with the single photoelectron pulse of very high gain in the order of 106. The individual cells are being connected to each other by a polysilicon resistor that results in the current pulse, which is proportional to the number of illuminated cells. SiPMs' high gain and fast timing are also accompanied by their response to the very small dynamic range of detected radiation energies as they are limited, resulting in very low photon detection efficiency (PDE) and high dark count rate.

2.6 PET-MR

This is the newer hybrid imaging modality that is more precise and sensitive as compared to the PET-CT, and it is a combination of the PET with magnetic resonance imaging (MR) (Fig. 2.6). This imaging modality is more precise and had advantages due to the excellent soft tissue resolution of the MR. Now, MRI is being significantly developed with various numerous applications of anatomical, functional, and metabolic information. This is possible due to the magnetic fields in different angles like static, gradient, and dynamic due to their interactions with the protons of the tissues [42, 43]. MR has various sequences that provide specific information, and it has excellent soft tissue contrast and no radiation, making the MRI more attractive option in imaging as compared to CT. This is more required in the paediatric applications, neuroimaging (Fig. 2.7), and cardiac imaging. But the fusion of the PET and MR is faced with many hurdles due to hardware compatibility and fusion [44–47]. The biggest problem is with the PET systems that use the PMTs for the detection of the scintillation light, and this is more sensitive in the magnetic fields, and due to this reason, these cannot be integrated in one system. Due to these technical problems, the separate PET and MR systems were in combination and have the very active shielding of the photomultiplier tubes from the magnetic fields of the MR. Philips developed this whole-body PET-MR system in 2010 [48]. Solid-state photodetectors, like APDs or SiPMs, are seen as the alternatives [49–52]. These photodetectors make the PET-MR system to acquire simultaneous acquisition of PET and MR data in the same field of view. Today, the integrated systems of these properties are developed by Siemens Biograph mMR [53] and GE Signa PET-MR [54] and are working properly.

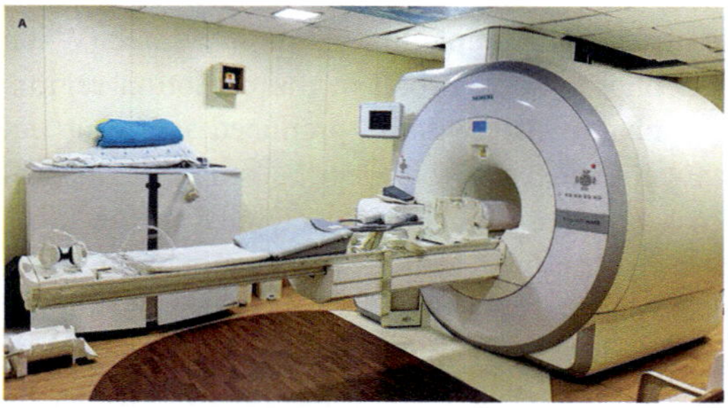

Fig. 2.6 PET-MR machine. (Courtesy Dr. Nidhi Goyal, Apollo Indraprastha Hospitals, New Delhi)

2.7 Detector Technology for CT, SPECT, and PET

The scintillation crystals are the important source of radiation detectors in CT, PET, and SPECT. These are very fast, having the capability of stopping the photons in the range of frequencies and emission energies leading to better detection of the detector materials (Diagram 2.2). Scintillation detector is a crystal that produces light when interaction with radiation and the amount of the scintillation light is converted

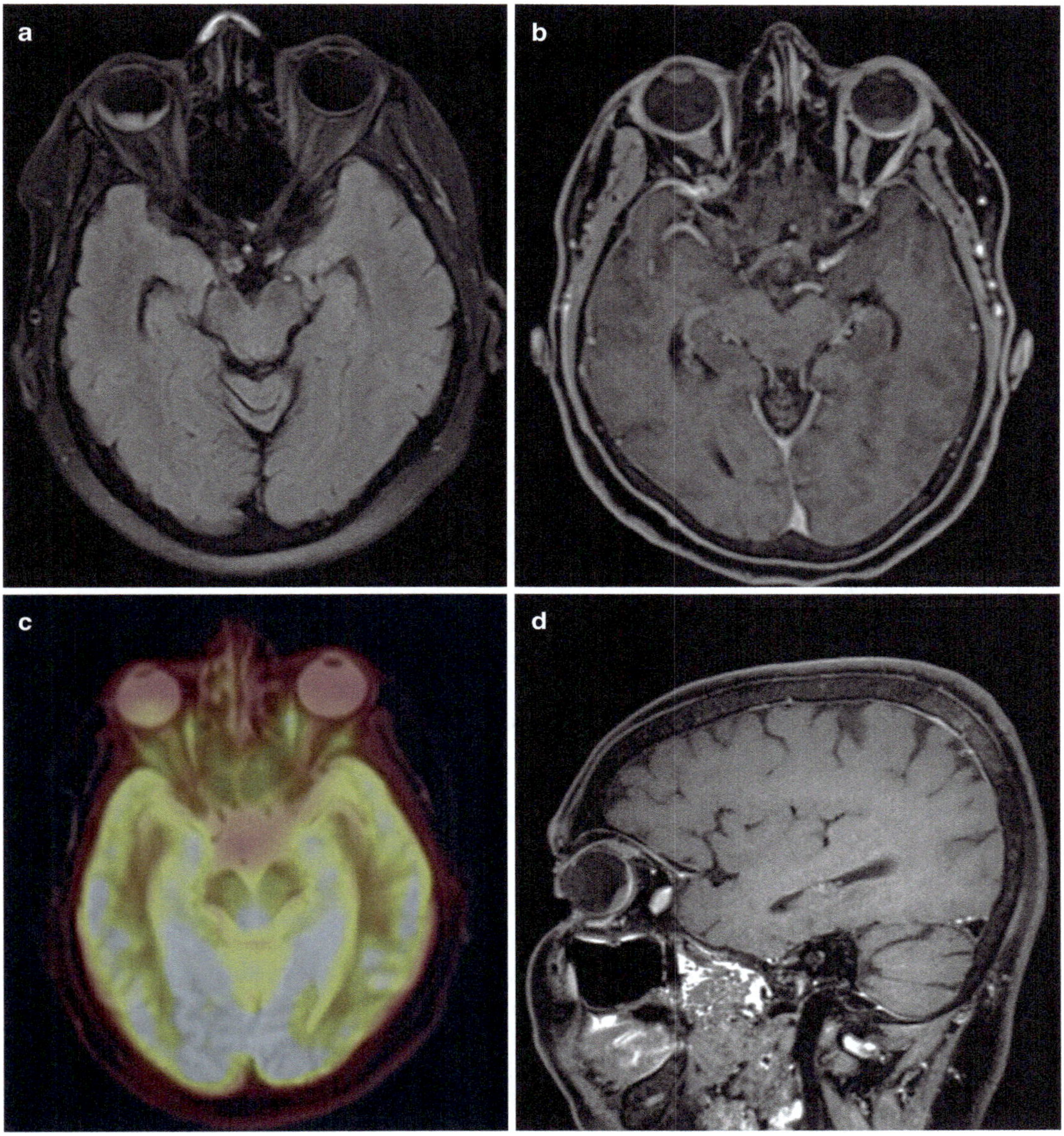

Fig. 2.7 PET-MR images showing the normal physiologic uptake in the brain parenchyma. (All figures courtesy Dr. Madhur Srivastava, Department of Nuclear Medicine and PET-CT, Nizams Institute of Medical Sciences, Hyderabad)

into an electrical signal [55], and this is being processed by the electronic system. Many newer scintillating materials are being developed and currently used. And they can be classified into organic or inorganic scintillators that are in the solid, liquid, or gaseous state. In the medical imaging applications, solid inorganic scintillators are usually preferred due to their higher density, which is needed for the high sensitivity imaging systems. The number of photons emitted per unit of deposited energy is directly related to the energy resolution based on the output. Most PET and SPECT systems have interaction position of the gamma photon [56] since the blocks comprise of continuous crystals [57, 58]. Some of the scintillators that are being used in

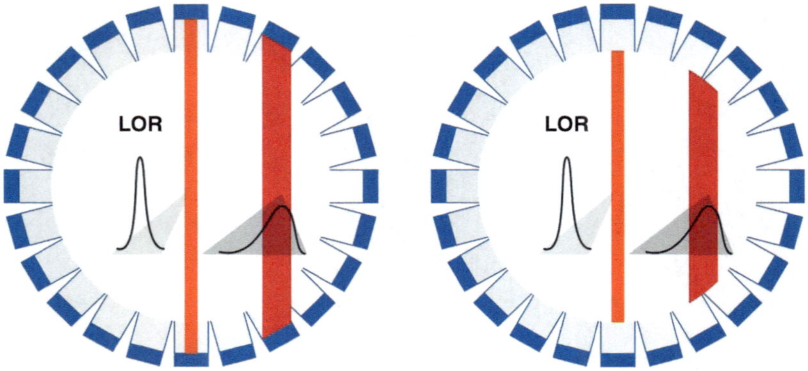

Diagram 2.2 PET scintillator crystals

CT, SPECT, and PET detector systems have similar properties [59–63]. Newer scintillator materials are the need of the hour due to technological advancements, and they are being developed continuously. Few newer scintillators are based on cerium doping of lanthanide and transition metal elements, such as LuAP:Ce, CeBr3, LuBO3:Ce, and others based on lead (Pb), tungsten (W), and gadolinium (Gd) [64].

2.7.1 Photomultiplier Tubes' (PMTs)

The main function of the PMTs is to measure and to detect the scintillation light that is emitted by the scintillator crystal. They have the vacuum enclosure in a thin photocathode layer at the entrance window with several electrodes called dynodes. These dynodes amplify the electrical signal that is created in the photocathode by means of secondary electron emissions. PMT produces an electrical pulse with amplitude. In this process, a number of scintillation photons reaching the photocathode are proportional to the energy that is being deposited. The high amplification capacity is the biggest advantage of PMTs as scintillation light. As they are sensitive to the magnetic fields, for this reason, they are not ideal for the combined PET-MR or SPECT-MR systems [65], and this is the major drawback. Another and better substitute to PMTs are solid-state detectors like the avalanche photodiodes (APDs) or silicon photomultipliers (SiPMs). The use of the solid-state detectors has more advantages like very high quantum efficiency, compact and flexible shape, ruggedness, and demonstrated insensitivity to magnetic fields with the potentially inexpensive mass production [66–68]. Various solid-state detectors are the semiconductor devices that have low-field depleted region where visible or near UV photons create the electron-hole pairs by photoelectric effect. These APDs are existing in very small devices like the monolithic arrays.

2.7.2 Silicon Photomultipliers (SiPMs)

As already described the SiPMs are made up of the densely packed matrix of small APD cells, which are biased to be operated above avalanche breakdown in the so-called Geiger mode. And the Geiger mode operation has more yield gain [69, 70]. The multicell structure is capable of providing the proportional output for moderate photon flux by adding the various signals of all cells that are being activated. In 2009, digital SiPMs, also known as Digital Photon Counter (DPC), was introduced by Philips where conventional array of Geiger mode photodiodes is combined with the fully digital electronic readout system, having the resolutions of up to 60 ps full width half maximum (FWHM) [70–73]. The semiconductor detectors are the main alternative for the scintillator-based detectors, which are used in the CT and SPECT imaging systems. The bigger advantage of the semiconductor detectors is they will directly convert the radiation to an electrical pulse, thus minimizing the degrading effects due to scintillation light production, propagation, and conversion to an electrical signal in the photodetector. But in the PET systems, they are not being used because they have lower stopping power for the high-energy 511 keV annihilation photons and are costly. Most commonly used semiconductors for nuclear medicine and CT imaging are CdTe and CdZnTe (CZT). These have high-stopping power that is similar to the NaI:Tl scintillator crystals, and they are capable of being operated at room temperature. With the use of highly granulated detectors, better quality, high spatial energy and time resolution can be achieved [74]. They have the important properties of some semiconductor materials are used for medical imaging applications [75].

Thus, the basic construction of the commonly used molecular imaging modalities shows the important principles of functioning.

References

1. Friedland GW, Thurber BD. The birth of CT. AJR Am J Roentgenol. 1996;167:1365–70. https://doi.org/10.2214/ajr.167.6.8956560.
2. Rinck PA. Magnetic resonance in medicine: the basic textbook of the European magnetic resonance forum. 12th revised and enlarged edition. Hoboken, NJ: Blackwell Scientific Publications; 2018.
3. Moser E, Laistler E, Schmitt F, Kontaxis G. Ultra-high field NMR and MRI— the role of magnet technology to increase sensitivity and specificity. Front Phys. 2017;5:33. https://doi.org/10.3389/fphy.2017.00033.
4. Beyer T, Freudenberg LS, Townsend DW, Czernin J. The future of hybrid imaging—part 1: hybrid imaging technologies and SPECT/CT. Insights Imaging. 2011;2:161–9. https://doi.org/10.1007/s13244-010-0063-2.
5. Beyer T, Townsend DW, Czernin J, Freudenberg LS. The future of hybrid imaging—part 2: PET/CT. Insights Imaging. 2011;2:225–34. https://doi.org/10.1007/s13244-011-0069-4.
6. Beyer T, Freundenberg LS, Czernin J, Townsend DW. The future of hybrid imaging-part 3: pet/mr, small-animal imaging and beyond. Insights Imaging. 2011;3:189. https://doi.org/10.1007/s13244-011-0136-x.
7. Jaszczak RJ. The early years of single photon emission computed tomography (SPECT): an anthology of selected reminiscences. Phys Med Biol. 2006 Jul 7;51(13):R99–115.
8. Madsen MT, Anderson JA, Halama JR, Kleck J, Simpkin DJ, Votaw JR, et al. AAPM task group 108: PET and PET/CT shielding requirements. Med Phys. 2006;33:4–15.
9. Lang TF, Hasegawa BH, Liew SC, Brown JK, Blankespoor SC, Reilly SM. Description of a prototype emission-transmission computed tomography imaging system. J Nucl Med. 1992;33:1881–7.
10. LaCroix KJ, Tsui BMW, Hasegawa BH, Brown JK. Investigation of the use of X-ray CT images for attenuation compensation in SPECT. IEEE Trans Nucl Sci. 1994;41:2793–9. https://doi.org/10.1109/23.340649.
11. Townsend DW. Multimodality imaging of structure and function. Phys Med Biol. 2008;53:R1–39. https://doi.org/10.1088/0031-9155/53/4/R01.
12. Kinahan PE, Hasegawa BH, Beyer T. X-ray-based attenuation correction for positron emission tomography/computed tomography scanners. Semin Nucl Med. 2003;33:166–79. https://doi.org/10.1053/snuc.2003.127307.
13. Goetze S, Wahl RL. Prevalence of misregistration between SPECT and CT for attenuation-corrected myocardial perfusion SPECT. J Nucl Cardiol. 2007;14:200–6.
14. Chen J, Caputlu-Wilson SF, Shi H, Galt JR, Faber TL, Garcia EV. Automated quality control of emission-transmission misalignment for attenuation correction in myocardial perfusion imaging with SPECT-CT systems. J Nucl Cardiol. 2006;13:43–9.
15. Seret A, Nguyen D, Bernard C. Quantitative capabilities of four state-of-the-art SPECT-CT cameras. EJNMMI Res. 2012;2:45. https://doi.org/10.1186/2191-219X-2-45.
16. Huellner MW, Strobel K. Clinical applications of SPECT/CT in imaging the extremities. Eur J Nucl Med Mol Imaging. 2014;41(Suppl. 1):S50–8. https://doi.org/10.1007/s00259-013-2533-5.
17. Buck AK, Nekolla S, Ziegler S, Beer A, Krause BJ, Herrmann K, et al. SPECT/CT. J Nucl Med. 2008;49:1305–19. https://doi.org/10.2967/jnumed.107.050195.
18. Anger HO. Scintillation camera. Rev Sci Instrum. 1958;29:27–33. https://doi.org/10.1063/1.1715998.
19. Erlandsson K, Buvat I, Pretorius PH, Thomas BA, Hutton BF. A review of partial volume correction techniques for emission tomography and their applications in neurology, cardiology and oncology. Phys Med Biol. 2012;57:R119–59. https://doi.org/10.1088/0031-9155/57/21/R119.
20. Yeo JM, Lim X, Khan Z, Pal S. Systematic review of the diagnostic utility of SPECT imaging in dementia. Eur Archiv Psychiatry Clin Neurosci. 2013;263:539–52. https://doi.org/10.1007/s00406-013-0426-z.
21. Finucane CM, Murray I, Sosabowski JK, Foster JM, Mather SJ. Quantitative accuracy of low-count SPECT imaging in phantom and in vivo mouse studies. Int J Mol Imaging. 2011;2011:8.

22. Huellner MW, Strobel K. Clinical applications of SPECT/CT in imaging the extremities. Eur J Nucl Med Mol Imaging. 2014;41(Suppl. 1):S50–8. https://doi.org/10.1007/s00259-013-2533-5.
23. Hobbs SB, Hamon BW, Oates ME. A spectrum of SPECT/CT image fusion applications in daily clinical practice. Clin Nucl Med. 2013;38:e336–41. https://doi.org/10.1097/RLU.0b013e318281625a.
24. Pretorius PH, Dahlberg ST, King MA. Investigation of respiratory motion compensation in a large population of patients undergoing Tc-99m cardiac perfusion SPECT/CT stress imaging. J Nucl Med. 2016;57:532.
25. Jackson PA, Beauregard JM, Hofman MS, Kron T, Hogg A, Hicks RJ. An automated voxelized dosimetry tool for radionuclide therapy based on serial quantitative SPECT/CT imaging. Med Phys. 2013;40:112503. https://doi.org/10.1118/1.4824318.
26. Beekman FJ, van der Have F, Vastenhouw B, van der Linden AJ, van Rijk PP, Burbach JP, Smidt MP. U-SPECT-I: a novel system for submillimeter-resolution tomography with radiolabeled molecules in mice. J Nucl Med. 2005;46:1194–200.
27. van der Meel R, Gallagher WM, Oliveira S, O'Connor AE, Schiffelers RM, Byrne AT. Recent advances in molecular imaging biomarkers in cancer: application of bench to bedside technologies. Drug Discov Today. 2010;15:102–14.
28. Labbe JP. SPECT/CT emerges from the shadow of PET/CT. Biophoton Int. 2003;10:50–7.
29. Hijnen NM, de Vries A, Nicolay K, Grüll H. Dual-isotope 111In/177Lu SPECT imaging as a tool in molecular imaging tracer design. Contrast Media Mol Imaging. 2012;7:214–22.
30. Even-Sapir E, Flusser G, Lerman H, Lievshitz G, Metser U. SPECT/multislice low-dose CT: a clinically relevant constituent in the imaging algorithm of nononcologic patients referred for bone scintigraphy. J Nucl Med. 2007;48:319–24.
31. Wu Y, Ren G, Meng F, Chen X, Ding D, Li H, et al. Ultralow-concentration Sm codoping in CsI:Tl scintillator: a case of little things can make a big difference. Opt Mater. 2014;38:297–300.
32. Wu Y, Ren G, Meng F, Chen X, Ding D, Li H, et al. Ultralow-concentration Sm codoping in CsI:Tl scintillator: a case of little things can make a big difference. Opt Mater. 2014;38:297–300.
33. Degenhardt C, Prescher G, Frach T, et al. The digital silicon photomultiplier—a novel sensor for the detection of scintillation light. In Proceedings of the IEEE Nuclear Science Symposium Conference Record (NSS/MIC '09); October 2009; pp. 2383–2386.
34. Photomultiplier Tubes (PMTs). Exp Methods Phys Sci. 2013;45:69–82.
35. Schug D, Wehner J, Dueppenbecker PM, et al. ToF performance evaluation of PET modules with digital silicon photomultiplier technology during MR operation. IEEE Trans Nucl Sci. 2015;62(3):658–63.
36. Moszynski M, Plettner C, Nassalski A, Szczesniak T, Swiderski L, Syntfeld-Kazuch A, et al. A comparative study of silicon drift detectors with photomultipliers, avalanche photodiodes and PIN photodiodes in gamma spectrometry with LaBr crystals. IEEE Trans Nucl Sci. 2009;56:1006–11.
37. Braga LHC, Gasparini L, Grant L, Henderson RK, Massari N, Perenzoni M, Stoppa D, Walker R. A fully digital 8 × 16 SiPM Array for PET applications with per-pixel TDCs and real-time energy output. IEEE J Solid State Circuits. 2014;49:301–14. https://doi.org/10.1109/JSSC.2013.2284351.
38. Gallivanoni A, Rech I, Ghioni M. Progress in quenching circuits for single photon avalanche diodes. IEEE Trans Nucl Sci. 2010;57:3815–26. https://doi.org/10.1109/TNS.2010.2074213.
39. Palubiak DP, Li Z, Deen MJ. Afterpulsing characteristics of free-running and time-gated single-photon avalanche diodes in 130-nm CMOS. IEEE Trans Electron Devices. 2015;62:3727–33. https://doi.org/10.1109/TED.2015.2475126.
40. Bonanno G, Finocchiaro P, Pappalardo A, Billotta S, Cosentino L, Belluso M, Di Mauro S, Occhipinti G. Precision measurements of photon detection efficiency for SiPM detectors. Nucl Instruments Methods Phys Res Sect A Accel Spectrometers Detect Assoc Equip. 2009;610:93–7. https://doi.org/10.1016/j.nima.2009.05.117.
41. Yoon HS, Ko GB, Kwon SI, Lee CM, Ito M, Chan SI, Lee DS, Hong SJ, Lee JS. Initial results of simultaneous PET/MRI experiments with an MRI-compatible silicon photomultiplier PET scanner. J Nucl Med. 2012;53:608–14. https://doi.org/10.2967/jnumed.111.097501.
42. Pro T, Ferri A, Gola A, Serra N, Tarolli A, Zorzi N, Piemonte C. New developments of near-UV SiPMs at FBK. IEEE Trans Nucl Sci. 2013;60:2247–53. https://doi.org/10.1109/TNS.2013.2259505.
43. Hartwig V, Giovannetti G, Vanello N, Lombardi M, Landini L, Simi S. Biological effects and safety in magnetic resonance imaging: a review. Int J Environ Res Public Health. 2009;6(6):1778–98.
44. Dini L, Abbro L. Bioeffects of moderate-intensity static magnetic fields on cell cultures. Micron. 2005;36(3):195–217.
45. Herzog H, Lerche C. Advances in clinical PET/MRI instrumentation. PET Clin. 2016;11:95–103. https://doi.org/10.1016/j.cpet.2015.09.001.
46. Vandenberghe S, Marsden PK. PET-MRI: a review of challenges and solutions in the development of integrated multimodality imaging. Phys Med Biol. 2015;60:R115–54. https://doi.org/10.1088/0031-9155/60/4/R115.
47. Zaidi H, Del Guerra A. An outlook on future design of hybrid PET/MRI systems. Med Phys. 2011;38:5667–89. https://doi.org/10.1118/1.3633909.
48. Cabello J, Ziegler SI. Advances in PET/MR instrumentation and image reconstruction. Br J Radiol.

2018;91:20160363. https://doi.org/10.1259/bjr.20160363.
49. Zaidi H, Ojha N, Morich M, Griesmer J, Hu Z, Maniawski P. Design and performance evaluation of a whole-body ingenuity TF PET-MRI system. Phys Med Biol. 2011;56:3091–106. https://doi.org/10.1088/0031-9155/56/10/013.
50. Pichler BJ, Judenhofer MS, Catana C, Walton JH, Kneilling M, Nutt RE. Performance test of an LSO-APD detector in a 7-T MRI scanner for simultaneous PET/MRI. J Nucl Med. 2006;47:639–47.
51. Spanoudaki VC, Mann AB, Otte AN, Konorov I, Torres-Espallardo I, Paul S, et al. Use of single photon counting detector arrays in combined PET/MR: characterization of LYSO-SiPM detector modules and comparison with a LSO-APD detector. J Instrum. 2007;2:P12002. https://doi.org/10.1088/1748-0221/2/12/P12002.
52. Judenhofer MS, Wehrl HF, Newport DF, Catana C, Siegel SB, Becker M. Simultaneous PET-MRI: a new approach for functional and morphological imaging. Nat Med. 2008;14:459–65. https://doi.org/10.1038/nm1700.
53. Spanoudaki VC, Levin CS. Photo-detectors for time of flight positron emission tomography (ToF-PET). Sensors. 2010;10:10484–505. https://doi.org/10.3390/s101110484.
54. Delso G, Fürst S, Jakoby B, Ladebeck R, Ganter C, Nekolla SG. Performance measurements of the siemens mMR integrated whole-body PET/MR scanner. J Nucl Med. 2011;52:1914–22. https://doi.org/10.2967/jnumed.111.092726.
55. Grant AM, Deller TW, Khalighi MM, Maramraju SH, Delso G, Levin CS. NEMA NU 2-2012 performance studies for the SiPM-based ToFPET component of the GE SIGNA PET/MR system. Med Phys. 2016;43:2334–43. https://doi.org/10.1118/1.4945416.
56. Mandai S, Jain V, Charbon E. A 780×800 μm^2 multichannel digital silicon photomultiplier with column-parallel time-to-digital converter and basic characterization. IEEE Trans Nucl Sci. 2014;61:44–52. https://doi.org/10.1109/TNS.2013.2294022.
57. Lecoq P, Auffray E, Brunner S, Hillemanns H, Jarron P, Knapitsch A, et al. Factors influencing time resolution of scintillators and ways to improve them. IEEE Trans Nucl Sci. 2010;57:2411–6. https://doi.org/10.1109/TNS.2010.2049860.
58. Hutton BF. The origins of SPECT and SPECT/CT. Eur J Nucl Med Mol Imaging. 2014;41:3–16.
59. Ritt P, Sanders J, Kuwert T. SPECT/CT technology. Clin Transl Imaging. 2014;2:445–57. https://doi.org/10.1007/s40336-014-0086-7.
60. Walrand S, Hesse M, Jamar F. Update on novel trends in PET/CT technology and its clinical applications. Br J Radiol. 2018;91:20160534.
61. Vandenberghe S, Marsden PK. PET-MRI: a review of challenges and solutions in the development of integrated multimodality imaging. Phys Med Biol. 2015;60:R115–54.
62. Gundacker S, Acerbi F, Auffray E, Ferri A, Gola A, Nemallapudi MV, et al. State of the art timing in TOF-PET detectors with LuAG, GAGG and L(Y)SO scintillators of various sizes coupled to FBK-SiPMs. J Instrum. 2016;11:P08008.
63. Chun SY. The use of anatomical information for molecular image reconstruction algorithms: attenuation/scatter correction, motion compensation, and noise reduction. Nucl Med Mol Imaging. 2016;50:13–23.
64. Beyer T, Freudenberg LS, Townsend DW, Czernin J. The future of hybrid imaging—part 1: hybrid imaging technologies and SPECT/CT. Insights Imaging. 2011;2:161–9.
65. Yamamoto S, Okumura S, Kato N, Yeom JY. Timing measurements of lutetium based scintillators combined with silicon photomultipliers for TOF-PET system. J Instrum. 2015;10:T09002.
66. Schug D, Wehner J, Dueppenbecker PM, Weissler B, Gebhardt P, Goldschmidt B, Solf T, Kiessling F, Schulz V. ToF performance evaluation of PET modules with digital silicon photomultiplier technology during MR operation. IEEE Trans Nucl Sci. 2015c;62:658–63.
67. Pichler BJ, Judenhofer MS, Catana C, Walton JH, Kneilling M, Nutt RE. Performance test of an LSO-APD detector in a 7-T MRI scanner for simultaneous PET/MRI. J Nucl Med. 2006;47:639–47.
68. Spanoudaki VC, Mann AB, Otte AN, Konorov I, Torres-Espallardo I, Paul S, et al. Use of single photon counting detector arrays in combined PET/MR: characterization of LYSO-SiPM detector modules and comparison with a LSO-APD detector. J Instrum. 2007;2:P12002. https://doi.org/10.1088/1748-0221/2/12/P12002.
69. Buzhan P, Dolgoshein B, Filatov L, Ilyin A, Kaplin V, Karakash A, Klemin S, Mirzoyan R, Otte AN, Popova E, Sosnovtsev V, Teshima M. Large area silicon photomultipliers: performance and applications. Nucl Instrum Methods Phys Res A. 2006;567:78–82.
70. Kolb A, Lorenz E, Judenhofer MS, Renker D, Lankes K, Pichler BJ. Evaluation of Geiger-mode APDs for PET block detector designs. Phys Med Biol. 2010;55:1815–32.
71. Aull BF, Loomis AH, Young DJ, Heinrichs RM, Felton BJ, Daniels PJ, Landers DJ. Geiger-mode avalanche photodiodes for three-dimensional imaging. Linc Lab J. 2002;13:335–50.
72. Schuette DR, Westhoff RC, Loomis AH, Young DJ, Ciampi JS, Aull BF, Reich RK. Hybridization process for back-illuminated silicon Geiger-mode avalanche photodiode arrays. Proc SPIE. 2010;7681(1):76810P.
73. Herbert DJ, Moehrs S, D'Ascenzo N, Belcari N, Del Guerra A, Morsani F. The silicon photomultiplier for application to high-resolution positron emis-

sion tomography. Nucl Instrum Methods Phys Res. 2007;A573:84–7.

74. Nguyen NC, Vercher-Conejero JL, Sattar A, Miller MA, Maniawski PJ, Jordan DW, et al. Image quality and diagnostic performance of a digital PET prototype in patients with oncologic diseases: initial experience and comparison with analog PET. J Nucl Med. 2015;56(9):1378–85.
75. Zhang J, Knopp MI, Knopp MV. Sparse detector configuration in SiPM digital photon counting PET: a feasibility study. Mol Imaging Biol. 2018. https://doi.org/10.1007/s11307-018-1250-7.

Molecular Imaging Biomarkers and Agents

3

Key Points (Abstracts)

Imaging biomarkers are defined as anatomic, physiologic, biochemical, or molecular parameters which are able to identify and diagnose by the use of the various imaging modalities the presence and severity of the particular disease. With the advent of the technology the biomarker concept and their applications are very important for the diagnosis and evaluation of the various pathologies. By the virtue of the small quantity doses of biomarkers still they are having very high sensitivity and specificity to evaluate various pathologies. And many of biomarkers are not much expensive and due to this they are being used very often in various preclinical and clinical studies. They are also useful for the detection and/or quantification of the biomarkers, and these biomarkers are capable of giving more important precise information which can be reproducible, and also give information at particular time; and also, to evaluate the therapeutic response as well as the effects.

The biomarkers can characterize the particular disease entity with the particular pattern of behaviour. Biomarkers which are being used in the cancer are primarily based on the various assays of blood or tissue.

Keywords

Biomarkers · CEST Imaging · PET-CT · Nano particles imaging · Monoclonal antibodies

3.1 Introduction

The term ***biomarker*** is used to for describing the biologic measure in the tissues and cells which will characterize the disease status and also for the prediction of the disease behaviour.

The biomarker components are being studied based on the various guidelines which can be used for the various cancer clinical trials and also for the clinical care [1, 2]. The REMARK guidelines (Reporting Recommendations for Tumor Marker Prognostic Studies) reporting criteria is now most commonly used in the cancer biomarker trials [2]. The important guidelines and trial reporting on the biomarkers are based on the various aspects like [1, 2]: to determine validity of the biomarkers in various aspects like the calibration, precision, and accuracy of the measurement; cancer therapeutics evaluation; and clinical value supporting the biomarker. Various measurements of the calibration, like positive or negative, and quantitative measurements can be measured by these biomarkers. The prospective evaluation of the biomarkers to access their efficiency and the final outcome which is based on the various factors and will be impacting on disease outcome can also be studied [1–3]. Evaluation of the multigene assays for various tumours like breast cancer which can be used for the adjuvant therapy trials and also for the validation for their use in the chemotherapy where there will be validation of the biomarkers [4] Diagram 3.1.

S. Shaikh, *Advances in Imaging*, https://doi.org/10.1007/978-981-16-9535-3_3

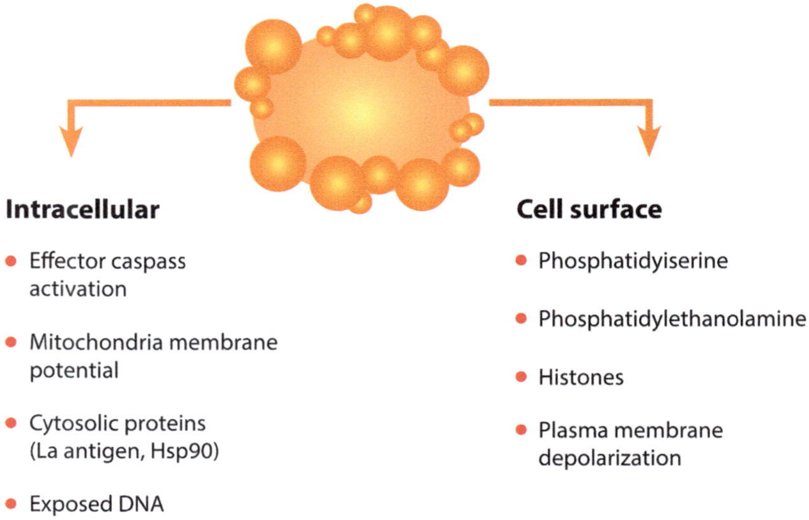

Diagram 3.1 Showing the intracellular and extracellular biomarkers for cell death imaging

These molecular biomarkers are of great potential and also very helpful for the use in the anatomical imaging, evaluate various pathological tissue characteristics in subclinical stages of the diseases and also for final outcome evaluation [5]. The use of these Biomarkers is different modalities, and is purely based on the kinetics and pharmacodynamics of those modalities. Magnetic resonance imaging (MRI) biomarkers are mostly used in the molecular imaging of various diseases. For the evaluation very low sensitivity is needed ~10 μM to ~10 mM for the contrast agent, and also on the MRI contrast [6–9]. These MRI contrast agents are being used for the targeting various biomarkers with the ~10 μM to ~10 mM concentrations in vivo. The metallic contrast agents which are delivered into cells at ~10 μM to ~10 mM are having potential to alter the cell behaviour and result in the cell death [10, 11]. MRI contrast agents are more useful in the extracellular compartment by using various biomarkers. These biomarkers are atomic or molecular targets, in the extracellular matrix which are made up of the various proteins and focussed on various ions, and metabolites causing one to one interaction between the agent and the target [12, 13]. MRI contrast agents are in different components of the various cells, liposomes, and nanoparticles [14–17] Diagram 3.2. They are capable of tracking the pharmacokinetic transport and also used for the nanoparticle drug delivery by the cell tracking mechanism. Also, it is very effective to analyse the various vascular permeability, perfusion, and also the blood-brain barrier [18, 19]. They can easily differentiate between the normal and the pathological tissues. T2 contrast agents are more relevant in this aspect and seen as the more advance potentials. The use of the exogenous chemical exchange saturation transfer (CEST) MRI contrast agents along with the hyperpolarized 13C MRI contrast agents are being developed in the recent years [2].

3.2 T1 and T2 MRI Contrast Agents

Technically MR sequences are capable of developing the image contrast based on the different T1 or T2 relaxation times [20]. Exogenous T1 and T2 contrast agents are having more affinity to accumulate in the pathological tissues which can identify more abnormalities [21, 22]. The contrast agents used for MRI studies need to have the excited magnetic resonance (MR) states from the relaxed stage to the equilibrium stage. The most commonly used are the gadolinium or manganese having unpaired electrons, for the relaxation of the excited signals of the MR signal [23, 24]. The factors affecting the micro chelates also

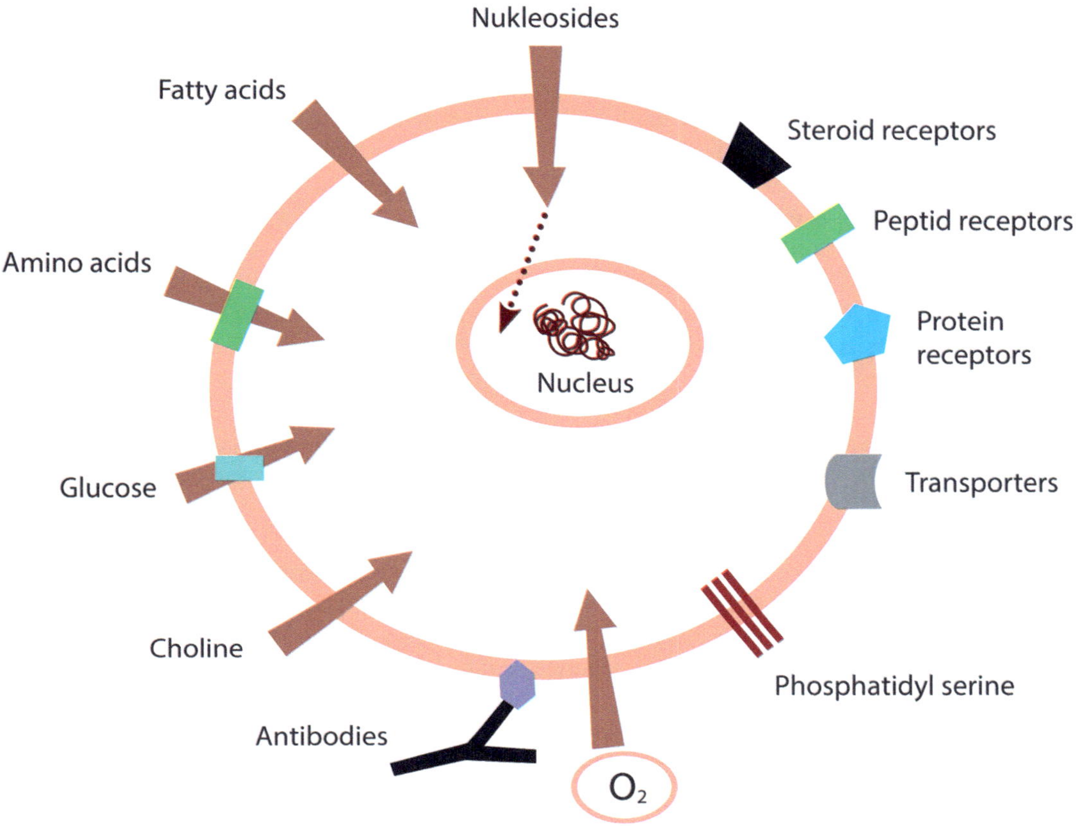

Diagram 3.2 The different biomarkers are having different targets. Various labels are conjugated to target moieties for stronger signals for the better evaluation

affect the various T1 relaxation of the tissues [12, 13]. The protons capacity on the water molecules will possess the same MR frequency depending on the various aspects of the chemical shift in the tissues.

3.2.1 Pharmacokinetic Relaxation-Based Agents

Many newer T1 and T2 MRI contrast agents are being developed and nanoparticles is one of them [25]. These agents are insensitivity to the T1 and T2 MRI contrast agents in nanoparticle. The tumbling time of the nanoparticle will be slower as compared with the small molecule MRI contrast agents, causing the enhancement of the relaxation properties of these agents. These two effects will be resulting in the increased T1 or T2 relaxation effects which are based on the size of the nanoparticle. The wash out is very slow of more than the 24 hours, and this is leading to the toxicity, of all these containing the Gd^{3+} or Mn^{2+} ions, or iron-based particles other than iron oxides [26, 27]. These multimodal agents are easily detected by MRI and positron emission tomography and optical imaging [28, 29]. Contrast agents for MRI and other imaging modalities will be having significant difference [30].

3.2.2 Responsive Relaxation-Based Agents

Biomarker-responsive T1 and T2 agents for the evaluation of the molecular conditions of the tissue environment. The poor sensitivity of MRI will require a greater number of the contrast biomarkers. T2 relaxation of the water is based on the concept of the water protons having the MR frequencies which will be able to accelerate or decelerate for the exchanges with a proton on a contrast agent. The use of the Glucose for the management of the carbohydrate and fluid depletion is also there [31]. The use of the various pharmacokinetics of CT can be done easily as the angiography and tissue perfusion are very simple, otherwise there will be increased pharmacokinetics of glucose leading to the vascular permeability to be accessed.

3.3 CEST MRI Contrast Agents

CEST MRI contrast agents have the slowest chemical exchange rates relative to T1, T2, and T2ex contrast agents [32]. As a result, these agents have the least-sensitive detection, requiring a minimum concentration in the single-millimolar range. CEST agents are the important specific extracellular biomarkers and are never used for the anatomical imaging. Paramagnetic CEST agents, which are known as paraCEST agents, combines the paramagnetic ion within a macrocyclic chelate to shift the MR frequency of +500 to −720 ppm from the MR frequency of water [33]. The use of the larger frequencies will result in selective saturation of the labile proton agent along with the direct saturation of water. The CEST Agents pharmacokinetically are the exogenous biomaterials like the various hydrogels which are being used in the stem cell therapy, as they are the non-invasive, very site-specific delivery into the various tissues. CEST MRI-based reporter genes are biocompatible and are not interfering with the T1 or T2 MRI mechanisms, which are capable of highlighting the multiple genes of the CEST MR image. Responsive CEST Contrast agents are called responsive agents to differentiate them from the non-responsive agents. These responsive agents are also called as the activatable agents.

3.4 Detection of Metabolites

CEST MRI is being used for the evaluation of the various metabolites, which will be including the glucose, glutamate, myo-inositol, creatinine, and hydrogen peroxide. The detection of all these components will lead to the detection and uptake of the various metabolically active compounds in the physiological amounts. The uptake in the glucose in a tumour tissue can be monitored by the glucoCEST. This GlucoCEST MRI will be able to monitor the CEST effect from the glutamate amine proton measuring the glutamate concentrations in the brain and also for the potential as a biomarker for the central nervous system disorders [34].

3.4.1 Measurement of pH

Extracellular pH measurement and monitoring will be helpful in the evaluation of the pH alterations which can be used for the clinical diagnoses many pathologies and conditions such as the renal failure, ischemia, and chronic obstructive pulmonary disease. The increased lactic acid secretion along with the reduced bicarbonate levels in the tumour tissues will result in the higher acidity of the various tissues.

3.4.2 Measurement of Temperature

The temperature evaluation of the tissues will lead in the increase chemical exchange rates. With the chemical exchange rate nearing the difference in MR frequency of the water and the amide's proton, then this process of the MR coalescence will cause the frequency of the agent to decrease.

3.5 Advances in Magnetic Resonance Imaging

The use of the Gd^{3+} ions for the promotion of the rapid T1 relaxation of the electron and for the acceleration of the various transfer rate of dynamic nuclear polarization, causing the significant improvement in the hyperpolarization by 1.5- to ten-fold [35]. The tumour pH can be measured by the hyperpolarized bicarbonate, which gets converted to the carbon dioxide, through the carbonic anhydrase enzyme activity [36]. Here MRS can be used for the quantification of the ratio of bicarbonate to carbon dioxide concentrations by the Henderson–Hasselbalch equation.

T1 and T2 $*$ contrast agents are basically used for the anatomical imaging, but the recent developments lead to the newer T2ex agents having the slower chemical exchange. CEST MRI contrast agents have a slow chemical exchange rate modulated by the various molecular biomarkers, thus significantly increasing the specificity for biomarker detection. The use of the molecular imaging agent has two components targeting component and a signalling component. The role of the agent is to evaluate the specific target (or targets) of interest for the various studies. Some molecular imaging techniques such as MRS [37], RS [38], and coherent anti stokes Raman scattering microscopy [39] they do not need the exogenous agent for visualizing biochemical targets and pathologies. The various imaging agents are in the form of the probes, imaging probes, agents, molecular beacons, molecular spies, molecular detectives, radiopharmaceuticals, tracers, radioligands, and radiolabelled probes. The radioactive agents are usually tagged/labelled with a radioisotope. Ideal molecular imaging agent should be having the very good ratio of specific to non-specific binding, various high selectivity of the various biochemical target/process of interest, suitable pharmacokinetics, excellent in vivo stability, good safety profile, potential for clinical translation, time and cost-effective synthesis, signal amplification, and multiplexing capabilities. The rate of absorption and delivery of the imaging agent to the target site, metabolism, excretion, and enterohepatic circulation are important. Ideal imaging agent also has rapid binding to or interaction with its target, fast blood clearance, urinary excretion, and persistent, high accumulation at the target site. The size criteria is an important along with the charge, and lipophilicity, again this is depending on the type of imaging agent [40–43]. The half-life of an imaging agent's signalling component, pharmacokinetics, and also the pharmacokinetics of the area of interest needs to be evaluated. The imaging agent should also have very good metabolic stability in vivo. The metabolic stability is important to prevent the breakdown of the various imaging agents by the various metabolic pathways, Enzyme substrate imaging agents are the imaging agents which will be undergoing the chemical modification so that they can't leave the cell. Various forms of the fluorophores, fluorescent proteins, luciferases, SERS nanoparticles can be used to target the various processes and can be used for the imaging at same time. Various categories of molecular imaging agents are the various small molecules, peptides, aptamers, high-molecular-weight antibodies, engineered protein fragments, and also various nanoparticles.

Bioluminescence imaging is also the important component of the molecular imaging where the luciferase is being used for the various smart/activatable signal components from the luciferase enzyme gene which is expressed.

There are two main types of small molecule imaging agents: 1) molecules that bind specific receptors, transporters, or ion channels, like the [11C]PK11195 which is the PET radioligand capable of binding the peripheral benzodiazepine receptor (PBR) for the evaluation of the microglia and neuroinflammation for the various neurological pathologies [44, 45]. Fluorine-18 radiolabelled fluorodeoxyglucose ([18F]FDG) is the most commonly used positron emission tomography (PET) imaging agent based on the hexokinase type II and glucose transporter I for the evaluation of the glucose metabolism. Various PET radiotracers like the 11C and 18F are used for the labelling smaller molecules due to their smaller size. The use of the small molecule agents can be helpful for the imaging of the glucose metabolism, hypoxia, fatty acid synthase, reporter genes, and biochemical targets involved in brain disease. Peptide imaging agents for the evaluation of the various targets, including integrins [46–48], matrix metalloproteinases [49, 50], caspases [51, 52], somatostatin receptors [53–55], neuropeptide Y receptor [56, 57], and gastrin releasing peptide receptor [58–60]. Peptides are more prone for the rapid proteolytic degradation in vivo and having the smaller plasma half-life.

3.6 Aptamers

Aptamers are the single-stranded DNA or RNA oligonucleotides which binds to the target site with a high degree of specificity and selectivity [61]. For in vitro setting, aptamers are being used more precisely for the various applications [62] replacing antibodies in various traditional in vitro diagnostic assays [63]. In Aptamers, the first aptamer (Pegaptanib) is the approved by the United States Food and Drug Administration (FDA) in 2004 for treatment of macular degeneration [64]. They are having excellent targeting capabilities as compared to the antibodies, as well that they can be synthesized easily [65–67], high diversity, not expensive. Thus the aptamers are having the important feature to distinguish between similar molecules, for the diagnosing and differentiating various diseases at early stages.

3.6.1 Antibodies and Engineered Proteins

Monoclonal antibodies (mAbs) are also called as the immunoglobulins which are the 150 kDa, Y-shaped proteins. The mAbs interacts with the binding pockets or active sites and also for binding the adhesion molecules, activation markers, antigens, and receptors [68].

mAbs therapy is very expensive affair but the predicting responders/nonresponders before the treatment is of great value. The overall versatility and usefulness is due to more time in the blood circulation along with the various transverse biological barriers (e.g., the blood-brain barrier and cell membranes). 125I, 111In, and 99mTc, are more helpful with the high-contrast images of tumours seen early in post-injection [69].

3.7 Nanoparticles

The nanotechnology in biomedical applications is being evolved which will be used for the translation of these nanomaterials and technologies into the clinical use [70]. As they are having high surface area-to-volume ratio due to which the various nanoparticles can carry the substantial amount of the targeting and/or signalling moieties and therapeutic drug. Nanoparticle targets can be used for the various applications like to determine the amount of the signal generated from each small molecule imaging agent which is bound to the target. This multivalent mode of attachment is crucial in the cases where the sensitivity of the imaging modality is an issue. The use of the large number of targeting moieties attached to the surface of nanoparticles is an advantage. The therapeutic payload means that nanoparticles can reduce various side effects like the chemotherapeutics. The therapeutic and diagnostic capabilities of nanoparticles make them more for their "theranostic potential", where the nanoparticle-based imaging agents can be detecting, monitoring, and treating pathologies. SWNTs for imaging molecular phenomena, targeting moieties (e.g., small molecules, peptides, aptamers, or engineered proteins), specific for the biochemical process of interest, need to be conjugated to their surface, transforming them into targeted SWNTs. The EPR effect principle is that the various macromolecules, including drugs and nanoparticles, can pass thought the various tumour tissue to the greater extent than normal tissue as they are having the increased vascular permeability based on the various tumour tissue types Diagram 3.3.

3.8 QDots

QDots are the small nanoparticles of the size 10 nm made up of the semiconductor materials like the cadmium and selenium. With the conducting properties of the QDots the quantum effect will have the various size and shape of individual crystals [71]. The emission wavelength of QDots can be altered by its size. QDots can be used in multiplexing by which it can be synthesized, with the emission wavelengths and concurrent excita-

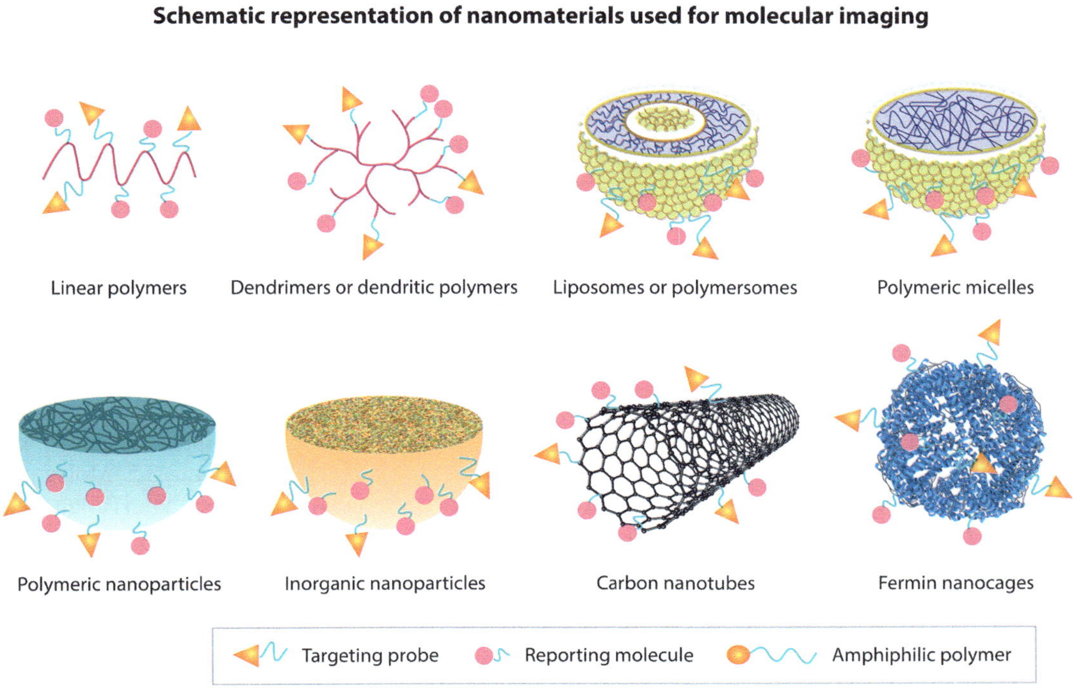

Diagram 3.3 Various nanoparticles used in molecular imaging

tion and several target imaging [72]. QDots can increase the size to 20–30 nm by adding the polymer coat and/or functionalization. QDots are brighter due to their high quantum yield, and are more photostable (i.e., they undergo significantly less photobleaching). Semiconductor nanocrystals are believed to be 20 times brighter and 100 times more photostable than standard fluorescent reporters [73], meaning images can be acquired over longer periods of time in a more sensitive manner. Biggest disadvantage of QDots is toxic core (made of cadmium), although adding a silica coating to cadmium QDots [74] or the development of new generation cadmium-free QDots [75] could help address toxicity concerns.

3.9 Gold Nanoparticles

As the colloidal gold is inert and approved by the FDA for the treatment of arthritis [76], it is believed that nanoparticles made from gold could be a safer alternative to SWNTs and QDots. The FDA has approved various therapy-based gold nanoparticles (AuNPs) for human administration [77], such as Auramine for the treatment of solid tumours. Two common types of AuNPs used as imaging agents are spherical AuNPs and gold nanorods. Aging which is based on the size, composition, and preparation, it can be used in various anatomical imaging modalities like the MRI, CT, radionuclide, and optical techniques. This phenomenon is known as the SERS effect due to a plasmonic resonance that occurs on the AuNP's surface when excited with a laser. The Gold nanorods are capable of converting the optical energy into heat causing changes in the local photothermal effects. Due to this the gold nanorods are serving the diagnostic as well as therapeutic options. Limitation is that the size of 100 nm spherical nanoparticles may cause problem to extravasate and reach their target site.

3.10 Superparamagnetic Iron Oxide Nanoparticles

Superparamagnetic iron oxide nanoparticles (SPIOs) for imaging with MRI are made up of the iron oxide (magnetite) core coated with a hydrophilic matrix material. The contrast is produced due to the changes in the local magnetic field. This contrast change will result in the ultrafast dephasing of neighbouring protons (shortened T2), causing the alteration in the MR signal [78]; The size of SPIOs changes from the 2–3 nm up to micrometres [78]. SPIOs used for molecular imaging are in tens of nanometres size range, dextran coat for stabilization, directly targeted to membrane receptors. SPIOs important for their biodegradability [79], also the targeting (and cell-loading/tracking) abilities, and low toxicity, but also due to the fact that nontargeted SPIOs have been used in the clinic for some time now (making clinical translation of targeted-SPIOs easier). Limitations of the SPIOs, are the requirements in larger numbers for the MR signal, and due to larger size, they can't permeate the intravascular sites [80]. Also, the slow clearance times, cannot distinguish targeted nanoparticle bound to the target(s) of interest from non-bound nanoparticle.

3.11 Multimodality Probes

Multimodality probes are imaging agents which can be detected by different imaging modalities simultaneously. These probes are capable of generating the multiple readouts for the same biological phenomenon. The various multimodality probes are mainly nanoparticle based like SPIOs, gold nanospheres/nanorods, SWNTs, QDots, engineered proteins [81], peptides [82], and small molecule-type multimodality probes [83] Diagram 3.4. Multimodality imaging probes are MRI/ optical, MRI/PET, MRI/SPECT, PET/optical, SPECT/optical, PAI/Raman, and PAI/ Raman/IVM imaging. Diagram 3.5 Molecular imaging of angiogenesis is 99mTc-labelled gadolinium-containing v3-targeted nanoparticles. SPECT and MRI nanoparticles imaging in the tumour-bearing rabbits [84] accumulation in tumour neo vasculature is demonstrated. 3D mapping of angiogenesis in the tumour can be done where some of the limitations of the modal-

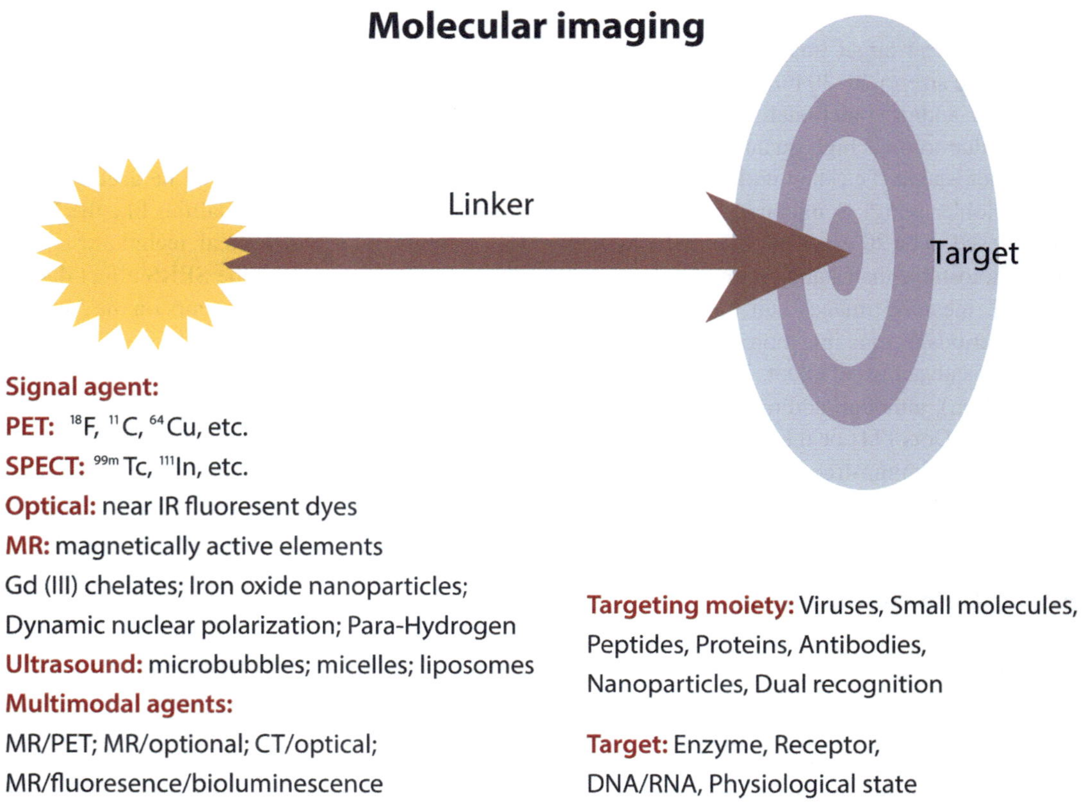

Diagram 3.4 Various representations of the molecular probes

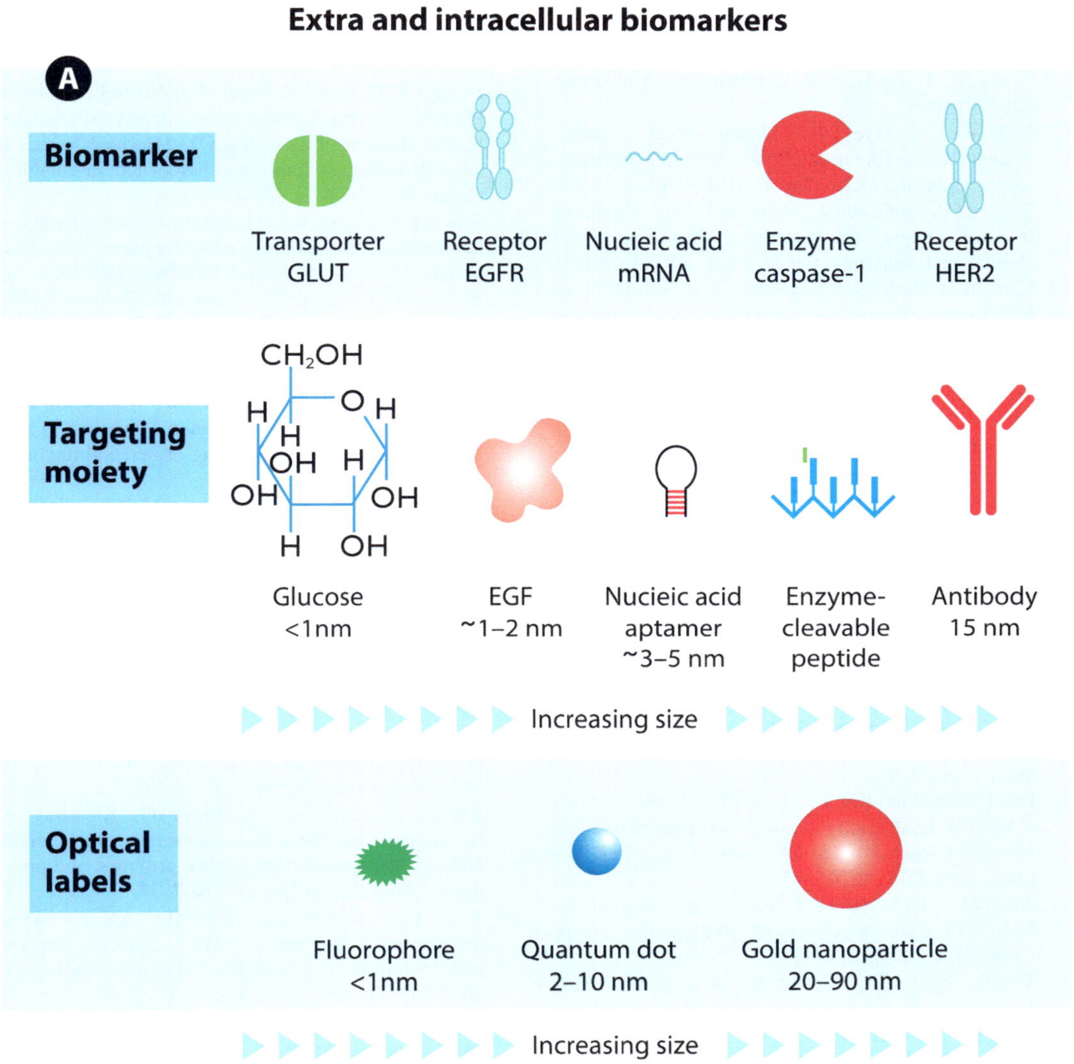

Diagram 3.5 Radiopharmaceutical targets on the cell surface

ities like CT cannot sometimes differentiate between the tumour and lymph node, thus SPECT/MRI multimodality probe in comparison with the SPECT probe and SPECT/CT. Another multimodality imaging probe is the imaging modalities (MRI, PAI, and Raman imaging) is the MPR nanoparticle [85]. This triple-modality probe can identify tumour margins in mice bearing orthotopic human glioblastoma tumours in the intact skull. The strengths of MRI, PAI, and Raman imaging, as the MPR nanoparticle are highly sensitively and accurately detect tumour margins at high spatial resolution. Advantages of the multimodality probe are less time, single injection is needed, 3) complementary to each other like the PET/MRI multimodality probes, and the pharmacokinetics will be kept constant [86]. The biggest challenge is the developing and using multimodality imaging probes is that some modalities (such as PET and MRI) differ in their sensitivities by more than three orders of magnitude [86].

Imaging agents The Achilles' heel of most molecular imaging techniques can be done after the administration of the exogenous imaging agent.

References

1. Henry NL, Hayes DF. Cancer biomarkers. Mol Oncol. 2012;6:140–6.
2. McShane LM, Hayes DF. Publication of tumor marker research results: the necessity for complete and transparent reporting. J Clin Oncol. 2012;30:4223–32.
3. Sargent DJ, Rubinstein L, Schwartz L, et al. Validation of novel imaging methodologies for use as cancer clinical trial endpoints. Eur J Cancer. 2009;45:290–9.
4. Carlson JJ, Roth JA. The impact of the Oncotype dx breast cancer assay in clinical practice: a systematic review and meta-analysis. Breast Cancer Res Treat. 2013;141:13–22.
5. Weissleder R, Ross BD, Rehemtulla R, Gambhir SS, editors. Molecular imaging: principles and practice. Shelton, CT: People's Med. Pub. House; 2010.
6. Ahrens ET, Rothbacher U, Jacobs RE, Fraser SE. A model for MRI contrast enhancement using T1 agents. PNAS. 1998;95:8443–8.
7. Mills PH, Ahrens ET. Theoretical MRI contrast model for T2 agents. Magn Reson Med. 2007;57:442–7.
8. Ali MM, Liu G, Shah T, Flask CA, Pagel MD. Using two chemical exchange saturation transfer magnetic resonance imaging contrast agents for molecular imaging studies. Acc Chem Res. 2008;42:915–24.
9. Nelson SJ, Ozhinsky E, Li Y, Park IW, Crane J. Strategies for rapid in vivo 1H and hyperpolarized 13C MR spectroscopic imaging. J Magn Reson. 2013;229:187–97.
10. Dua P, Chaudhari KN, Lee C-H, Chaudhari NK, Song S-W, et al. Evaluation of toxicity and gene expression changes triggered by oxide nanoparticles. Bull Kor Chem Soc. 2011;32:2051–7.
11. Allen MJ, MacRenaris KW, Venkatasubramanian PN, Meade TJ. Cellular delivery of MRI contrast agents. Chem Biol. 2004;11:301–7.
12. Yoo B, Pagel MD. An overview of responsive MRI contrast agents for molecular imaging. Front Biosci. 2008;13:1733–52.
13. Hingorani DV, Bernstein AS, Pagel MD. A review of responsive MRI contrast agents: 2005–2014. Contrast Media Mol Imaging. 2014;10:245–65.
14. Bulte JWM, Kraitchman DL, Ben-Hur T. Use of iron oxide MR contrast agents for monitoring stem cell therapy. In: Greer DA, editor. Focus on stem cell research. Hauppauge, NY: Nova Sci; 2004. p. 1–32.
15. Ferrauto G, Delli Castelli D, Di Gregorio E, Langereis S, Burdinski D, et al. Lanthanide-loaded erythrocytes as highly sensitive chemical exchange saturation transfer MRI contrast agents. J Am Chem Soc. 2014;136:638–41.
16. Terreno E, Cabella C, Carrera C, Delli Castelli D, Mazzon R, et al. From spherical to osmotically shrunken paramagnetic liposomes: an improved generation of LIPOCEST MRI agents with highly shifted water protons. Angew Chem Int Ed. 2007;46:966–8.
17. Ali MM, Yoo B, Pagel MD. Tracking the relative in vivo pharmacokinetics of nanoparticles with PARACEST MRI. Mol Pharm. 2009;6:1409–16.
18. Davis TW, O'Neal JM, Pagel MD, Zweifel BS, Mehta PP, et al. Synergy between celecoxib and radiotherapy results from inhibition of COX-2-derived PGE2, a survival factor for tumor and associated vasculature. Cancer Res. 2004;64:279–85.
19. Kassner A, Thornhill R. Measuring the integrity of the human blood-brain barrier using magnetic resonance imaging. Methods Mol Biol. 2011;686:229–45.
20. Brown RW, Cheng Y-CN, Haake EM, Thompson MR, Venkatesan R, editors. Magnetic resonance imaging: physical principles and sequence design. 2nd ed. Hoboken NJ: Wiley; 2014.
21. Carr DH, Brown J, Bydder GM, Weinmann H-J, Speck U, et al. Intravenous chelated gadolinium as a contrast agent in NMR imaging of cerebral tumours. Lancet. 1984;1:484–6.
22. Edelman RR, Mattle HP, Atkinson DJ, Hill T, Finn JP, et al. Cerebral blood flow: assessment with dynamic contrast-enhanced T2 ∗-weighted MR imaging at 1.5 T. Radiologica. 1990;176:211–20.
23. Carr DH, Brown J, Bydder GM, Steiner RH, Weinmann HJ, et al. Gadolinium-DTPA as a contrast agent in MRI: initial clinical experience in 20 patients. Am J Roentgenol. 1984;143:215–24.
24. Fiel RJ, Button TM, Gilani S, Mark EH, Musser DA, et al. Proton relaxation enhancement by manganese(III)TPPS4 in a model tumor system. Magn Reson Imaging. 1987;5:149–56.
25. Kunjachan S, Ehling J, Storm G, Kiessling F, Lammers T. Noninvasive imaging of nanomedicines and nanotheranostics: principles, progress, and prospects. Chem Rev. 2015;115:10907–37.
26. Kuo PH, Kanal E, Abu-Alfa AK, Cowper SE. Gadolinium-based MR contrast agents and nephrogenic systemic fibrosis. Radiology. 2007;242:647–9.
27. Dydak U, Criswell SR. Imaging modalities for manganese toxicity. Issues Toxicol. 2015;22:477–512.
28. Frullano L, Catana C, Benner T, Sherry AD, Caravan P. Bimodal MRI-PET agent for quantitative pH imaging. Angew Chem Int Ed. 2010;49:2382–4.
29. Jing L, Ding K, Kershaw SV, Kempson IM, Rogach AL, Gao M. Magnetically engineered semiconductor quantum dots as multimodal imaging probes. Adv Mater. 2014;26:6367–86.
30. Lee S, Chen X. Dual-modality probes for molecular imaging. Mol Imaging. 2009;8(2):87–100.
31. Yadav NN, Xu J, Bar-Shir A, Qin Q, Chan KWY, et al. Natural D-glucose as a biodegradable MRI relaxation agent. Magn Reson Med. 2014;72:823–8.
32. Sherry AD, Wu Y. The importance of water exchange rates in the design of responsive agents for MRI. Curr Opin Chem Biol. 2013;17:167–74.
33. Viswanathan S, Kovacs Z, Green KN, Ratnakar SJ, Sherry AD. Alternatives to gadolinium-based metal chelates for magnetic resonance imaging. Chem Rev. 2010;110:2960–3018.

34. Cai K, Haris M, Kogan F, Greenberg JH, Hariharan H, et al. Magnetic resonance imaging of glutamate. Nat Med. 2012;18:302–6.
35. Ardenkjær-Larsen JH, Macholl S, Johannesson H. Dynamic nuclear polarization with trityls at 1.2 K. Appl Magn Reson. 2008;34:509–22.
36. Gallagher FA, Kettunen MI, Day SE, Hu E-D, Ardenkjær-Larsen JH, et al. Magnetic resonance imaging of pH in vivo using hyperpolarized 13C-labelled bicarbonate. Nature. 2008;453:940–3.
37. Mullins ME. MR spectroscopy: truly molecular imaging; past, present and future. Neuroimaging Clin N Am. 2006;16:605–18.
38. Wachsmann-Hogiu S, Weeks T, Huser T. Chemical analysis in vivo and in vitro by Raman spectroscopy–from single cells to humans. Curr Opin Biotechnol. 2009;20:63–73.
39. Cheng JX, Xie S. Coherent anti-stokes raman scattering microscopy: instrumentation, theory, and applications. J Phys Chem B. 2004;108:827–40.
40. Longmire M, Choyke PL, Kobayashi H. Clearance properties of nano-sized particles and molecules as imaging agents: considerations and caveats. Nanomedicine. 2008;3:703–17.
41. Ogawa M, Kosaka N, Choyke PL, Kobayashi H. In vivo molecular imaging of cancer with a quenching near-infrared fluorescent probe using conjugates of monoclonal antibodies and indocyanine green. Cancer Res. 2009;69:1268–72.
42. Schmidt MM, Wittrup KD. A modeling analysis of the effects of molecular size and binding affinity on tumor targeting. Mol Cancer Ther. 2009;8:2861–71.
43. Torchilin VP. Handbook of targeted delivery of imaging agents. Boca Raton, FL: CRC; 1995.
44. Venneti S, Lopresti BJ, Wang G, Hamilton RL, Mathis CA, Klunk WE, Apte UM, Wiley CA. PK11195 labels activated microglia in Alzheimer's disease and in vivo in a mouse model using PET. Neurobiol Aging. 2009;30:1217–26.
45. Versijpt JJ, Dumont F, Van Laere KJ, Decoo D, Santens P, Audenaert K, Achten E, Slegers G, Dierckx RA, Korf J. Assessment of neuroinflammation and microglial activation in Alzheimer's disease with radiolabelled PK11195 and single photon emission computed tomography. A pilot study Eur Neurol. 2003;50:39–47.
46. Beer AJ, Lorenzen S, Metz S, Herrmann K, Watzlowik P, Wester HJ, Peschel C, Lordick F, Schwaiger M. Comparison of integrin alphaVbeta3 expression and glucose metabolism in primary and metastatic lesions in cancer patients: a PET study using 18F-galacto-RGD and 18F-FDG. J Nucl Med. 2008;49:22–9.
47. Chen X, Conti PS, Moats RA. In vivo near-infrared fluorescence imaging of integrin alphavbeta3 in brain tumor xenografts. Cancer Res. 2004;64:8009–14.
48. Mittra E, Goris M, Iagaru A, Kardan A, Liu S, Shen B, Chin FT, Chen X, Gambhir SS. First in man studies of [18F]FPPRGD2: a novel PET radiopharmaceutical for imaging v3 integrin levels. J Nucl Med. 2010;51:1433.
49. Bremer C, Tung CH, Weissleder R. In vivo molecular target assessment of matrix metalloproteinase inhibition. Nat Med. 2001;7:743–8.
50. Jiang T, Olson ES, Nguyen QT, Roy M, Jennings PA, Tsien RY. Tumor imaging by means of proteolytic activation of cell-penetrating peptides. Proc Natl Acad Sci U S A. 2004;101:17867–72.
51. Drew SC, Haigh CL, Klemm HM, Masters CL, Collins SJ, Barnham KJ, Lawson VA. Optical imaging detects apoptosis in the brain and peripheral organs of prion-infected mice. J Neuropathol Exp Neurol. 2011;70:143–50.
52. Edgington LE, Berger AB, Blum G, Albrow VE, Paulick MG, Lineberry N, Bogyo M. Noninvasive optical imaging of apoptosis by caspase-targeted activity-based probes. Nat Med. 2009;15:967–73.
53. Decristoforo C, Melendez-Alafort L, Sosabowski JK, Mather SJ. 99mTc-HYNIC- [Tyr3]-octreotide for imaging somatostatin-receptor-positive tumors: preclinical evaluation and comparison with 111In-octreotide. J Nucl Med. 2000;41:1114–9.
54. Guhlke S, Wester HJ, Bruns C, Stocklin G. (2-[18F] fluoropropionyl-(D)phe1)-octreotide, a potential radiopharmaceutical for quantitative somatostatin receptor imaging with PET: synthesis, radiolabeling, in vitro validation and biodistribution in mice. Nucl Med Biol. 1994;21:819–25.
55. Pearson DA, Lister-James J, McBride WJ, Wilson DM, Martel LJ, Civitello ER, Taylor JE, Moyer BR, Dean RT. Somatostatin receptor-binding peptides labelled with technetium-99m: chemistry and initial biological studies. J Med Chem. 1996;39:1361–71.
56. Liu JT, Mandella MJ, Ra H, Wong LK, Solgaard O, Kino GS, Piyawattanametha W, Contag CH, Wang TD. Miniature near-infrared dual-axes confocal microscope utilizing a two-dimensional microelectromechanical systems scanner. Opt Lett. 2007;32:256–8.
57. Zwanziger D, Khan IU, Neundorf I, Sieger S, Lehmann L, Friebe M, Dinkelborg L, Beck-Sickinger AG. Novel chemically modified analogues of neuropeptide Y for tumor targeting. Bioconjug Chem. 2008;19:1430–8.
58. Schuhmacher J, Zhang H, Doll J, Macke HR, Matys R, Hauser H, Henze M, Haberkorn U, Eisenhut M. GRP receptor-targeted PET of a rat pancreas carcinoma xenograft in nude mice with a 68Ga-labeled bombesin(6–14) analog. J Nucl Med. 2005;46:691–9.
59. Van de Wiele C, Dumont F, Vanden Broecke R, Oosterlinck W, Cocquyt V, Serreyn R, Peers S, Thornback J, Slegers G, Dierckx RA. Technetium-99m RP527, a GRP analogue for visualisation of GRP receptor-expressing malignancies: a feasibility study. Eur J Nucl Med. 2000;27:1694–9.
60. Van de Wiele C, Phonteyne P, Pauwels P, Goethals I, Van den Broecke R, Cocquyt V, Dierckx RA. Gastrin-releasing peptide receptor imaging in human breast carcinoma versus immunohistochemistry. J Nucl Med. 2008;49:260–4.

61. Bouchard PR, Hutabarat RM, Thompson KM. Discovery and development of therapeutic aptamers. Annu Rev PharmacolToxicol. 2010;50:237–57.
62. Tavitian B. In vivo imaging with oligonucleotides for diagnosis and drug development. Gut. 2003;52(Suppl 4):iv40–7.
63. Jayasena SD. Aptamers: an emerging class of molecules that rival antibodies in diagnostics. Clin Chem. 1999;45:1628–50.
64. Doggrell SA. Pegaptanib: the first antiangiogenic agent approved for neovascular macular degeneration. Expert Opin Pharmacother. 2005;6:1421–3.
65. Friedman M, Stahl S. Engineered affinity proteins for tumour-targeting applications. Biotechnol Appl Biochem. 2009;53:1–29.
66. Levine HA, Nilsen-Hamilton M. A mathematical analysis of SELEX. Comput Biol Chem. 2007;31:11–35.
67. Thiel KW, Giangrande PH. Therapeutic applications of DNA and RNA aptamers. Oligonucleotides. 2009;19:209–22.
68. Malviya G, Conti F, Chianelli M, Scopinaro F, Dierckx RA, Signore A. Molecular imaging of rheumatoid arthritis by radiolabelled monoclonal antibodies: new imaging strategies to guide molecular therapies. Eur J Nucl Med Mol Imaging. 2010;37:386–98.
69. Olafsen T, Wu AM. Antibody vectors for imaging. Semin Nucl Med. 2010;40:167–81.
70. Xia Y. Nanomaterials at work in biomedical research. Nat Mater. 2008;7:758–60.
71. Debbage P, Jaschke W. Molecular imaging with nanoparticles: giant roles for dwarf actors. Histochem Cell Biol. 2008;130:845–75.
72. Wang X, Yang L, Chen ZG, Shin DM. Application of nanotechnology in cancer therapy and imaging. Cancer J Clin. 2008;58:97–110.
73. Walling MA, Novak JA, Shepard JR. Quantum dots for live cell and in vivo imaging. Int J Mol Sci. 2009;10:441–91.
74. Chen Z, Chen H, Meng H, Xing G, Gao X, Sun B, Shi X, Yuan H, Zhang C, Liu R, Zhao F, Zhao Y, Fang X. Bio-distribution and metabolic paths of silica coated CdSeS quantum dots. Toxicol Appl Pharmacol. 2008;230:364–71.
75. Wang K, Shen B, Huang T, Sun X, Li W, Jin G, Li L, Bu L, Li R, Wang D, Chen X. MR reporter gene imaging of endostatin expression and therapy. Mol Imaging Biol. 2010;12(5):520–9.
76. Abrams MJ, Murrer BA. Metal compounds in therapy and diagnosis. Science. 1993;261:725–30.
77. McNeil SE. Nanoparticle therapeutics: a personal perspective. Wiley Interdiscip Rev Nanomed Nanobiotechnol. 2009;1:264–71.
78. Thorek DL, Chen AK, Czupryna J, Tsourkas A. Superparamagnetic iron oxide nanoparticle probes for molecular imaging. Ann Biomed Eng. 2006;34:23–38.
79. Elias A, Tsourkas A. Imaging circulating cells and lymphoid tissues with iron oxide nanoparticles. Hematology Am Soc Hematol Educ Program. 2009;2009:720–6.
80. Albers MJ, Bok R, Chen AP, Cunningham CH, Zierhut ML, Zhang VY, Kohler SJ, Tropp J, Hurd RE, Yen YF, Nelson SJ, Vigneron DB, Kurhanewicz J. Hyperpolarized 13C lactate, pyruvate, and alanine: noninvasive biomarkers for prostate cancer detection and grading. Cancer Res. 2008;68:8607–15.
81. Ogawa M, Regino CA, Seidel J, Green MV, Xi W, Williams M, Kosaka N, Choyke PL, Kobayashi H. Dual-modality molecular imaging using antibodies labelled with activatable fluorescence and a radionuclide for specific and quantitative targeted cancer detection. Bioconjug Chem. 2009;20:2177–84.
82. Edwards WB, Xu B, Akers W, Cheney PP, Liang K, Rogers BE, Anderson CJ, Achilefu S. Agonist-antagonist dilemma in molecular imaging: evaluation of a monomolecular multimodal imaging agent for the somatostatin receptor. Bioconjug Chem. 2008;19:192–200.
83. Mishra A, Pfeuffer J, Mishra R, Engelmann J, Mishra AK, Ugurbil K, Logothetis NK. A new class of Gd-based DO3A-ethylamine-derived targeted contrast agents for MR and optical imaging. Bioconjug Chem. 2006;17:773–80.
84. Lijowski M, Caruthers S, Hu G, Zhang H, Scott MJ, Williams T, Erpelding T, Schmieder AH, Kiefer G, Gulyas G, Athey PS, Gaffney PJ, Wickline SA, Lanza GM. High sensitivity: high-resolution SPECT-CT/MR molecular imaging of angiogenesis in the Vx2 model. Investig Radiol. 2009;44:15–22.
85. Kircher MF, de la Zerda A, Jokerst JV, Zavaleta C, Kempen P, Mittra E, Habte F, Sinclair R, Gambhir SS. A brain tumor molecular imaging strategy using a novel triple modality nanoparticle. Nat Med. 2012;18(5):829–34. https://doi.org/10.1038/nm.2721.
86. Louie A. Multimodality imaging probes: design and challenges. Chem Rev. 2010;110:3146–95.

4 Molecular Imaging in Oncology

Key Points (Abstract)

Various aspects of the metabolic and molecular imaging of tumour are undergoing significant changes based on various technological and physiological aspects for tumour grading, tissue characterization, to define the extent and infiltration of tumours, and planning as well as monitoring the response to therapy. MRI and associated molecular tracer imaging techniques are having potential applications. Significant advances are seen based on MRI, PET, and single-photon emission computed tomography, which are being used for tumour blood flow and microvasculature characterizations.

The use of various biomolecules for the evaluation of various malignancies is based on different malignancies, for post-therapeutic evaluation of these targets. Molecular MR techniques are more preferable due to easy availability of MRI, no radiation, and excellent soft tissue contrast which has motivated more use of MRI for the evaluation of various cellular and gene expression levels.

PET scan is used by the use of the glucose metabolism to evaluate tumour metabolism, and various magnetic resonance spectroscopy can also give more precise information on the metabolism. Protein and DNA synthesis changes can be evaluated by various labelled amino acids and nucleosides. With these available techniques, it will be more possible for the evaluation of tumour size, extent, and infiltration, and also for the characterization of different lesions and also to distinguish between the recurrent tumour and necrosis. Another aspect is to identify the most viable tumour and for taking biopsy from the most viable tumour This will be more helpful for planning and monitoring response to therapy post radiation and chemotherapy.

Various aspects of genomic analysis, targeted drugs, cancer therapeutics, and molecular diagnostics are the upcoming trends in molecular imaging. The role of biomarkers is crucial in the evaluation of various pathologies. Other concepts are by using other biomarkers like genes, genetic expressions, proteins, and metabolites which are commonly used.

Keywords

Cancer · Magnetic resonance imaging · Magnetic resonance spectroscopy · Hyperpolarization · Chemical Exchange Saturation Transfer (CEST) imaging · Reporter genes · Cancer immunotherapy

4.1 Introduction

Personalized medicine is defined by the US President's Council of Advisors on Science and Technology as referring to "...the tailoring of medical treatment to the individual characteris-

S. Shaikh, *Advances in Imaging*, https://doi.org/10.1007/978-981-16-9535-3_4

tics of each patient; to classify individuals into subpopulations that differ in their susceptibility to a particular disease or their response to a specific treatment so that preventive or therapeutic interventions can then be concentrated on those who will benefit, sparing expense and side effects for those who will not" [1, 2]. The Personalized Medicine Coalition has added "...that the molecular methods which will make the personalized medicine reality is the variations in genes, gene expression, proteins, and metabolites, and also the new treatments which will, be targeting the molecular mechanism like the disease state, prediction of future disease states, drug response, and treatment prognosis – to help physicians individualize treatment for each patient" [2, 3]. There are significant changes in the personalized treatment concept of the two important scientific developments: (1) genomic analysis has shown the combination of various molecular moieties like in carcinoma breast and (2) "targeted" drugs which are having focussed action and are capable for the inhibition of the various biochemical pathways. These advances in genomics along with the application of genetic testing is now being evaluated meticulously and having the significant influence on cancer risk assessment, determination of prognosis, and selection of treatment [4]. Various clinical applications of genetic tools are sequencing and analysis of germline genomic rearrangements of various cancer genes like *BRCA1*, *BRCA2*, and *TP53* [5]; mismatched repair of various genes such as *MLH1*, *MSH2*, *MSH6*, and *PMS2* [6]; the development and use of clinical karyotyping for various hematologic malignancies [7]; analysis of ERBB2 overexpression in breast cancer [8]; KRAS gene mutations in colorectal cancer [9], and gene expression analysis in breast cancer as a form of molecular pathology [10] (Diagram 4.1). New technologies comprise genomic, proteomic, single-cell analyses and high-throughput phenotypic assays and also the powerful computational methods for the biological networks related to cellular and molecular origins of cancer. The new paradigm (P4) in systems medicine which has evolved is the "predictive, preventive, personalized and participatory (P4)" medicine and also associated with various social challenges, along with the concept of oncology [11]. Here various scientific, organizational, and wellness strategies are being used for personalized medicine [11].

Predictive biomarkers along with genetic testing are capable of evaluating the total outcome of cancer and will be helpful for the use of the new drugs which will have more efficacy to a specific therapy [12, 13]. Patients are selected based on the biomarker levels which is important for post-treatment efficacy involvement evaluation. These biomarkers will be helpful in the selection of various optimal drug doses and will also be able to identify toxic effects. With this, it will cause significant reduction in healthcare costs and increase the quality of life of patients [14]. These predictive biomarkers are the direct targets of drugs and molecules which are capable of DNA repair or polymorphisms in genes which are associated with various drug metabolism [13]. Various prognostic biomarkers are capable of predicting the course of these specific diseases and also for the good vs. poor results for these diseases [15]. Various examples of prognostic oncology markers are various molecules which are involved in tumour cell proliferation, dedifferentiation, angiogenesis, invasion, or metastasis.

Genetic testing is used to identify the correct drug for the correct patient [2] from these mentioned categories: (1) diagnostics: the role of genetic sequences to confirm the presence of disease; (2) prognostics: by the evaluation of genetic mutations, it will be possible to identify diseases like cystic fibrosis genotype testing; (3) pharmacogenomics: evaluation of genetic variations for the identification of these markers especially the focussed therapy [2]. The identification of specific features of individual patients like the gene sequences and their use for the tailoring medical treatment is more focussed.

The concept of imaging is to have influence in all the stages of disease processes. CT for the diagnosis or detection of the several cancers has increased sensitivity [16, 17]. Molecular imaging with 18F-2-fluoro-deoxy-D-glucose (FDG)-PET and PET-CT in cancer has also revolutionized the management of cancer patients. The coming decade has been significant for the advances in

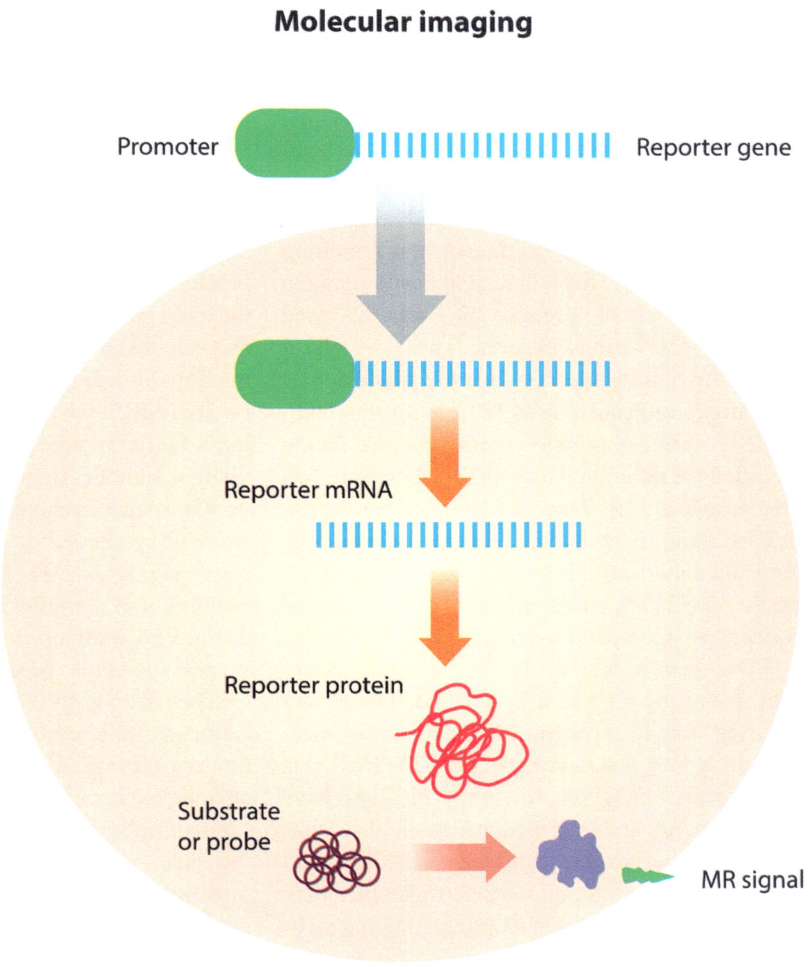

Diagram 4.1 The use of the micro-sized and nano-sized particles for the molecular imaging of the ultrasound. Both intracellular and extracellular interactions

molecular imaging, their integrated diagnostics, which are being biology-driven interventional radiology and theranostics [18].

4.2 Molecular Diagnostics

Molecular diagnostics is an individualized form of diagnosis like for cancer patients who are likely to the responding to the targeted chemotherapies [2]. Biological role of biomarker ER is seen on the basis of various oestrogen receptors. Availability of the biological predictive and putative predictive marker is very crucial for the analysis of various diseases. Thus, molecular diagnostics is in the rapid state of evolution based on various aspects of drug selection, predicting its efficacy and toxicity, and also for monitoring disease response. Classification of disease processes of various cancers is based on molecular characterization which will be helpful for the management [19–21]. These various molecular changes will also sub-classify malignant tumours into various homogenous molecular subtypes [22].

4.3 Personalized Oncology

"Personalized oncology is the important concept that each individual solid tumor and hematologic malignancy in each person is unique in cause, rate of progression and responsiveness to surgery, chemotherapy and radiation therapy" [23, 24]. The use of advanced genomic and proteomic technologies had made it easier to sub-classify various diseases with molecular imaging. Different gene sequences and/or gene expressions are being used in various malignancies like breast cancer (HER2), colorectal cancer (KRAS and BRAF), lung cancer (EGF receptor gene [EGFR]) melanoma (BRAF), and malignant lymphoma (both lymphoid and non-lymphoid leukaemias) [23]. This will lead to developing the future concept of precise biomarker-assisted diagnosis for various cancers. There will be a possibility of integration, with more added values for various molecular tests [23]. With this technique, various genomic alterations are being recorded for individual tumours, and they are further growing [22]. Thus, molecular characteristics of tumours will characterize the patient's clinical characteristics. Various companion diagnostics are being more profitable based on the concept of "Companion diagnostics".

FDG is now widely used imaging modality [25]. Many newer positron-labelled tracers will be used for in vivo metabolic imaging with PET. Magnetic resonance spectroscopy (MRS) is also a form of metabolic imaging which will have various energy and intermediary metabolism patterns [26], and newer techniques are being used for gene expression and various molecular processes [27]. These MRI and optical imaging techniques are used for various molecular processes, for the analysis of metabolic and molecular imaging. Tumour perfusion and water diffusions by MRI will give detailed information about various metabolic and molecular changes seen in brain tumours [28].

4.4 Tomographic Imaging

There are various tomographic imaging methods for the evaluation of various physiological and structural targets. Multidetector CT will give the important aspects of information in seconds based on the pattern of enhancement and the use of iodinated contrast media for functional images; MRI will give information regarding blood flow measurement parameters like fluid flow, free water diffusion, or molecular transfer of magnetization in tissues. Functional MRI (fMRI) principle is based on the property of paramagnetic deoxyhaemoglobin by blood oxygen level-dependent [BOLD] imaging and is a common technique for functional imaging. One of the important aspects of BOLD imaging is in the cognitive neuroscience evaluation for the neuronal activation assessment and identification same is also seen in the oncology based on the areas of the brain parenchyma involved due to the tumours and also due to the post chemotherapy and radiotherapy. Molecular resonance frequencies are the basis of MRS, where protons (1 H) or 31P are the important components of water, lipids, and the main metabolic intermediates. MRS is having very less spatial resolution, and enough larger tissue will be needed of several millilitres for efficient signals. This forms the basis of the evaluation of the other nuclei, like 13C, 19F, and 23Na. PET imaging is more specific for imaging various molecular processes.

This is done by short-lived positron-emitting isotopes at micromolar or nanomolar concentrations by biological tissues. With specific physical characteristics of isotopes and molecules, the evaluation by PET scanners will be more sensitive as compared with other imaging techniques.

Single-photon emission computed tomography (SPECT) uses gamma-emitting isotopes for the detection of tracers like 99mTc and 123I, by the rotating scintillation detectors (gamma cameras). SPECT is less expensive as compared to PET but not as much sensitive for the evaluation of molecular processes. Experimental molecular imaging is based on the use of various macromolecules, like proteins, peptides, and oligonucleotides, all these can be tagged to fluorescent markers which can be used in optical imaging, paramagnetic or ferromagnetic markers for MRI, or radiation-emitting markers for PET and SPECT [29, 30]. But an important fact is that most of the macromolecules are not crossing the blood–brain barrier. Optical imaging will enable more molecular processes, from nanometre size. Tumour grading of WHO grading of tumours is commonly accepted [31], and based on these classifications, four histological grades are seen. Grade I tumours are mostly meningiomas, neurinomas, or schwannomas and can be cured. Grade II tumours are astrocytomas and oligodendrogliomas and are low-grade tumours due to their low proliferation rates and lack of histological features of malignancy. But these tumours have the capacity to infiltrate the healthy brain are the anaplastic astrocytoma's and oligodendrogliomas, with survival rates of only few years, grade IV tumours like glioblastomas, which recur after the treatment and has very short life span. As per the management protocols, high-grade tumours will need irradiation and chemotherapy, as low-grade gliomas are individualized and conservative. These metabolic and molecular imaging can help in tumour grading also. With the breach of blood–brain barrier, it will show the malignant breakdown of tumours. Diffusion-weighted imaging is based on the changes in cellular tissue and related as we all know that the extracellular space will show the changes in preferential direction of water diffusion and fractional anisotropy. These are related to tumour cellularity and also peripheral tumour invasion, especially for the white matter due to its structure and significant white matter loss during the disease processes [32–34] (Diagram 4.2).

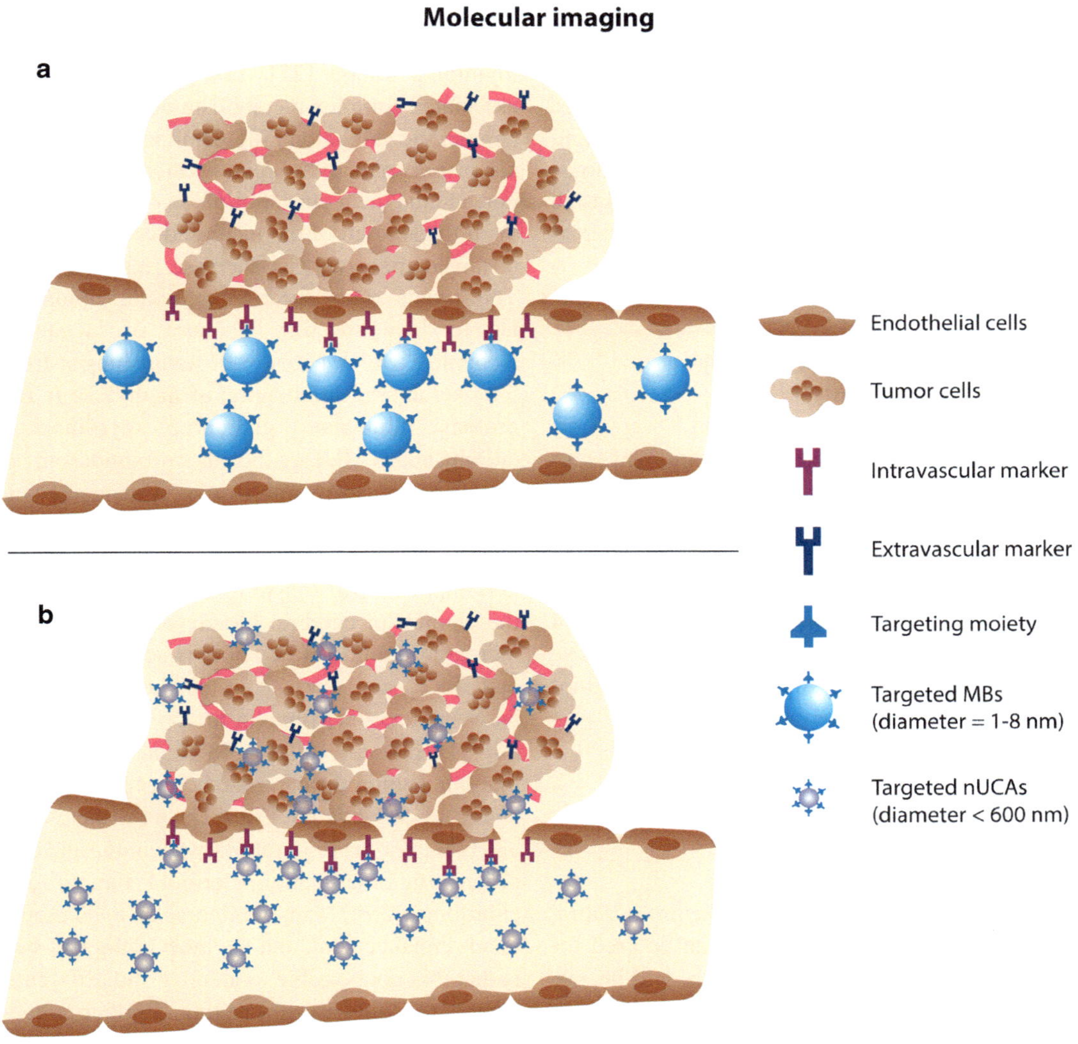

Diagram 4.2 Various mechanisms of intravascular and extravascular markers and relation to the normal and cancer cells. (**a**) Targeting of the MBs and (**b**) nUCAs

4.5 Blood Flow Measurement

Blood flow measurement in brain is done by two ways. The techniques will use diffusible tracers for the measurement of blood flow which will be supplying oxygen and all the nutrients for various microvascular substrate exchanges like 15O-water PET and MRI using arterial spin-labelling (ASL). The other technique is to quantify the total regional body blood flow. The use of dynamic imaging by injecting the contrast which will not pass through the intact blood–brain barrier. The dynamic MRI and CT techniques can cause leakage of contrast media into the interstitial space; these dynamic imaging techniques will provide the movement of the contrast through capillary endothelium and extravascular, extracellular, and cellular spaces. [35, 36]. Increased blood flow and blood volume are noted in high-grade tumours rather than low-grade tumours [37]. The basis of blood flow and permeability of vessels as well as the blood–brain barrier is important for the delivery of drugs.

4.6 FDG-PET and Energy Metabolism

The metabolism of energy is the important component for the functioning of all the tissues, which can be easily measured by PET. Glucose analogue is the most commonly used in glucose metabolism and the malignant tumours usually showing high FDG uptake. For the diagnosis of tumours in brain, there is very high glucose metabolism of normal grey matter; FDG methionine is another evolving radiotracer.

4.7 Amino Acid PET and Protein Synthesis

Protein synthesis will be more in the proliferating brain tumours, and this concept can be used for in vivo imaging, and with this, there will be significantly increased uptake of labelled amino acids in brain tumours. The increased amount of the methionine in gliomas with blood–brain barrier damage can be inhibited by various branched-chain amino acids [38] and can be done by the activated carrier-mediated transport [39, 40] as seen in low-grade gliomas due to the absence of damage to blood–brain barrier. The use of SPECT has shown significant increased uptake of 123I-iodo-αmethyl tyrosine in gliomas [41, 42]. The amount of amino acid uptake correlates with the tumour grade [43–45] and is most important for survival [46, 47]. The use of thymidine PET and DNA synthesis will show the features of malignant tumours based on cellular proliferation. And this measurement of cellular proliferation will define the quantity of the DNA synthesis. Thymidine uptake will define the amount of thymidine transport into tissue and is based on the phosphorylation of various cell-cycle-dependent thymidine kinase [25]. 11C-labelled CO_2 and associated complex metabolism of the tracer will hamper the validation [48]. Choline is the precursor of phosphatidyl choline, which is an important and the main phospholipid in cell membrane. With the amount of the increased cell membrane turnover, there will be increase in the choline. The signals can be the combination of lipids and lactate. The spectral signature of lactate is J-coupled, which helps in distinguishing it from the overlapping lipid signal of methylene (CH_2) protons. Glutamate, glutamine, myo-inositol, taurine, and GABA are the other proton resources having higher acquisition times. Various associated things like tumour vascularity, metabolism, invasiveness, and malignancy are having important impact. Diffusion-weighted MRI along with the amount of cerebral blood volume mapping, increased amino acid uptake, is seen in SPECT and PET, and these can easily differentiate between tumours from non-tumorous lesions [49, 50]. Diffusion-weighted MRI and perfusion imaging cannot differentiate between lymphoma and glial cell tumour [51, 52], dural metastasis and meningioma [53], pituitary adenoma and craniopharyngioma, and epidermoid tumour and chordoma [54]. Many tumours have heterogeneous enhancement, and the most malignant part is that it is not possible to identify and differentiate them by anatomical imaging. Tumour boundaries cannot be completely diagnosed in cases of the low-grade gliomas, and reverse is that high-grade gliomas are mostly heterogeneous and may not show significant contrast enhancement. Blood flow and glucose metabolism which will be of low uptake will be surrounding most of the malignant brain tumours. Some of the factors like local pressure, oedema, and reduced neuronal activity will impact this. Various protocols of metabolic and molecular imaging can monitor various treatment targets directly and can guide therapy with significant amount of sensitivity.

4.8 Radiation Therapy

Radiation therapy is an important mode of management of cancers which will have the capacity to kill tumour cells, but along with this, the tumour cells in the surrounding area will be crucial in preventing early recurrence. Advanced MRI techniques and amino acid PET can depict glioma invasion which can be seen in the routine conventional MRI sequences [55, 56]. Tissue hypoxia is important for the evaluation of relative resistance to irradiation and can increase vascular proliferation to vary higher extent. Sometimes, the amount of oxygen consumption is lower in normal brain than which can be seen in normal brain [57, 58] in which glucose consumption is significantly increased. Misonidazole can be used for the evaluation of hypoxic tissue as its diffusion in brain parenchyma is very slow but uniformly distributed. 11C-Methionine is another metabolite which has significant radiosensitivity for low-grade gliomas [59].

MRI is useful for the evaluation of radiotherapy response and also for the measurement of contrast agent transfer coefficients which can identify the homogenous grade IV gliomas after partial resection and radiotherapy [60]. Various advanced imaging techniques, like the FDG-PET and diffusion tensor imaging, can be used for the evaluation of healthy brain tissue damage which can be seen due to irradiation [61, 62]. Necrosis versus residual tumour is always very difficult to identify with various anatomical modalities and due to this drawback many newer molecular imaging modalities are coming up. The use of therapeutic intervention, especially radiation therapy, will result in delayed necrosis in brain tumours. Thus, MRS is more helpful for differentiating between the residual or recurrent tumours and pure radiation necrosis. Apparent-diffusion coefficient is higher in necrotic tissue as compared to the recurrent tumour tissue [63, 64], and as mentioned here, diffusion-weighted MRI has very less specificity as compared to MRS [65].

4.9 Chemotherapy

The amount of the blood flow to a particular organ will define the amount of chemotherapeutic agent delivery to the tumour tissue, and this can be measured with SPECT, PET, dynamic MRI, and CT. In some situations, the amount of blood inflow to and outflow from the tumour will be based on the global and regional blood flow, and the difference will not be much in total delivery in the area under the curve. Contrast-enhanced MRI and CT with their dynamic MRI techniques can calculate the capillary endothelial permeability surface area [35] or can also be done with PET imaging 68GaEDTA [66, 67].

The chemotherapeutics transfer to brain and brain tumours can be measured by tagging the drug, which is seen in the possible cases of the nitrosoureas carmustine (BCNU), limousine (CCNU), SarCNU, [68, 69] and temozolomide [70]. PET and temozolomide labelled with 11C can be used in two different positions for the chemotherapeutic evaluation in vivo in human gliomas.

Evaluation of vascular endothelial growth factor will be the potential targets for antiangiogenic treatments. Labelling of various monoclonal antibodies against avascular endothelial growth factor along with PET markers is being assessed in various studies. Molecular imaging is also used for the evaluation of the delivery of gene as to assess the efficacy of various vectors.

Monitoring of cell-based therapies can be done by cell labelling. The stem cells also use the same gene strategy for human mesenchymal cells expressing HSV-1-tk 3–4 days after the transplantation of cells in mice from a colon cancer cell line. Various validated parameters like various blood flow and volume, apparent-diffusion coefficient, choline-to-N-acetyl aspartate ratio, and also local uptake of 18F-labelled tracers, such as FDG, FET, and FLT, are being used. The combination of imaging modalities for the planning of individual radiotherapy and various neurosurgical interventions can also be used for the assessment of efficacy, safety, and preservation of brain function.

Here, the use of various molecular imaging will provide a new approach to image and for the characterization of biomolecules and molecular changes due to cancer malignancy [71]. As we all know, molecular imaging is used for monitoring structural, functional, and molecular changes in cancer tissues which are being depicted both clinically and pre-clinically [72–82]. The use of optical imaging is also there for various image-specific molecular imaging of cancer by using various molecular targeted contrast agents [77, 83]. The optical-based method is capable of providing the early information about the changes in various post-treatment evaluations [84, 85]. Imaging of cancer metabolism will have the altered cellular metabolism which will be an important factor for cancer growth and malignancy [86, 87]. Glycolysis, pentose phosphate pathway (PPP), and TCA cycle, and other pathways, are being used for the evaluation of the regulation in cancer cells [88–93]. Otto Warburg showed the concept of high glucose consumption and lactate production in cancer for tumour metabolism which is different from the baseline normal tissue [94, 95]. Magnetic resonance spectroscopy as we all know detects metabolic changes in cancerous as well as in normal tissues [96]. Various metabolic markers which are being detectable by MRS give the information about biochemical changes that happen due to tumour growth and are also based on various metabolic tumour phenotypes. Proton MRS (1 H MRS) is most commonly used to evaluate the metabolic changes in cancer tissue [97–103]. 31P (phosphorus), 13C (carbon), and 19F (fluorine) can also be used for monitoring various bioenergetics and metabolic changes in malignant cells [104–117]. 1 H signal from total choline (Cho) is elevated in cellular proliferation in cancer showing the malignant potential [118–121]. Magnetic resonance spectroscopic imaging (MRSI) will give spatial information of various metabolites in the cancer tissue [122, 123]. These spatial mapping of Cho proton signal will be helpful for tumour tissue evaluation and to monitor therapeutic responses [124, 125]. Various 31P MRS will detect the phosphorous metabolites [126].

Hyperpolarized MRI in cancer is being done by the 13C-labelled pyruvate infusion for the evaluation of the increased tumour glycolysis in cancer. Tumour mapping of pH changes in tumour is used as the marker for treatment efficacy evaluation and for setting the cancer treatment protocols.

4.10 Chemical Exchange Saturation Transfer (CEST) Imaging

Chemical exchange saturation transfer (CEST) is a new contrast enhancement technique used for the detection of various molecules and macromolecules having the exchangeable protons [127–129]. Various exchangeable protons are used for the saturated frequency selective radiofrequency (RF) saturation pulse which will have zero magnetization on exchangeable protons, and this is based on the exchange of the bulk water protons which will be decreasing as there will be decrease in the bulk water signal [128, 129].

4.10.1 Imaging of Mobile Protein and Peptide in Cancer

Amide proton transfer (APT) imaging is based on the use of mobile protein and peptides in cancers in vivo [130–134]. It is based on the exchange between protons of free water and amide groups (–NH) of endogenous mobile proteins and peptides [135]. There will be increased APT in tumour as compared to the adjacent and contralateral normal brain parenchyma [131, 136–138]. This will show higher APT contrast in high-grade tumour in comparison to low-grade tumour [131]. This is being used in breast cancer, prostate cancer, bladder cancer, etc.

The basis of imaging is the use of various endogenous mobile proteins and peptides for signal measurement. CEST imaging of protease enzyme expression is based on enzyme inhibitors.

Gene expression in cancer cell can also be used with the reporter genes. These genes can also be used for the evaluation of gene therapy and also for the assessment of various functions like cellular differentiation, cell trafficking, and specific metabolic activity and also to assess changes in microenvironment [139]. Here, gadolinium-based contrast will be able to maintain gadolinium ion in water, which will be inaccessible unless the β-galactosidase enzyme expression can be done. Various reporter gene is being inserted in the downstream of a gene promoter producing the reporter protein after translation.

4.11 Molecular MR Imaging in Cancer Immunotherapy

Cell-based cancer immunotherapy is the newer approach for the evaluation of cancer by triggering the patients' own immune system to produce anti-tumour response. Different cell types, like lymphocytes ($CD4^+$ and $CD8^+$ T cells), dendritic cells (DCs) and natural killer cells (NK cells) will show their efficacy, so that the cancerous cells will be targeted more than the adjacent normal tissues. Various markers may need the time from the weeks to months for their actions.

The cells labelled with nanoparticles are used for the direct clinical translation. Non-invasive MRI can offer the real-time immune cell tracking by using the markers for tumour response as early as 24 h after start of therapy (Diagram 4.3).

4.12 Lymphotropic Imaging

Correct nodal staging is important for the use in various primary malignancy. Lymphotropic nanoparticles like the inverse spinel, superparamagnetic iron oxide core containing various packing of dextrans for the circulation time can be used. After administration, they pass through the extravasated vasculature into the interstitial space, then into the lymph nodes via the lymphatic system. The nanoparticles can be detected

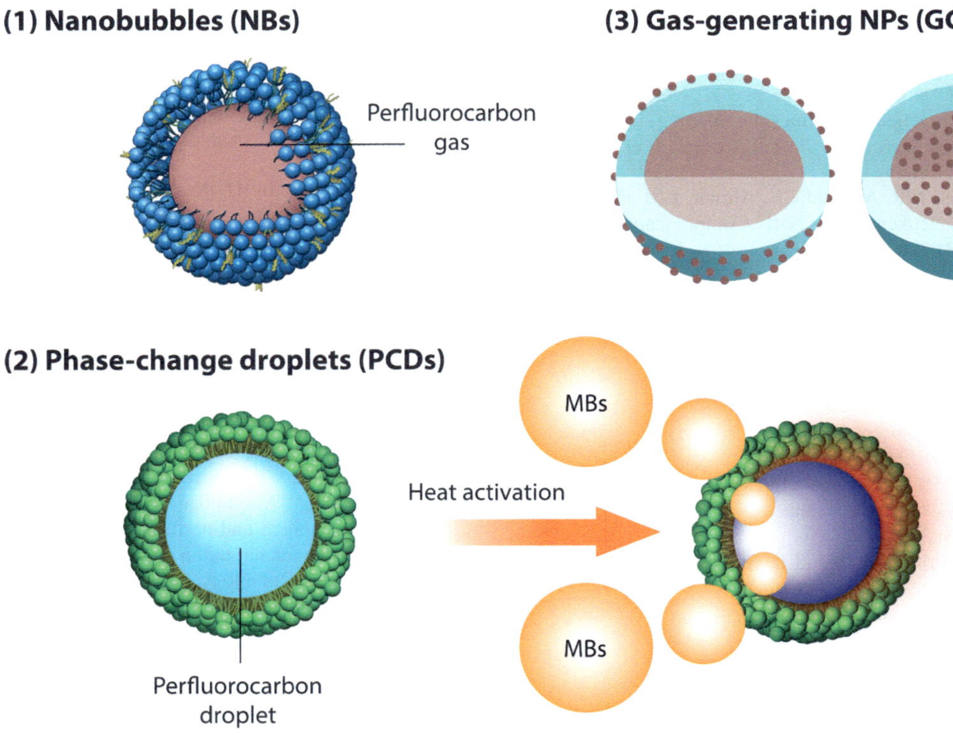

Diagram 4.3 Various types of nanoparticles

as the drop of the signal on T2- and T2-weighted MR images for these various nanoparticles applications. Node infiltrated by malignant cells will show no nanoparticle uptake due to the absence of functioning macrophages. Images are to be obtained at 24 h after the administration of the nanoparticles, as this is the time required for the nanoparticles to be internalized by the macrophages.

References

1. President's Council of Advisors on Science and Technology. Priorities for personalized medicine [online]. Available from URL: http://www.whitehouse.gov/files/documents/ostp/PCAST/pcast_report_v2.pdf Accessed 2011 Feb 18.
2. Hoggart J. Personalized medicine — trends in molecular diagnostics. Exponential growth expected in the next ten years. Mol Diagn Ther. 2011;15(1):53–5.
3. Personalized Medicine Coalition. The case for personalized medicine. Washington, DC: Personalized Medicine Coalition; 2006.
4. Pasche B, Absher D. Whole-genome sequencing. A step closer to personalized medicine. JAMA. 2011;305(15):1596–7.
5. Daly MB, Axilbund JE, Buys S, et al. National comprehensive cancer network. Genetic/familial high-risk assessment: breast and ovarian. J Natl ComprCancNetw. 2010;8(5):562–94.
6. Burt RW, Barthel JS, Dunn KB, et al., NCCN. NCCN clinical practice guidelines in oncology: colorectal cancer screening. J Natl Compr Canc Netw 2010;8(1):8–61.
7. O'Donnell MR, Abboud CH, Altman J, et al. Acute myeloid leukemia. J Natl Compr Canc Netw. 2011;9(3):280–317.
8. Yaziji H, Goldstein LC, Barry TS, et al. HER-2 testing in breast cancer using parallel tissue-based methods. JAMA. 2004;291(16):1972–7.
9. De Roock W, Jonker DJ, Di Nicoantonio F, et al. Association of KRAS p. G13D mutation with outcome in patients with chemotherapy-refractory metastatic colorectal cancer treated with cetuximab. JAMA. 2010;304(16):1812–20.
10. Kim C, Paik S. Gene-expression-based prognostic assays for breast cancer. Nat Rev Clin Oncol. 2010;7(6):340–7.
11. Tian Q, Price ND, Hood L. Systems cancer medicine: towards realization of predictive, preventive, personalized and participatory (P4) medicine. J Intern Med. 2012;271:111–21.
12. Walgren RA, Meucci MA, McLeod HL. Pharmacogenomics discovery approaches : will the real genes please stand up? J Clin Oncol. 2005;23:7342–9.
13. Duffy MJ, O'Donovan N, Crown J. Use of molecular markers for predicting therapy response in cancer patients. Cancer Treat Rev. 2011;37:151–9.
14. Huang RS, Ratain MJ. Pharmacogenetics and pharmacogenomics of anticancer agents. CA Cancer J Clin. 2009;59:42–55.
15. Sawyers CL. The cancer biomarker problem. Nature. 2008;452:548–52.
16. Hricak H. Oncologic imaging: a guiding hand of personalized cancer care. Radiology. 2011;259(3):633–40.
17. Hellquist BN, Duffy SW, Abdsaleh S, et al. Effectiveness of population-based service screening with mammography for women ages 40–49 years: evaluation of the Swedish mammography screening in young women (SCRY) cohort. Cancer. 2010;117(4):714–22.
18. Basu S. Personalized versus evidence-based medicine with PET-based imaging. Nat Rev Clin Oncol. 2010;7:665–8.
19. Stephen PJ, McBride DJ, Lin ML, et al. Complex landscapes of somatic rearrangement in human breast cancer genomes. Nature. 2009;462:1005–10.
20. Pao W, Chemielecki J. Rational, biologically based treatment of EGFR-mutant non-small-cell lung cancer. Nat Rev Cancer. 2010;10:760–74.
21. Casali PG, Blay JY. On behalf of the ESMO/CONTICANET/EURONET consensus panel of experts. Gastrointestinal stromal tumors: ESMO clinical practice guidelines for diagnosis, treatment and follow-up. Ann Oncol. 2010;21(Suppl 5):v98–102.
22. Blay J-Y, Lacombe D, Meunier F, Stupp R. Personalized medicine in oncology: questions for the next 20 years. Lancet. 2012;13:448–9.
23. Ross JS. Cancer biomarkers, companion diagnostics and personalized oncology. Biomark Med. 2011;5(3):277–9.
24. Ginsburg GS, McCarthy JJ. Personalized medicine: revolutionizing drug discovery and patient care. Trends Biotechnol. 2001;19:491–6.
25. Reivich M, Kuhl D, Wolf A, et al. Measurement of local cerebral glucose metabolism in man with 18F-2-fl uoro-2-deoxy-D-glucose. Acta NeurolScand. 1977;64(suppl):190–1.
26. Negendank W. Studies of human tumors by MRS: a review. NMR Biomed. 1992;5:303–24.
27. Gelovani TJ, Blasberg RG. In vivo imaging of molecular-genetic targets for cancer therapy. Cancer Cell. 2003;3:327–32.
28. Provenzale JM, Mukundan S, Barboriak DP. Diffusion-weighted and perfusion MR imaging for brain tumor characterization and assessment of treatment response. Radiology. 2006;239:632–49.
29. Weissleder R. Molecular imaging in cancer. Science. 2006;312:1168–71.
30. Massoud TF, Gambhir SS. Molecular imaging in living subjects: seeing fundamental biological processes in a new light. Genes Dev. 2003;17:545–80.

31. Kleihues P, Louis DN, Scheithauer BW, et al. The WHO classification of tumors of the nervous system. J Neuropathol Exp Neurol. 2002;61:215–25.
32. Stadlbauer A, Ganslandt O, Buslei R, et al. Gliomas: histopathologic evaluation of changes in directionality and magnitude of water diffusion at diffusion-tensor MR imaging. Radiology. 2006;240:803–10.
33. Sugahara T, Korogi Y, Kochi M, et al. Usefulness of diffusion weighted MRI with echo-planar technique in the evaluation of cellularity in gliomas. J Magn Reson Imaging. 1999;9:53–60.
34. Bode MK, Ruohonen J, Nieminen MT, Pyhtinen J. Potential of diffusion imaging in brain tumors: a review. Acta Radiol. 2006;47:585–94.
35. Tofts PS. Modeling tracer kinetics in dynamic Gd-DTPA MR imaging. J Magn Reson Imaging. 1997;7:91–101.
36. Jackson A. Analysis of dynamic contrast enhanced MRI. Br J Radiol. 2004;77:S154–66.
37. Law M, Yang S, Wang H, et al. Glioma grading: sensitivity, specificity, and predictive values of perfusion MR imaging and proton MR spectroscopic imaging compared with conventional MR imaging. AJNR Am J Neuroradiol. 2003;24:1989–98.
38. Bergstrom M, Ericson K, Hagenfeldt L, et al. PET study of methionine accumulation in glioma and normal brain tissue: competition with branched chain amino acids. J Comput Assist Tomogr. 1987;11:208–13.
39. Killian DM, Chikhale PJ. Predominant functional activity of the large, neutral amino acid transporter (LAT1) isoform at the cerebrovasculature. Neurosci Lett. 2001;306:1–4.
40. Miyagawa T, Oku T, Uehara H, et al. "Facilitated" amino acid transport is upregulated in brain tumors. J Comput Assist Tomogr 1998; 18: 500–509, 722. http://neurology.thelancet.com, vol 6 August 2007 Review.
41. Langen KJ, Ziemons K, Kiwit JC, et al. 3-[123I] iodo-alphamethyltyrosine and [methyl-11C]-L-methionine uptake in cerebral gliomas: a comparative study using SPECT and PET. J Nucl Med. 1997;38:517–22.
42. Plotkin M, Eisenacher J, Bruhn H, et al. 123I-IMT SPECT and 1 H MR-spectroscopy at 3.0 T in the differential diagnosis of recurrent or residual gliomas: a comparative study. J Neuro-Oncol. 2004;70:49–58.
43. Sato N, Suzuki M, Kuwata N, et al. Evaluation of the malignancy of glioma using 11C-methionine positron emission tomography and proliferating cell nuclear antigen staining. Neurosurg Rev. 1999;22:210–4.
44. Derlon JM, Chapon F, Noel MH, et al. Non-invasive grading of oligodendrogliomas: correlation between in vivo metabolic pattern and histopathology. Eur J Nucl Med. 2000;27:778–87.
45. Popperl G, Kreth FW, Herms J, et al. Analysis of 18F-FET PET for grading of recurrent gliomas: is evaluation of uptake kinetics superior to standard methods? J Nucl Med. 2006;47:393–403.
46. De Witte O, Goldberg I, Wikler D, et al. Positron emission tomography with injection of methionine as a prognostic factor in glioma. J Neurosurg. 2001;95:746–50.
47. Ribom D, Eriksson A, Hartman M, et al. Positron emission tomography (11)C-methionine and survival in patients with lowgrade gliomas. Cancer. 2001;92:1541–9.
48. Mankoff DA, Shields AF, Link JM, et al. Kinetic analysis of 2-[11C]thymidine PET imaging studies: validation studies. J Nucl Med. 1999;40:614–24.
49. Herholz K, Holzer T, Bauer B, et al. 11C-methionine PET for differential diagnosis of low-grade gliomas. Neurology. 1998;50:1316–22.
50. Chung JK, Kim YK, Kim SK, et al. Usefulness of 11C-methionine PET in the evaluation of brain lesions that are hypo- or isometabolic on 18F-FDG PET. Eur J Nucl Med Mol Imaging. 2002;29:176–82.
51. Calli C, Kitis O, Yunten N, Yurtseven T, Islekel S, Akalin T. Perfusion and diffusion MR imaging in enhancing malignant cerebral tumors. Eur J Radiol. 2006;58:394–403.
52. Hartmann M, Heiland S, Harting I, et al. Distinguishing of primary cerebral lymphoma from high-grade glioma with perfusionweighted magnetic resonance imaging. Neurosci Lett. 2003;338:119–22.
53. Kremer S, Grand S, Remy C, et al. Contribution of dynamic contrast MR imaging to the differentiation between dural metastasis and meningioma. Neuroradiology. 2004;46:642–8.
54. Yamasaki F, Kurisu K, Satoh K, et al. Apparent diffusion coefficient of human brain tumors at MR imaging. Radiology. 2005;235:985–91.
55. Grosu AL, Weber WA, Riedel E, et al. L-(methyl-11C) methionine positron emission tomography for target delineation in resected high-grade gliomas before radiotherapy. Int J Radiat Oncol Biol Phys. 2005;63:64–74.
56. Jena R, Price SJ, Baker C, et al. Diffusion tensor imaging: possible implications for radiotherapy treatment planning of patients with high-grade glioma. Clin Oncol (R Coll Radiol). 2005;17:581–90.
57. Tyler JL, Diksic M, Villemure JG, et al. Metabolic and hemodynamic evaluation of gliomas using positron emission tomography. J Nucl Med. 1987;28:1123–33.
58. Rhodes CG, Wise RJ, Gibbs JM, et al. In vivo disturbance of the oxidative metabolism of glucose in human cerebral gliomas. Ann Neurol. 1983;14:614–26.
59. Ribom D, Engler H, Blomquist E, Smits A. Potential significance of (11)C-methionine PET as a marker for the radiosensitivity of lowgrade gliomas. Eur J Nucl Med. 2002;29:632–40.
60. Mills SJ, Patankar TA, Haroon HA, Baleriaux D, Swindell R, Jackson A. Do cerebral blood volume and contrast transfer coefficient predict prognosis in human glioma? Am J Neuroradiol. 2006;27:853–8.
61. Mabbott DJ, Noseworthy MD, Bouff E, Rockel C, Laughlin S. Diffusion tensor imaging of white

matter after cranial radiation in children for medulloblastoma: correlation with IQ. Neuro Oncol. 2006;8:244–52.
62. Kahkonen M, Metsahonkala L, Minn H, et al. Cerebral glucose metabolism in survivors of childhood acute lymphoblastic leukemia. Cancer. 2000;88:693–700.
63. Chan YL, Yeung DK, Leung SF, Chan PN. Diffusion-weighted magnetic resonance imaging in radiation-induced cerebral necrosis. Apparent diffusion coefficient in lesion components. J Comput Assist Tomogr. 2003;27(674):80.
64. Hein PA, Eskey CJ, Dunn JF, Hug EB. Diffusion-weighted imaging in the follow-up of treated high-grade gliomas: tumor recurrence versus radiation injury. AJNR Am J Neuroradiol. 2004;25:201–9.
65. Rock JP, Scarpace L, Hearshen D, et al. Associations among magnetic resonance spectroscopy, apparent diffusion coefficients, and image-guided histopathology with special attention to radiation necrosis. Neurosurgery. 2004;54:1111–7.
66. Iannotti F, Fieschi C, Alfano B, et al. Simplified, noninvasive PET measurement of blood–brain barrier permeability. J Comput Assist Tomogr. 1987;11:390–7.
67. Hawkins RA, Phelps ME, Huang SC, et al. A kinetic evaluation of blood–brain barrier permeability in human brain tumors with [68Ga]EDTA and positron computed tomography. J Cereb Blood Flow Metab. 1984;4:507–15.
68. Mitsuki S, Diksic M, Conway T, Yamamoto YL, Villemure JG, Feindel W. Pharmacokinetics of 11C-labelled BCNU and SarCNU in gliomas studied by PET. J Neuro-Oncol. 1991;10:47–55.
69. Diksic M, Sako K, Feindel W, et al. Pharmacokinetics of positronlabeled 1,3-bis(2- chloroethyl)nitrosourea in human brain tumors using positron emission tomography. Cancer Res. 1984;44:3120–4.
70. Meikle SR, Matthews JC, Brock CS, et al. Pharmacokinetic assessment of novel anti-cancer drugs using spectral analysis and positron emission tomography: a feasibility study. Cancer Chemother Pharmacol. 1998;42:183–93.
71. Weissleder R. Molecular imaging in cancer. Science. 2006;312:1168–71.
72. Schillaci O. Single-photon emission computed tomography/computed tomography in lung cancer and malignant lymphoma. Semin Nucl Med. 2006;36:275–85.
73. Vangestel C, Van de Wiele C, Mees G, Mertens K, Staelens S, Reutelingsperger C, Pauwels P, Van Damme N, Peeters M. Single-photon emission computed tomographic imaging of the early time course of therapyinduced cell death using technetium 99 m tricarbonyl his-annexin A5 in a colorectal cancer xenograft model. Mol Imaging. 2012;11:135–47.
74. Gambhir SS. Molecular imaging of cancer with positron emission tomography. Nat Rev Cancer. 2002;2:683–93.
75. Weber WA. Use of PET for monitoring cancer therapy and for predicting outcome. J Nucl Med. 2005;46:983–95.
76. Aliaga A, Rousseau JA, Cadorette J, Croteau E, van Lier JE, Lecomte R, Benard F. A small animal positron emission tomography study of the effect of chemotherapy and hormonal therapy on the uptake of 2-deoxy-2-[F-18]fluoro-d-glucose in murine models of breast cancer. Mol Imaging Biol. 2007;9:144–50.
77. Hadjipanayis CG, Jiang H, Roberts DW, Yang L. Current and future clinical applications for optical imaging of cancer: from intraoperative surgical guidance to cancer screening. Semin Oncol. 2011;38:109–18.
78. Kaijzel EL, van der Pluijm G, Lowik CW. Whole-body optical imaging in animal models to assess cancer development and progression. Clin Cancer Res. 2007;13:3490–7.
79. Peldschus K, Ittrich H. Magnetic resonance imaging of metastases in xenograft mouse models of cancer. Methods Mol Biol. 2014;1070:213–22.
80. Hoeks CM, Barentsz JO, Hambrock T, Yakar D, Somford DM, Heijmink SW, Scheenen TW, Vos PC, Huisman H, van Oort IM, et al. Prostate cancer: multiparametric MR imaging for detection, localization, and staging. Radiology. 2011;261:46–66.
81. Orel SG, Schnall MD. MR imaging of the breast for the detection, diagnosis, and staging of breast cancer. Radiology. 2001;220:13–30.
82. Padhani AR, Liu G, Koh DM, Chenevert TL, Thoeny HC, Takahara T, DzikJurasz A, Ross BD, Van Cauteren M, Collins D, et al. Diffusion-weighted magnetic resonance imaging as a cancer biomarker: consensus and recommendations. Neoplasia. 2009;11:102–25.
83. Yhee JY, Kim SA, Koo H, Son S, Ryu JH, Youn IC, Choi K, Kwon IC, Kim K. Optical imaging of cancer-related proteases using near-infrared fluorescence matrix metalloproteinase-sensitive and cathepsin B-sensitive probes. Theranostics. 2012;2:179–89.
84. Shah AT, DemoryBeckler M, Walsh AJ, Jones WP, Pohlmann PR, Skala MC. Optical metabolic imaging of treatment response in human head and neck squamous cell carcinoma. PLoS One. 2014;9:e90746.
85. Harada H, Kizaka-Kondoh S, Hiraoka M. Optical imaging of tumor hypoxia and evaluation of efficacy of a hypoxia-targeting drug in living animals. Mol Imaging. 2005;4:182–93.
86. Cairns RA, Harris IS, Mak TW. Regulation of cancer cell metabolism. Nat Rev Cancer. 2011;11:85–95.
87. DeBerardinis RJ. Is cancer a disease of abnormal cellular metabolism? New angles on an old idea. Genet Med. 2008;10:767–77.
88. Ganapathy-Kanniappan S, Geschwind JF. Tumor glycolysis as a target for cancer therapy: progress and prospects. Mol Cancer. 2013;12:152.
89. Warmoes MO, Locasale JW. Heterogeneity of glycolysis in cancers and therapeutic opportunities. Biochem Pharmacol. 2014;92:12–21.

90. Jiang P, Du W, Wu M. Regulation of the pentose phosphate pathway in cancer. Protein Cell. 2014;5:592–602.
91. Chen JQ, Russo J. Dysregulation of glucose transport, glycolysis, TCA cycle and glutaminolysis by oncogenes and tumor suppressors in cancer cells. Biochim Biophys Acta. 2012;1826:370–84.
92. Gaude E, Frezza C. Defects in mitochondrial metabolism and cancer. Cancer Metab. 2014;2:10.
93. Galluzzi L, Kepp O, Vander Heiden MG, Kroemer G. Metabolic targets for cancer therapy. Nat Rev Drug Discov. 2013;12:829–46.
94. Warburg OPK, Negelein E. üeber den Stoffwechsel der Tumoren. Biochem Z. 1924;152:319–44.
95. Warburg O. On the origin of cancer cells. Science. 1956;123:309–14.
96. Gillies RJ, Morse DL. In vivo magnetic resonance spectroscopy in cancer. Annu Rev Biomed Eng. 2005;7:287–326.
97. Mahon MM, Williams AD, Soutter WP, Cox IJ, McIndoe GA, Coutts GA, Dina R, deSouza NM. 1H magnetic resonance spectroscopy of invasive cervical cancer: an in vivo study with ex vivo corroboration. NMR Biomed. 2004;17:1–9.
98. Kim JK, Kim DY, Lee YH, Sung NK, Chung DS, Kim OD, Kim KB. In vivo differential diagnosis of prostate cancer and benign prostatic hyperplasia: localized proton magnetic resonance spectroscopy using externalbody surface coil. Magn Reson Imaging. 1998;16:1281–8.
99. Le HC, Lupu M, Kotedia K, Rosen N, Solit D, Koutcher JA. Proton MRS detects metabolic changes in hormone sensitive and resistant human prostate cancer models CWR22 and CWR22r. Magn Reson Med. 2009;62:1112–9.
100. Haris M, et al. Molecular magnetic resonance imaging in cancer. J Transl Med. 2015;13:313.
101. Kinoshita Y, Yokota A. Absolute concentrations of metabolites in human brain tumors using in vitro proton magnetic resonance spectroscopy. NMR Biomed. 1997;10:2–12.
102. Dowling C, Bollen AW, Noworolski SM, McDermott MW, Barbaro NM, Day MR, Henry RG, Chang SM, Dillon WP, Nelson SJ, Vigneron DB. Preoperative proton MR spectroscopic imaging of brain tumors: correlation with histopathologic analysis of resection specimens. AJNR Am J Neuroradiol. 2001;22:604–12.
103. Majos C, Julia-Sape M, Alonso J, Serrallonga M, Aguilera C, Acebes JJ, Arus C, Gili J. Brain tumor classification by proton MR spectroscopy: comparison of diagnostic accuracy at short and long TE. AJNR Am J Neuroradiol. 2004;25:1696–704.
104. Albers MJ, Krieger MD, Gonzalez-Gomez I, Gilles FH, McComb JG, Nelson MD Jr, Bluml S. Proton-decoupled 31P MRS in untreated pediatric brain tumors. Magn Reson Med. 2005;53:22–9.
105. Bluml S, Seymour KJ, Ross BD. Developmental changes in choline and ethanolamine-containing compounds measured with proton decoupled (31) P MRS in in vivo human brain. Magn Reson Med. 1999;42:643–54.
106. Glaholm J, Leach MO, Collins DJ, Mansi J, Sharp JC, Madden A, Smith IE, McCready VR. In-vivo 31P magnetic resonance spectroscopy for monitoring treatment response in breast cancer. Lancet. 1989;1:1326–7.
107. Kristjansen PE, Spang-Thomsen M, Quistorff B. Different energy metabolism in two human small cell lung cancer subpopulations examined by 31P magnetic resonance spectroscopy and biochemical analysis in vivo and in vitro. Cancer Res. 1991;51:5160–4.
108. Kalra R, Wade KE, Hands L, Styles P, Camplejohn R, Greenall M, Adams GE, Harris AL, Radda GK. Phosphomonoester is associated with proliferation in human breast cancer: a 31P MRS study. Br J Cancer. 1993;67:1145–53.
109. Al-Saffar NM, Troy H, de Ramirez MA, Jackson LE, Madhu B, Griffiths JR, Leach MO, Workman P, Lacal JC, Judson IR, Chung YL. Noninvasive magnetic resonance spectroscopic pharmacodynamic markers of the choline kinase inhibitor MN58b in human carcinoma models. Cancer Res. 2006;66:427–34.
110. Kurhanewicz J, Bok R, Nelson SJ, Vigneron DB. Current and potential applications of clinical 13C MR spectroscopy. J Nucl Med. 2008;49:341–4.
111. Rivenzon-Segal D, Margalit R, Degani H. Glycolysis as a metabolic marker in orthotopic breast cancer, monitored by in vivo (13)C MRS. Am J Physiol Endocrinol Metab. 2002;283:E623–30.
112. Halliday KR, Fenoglio-Preiser C, Sillerud LO. Differentiation of human tumors from nonmalignant tissue by natural-abundance 13C NMR spectroscopy. Magn Reson Med. 1988;7:384–411.
113. Sillerud LO, Halliday KR, Griffey RH, Fenoglio-Preiser C, Sheppard S. In vivo 13C NMR spectroscopy of the human prostate. Magn Reson Med. 1988;8:224–30.
114. Findlay MP, Leach MO, Cunningham D, Collins DJ, Payne GS, Glaholm J, Mansi JL, McCready VR. The non-invasive monitoring of low dose, infusional 5-fluorouracil and its modulation by interferon-alpha using in vivo 19F magnetic resonance spectroscopy in patients with colorectal cancer: a pilot study. Ann Oncol. 1993;4:597–602.
115. Kristjansen PE, Quistorff B, Spang-Thomsen M, Hansen HH. Intratumoral pharmacokinetic analysis by 19F-magnetic resonance spectroscopy and cytostatic in vivo activity of gemcitabine (dFdC) in two small cell lung cancer xenografts. Ann Oncol. 1993;4:157–60.
116. McIntyre DJ, Howe FA, Ladroue C, Lofts F, Stubbs M, Griffiths JR. Can localised (19)F magnetic resonance spectroscopy pharmacokinetics of 5FU in colorectal metastases predict clinical response? Cancer Chemother Pharmacol. 2011;68:29–36.
117. Kamm YJ, Heerschap A, van den Bergh EJ, Wagener DJ. 19F-magnetic resonance spectroscopy in patients with liver metastases of colorectal can-

cer treated with 5-fluorouracil. Anti-Cancer Drugs. 2004;15:229–33.
118. Shimizu H, Kumabe T, Shirane R, Yoshimoto T. Correlation between choline level measured by proton MR spectroscopy and Ki-67 labeling index in gliomas. AJNR Am J Neuroradiol. 2000;21:659–65.
119. Kwock L, Smith JK, Castillo M, Ewend MG, Collichio F, Morris DE, Bouldin TW, Cush S. Clinical role of proton magnetic resonance spectroscopy in oncology: brain, breast, and prostate cancer. Lancet Oncol. 2006;7:859–68.
120. Bartella L, Morris EA, Dershaw DD, Liberman L, Thakur SB, Moskowitz C, Guido J, Huang W. Proton MR spectroscopy with choline peak as malignancy marker improves positive predictive value for breast cancer diagnosis: preliminary study. Radiology. 2006;239:686–92.
121. Bolan PJ, Meisamy S, Baker EH, Lin J, Emory T, Nelson M, Everson LI, Yee D, Garwood M. In vivo quantification of choline compounds in the breast with 1H MR spectroscopy. Magn Reson Med. 2003;50:1134–43.
122. Kurhanewicz J, Vigneron DB, Nelson SJ. Three-dimensional magnetic resonance spectroscopic imaging of brain and prostate cancer. Neoplasia. 2000;2:166–89.
123. Posse S, Otazo R, Dager SR, Alger J. MR spectroscopic imaging: principles and recent advances. J Magn Reson Imaging. 2013;37:1301–25.
124. Gruber S, Debski BK, Pinker K, Chmelik M, Grabner G, Helbich T, Trattnig S, Bogner W. Three-dimensional proton MR spectroscopic imaging at 3T for the differentiation of benign and malignant breast lesions. Radiology. 2011;261:752–61.
125. Jacobs MA, Barker PB, Bottomley PA, Bhujwalla Z, Bluemke DA. Proton magnetic resonance spectroscopic imaging of human breast cancer: a preliminary study. J Magn Reson Imaging. 2004;19:68–75.
126. Kemp GJ, Meyerspeer M, Moser E. Absolute quantification of phosphorus metabolite concentrations in human muscle in vivo by 31P MRS: a quantitative review. NMR Biomed. 2007;20:555–65.
127. Sherry AD, Woods M. Chemical exchange saturation transfer contrast agents for magnetic resonance imaging. Annu Rev Biomed Eng. 2008;10:391–411.
128. Kogan F, Hariharan H, Reddy R. Chemical exchange saturation transfer (CEST) imaging: description of technique and potential clinical applications. Curr Radiol Rep. 2013;1:102–14.
129. Ward KM, Aletras AH, Balaban RS. A new class of contrast agents for MRI based on proton chemical exchange dependent saturation transfer (CEST). J Magn Reson. 2000;143:79–87.
130. Jia G, Abaza R, Williams JD, Zynger DL, Zhou J, Shah ZK, Patel M, Sammet S, Wei L, Bahnson RR, Knopp MV. Amide proton transfer MR imaging of prostate cancer: a preliminary study. J Magn Reson Imaging. 2011;33:647–54.
131. Togao O, Yoshiura T, Keupp J, Hiwatashi A, Yamashita K, Kikuchi K, Suzuki Y, Suzuki SO, Iwaki T, Hata N, et al. Amide proton transfer imaging of adult diffuse gliomas: correlation with histopathological grades. Neuro-Oncology. 2014;16:441–8.
132. Togao O, Kessinger CW, Huang G, Soesbe TC, Sagiyama K, Dimitrov I, Sherry AD, Gao J, Takahashi M. Characterization of lung cancer by amide proton transfer (APT) imaging: an in vivo study in an orthotopic mouse model. PLoS One. 2013;8:e77019.
133. Yuan J, Chen S, King AD, Zhou J, Bhatia KS, Zhang Q, Yeung DK, Wei J, Mok GS, Wang YX. Amide proton transfer-weighted imaging of the head and neck at 3 T: a feasibility study on healthy human subjects and patients with head and neck cancer. NMR Biomed. 2014;27:1239–47.
134. Klomp DW, Dula AN, Arlinghaus LR, Italiaander M, Dortch RD, Zu Z, Williams JM, Gochberg DF, Luijten PR, Gore JC, et al. Amide proton transfer imaging of the human breast at 7T: development and reproducibility. NMR Biomed. 2013;26:1271–7.
135. Zhou J, Payen JF, Wilson DA, Traystman RJ, van Zijl PC. Using the amide proton signals of intracellular proteins and peptides to detect pH effects in MRI. Nat Med. 2003;9:1085–90.
136. Jones CK, Schlosser MJ, van Zijl PC, Pomper MG, Golay X, Zhou J. Amide proton transfer imaging of human brain tumors at 3T. Magn Reson Med. 2006;56:585–92.
137. Zhou J, Tryggestad E, Wen Z, Lal B, Zhou T, Grossman R, Wang S, Yan K, Fu DX, Ford E, et al. Differentiation between glioma and radiation necrosis using molecular magnetic resonance imaging of endogenous proteins and peptides. Nat Med. 2011;17:130–4.
138. Sagiyama K, Mashimo T, Togao O, Vemireddy V, Hatanpaa KJ, Maher EA, Mickey BE, Pan E, Sherry AD, Bachoo RM, Takahashi M. In vivo chemical exchange saturation transfer imaging allows early detection of a therapeutic response in glioblastoma. Proc Natl Acad Sci U S A. 2014;111:4542–7.
139. Gilad AA, Ziv K, McMahon MT, van Zijl PC, Neeman M, Bulte JW. MRI reporter genes. J Nucl Med. 2008;49:1905–8.

Molecular Imaging in Infection and Inflammation

5

Key Points (Abstract)

Inflammation is an important mechanism for various acute physiologic defence mechanisms against various pathogens, and thus the excessive, uncontrolled, or chronic inflammatory reactions can result in various pathologic changes. They are rheumatic and autoimmune diseases, like rheumatoid arthritis (RA) or vasculitis, and many cardiovascular and neurologic disorders. One of the routinely used mechanisms is the use of various traditional 67Gacitrate scintigraphy or white blood cell scintigraphy used in nuclear medicine for the imaging of inflammation and infection.

Keywords

Infection · Inflammation · Rheumatoid arthritis · PET · Scintigraphy

5.1 Introduction

Now PET imaging with the use for 18F-FDG is based on increased glucose metabolism in various proinflammatory cells [1] and is now being established as an important non-invasive modality for the diagnosis, evaluation, and monitoring of these inflammatory processes. It is non-specific and also based on various physiological components like blood glucose levels or renal function which will prevent its use.

5.2 Infection Inflammation Imaging

5.2.1 PET Molecular Imaging

18F-FDG PET/CT is an important modality for the evaluation of various infections and inflammations without specificity. Various receptor tracers which are targeting the somatostatin and chemokine receptors in these proinflammatory cells are being used widely in myocardial inflammation. Various PET and SPECT probes are being evaluated for various inflammatory cell receptors, various cell adhesion molecules, and proinflammatory cytokines and enzymes. There is a reduced sensitivity in the imaging of cardiac inflammation by the FDG PET which requires a specific approach for the evaluation of the physiological myocardial FDG uptake. The use of SSTR-directed PET is used for the evaluation of postinfarction myocardial inflammation in myocardium infarction cases which is in correlation with CXCR4 expression in bone marrow with different systemic inflammatory response [2] and also in the case which are having higher myocardial tracer uptake associated with lesser scar tissue in the infarcted area [2]. PET signal is from macrophages, which are having the capabilities related with chemokine receptor on their surface T cells, B cells, and/or progenitor cells which will add to the associated pathology and also for various clinical implications [3]. CXCR4 axis

S. Shaikh, *Advances in Imaging*, https://doi.org/10.1007/978-981-16-9535-3_5

will show both atheroprotective atherogenic and proinflammatory effects [4, 5]. There will be an imbalance in the highly inflammatory CCR21 macrophages and monocytes leading to various pathological changes and inflammatory conditions, such as atherosclerosis and RA [6]. The use of various transmembrane receptor alpha-v beta-3 integrin (avb3) will be mediating the cell adhesion which will be having important role in angiogenesis, and also crucial for the analysis of various inflammatory and oncological conditions [7, 8].

The pathogenesis of atherosclerosis, where both macrophages and activated endothelial cells are being used for the high levels of the avb3 receptor [9]. The distribution of mitochondrial translocator protein (TSPO) ligand 18F-GE180 will denote various phases of inflammation in heart and brain resulting after acute myocardial infarction. Various newer imaging probes will be of much use for bacterial imaging in humans. Newer other imaging probes along with various receptor-directed tracers which will be targeting the immune cells, like T lymphocytes (CD3 and CD4) and B lymphocytes (CD20), or granulocytes (BW250/183), [10] along with various tracers are used for specific non-invasive imaging of bacterial infections.

5.3 Targeting Cell Proliferation and Cell Metabolism

Various tracers which will be used for targeting increased inflammatory cell metabolism are also being evaluated. As most of them are not infection specific, they will be offering various other advantages like the evaluation of inflammatory heart pathologies like myocarditis or sarcoidosis. The use of radiolabelled amino acid 11C-methionine as the marker of amino acid transport and protein synthesis is widely used in oncology especially for the imaging of brain tumours and multiple myeloma [11–15]. Here the methionine uptake is significantly increased in monocytes and macrophages that migrate to the sites of inflammatory activity [16, 17].

5.3.1 Fluorothymidine

18F-fluorothymidine (FLT) is an important marker for the evaluation of tumour proliferation. This is being transported into the cell by nucleoside transporters, phosphorylated by thymidine kinase 1 which is active between the late G1 and early G2 phase of the cell cycle, and is trapped within the cell [18]. With this concept, the use of FLT is important for the imaging of inflammation by cell proliferation.

5.3.2 Sodium Fluoride

PET imaging with sodium 18F-fluoride (NaF) is used for the analysis of bone metabolism and osteogenic activity [19] (Diagram 5.1). This is also used to identify various microcalcifications, so this is used to mark the amount of calcium activity in cardiovascular disorders like aortic stenosis or atherosclerosis and other various inflammatory conditions such as RA. In the experimental mouse model of RA, this NaF is used for the evaluation of various enhanced bone metabolisms. PET signal will be useful for various correlations; one of this is with the degree of bone destruction [20]. One of the studies that compared the NaF and FDG PET in 12 patients with RA finds the similar pattern in both tracers, with NaF PET being able to successfully identify RA-affected joints [21] (Diagram 5.2). Various studies are being used for the characterization of vascular wall microcalcifications especially for the evaluation of large aorta, carotid, and even coronary arteries [22–25]. In incidental oncology patients who underwent NaF PET/CT, tracer accumulation in common carotid arteries is proportional to cardiovascular risk factors and carotid calcified plaque burden [22].

5.3.3 Other Tracers

Newer PET radiotracers are being developed, which shows the infection and inflammation imaging, along with the targeting tracers like anti-

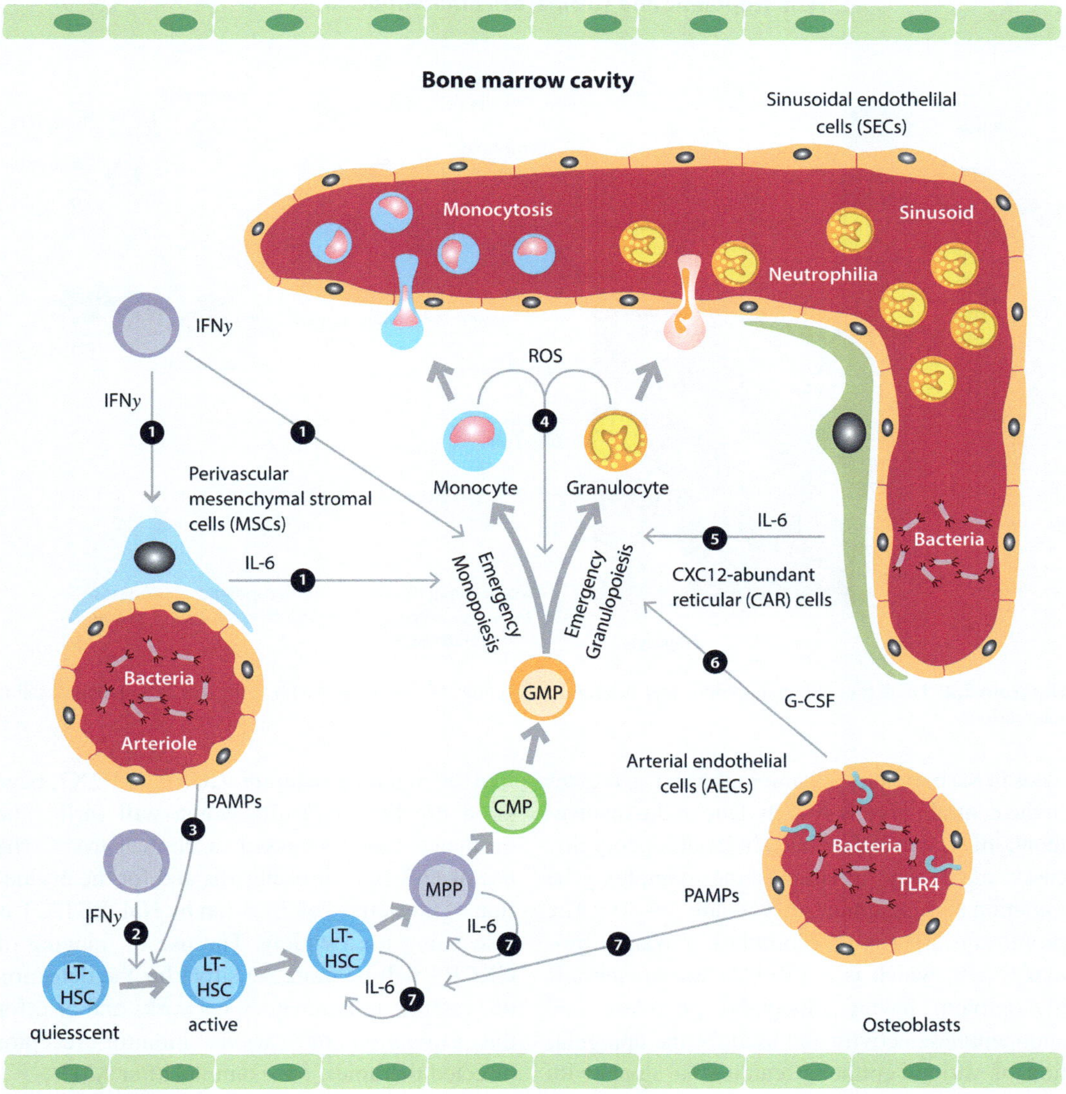

Diagram 5.1 Various reactions happening in bone marrow with different components of molecular cells interacting with each other

biotics, adhesion molecules, integrin and selectin, immunoglobulin, or cytokines and enzymes, for example, matrix metalloproteinase or tumour necrosis factor alpha [10]. The various adhesion protein-1 are glycoprotein on endothelial cells and important is that the transferring of leukocytes from blood to tissues in inflammation [26]. Various newer promising radiolabelled antibodies and peptides have also been evaluated [26–30]. Three single-chain transmembrane glycoproteins are further classifieds into L-, E, and P-selectins again depending on the cell type of origin [31]. The use of P-selectin in a-granules of platelets and expression is being done by the activated endothelia [32]. Due to this, it can be used for imaging atherosclerosis and radiolabelled probes along with the preclinical models [33–35]. The purinergic family of receptors are the adenosine triphosphate-gated ion channel which will be predominantly expressed on macrophages and mono-

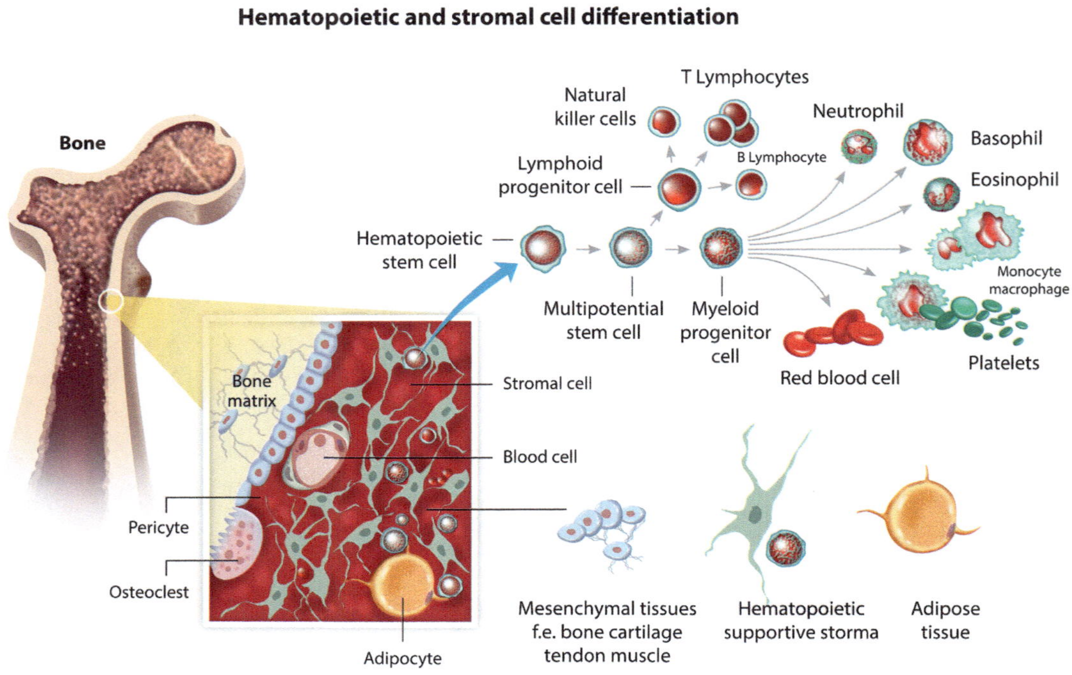

Diagram 5.2 Depiction of hematopoietic and stem cell differentiations associated with various cells and their possible interactions

cytes in the periphery and microglia and astrocytes in the central nervous system. Due to the involvement, this is more often used in inflammatory diseases as a key inflammasome complex, the initiation and inflammatory cascade [36–41]. The promising target is the fibroblast activation protein (FAP), which is a 170-kDa transmembrane glycoprotein having dipeptidyl peptidase and endopeptidase activity and used for the upregulation of various epithelial carcinoma along with the region of tissue remodelling, including fibrosis and arthritis [42]. The small molecular based PET tracers are also clinically available [43, 44].

Thus, with the use of 18F-FDG PET/CT which is an established tracer in nuclear medicine and the infection and inflammation imaging has proved that the various clinical settings may or may not be having fever. Various disease pathologies which will be able to evaluate the fever of unknown origin, [45] endocarditis, [46] or sarcoidosis [47] can also be evaluated. In all these, glucose analogue is having the small specificity for detecting inflammatory cells. Various other monocyte-/macrophage-targeting tracers, like the mannose receptor, CCR2, or P2X7, have good preclinical results which will further be evaluated based assessed in clinical trials. The use of PET in atherosclerosis and for the evaluation of the active calcification by NaF PET/CT is also being used widely. The use of imaging of CXCR4 will be more sensitive for the detection of systemic inflammatory networks and also for the evaluation of various monitor receptor directed therapies, for example, after AMI.

The interest in the use of the molecular imaging of infections and inflammation is having significant impact of overtreatment (e.g., immune suppression in inflammation) and the induction of resistance (i.e., patterns of increasing antibiotic resistance in infections). Similarities and differences in the pathophysiology of infectious and inflammatory diseases have significantly improved. Molecular imaging is capable of more separating inflammatory processes from infection-related processes. The advent of hybrid multimodality imaging techniques, accompanied by new radiopharmaceuticals and smart chemistry, the use for the inflammation.

5.4 Presumed or Established Infectious or Inflammatory Disorders

If there is an infectious focus, is it an inflammatory sign? Extent of the lesion? Infectious metastases? Therapeutic evaluation of drugs entering and penetrating the infection site? Is the therapy successful? To give more specific therapeutic options. 18F-FDG PET/CT is the most used radiotracer for the evaluation of diagnostic imaging for infection and inflammation. Presence of leukocytes, macrophages, monocytes, lymphocytes, and giant cells will directly correlate with the amount of injury and infection. The commonly used modalities of the 18F-FDG PET/CT in infection and inflammation are sarcoidosis, peripheral bone osteomyelitis, spinal infection, fever of unknown origin, metastatic infection, bacteraemia in high-risk patients, and vasculitis [48]. Other important applications are fungal infections, vascular graft infections, joint prosthesis infections, diabetic foot infections, like endocarditis, inflammatory bowel diseases, and various infectious and inflammatory diseases in children.

5.5 Molecular Imaging of Infectious Diseases

18F-FDG PET/CT use had led to a significant change in patient management. Various existing imaging modalities are invasive in nature and will be carrying the increased risk of infection like vascular-access ports, vascular and orthopaedic inserts, and various cardiac devices which are implanted in elective or emergency settings where there is chance of contamination. The role of the PET-CT is very high in the evaluation of diagnosis, staging, and post therapy evaluation of various infections, and further, the clinical impact will be increasing more in future [49]. Due to various conditions which overlap, various protocols are being evaluated for the differentiation of the inflammation, malignancies, and also for wound healing. The use of labelled white blood cells is more specific for the evaluation of various infections and is preferred for the diagnosis of osteomyelitis, joint prosthesis infections, and diabetic foot infections. The use of 99mTc-labeled interleukin-2, which is specific for inflammation due to the interleukin-2 receptor, overexpressed by activated T lymphocytes during inflammation, shows excellent results in various autoimmune and inflammatory diseases [50]. Various tracers are not safe for evaluation [51]. Therapeutic agents or humanized antibodies like bevacizumab or trastuzumab [52] are being used. The tracer should have high sensitivity and specificity, shorter half-life for easy preparation and application, and also low cost. The use of antibiotic-based tracers is more specific for the problem-solving aspects questions related with the particular infection. Agents with more promising aspects for the evaluation of infection-specific imaging are antimicrobial peptides, antigen-specific antibodies and antibody fragments, and prokaryotic compounds. In the coming days, the role of imaging will be not only to distinguish inflammation from infection but can also confirm the microorganism which is causing it. The necrotizing fasciitis is notorious and may need surgical procedures. Same with *Pseudomonas aeruginosa*, where the early diagnosis will improve the final outcome. Now the concept of molecular imaging is not confined to radionuclides, but newer concepts of optical imaging are also evaluated as well [53]. In optical imaging, the use of various fluorophores is to generate optical signal on excitation by an external light source of a specific wavelength, such as a laser. The use of unconjugated fluorophore indocyanine green will be conjugated to a targeting molecule for the specific area of interest. This emitted signal is captured, and the main advantage of fast imaging is having very high resolution. Optical imaging is now used for superficial imaging, for endoscopic and intraoperative. Optoacoustic or photoacoustic imaging is newer imaging technique used for the evaluation of maximum penetration depth and also for various potential clinical applications. Optoacoustic imaging principle is thermal expansion of a tissue by the absorption of short laser pulses due to intrinsic fluorophores which are administered in the body. Ultrasonic pressures have shorter wavelength than optical waves, with deeper penetration than that of the ultrasound imaging (3–5 cm). So, these molecular optical and optoacoustic imaging techniques are in close synergy with various radionuclide imaging (PET and SPECT), MR imaging, and ultrasound.

MR imaging is not radiation safe in children and in those who require serial scans for the success of therapy. PET/MR imaging is ideal for the evaluation of inflammatory diseases, such as insulitis, spondylodiskitis, inflammatory bowel diseases, soft tissue infection, neurologic inflammation and infection, infected diabetic foot, and infectious and inflammatory diseases in children.

Ultrasound is a non-invasive modality for the diagnosis of infectious abscesses. Therapeutic ultrasound is based on thermal or mechanical effects. Nonthermal ultrasound along with drugs is being used for a number of diseases. Microbubbles, molecule targeted echo contrast agents, and various carriers or enhancers of drugs are added to these newer dimensions for the diagnosis and therapy. Translational medicine advances along with molecular imaging will result in the new era. Oncology is the forefront where the trials are being done in many conditions leading to the role of personalized or precision medicine. These various molecular imaging techniques will highlight various pathophysiologic processes, various cell types, and different pathogens involved, for the detection of potential target, and pathogenic bacteria and biologically active molecules which will be used for the diagnosis and treatment monitoring.

References

1. Meller J, Sahlmann CO, Scheel AK. 18F-FDG PET and PET/CT in fever of unknown origin. J Nucl Med. 2007;48(1):35–45.
2. Reiter T, Kircher M, Schirbel A, et al. Imaging of C-X-C motif chemokine receptor CXCR4 expression after myocardial infarction with [(68)Ga] Pentixafor-PET/CT in correlation with cardiac MRI. JACC Cardiovasc Imaging. 2018;11(10):1541–3.
3. Pawig L, Klasen C, Weber C, et al. Diversity and inter-connections in the CXCR4 chemokine receptor/ligand family: molecular perspectives. Front Immunol. 2015;6:429.
4. van der Vorst EP, Doring Y, Weber C. MIF and CXCL12 in cardiovascular diseases: functional differences and similarities. Front Immunol. 2015;6:373.
5. Doring Y, Pawig L, Weber C, et al. The CXCL12/CXCR4 chemokine ligand/receptor axis in cardiovascular disease. Front Physiol. 2014;5:212.
6. Raghu H, Lepus CM, Wang Q, et al. CCL2/CCR2, but not CCL5/CCR5, mediates monocyte recruitment, inflammation and cartilage destruction in osteoarthritis. Ann Rheum Dis. 2017;76(5):914–22.
7. Brooks PC, Clark RA, Cheresh DA. Requirement of vascular integrin alpha v beta 3 for angiogenesis. Science. 1994;264(5158):569–71.
8. Brooks PC, Montgomery AM, Rosenfeld M, et al. Integrin alpha v beta 3 antagonists promote tumor regression by inducing apoptosis of angiogenic blood vessels. Cell. 1994;79(7):1157–64.
9. Hoshiga M, Alpers CE, Smith LL, et al. Alpha-v beta-3 integrin expression in normal and atherosclerotic artery. Circ Res. 1995;77(6):1129–35.
10. Lee HJ, Ehlerding EB, Cai W. Antibody-based tracers for PET/SPECT imaging of chronic inflammatory diseases. Chembiochem. 2019;20(4):422–36.
11. Herholz K, Holzer T, Bauer B, et al. 11C-methionine PET for differential diagnosis of low-grade gliomas. Neurology. 1998;50(5):1316–22.
12. Kracht LW, Miletic H, Busch S, et al. Delineation of brain tumor extent with [11C]L-methionine positron emission tomography: local comparison with stereotactic histopathology. Clin Cancer Res. 2004;10(21):7163–70.
13. Lapa C, Garcia-Velloso MJ, Luckerath K, et al. (11) CMethionine-PET in multiple myeloma: a combined study from two different institutions. Theranostics. 2017;7(11):2956–64.
14. Luckerath K, Lapa C, Albert C, et al. 11C-methionine-PET: a novel and sensitive tool for monitoring of early response to treatment in multiple myeloma. Oncotarget. 2015;6(10):8418–29.
15. Luckerath K, Lapa C, Spahmann A, et al. Targeting paraprotein biosynthesis for non-invasive characterization of myeloma biology. PLoS One. 2013;8(12):e84840.
16. Swirski FK, Nahrendorf M. Leukocyte behavior in atherosclerosis, myocardial infarction, and heart failure. Science. 2013;339(6116):161–6.
17. Nahrendorf M. Myeloid cell contributions to cardiovascular health and disease. Nat Med. 2018;24(6):711–20.
18. Herrmann K, Buck AK. Proliferation imaging with (1)(8)F-fluorothymidine PET/computed tomography: physiologic uptake, variants, and pitfalls. PET Clin. 2014;9(3):331–8.
19. Blau M, Nagler W, Bender MA. Fluorine-18: a new isotope for bone scanning. J Nucl Med. 1962;3:332–4.

20. Irmler IM, Gebhardt P, Hoffmann B, et al. 18F-fluoride positron emission tomography/computed tomography infection and inflammation imaging 13 for noninvasive in vivo quantification of pathophysiological bone metabolism in experimental murine arthritis. Arthritis Res Ther. 2014;16(4):R155.
21. Watanabe T, Takase-Minegishi K, Ihata A, et al. (18) F-FDG and (18)F-NaF PET/CT demonstrate coupling of inflammation and accelerated bone turnover in rheumatoid arthritis. Mod Rheumatol. 2016;26(2):180–7.
22. Derlin T, Wisotzki C, Richter U, et al. In vivo imaging of mineral deposition in carotid plaque using 18F-sodium fluoride PET/CT: correlation with atherogenic risk factors. J Nucl Med. 2011;52(3):362–8.
23. Derlin T, Richter U, Bannas P, et al. Feasibility of 18F-sodium fluoride PET/CT for imaging of atherosclerotic plaque. J Nucl Med. 2010;51(6):862–5.
24. Li Y, Berenji GR, Shaba WF, et al. Association of vascular fluoride uptake with vascular calcification and coronary artery disease. Nucl Med Commun. 2012;33(1):14–20.
25. Dweck MR, Chow MW, Joshi NV, et al. Coronary arterial 18F-sodium fluoride uptake: a novel marker of plaque biology. J Am Coll Cardiol. 2012;59(17):1539–48.
26. Moisio O, Siitonen R, Liljenback H, et al. Exploring alternative radiolabeling strategies for sialic acid-binding immunoglobulin-like lectin 9 peptide: [(68) Ga]Ga- and [(18)F]AlF-NOTA-Siglec-9. Molecules 2018;23(2) [pii:E305].
27. Lankinen P, Makinen TJ, Poyhonen TA, et al. (68) Ga-DOTAVAP-P1 PET imaging capable of demonstrating the phase of inflammation in healing bones and the progress of infection in osteomyelitic bones. Eur J Nucl Med Mol Imaging. 2008;35(2):352–64.
28. Autio A, Vainio PJ, Suilamo S, et al. Preclinical evaluation of a radioiodinated fully human antibody for in vivo imaging of vascular adhesion protein-1-positive vasculature in inflammation. J Nucl Med. 2013;54(8):1315–9.
29. Autio A, Henttinen T, Sipila HJ, et al. Mini-PEG spacering of VAP-1-targeting 68Ga-DOTAVAP-P1 peptide improves PET imaging of inflammation. EJNMMI Res. 2011;1(1):10.
30. Aalto K, Autio A, Kiss EA, et al. Siglec-9 is a novel leukocyte ligand for vascular adhesion protein-1 and can be used in PET imaging of inflammation and cancer. Blood. 2011;118(13):3725–33.
31. McMurray RW. Adhesion molecules in autoimmune disease. Semin Arthritis Rheum. 1996;25(4):215–33.
32. Ley K. The role of selectins in inflammation and disease. Trends Mol Med. 2003;9(6):263–8.
33. Li X, Bauer W, Israel I, et al. Targeting P-selectin by gallium-68-labeled fucoidan positron emission tomography for noninvasive characterization of vulnerable plaques: correlation with in vivo 17.6T MRI. Arterioscler Thromb Vasc Biol. 2014;34(8):1661–7.
34. Nakamura I, Hasegawa K, Wada Y, et al. Detection of early stage atherosclerotic plaques using PET and CT fusion imaging targeting P-selectin in low density lipoprotein receptor-deficient mice. Biochem Biophys Res Commun. 2013;433(1):47–51.
35. Xu Y, Li J, Fang W, et al. A potential thrombus diagnosis reagent based on P-selectin monoclonal antibody SZ-51 light chain. Thromb Res. 2008;123(2):306–15.
36. Kolb HC, Barret O, Bhattacharya A, et al. Preclinical evaluation and nonhuman primate receptor occupancy study of (18)F-JNJ-64413739, a PET radioligand for P2X7 receptors. J Nucl Med. 2019;60(8):1154–9.
37. Territo PR, Meyer JA, Peters JS, et al. Characterization of (11)C-GSK1482160 for targeting the P2X7 receptor as a biomarker for neuroinflammation. J Nucl Med. 2017;58(3):458–65.
38. Ory D, Celen S, Gijsbers R, et al. Preclinical evaluation of a P2X7 receptor-selective radiotracer: PET studies in a rat model with local overexpression of the human P2X7 receptor and in nonhuman primates. J Nucl Med. 2016;57(9):1436–41.
39. Fantoni ER, Dal Ben D, Falzoni S, et al. Design, synthesis and evaluation in an LPS rodent model of neuroinflammation of a novel (18)F-labelled PET tracer targeting P2X7. EJNMMI Res. 2017;7(1):31.
40. Jin H, Han J, Resing D, et al. Synthesis and in vitro characterization of a P2X7 radioligand [(123)I] TZ6019 and its response to neuroinflammation in a mouse model of Alzheimer disease. Eur J Pharmacol. 2018;820:8–17.
41. Janssen B, Vugts DJ, Wilkinson SM, et al. Identification of the allosteric P2X7 receptor antagonist [(11)C]SMW139 as a PET tracer of microglial activation. Sci Rep. 2018;8(1):6580.
42. Hamson EJ, Keane FM, Tholen S, et al. Understanding fibroblast activation protein (FAP): substrates, activities, expression and targeting for cancer therapy. Proteomics Clin Appl. 2014;8(5–6):454–63.
43. Loktev A, Lindner T, Mier W, et al. A tumor-imaging method targeting cancer-associated fibroblasts. J Nucl Med. 2018;59(9):1423–9.
44. Lindner T, Loktev A, Altmann A, et al. Development of quinoline-based theranostic ligands for the targeting of fibroblast activation protein. J Nucl Med. 2018;59(9):1415–22.
45. Kouijzer IJE, Mulders-Manders CM, BleekerRovers CP, et al. Fever of unknown origin: the value of FDG-PET/CT. Semin Nucl Med. 2018;48(2):100–7.
46. Mahmood M, Kendi AT, Ajmal S, et al. Meta-analysis of 18F-FDG PET/CT in the diagnosis of infective endocarditis. J NuclCardiol. 2019;26(3):922–35.
47. Piekarski E, Benali K, Rouzet F. Nuclear imaging in sarcoidosis. Semin Nucl Med. 2018;48(3):246–60.
48. Jamar F, Buscombe J, Chiti A, et al. EANM/SNMMI guideline for 18F-FDG use in inflammation and infection. J Nucl Med. 2013;54:647–58.
49. Glaudemans AW, Signore A. FDG-PET/CT in infections: the imaging method of choice? Eur J Nucl Med Mol Imaging. 2010;37:1986–91.
50. Glaudemans AW, Bonanno E, Galli F, et al. In vivo and in vitro evidence that 99mTc-HYNIC-interleukin-2 is

able to detect T lymphocytes in vulnerable atherosclerotic plaques of the carotid artery. Eur J Nucl Med Mol Imaging. 2014;41:1710–9.

51. Scheuer W, van Dam GM, Dobosz M, Schwaiger M, Ntziachristos V. Drugbased optical agents: infiltrating clinics at lower risk. Sci Transl Med. 2012;4:134ps11.
52. Gaykema SB, Schroder CP, Vitfell-Rasmussen J, et al. ¨ 89Zr-trastuzumab and 89Zr-bevacizumab PET to evaluate the effect of the HSP90 inhibitor NVPAUY922 in metastatic breast cancer patients. Clin Cancer Res. 2014;20:3945–54.
53. van Oosten M, Schafer T, Gazendam JA, et al. Real-time in vivo imaging of ¨ invasive- and biomaterial-associated bacterial infections using fluorescently labelled vancomycin. Nat Commun. 2013;4:2584.

Functional Molecular Imaging: I

6

Key Points (Abstract)

Molecular imaging is defined as non-invasive imaging of cellular and subcellular events; this is having significant changes in the research and clinical disciplines in this era. The combination of the various advances in the fields of engineering, molecular biology, chemistry, immunology, and genetics has resulted in many multi- and interdisciplinary innovations with the goals of the various non-invasive strategies which will be used for the easy identification, risk stratification, and monitoring response to the therapy with very high sensitivity and specificity. Imaging of molecular and cellular functions will go hand in hand with molecular therapies, resulting in a significant increase in the combination of imaging with therapy. Positron emission tomography (PET), PET combined with computed tomography (CT), and single-photon emission computed tomography are having significant advances in recent days. These along with magnetic resonance (MR), optical, CT, and ultrasonographic (US) imaging.

Keywords

Molecular imaging · Optical imaging · MRI PET-CT · PARACEST · Molecular CT Molecular ultrasound

6.1 Molecular Imaging

The preference for non-invasive imaging for various disease processes has seen a significant increase in the growth in the form of clinical practice. The advancements in the various aspects of computed tomography (CT), magnetic resonance (MR) imaging, and ultrasonography (US) has evolved the imaging to the newer heights [1]. CT is usually offering the various patient throughput and these high-resolution images, with this the molecular images with the CT images, are difficult for evaluation. US currently is without radiation exposure, but the sound wave reflection and perturbation will not be able to perform the better way along the molecular composition of tissue. The basis of the MR imaging is molecular but the recent molecular imaging protocols will provide more anatomic as well as functional information. The recent advances in the pulse sequences and protocols have resulted in the evaluation of the various cellular or subcellular events, like the MR spectroscopy and diffusion-weighted imaging, providing information on the molecular composition of the tissue and water diffusion, respectively [2, 3]. Positron emission tomography (PET), with the available radiotracers, is the established molecular imaging technique that is being used for many years. PET scanners disadvantage is the very low spatial resolution as compared to the CT, MR imaging, and US; for this, PET is combined with CT or MR imaging for anatomic detail. New molecular imaging techniques and various imag-

S. Shaikh, *Advances in Imaging*, https://doi.org/10.1007/978-981-16-9535-3_6

ing molecular probes are being tested for preclinical or clinical trials, and some are being used for clinical evaluation [1, 4–9]. Examples of the molecular probes are nontargeted and targeted [10], Activatable MR [11–14] and Optical probes [15]; Endoscopic [16, 17] and Intraoperative optical devices [18–20]; Ultrasonic molecular imaging [21]; Photoacoustic imaging [22]; and Raman spectroscopy [9, 23]. The target-specific imaging has increased sensitivity (1023–1025 M for most contrast agents) [24] contrast agent detection which is superior (not well characterized, approximate estimation) [24, 25]; it is orders of magnitude lower than that of PET [24] or US detection of microbubbles [26]. With the advances in the newer designs and chemistry of MR imaging contrast agents, the concept of molecular imaging with the use of MR is a reality [27]. Molecular MR imaging contrast agents nanoparticulate probes are made up of the contrast-generating metal iron oxide nanoparticles or nano scaffolds which are loaded with gadolinium chelates [Gd^{3+}] and at the molecular target with the binding of the ligand to the contrast agent. Target-specific contrast agents in MR imaging is a problem with low sensitivity, but recent advances will overcome this.

6.2 Principles of MR Contrast Agents, T2 and T1 Contrast Agents

Contrast enhancement on T2-weighted images agents is superparamagnetic iron oxide nanoparticles, comprising of the score of iron oxide measuring 3–5 nm, and coated with dextran, starch, polymer, or citrate [28]. Thin dextran coatings with the more extensive polymer coating will result in the monodisperse in vivo (monodisperse iron oxide nanoparticles, or MION) [29]. These are the hydrodynamic diameter, leading to the ultrasmall superparamagnetic iron oxide (USPIO) iron oxide nanoparticles of the size of less than 50 nm. The particle stabilization via crosslinking of its dextran coating will be resulting in nanoparticle cross-linked iron oxide (CLIO) [30]. USPIO and CLIO are the long-circulating particles with an average blood half-life of approximately 24 hours which is being removed from the circulation by the reticuloendothelial system [31]. The long half-life and small size of approximately 30 nm can penetrate tissues of interest like myocardium, atherosclerotic plaques, neurological conditions, or tumours. They can be targeted towards a specific receptor or molecule of interest by binding the various ligands like the various antibodies, peptides, or small molecules to their surface. T1 contrast agents are the chelates of paramagnetic metal ions, most commonly Gd^{3+}, which will be exhibiting the very high magnetic moment due to its seven unpaired electrons. Gadolinium-containing dendrimers [32] are the particles having the core and tree-like surface structure, micelles [33], gadolinium containing liposomes [34], and gadolinium-containing perfluorocarbon emulsions [35] or high-density lipoprotein like nanoparticles [36].

6.3 Contrast Agents Based on Fluorine 19

MR imaging applications with the water protons (hydrogen 1 [1H]) will be able to create the contrast by the enhancement, on MR images. Low natural abundance and a very high gyromagnetic ratio, fluorine 19 [19F] is best suited for this purpose. For this, the nanoparticles which will have the high numbers of 19F atoms can be used as contrast agents [37].

6.4 Chemical Exchange Saturation Transfer Agents

Paramagnetic contrast agents are based on the magnetization transfer method. The various contrast agents used are known as the chemical exchange saturation transfer, or CEST, agents. MR imaging based on the magnetic transfer method is reviewed [38]. These agents will produce the MR imaging contrast enhancement which is based on the way that the contrast enhancement is not solely based on proton relaxation, instead on the select magnetization of the water signal, causing the minimal effect on its longitudinal relaxation rate. These CEST agents are seen on the two pools of protons having different nuclear MR chemical shifts. One pool has the contrast agent with its exchangeable protons; and another one has the bulk water. When these agents contain paramagnetic lanthanides like dysprosium ion (Dy^{3+}), terbium ion (Tb^{3+}), thulium ion (Tm^{3+}), or ytterbium ion (Yb^{3+}), they are called PARACEST agents [38–40]. PARACEST agents will be enhancing more specifically. PARACEST agents which are based on liposomes with paramagnetic lanthanide complex Tm-DOTMA are there. Activatable MR Contrast Agents of MR molecular imaging contrast agents known as the MR imaging probes, which will be able to change the response to the local environment. "Smart" contrast agents are called due to the imaging signal which is being induced due to the particular disease [41]. Enzyme-sensing probes like b-galactosidase-sensitive paramagnetic substrates are being described by Louie et al. [12]; the b-galactosidase-sensitive probe is also inactive in its native form. Superparamagnetic iron oxide particles are being used to design activatable MR probes which have the unique magnetic phenomenon, known as the magnetic relaxation. This technique is for the evaluation of the detecting biomolecules in homogeneous assays with very low detection levels, as low as 500 mmol [42–45]. The design of these probes, enzymatic substrate will cause the loss of the PARACEST signal [46] or the appearance of the PARACEST signal [47]. These phenomena are known as switch off and switch on, respectively.

6.5 Multimodality Probes

Multimodality imaging probes have significant advantages in the form of the various complimentary modalities. Here the goal is to achieve a very high spatial resolution and very high sensitivity (e.g., by combining MR imaging with nuclear imaging) for the preoperative staging and intraoperative molecular imaging [23, 48].

6.5.1 Multimodal Probe

The use of the multimodal probe in MR imaging is for preoperative staging and in the optical imaging is for Raman spectroscopic imaging [23]. The basic principle of MR imaging is due to the various interactions of atomic nuclei with the external magnetic field. Nuclear spins will be oriented in two possible directions: parallel ("spin-up") or antiparallel ("spin-down") to the external field (B0). Very small number of unequally oriented spins will have very low sensitivity [49]. This signal enhancement will result in the protons, for example, carbon 13 (13C) and nitrogen 15, with low abundance with their molecular distribution for the short imaging times [50], causing the metabolic processes in vivo [51]. The hyperpolarized state of molecules will be created by the two dynamic nuclear polarization techniques, such as the so-called Overhauser effect, along with the contrast agent [52].

6.6 Molecular CT Imaging

CT is widely available, relatively cost-effective, and enables high-resolution whole-body imaging with excellent speed. CT in principle should be a very suitable platform for molecular imaging. The biggest limitation is very less sensitivity and very low soft-tissue contrast. Soft tissue contrast in CT is based on the mass attenuation coefficient of the tissue and will be more increased by injecting a contrast agent. All CT contrast agents are small, iodinated molecules that are very effective in absorbing X-rays.

6.6.1 Principles of Molecular CT Contrast Agents

The principle of CT for measuring X-ray absorption will require the use of materials with very high atomic numbers (Z) for increasing the image contrast and ultimately the sensitivity of CT imaging for the contrast agents. These CT molecular contrast agents have the maximum number of X-ray-absorbing atoms into a nanoparticle, like the emulsions [53–55], liposomes [56], and lipoproteins [36] to polymeric nanoparticles [57, 58]. The important feature of this nanoparticle design is the pharmacokinetics. The circulation time can be increased as for the bismuth sulphide nanoparticle agent [59]; here the circulation time is longer than 2 h. Longer circulation times will increase the interaction and binding of a contrast agent to a target.

6.6.2 Applications of Molecular CT Imaging

The development of molecular CT imaging agents is in infancy, with very few being used in the in vivo models. Since gold is a safe material, gold-based nanoparticle contrast agents can be used for the in vivo CT imaging. These gold nanoparticles do not have the match of these agents where the conventional iodinated contrast agents are relevant for CT [60]. The targeted gold nanoparticles for cancer imaging are being used in vitro cell samples [61, 62]. Gold embedded in liposomes can be used for the in vivo imaging of macrophages in atherosclerotic plaques [63]. Multispectral (multicolours) of the CT will be allowing the gold nanoparticles to be differentiated from the X-ray-absorbing materials, like iodine and calcium, and can be used for the plaque characterization at CT [62]. Late development of CT molecular imaging will be the major hurdle that CT will have less sensitivity. Here, the CT requires very high concentrations of high-atomic-number materials for the development of the high contrast. Iodine is not well characterized but is estimated to have significant increase in the range of hundreds of millimolar to molar [64, 65]. Due to the intrinsic principle of CT measuring X-ray absorption, the CT attenuation of the contrast agent will have a more specific value.

6.7 Molecular US Imaging

The use of the targeted contrast-enhanced US imaging is the emerging newer molecular imaging modality. Molecular US is a semiquantitative and quantitative assessment of molecular target expression having the very high sensitivity, along with the advances in contrast agent design for the clinical translation in the near future [66, 67].

6.7.1 Principles of Molecular US Contrast Agents

Two main types of the US contrast agents are: (a) microbubble-based agents and (b) non-microbubble-based agents [66, 68]. Microbubbles are the gas-liquid emulsions, containing the gaseous core which is surrounded by the shell with a size of approximately 1–4 mm. The gaseous core will cause a very high echogenic response causing a very high contrast-to-background tissue ratio [66]. The US detection of microbubbles has the nonlinear behaviour of microbubbles, causing the compression to expand the acoustic field, which is very close to the resonance frequency, ultimately resulting in nonlinear scattering of sound to frequencies two times or more above like the harmonics or below known as subharmonics the input frequency [5] (Diagram 6.1). The frequency filtering of the nonlinear resonance of the microbubbles and linear signals allow the detection of the signals by the microbubbles, as compared with background tissue signal which is suppressed. The microbubbles with different characteristics are being synthesized with the different shell compositions of different gaseous cores. The microbubble shells consist of various polymers, albumin, galactose [69], or lipids, air or high-molecular-weight gases like the perfluorocarbon or sulphur hexafluoride are being used as gas cores [70]. Microbubbles have a large size, preventing them to be leaked from the surrounding extravascular space. This is seen in the imaging by targeting the various microbubbles to disease processes causing the vascular endothelial cells lining to be reflected in the luminal surface of capillaries and vessels, due to inflammation and angiogenesis [66, 67]. Non-microbubble-based contrast agents are smaller in size and can enter the extravascular space, and can image the extracellular space vascular compartment. The different types of non-microbubble particles will be varying in size and

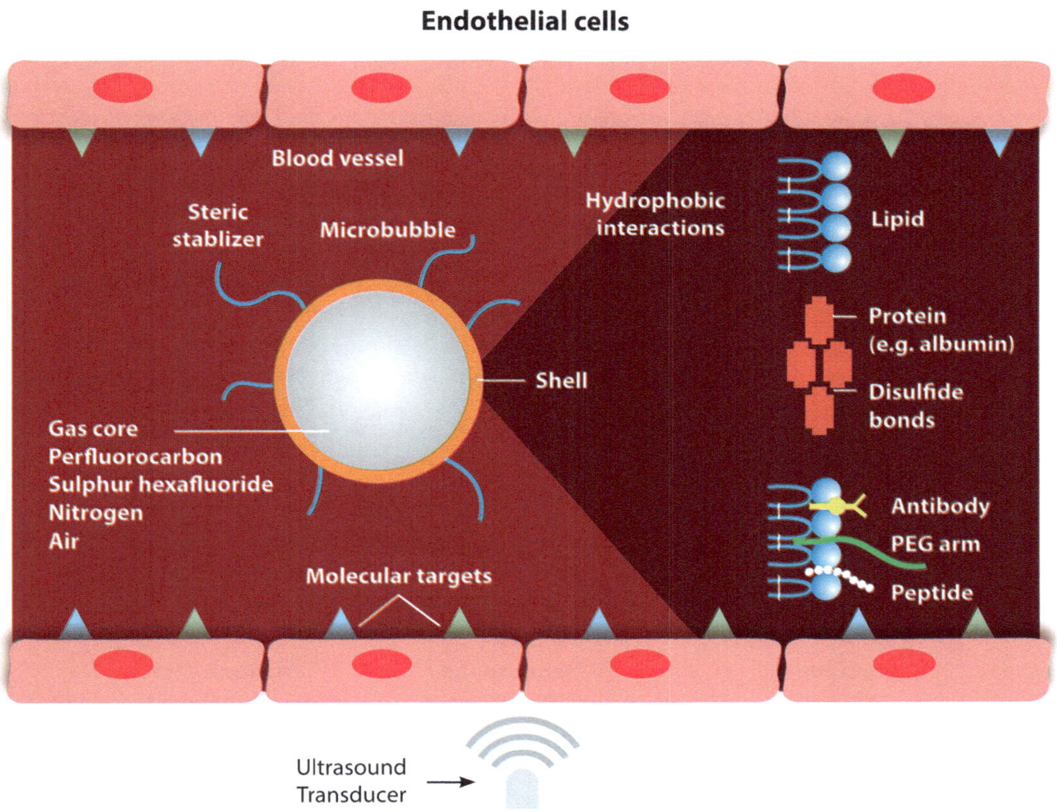

Diagram 6.1 Various interactions happening in the cell after injection of the microbubbles

composition [66]. Echogenic liposomes will be made up of the aqueous core which will be surrounded by the lipid bilayer. The various perfluorocarbon (PFC) emulsion nanodroplets are liquid-liquid emulsions which consist of the perfluorocarbon core and a phospholipid monolayer capsule. Liquid core of PFC nanodroplets will be vaporized into gas with this acoustic energy, causing a significant increase in the echogenicity of the particles [66] (Diagram 6.2). Nanobubbles are smaller as-liquid emulsions having the biodegradable polymer shell having the nontargeted passive drug delivery. The solid nanoparticles will be the amorphous particles made up of the silica or iron oxide and containing the many gas pockets to detect the backscatter for US imaging. The Quantification of Molecular US Imaging Signal by the use of the various contrast Microbubbles due to the contrast enhanced US is directly proportional to the concentration or number of the injected microbubbles [71]; with this, the quantification of the microbubbles in molecular US imaging is easier [66] (Diagram 6.3). The imaging beam may not be seen in all the scenarios. The nonspecific binding of targeted microbubbles to endothelial cells can be seen due to the interaction between the microbubble and vascular endothelial cells and can be due to the small cellular expression known as the microbubbles per cell surface marker.

The use of the dual-targeted microbubbles will mimic the features of the leukocytes in vivo. The dual-targeted microbubble targeted with the P-selectin and vascular cell adhesion molecule-1 (VCAM-1) can see the attachment of a leukocyte at various sites of the inflammation due to the interaction with P-selectin and then firmly attaching via VCAM1 [66].

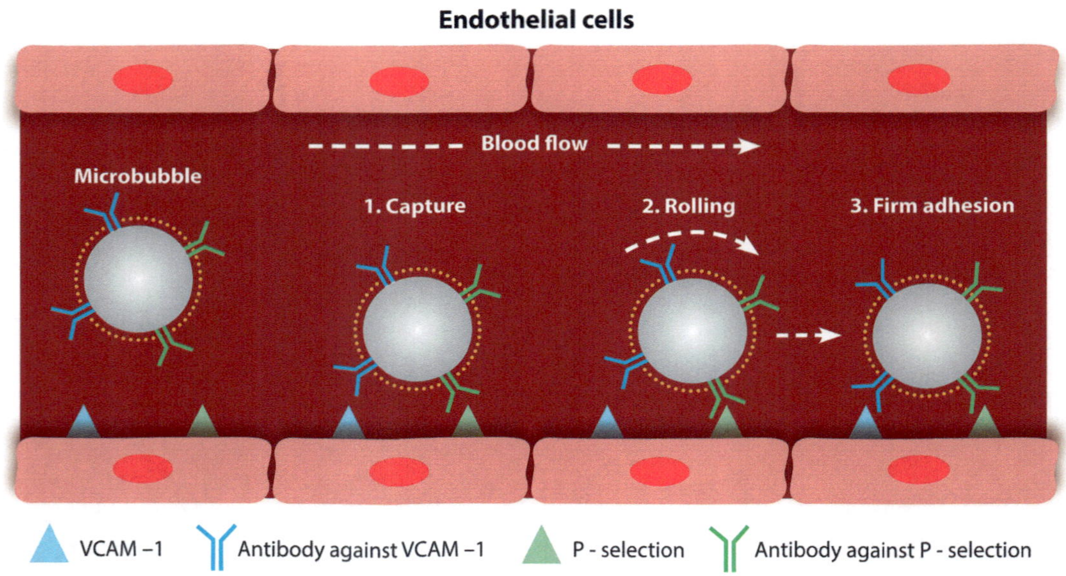

Diagram 6.2 Microbubble interaction in the vessel after injection

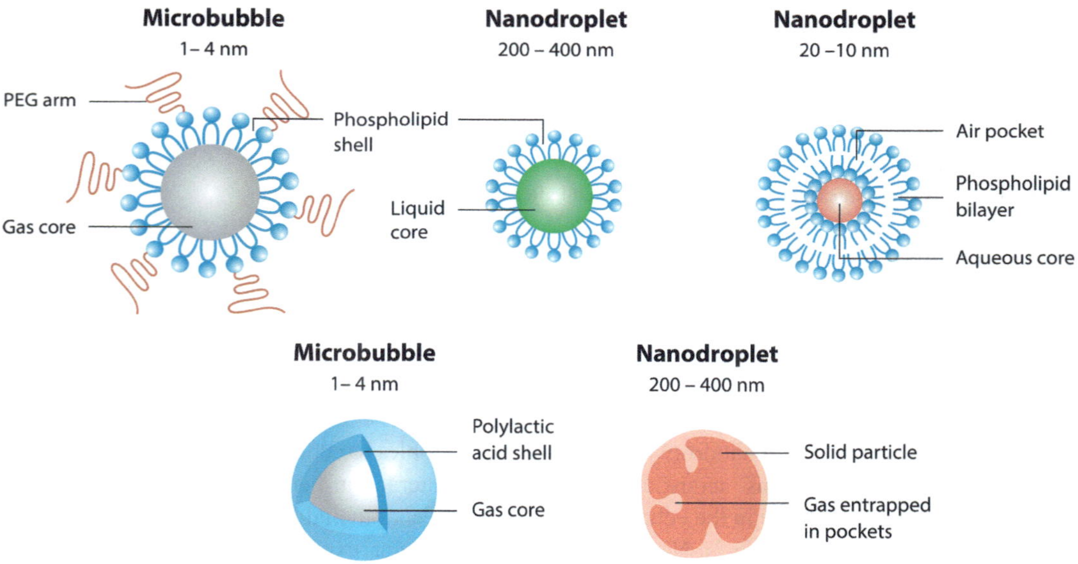

Diagram 6.3 Various nanoparticles and microbubbles with sizes and their interactions

References

1. Weissleder R, Pittet MJ. Imaging in the era of molecular oncology. Nature. 2008;452(7187):580–9.
2. Mazaheri Y, Shukla-Dave A, Muellner A, Hricak H. MRI of the prostate: clinical relevance and emerging applications. J Magn Reson Imaging. 2011;33(2):258–74.
3. Vargas HA, Akin O, Franiel T, et al. Diffusion-weighted endorectal MR imaging at 3 T for prostate cancer: tumor detection and assessment of aggressiveness. Radiology. 2011;259(3):775–84.
4. Biswal S, Resnick DL, Hoffman JM, Gambhir SS. Molecular imaging: integration of molecular imaging into the musculoskeletal imaging practice. Radiology. 2007;244(3):651–71.

5. Pysz MA, Willmann JK. Targeted contrastenhanced ultrasound: an emerging technology in abdominal and pelvic imaging. Gastroenterology. 2011;140(3):785–90.
6. Kircher MF, Gambhir SS, Grimm J. Noninvasive cell-tracking methods. Nat Rev Clin Oncol. 2011;8(11):677–88.
7. Pysz MA, Gambhir SS, Willmann JK. Molecular imaging: current status and emerging strategies. Clin Radiol. 2010;65(7):500–16.
8. Willmann JK, van Bruggen N, Dinkelborg LM, Gambhir SS. Molecular imaging in drug development. Nat Rev Drug Discov. 2008;7(7):591–607.
9. Zavaleta CL, Kircher MF, Gambhir SS. Raman's "effect" on molecular imaging. J Nucl Med. 2011;52(12):1839–44.
10. Islam T, Josephson L. Current state and future applications of active targeting in malignancies using superparamagnetic iron oxide nanoparticles. Cancer Biomark. 2009;5(2):99–107.
11. Chen JW, Querol Sans M, Bogdanov A Jr, Weissleder R. Imaging of myeloperoxidase in mice by using novel amplifiable paramagnetic substrates. Radiology. 2006;240(2):473–81.
12. Louie AY, Hüber MM, Ahrens ET, et al. In vivo visualization of gene expression using magnetic resonance imaging. Nat Biotechnol. 2000;18(3):321–5.
13. Nahrendorf M, Sosnovik D, Chen JW, et al. Activatable magnetic resonance imaging agent reports myeloperoxidase activity in healing infarcts and noninvasively detects the antiinflammatory effects of atorvastatin on ischemia-reperfusion injury. Circulation. 2008;117(9):1153–60.
14. Ronald JA, Chen JW, Chen Y, et al. Enzymesensitive magnetic resonance imaging targeting myeloperoxidase identifies active inflammation in experimental rabbit atherosclerotic plaques. Circulation. 2009;120(7):592–9.
15. Elias DR, Thorek DL, Chen AK, Czupryna J, Tsourkas A. In vivo imaging of cancer biomarkers using activatable molecular probes. Cancer Biomark. 2008;4(6):287–305.
16. Buchner AM, Shahid MW, Heckman MG, et al. Comparison of probe-based confocal laser endomicroscopy with virtual chromoendoscopy for classification of colon polyps. Gastroenterology. 2010;138(3):834–42.
17. Wolfsen HC. New technologies for imaging of Barrett's esophagus. Surg Oncol Clin N Am. 2009;18(3):487–502.
18. Gibbs-Strauss SL, Rosenberg M, Clough BL, Troyan SL, Frangioni JV. First-in-human clinical trials of imaging devices: an example from optical imaging. Conf Proc IEEE Eng Med Biol Soc. 2009;2009:2001–4.
19. Matsui A, Tanaka E, Choi HS, et al. Realtime intraoperative near-infrared fluorescence identification of the extrahepatic bile ducts using clinically available contrast agents. Surgery. 2010;148(1):87–95.
20. Troyan SL, Kianzad V, Gibbs-Strauss SL, et al. The FLARE intraoperative near-infrared fluorescence imaging system: a first-in-human clinical trial in breast cancer sentinel lymph node mapping. Ann Surg Oncol. 2009;16(10):2943–52.
21. Willmann JK, Lutz AM, Paulmurugan R, et al. Dual-targeted contrast agent for US assessment of tumor angiogenesis in vivo. Radiology. 2008;248(3):936–44.
22. De la Zerda A, Zavaleta C, Keren S, et al. Carbon nanotubes as photoacoustic molecular imaging agents in living mice. Nat Nanotechnol. 2008;3(9):557–62.
23. Kircher MF, De la Zerda A, Jokerst J, et al. A brain tumor molecular imaging strategy using a novel triple-modality nanoparticle. Nat Med. (in press)
24. Massoud TF, Gambhir SS. Molecular imaging in living subjects: seeing fundamental biological processes in a new light. Genes Dev. 2003;17(5):545–80.
25. Frangioni JV, Hajjar RJ. In vivo tracking of stem cells for clinical trials in cardiovascular disease. Circulation. 2004;110(21):3378–83.
26. Klibanov AL, Rasche PT, Hughes MS, et al. Detection of individual microbubbles of ultrasound contrast agents: imaging of freefloating and targeted bubbles. Investig Radiol. 2004;39(3):187–95.
27. Aime S, Cabella C, Colombatto S, Geninatti Crich S, Gianolio E, Maggioni F. Insights into the use of paramagnetic Gd(III) complexes in MR-molecular imaging investigations. J Magn Reson Imaging. 2002;16(4):394–406.
28. Sosnovik DE, Nahrendorf M, Weissleder R. Molecular magnetic resonance imaging in cardiovascular medicine. Circulation. 2007;115(15):2076–86.
29. Shen T, Weissleder R, Papisov M, Bogdanov A Jr, Brady TJ. Monocrystalline iron oxide nanocompounds (MION): physicochemical properties. Magn Reson Med. 1993;29(5):599–604.
30. Wunderbaldinger P, Josephson L, Weissleder R. Crosslinked iron oxides (CLIO): a new platform for the development of targeted MR contrast agents. Acad Radiol. 2002;9(Suppl 2):S304–6.
31. Harisinghani MG, Barentsz J, Hahn PF, et al. Noninvasive detection of clinically occult lymph-node metastases in prostate cancer. N Engl J Med. 2003;348(25):2491–9.
32. Swanson SD, Kukowska-Latallo JF, Patri AK, et al. Targeted gadolinium-loaded dendrimer nanoparticles for tumor-specific magnetic resonance contrast enhancement. Int J Nanomedicine. 2008;3(2):201–10.
33. Mulder WJ, Strijkers GJ, van Tilborg GA, Griffioen AW, Nicolay K. Lipid-based nanoparticles for contrast-enhanced MRI and molecular imaging. NMR Biomed. 2006;19(1):142–64.
34. Ghaghada KB, Ravoori M, Sabapathy D, Bankson J, Kundra V, Annapragada A. New dual mode gadolinium nanoparticle contrast agent for magnetic resonance imaging. PLoS One. 2009;4(10):e7628.
35. Morawski AM, Winter PM, Crowder KC, et al. Targeted nanoparticles for quantitative imaging of

sparse molecular epitopes with MRI. Magn Reson Med. 2004;51(3):480–6.
36. Skajaa T, Cormode DP, Falk E, Mulder WJ, Fisher EA, Fayad ZA. High-density lipoprotein-based contrast agents for multimodal imaging of atherosclerosis. Arterioscler Thromb Vasc Biol. 2010;30(2):169–76.
37. Ahrens ET, Flores R, Xu H, Morel PA. In vivo imaging platform for tracking immunotherapeutic cells. Nat Biotechnol. 2005;23(8):983–7.
38. Hancu I, Dixon WT, Woods M, Vinogradov E, Sherry AD, Lenkinski RE. CEST and PARACEST MR contrast agents. Acta Radiol. 2010;51(8):910–23.
39. Woods M, Woessner DE, Sherry AD. Paramagnetic lanthanide complexes as PARACEST agents for medical imaging. Chem Soc Rev. 2006;35(6):500–11.
40. Zhang S, Merritt M, Woessner DE, Lenkinski RE, Sherry AD. PARACEST agents: modulating MRI contrast via water proton exchange. Acc Chem Res. 2003;36(10):783–90.
41. Querol M, Bogdanov A Jr. Environment-sensitive and enzyme-sensitive MR contrast agents. Handb Exp Pharmacol. 2008;185(Pt 2):37–57.
42. Perez JM, Josephson L, O'Loughlin T, Högemann D, Weissleder R. Magnetic relaxation switches capable of sensing molecular interactions. Nat Biotechnol. 2002;20(8):816–20.
43. Perez JM, Simeone FJ, Saeki Y, Josephson L, Weissleder R. Viral-induced self-assembly of magnetic nanoparticles allows the detection of viral particles in biological media. J Am Chem Soc. 2003;125(34):10192–3.
44. Grimm J, Perez JM, Josephson L, Weissleder R. Novel nanosensors for rapid analysis of telomerase activity. Cancer Res. 2004;64(2):639–43.
45. Perez JM, Grimm J, Josephson L, Weissleder R. Integrated nanosensors to determine levels and functional activity of human telomerase. Neoplasia. 2008;10(10):1066–72.
46. Yoo B, Pagel MDA. A PARACEST MRI contrast agent to detect enzyme activity. J Am Chem Soc. 2006;128(43):14032–3.
47. Chauvin T, Durand P, Bernier M, et al. Detection of enzymatic activity by PARACEST MRI: a general approach to target a large variety of enzymes. Angew Chem Int Ed Engl. 2008;47(23):4370–2.
48. Kircher MF, Mahmood U, King RS, Weissleder R, Josephson L. A multimodal nanoparticle for preoperative magnetic resonance imaging and intraoperative optical brain tumor delineation. Cancer Res. 2003;63(23):8122–5.
49. Golman K, Olsson LE, Axelsson O, Månsson S, Karlsson M, Petersson JS. Molecular imaging using hyperpolarized 13C. Br J Radiol 2003;76(Spec No 2):S118–S127.
50. Josephson L, Kircher MF, Mahmood U, Tang Y, Weissleder R. Near-infrared fluorescent nanoparticles as combined MR/optical imaging probes. Bioconjug Chem. 2002;13(3):554–60.
51. Viale A, Aime S. Current concepts on hyperpolarized molecules in MRI. Curr Opin Chem Biol. 2010;14(1):90–6.
52. Golman K, Petersson JS, Ardenkjaer-Larsen JH, et al. Dynamic in vivo oxymetry using overhauser enhanced MR imaging. J Magn Reson Imaging. 2000;12(6):929–38.
53. de Vries A, Custers E, Lub J, van den Bosch S, Nicolay K, Grüll H. Block-copolymer-stabilized iodinated emulsions for use as CT contrast agents. Biomaterials. 2010;31(25):6537–44.
54. Hyafil F, Cornily JC, Feig JE, et al. Noninvasive detection of macrophages using a nanoparticulate contrast agent for computed tomography. Nat Med. 2007;13(5):636–41.
55. Kong WH, Lee WJ, Cui ZY, et al. Nanoparticulate carrier containing water-insoluble iodinated oil as a multifunctional contrast agent for computed tomography imaging. Biomaterials. 2007;28(36):5555–61.
56. Elrod DB, Partha R, Danila D, Casscells SW, Conyers JL. An iodinated liposomal computed tomographic contrast agent prepared from a diiodophosphatidylcholine lipid. Nano medicine. 2009;5(1):42–5.
57. Aviv H, Bartling S, Kieslling F, Margel S. Radiopaque iodinated copolymeric nanoparticles for x-ray imaging applications. Biomaterials. 2009;30(29):5610–6.
58. Galperin A, Margel D, Baniel J, Dank G, Biton H, Margel S. Radiopaque iodinated polymeric nanoparticles for x-ray imaging applications. Biomaterials. 2007;28(30):4461–8.
59. Rabin O, Manuel Perez J, Grimm J, Wojtkiewicz G, Weissleder R. An x-ray computed tomography imaging agent based on long-circulating bismuth sulphide nanoparticles. Nat Mater. 2006;5(2):118–22.
60. Jackson PA, Rahman WN, Wong CJ, Ackerly T, Geso M. Potential dependent superiority of gold nanoparticles in comparison to iodinated contrast agents. Eur J Radiol. 2010;75(1):104–9.
61. Aydogan B, Li J, Rajh T, et al. AuNP-DG: deoxyglucose-labeled gold nanoparticles as x-ray computed tomography contrast agents for cancer imaging. Mol Imaging Biol. 2010;12(5):463–7.
62. Popovtzer R, Agrawal A, Kotov NA, et al. Targeted gold nanoparticles enable molecular CT imaging of cancer. Nano Lett. 2008;8(12):4593–6.
63. Cormode DP, Roessl E, Thran A, et al. Atherosclerotic plaque composition: analysis with multicolor CT and targeted gold nanoparticles. Radiology. 2010;256(3):774–82.
64. Frangioni JV, Hajjar RJ. In vivo tracking of stem cells for clinical trials in cardiovascular disease. Circulation. 2004;110(21):3378–83.
65. Massoud TF, Gambhir SS. Molecular imaging in living subjects: seeing fundamental biological processes in a new light. Genes Dev. 2003;17(5):545–80.
66. Deshpande N, Needles A, Willmann JK. Molecular ultrasound imaging: current status and future directions. Clin Radiol. 2010;65(7):567–81.

67. Kiessling F, Huppert J, Palmowski M. Functional and molecular ultrasound imaging: concepts and contrast agents. Curr Med Chem. 2009;16(5):627–42.
68. Deshpande N, Pysz MA, Willmann JK. Molecular ultrasound assessment of tumor angiogenesis. Angiogenesis. 2010;13(2):175–88.
69. Cheng KT. Sonicated human serum microspheres. In: Molecular imaging and contrast agent database. Bethesda, MD: MICAD; 2004.
70. Klibanov AL. Molecular imaging with targeted ultrasound contrast microbubbles. Ernst Schering Res Found Workshop. 2005;49:171–91.
71. de Jong N, Hoff L. Ultrasound scattering properties of Albunex microspheres. Ultrasonics. 1993;31(3):175–81.

7 Functional Molecular Imaging II

Key Points (Abstract)

Molecular imaging is already having major impact on the early diagnosis of diseases and disease monitoring and will also in the next decade. Nuclear imaging modalities are the main molecular imaging modalities. With the continuous development of various molecularly targeted contrast agents for the various imaging techniques such as magnetic resonance (MR), computed tomography (CT), and ultrasonography (US), the entire scenario of the clinical and the molecular imaging is increasing day by day. The various applications of the molecular MR imaging-, CT-, and US-based imaging are being successfully used for the translation of these techniques.

Keywords

Molecular imaging · Inflammation · Vascular-cell adhesion molecule · Intercellular adhesion molecule · Selectins · Leucocytes · USPIO · Microparticles · Endothelial cells · Endothelium · Platelets 1

7.1 Ultrasound Molecular Imaging

Molecular imaging involves the evaluation of the various biologic processes in the living subjects at the various cellular and subcellular levels [1]. Here the principle of molecular imaging is in contrast of the traditional medical imaging, magnetic resonance (MR) imaging, computed tomography (CT), and ultrasonography (US) are the commonly used techniques for the evaluation of the majority of the disease conditions. These will provide the different detailed quantitative information as well as the physiologic response of the tissue composition. Thus, the combination of these imaging modalities to the molecular imaging will be very active and focussed for the extensive ongoing research [1–4]. The principles of the MR-, CT-, and US-based molecular imaging are explained in detail along with the emerging applications for the clinical translation in oncology Diagram 7.1.

7.2 Applications of Molecular and Cellular MR Imaging Oncology Lymph Node Staging

MR-based molecular imaging uses various contrast agents and one of the important one is the intravenously injected iron oxide nanoparticles for lymph node staging [5]. The concept here is to have the differential uptake of the contrast agent by different cells and thus helpful for the evaluation of the various cellular composition in different pathological states. The existing imaging modalities are based on the size criteria for differentiating benign from malignant lymphadenopathy and are not consistent with the metastases

S. Shaikh, *Advances in Imaging*, https://doi.org/10.1007/978-981-16-9535-3_7

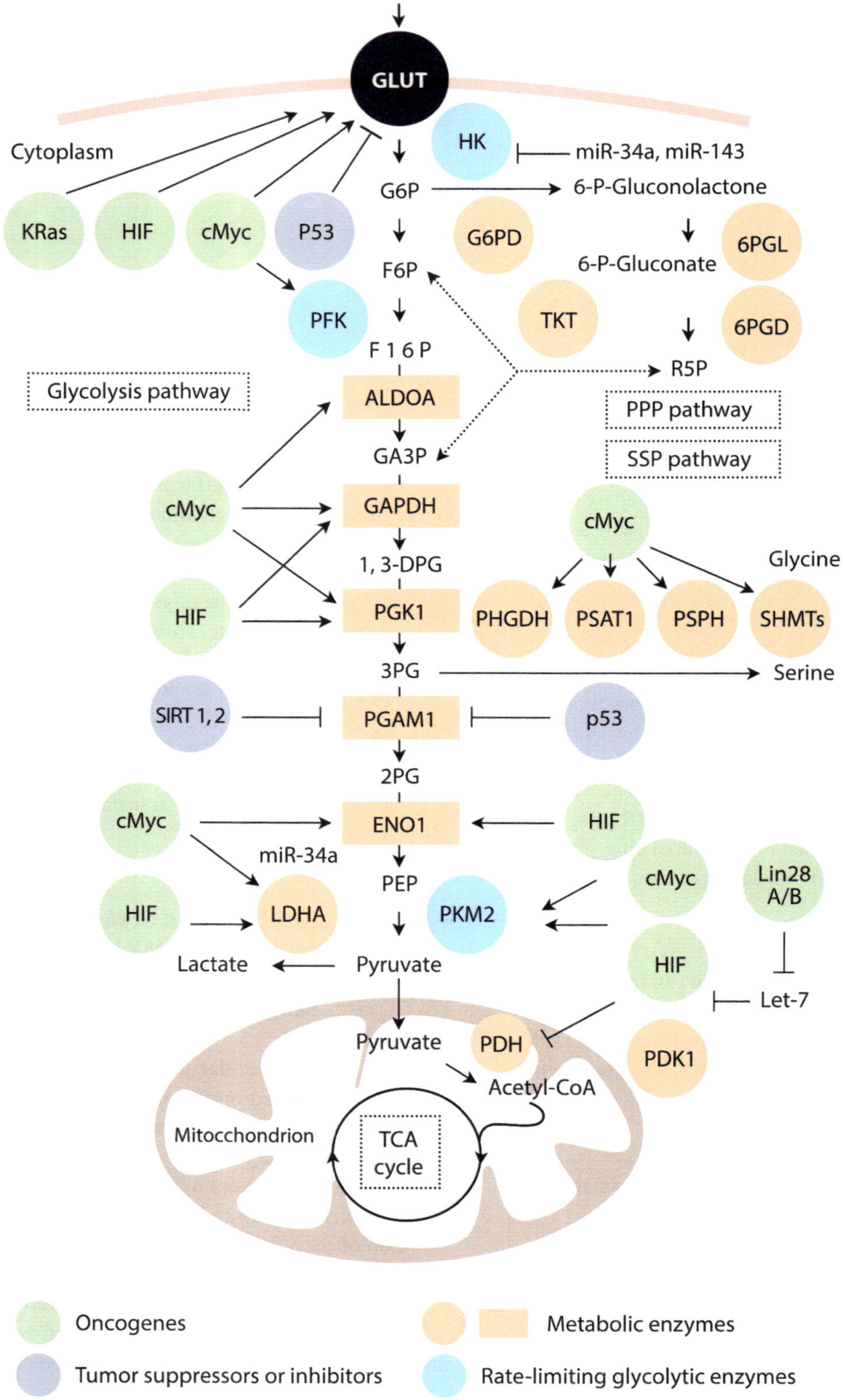

Diagram 7.1 Various interactions happening at the level of the cellular metabolism in various oncogenesis

evaluation. The smaller nodes can also be metastatic, and the nodal criteria are not purely on this for the evaluation of the various lymph nodes. Due to this the lymph node–specific MR contrast agent is developed for the more accurate evaluation of the nodal staging. Lymphotropic nanoparticle-enhanced MR imaging, or LNMRI, is the important tool for the exact characterization of lymph node metastases [6]. LNMRI is using the ultrasmall superparamagnetic iron oxide (USPIO) particles ranging from the 30 to 50 nm in size and composed of a crystalline iron oxide core which will be measuring between 4.3 and 6.0 nm which is made up of the low-molecular weight dextran [7]. Their advantage is the small size and prolonged blood half-life leading to easy passage through the capillary wall, into the lymphatic vessels, and to reticuloendothelial system of lymph nodes [8, 9]. Non-malignant lymph nodes will show the significant increased nanoparticle uptake in the presence of the phagocytotic reticuloendothelial cells, where there is the significant shortening of T2 causing the dark signal intensity on T2- and T2-weighted images. If the node is infiltrated by the tumour, then the nanoparticle will be more accumulated in the lymph node where the nodal tissue will be having the higher T2 relaxation time with signal retention [10, 11]. The multimodality approach is there for the evaluation of the lymph nodes. Thus, USPIOs will accumulate in lymph nodes, leading to the magneto-optical nanoparticle probes development [12–14]. These probes will be adding the different aspects of the probes which will add the different optical component due to the specific proteolytic enzymes. This optical component will give more information of the status of the lymph node in benign and malignant conditions especially in the intraoperative or endoscopic setting.

Imaging of angiogenesis—The MR imaging for the evaluation of the tumour angiogenesis, for the targeting integrin expression. Here the integrins are the transmembrane proteins which will be expressed on the basis of the endothelial cells and are also seen in the angiogenic response.

7.3 Imaging of Molecular Markers of Tumour Cells

The various development of imaging approaches will be using the nanoparticles which will be having the markers overexpressed on tumour cells on the concept of the angiogenesis, where the nanoparticles will be the first one to leave the vasculature. Prostate-specific membrane antigen (PSMA) is the marker used for the prostate cancer [15] and is targeted in a similar approach [16]. Various nanoparticles targeting with the folate receptor is showing promise on various cells [17–22].

7.4 Cardiovascular Application Atherosclerosis

The plaque evaluation is the important imaging concept for the earlier stage risk quantification for various complications for the plaques is needed. Development of atherosclerotic plaques is an inflammatory process which is attached to the arterial wall and can easily differentiate into macrophages, leading to the plaque progression by the complex interplay along with the other mediators [23–25].

7.5 Macrophages

Macrophages cells are having the highest phagocytotic activity and constitute 10–20% of cells within a plaque. Intravenously injected USPIOs are being phagocytosed by these macrophages, which forms the basis of the plaque formation. The different target-specific parameters use the paramagnetic and fluorescent micelles which will specifically target the scavenger receptor as an over expression of the various macrophages [26], or the Gd^{3+}–labelled peptides which will also bind to matrix metalloproteinases being expressed by the various activated macrophages [27].

7.6 Cell Adhesion Molecules

Cell adhesion molecules will be allowing the leukocytes for getting attached to the various inflamed vascular endothelial cells by the process of atherogenesis at an early stage and further promising molecular markers for the early diagnosis and treatment monitoring of atherosclerosis. The use of the dual-modality MR imaging/fluorescent will be allowing the imaging of VCAM-1 expression along with the ex vivo fluorescence imaging [28]. Radioactive tracer will also be seen along with the various trimodal nanoparticle for the MR imaging/positron emission tomography (PET)/near-infrared fluorescence imaging. The cross-linked iron oxide copper 64 along with the near-infrared fluorochrome VT 680 particle [29], will show the increased sensitivity and signal quantification.

7.7 Lipoproteins

MR imaging of atherosclerosis is by the various lipoproteins which has shown the impact of the imaging. Their biocompatibility and biodegradability will lead to them by recognition of reticuloendothelial system. The various aspects of the high-density lipoproteins (HDLs) will easily pass due to their smaller size through the vascular endothelium and will penetrate the underlying tissues [30].

7.8 Angiogenesis

Neovascularizing micro vessels are important in the formation of the atherosclerotic plaque and like in the various cancers these antiangiogenic therapies will be the best options. The one of best markers for plaque neo vasculature is the anb3 integrin, seen in the vascular endothelium at atherosclerotic regions. The activatable MR imaging probes in inflammation will be of important challenge. In the process of the atherosclerosis, there is also the inflammatory process, going on due to the myeloperoxidase enzyme secretion by activated macrophages and is also involved in plaque destabilization and clinical outcome.

Metabolic imaging of various metabolites in their specific pathways can be done by the various hyperpolarization techniques and in the research efforts [31–34]. The various aspects of the therapeutic options are due reduced conversion of pyruvate to lactate demonstrated by the lymphoma-bearing mice 24 h after chemotherapy [35]. Metabolic imaging is also having the clinical translation imaging of tissue pH by this novel hyperpolarization techniques. The diagnosis of the tissue pH is the most important factor for the evaluation of the various conditions with the associated pH changes. In the various tumours, the extracellular pH is very much lower than the normal tissue which will be serving as the biomarker for the various disease diagnosis and therapeutic monitoring.

7.9 Cell Tracking

The concept of the various tracking migration of the cells are an important application for the biological monitoring of the cell efficacy and also for the evaluation of the cell-based therapies [36]. The principle of MR imaging–based cell tracking can be used for the evaluation of the translation to label a cell population with the suitable MR contrast agents which will be, followed by reinjection locally or systemically [36, 37]. The sequential liver MR imaging is being performed up to 24 weeks after transplantation. The various aspects of the feasibility of the iron oxide–labelled cells can be done after the systemic injection. Pancreatic islet evaluation is more safe and more successful in all recipients. The significant islet destruction or impaired engraftment can be done by the various positively or negatively charged SPIOs which are being seen by the various non-phagocytic cells. As they will be requiring the long incubation times which will result in the intracellular iron oxide uptake for in vivo detection [38, 39]. Various coating of the iron oxide nanoparticles with antibodies [40, 41], peptides [42, 43], or other moieties can be evaluated [44] which will induce the various nanoparticle internalization have been explored.

7.10 Applications of Molecular US Imaging

7.10.1 Imaging of Inflammation

Inflammation is the important component of the various pathophysiologic bases of the various disease states, and for this the evaluation of the inflammatory processes in vivo at the cellular level is very important for both early diagnosis and monitoring the response to the treatment.

This imaging and quantification of inflammation can be done by the various contrast microbubbles used as the target molecular markers for the capturing and adhesion of leukocytes to vascular endothelial wall of capillaries. The use of the molecular ultrasound imaging techniques has also shown the significant results in the imaging and quantification of various inflammatory markers at the various molecular levels like in the inflammatory bowel disease [45, 46]. The in vivo US imaging signal will be able to do the ex vivo expression levels of P-selectin and the grade of inflammation. Thus, the molecular US is the very promising non-invasive imaging technique for the evaluation and monitoring the various inflammations.

7.10.2 Imaging of Thrombus Formation

The evaluation of the intravascular thrombus is very important for the management decision of the patients with stroke in high risk for the cerebral and the other embolic diseases. The imaging of tumour angiogenesis in the tumour evaluation should be done together for the formation of the newer blood vessels in the area of interest [47]. This is associated with the overexpression of the molecular markers on the tumour vascular endothelial cells. These dual-targeted microbubbles will improve the detection of tumour angiogenesis, and this is very important for the evaluation based on the different times along the tumour development [48]. The targeting of the molecular angiogenic markers is also done for the monitoring the efficacy of drug therapy. The imaging signals from the targeted microbubbles will be decreased in tumours which are undergoing therapy for the correlation shown by the various target expression levels and the micro vessel density. The newer advancements in the MR imaging-, CT-, and US-are used for the molecular imaging and are now showing the promising results and as well as for the interrogation of the various molecular and cellular events. The biggest challenges are the limitations in sensitivity, specificity, and clinical translatability. With this the MR and CT imaging will be having the higher sensitivity to compete with the PET. The sensitivity of MR imaging is based on the 1023–1025 mol/L for most clinical agents, and CT is less sensitive than the PET [49]. The increased sensitivity for MR imaging will include higher field strengths of the 3 T and 7 T, chemical exchange saturation transfer imaging, hyperpolarization, and various probes which will be exploiting principles of compartmentalization and/or hybridization. This information will be reflecting in the presence of macrophages which are involved in various inflammatory processes and can be seen in the arterial wall, which is diagnostic of the atherosclerosis. The identification and the validation of various disease-specific molecular targets along with the design of molecular contrast agents that will be accumulating in the targets [4]. Multi- and interdisciplinary team will be consisting of experts comprising of the radiologists, material scientists, chemists, biologists, pharmacologists, electrical engineers, mathematicians, and clinicians, who will be working for the MR imaging–, CT-, and US-based molecular imaging modalities making it to the reality.

7.10.3 Cellularity and Diffusion Imaging

Multiplication and significantly increased and unregulated rates of cell proliferation are the important characteristic features of the aggressive tumours. A direct molecular approach for assessing proliferation is the use of (18)F fluorothymidine PET, capable of the measuring the enzyme thymidine kinase 1 activity as cells undergo divisions. Another aspect of the imaging is the "indirect" MR approach imaging by diffusion imaging, measuring the results of the proliferation. Magnetic resonance imaging is more sensitive to the rate of diffusion of water molecules (diffusion-weighted imaging (DWI)) providing the novel information on tissue cellularity now being used for the tumours studies and their response to therapy. Conventional MRI detects signals by the principle of the random Brownian motion [50]. Apparent diffusion coefficient values can be evaluated by keep in the different parameters. DWI is done adding the extra magnetic field gradients to increase the MR signal based on the ADC and the gradient strength. Diffusion-weighted imaging is used for the evaluation of the amount of the cellularity [51, 52]. Density of the cells in a tumour, part of the tumour will be defining the amount of the malignant potential. ADC values quantified after the treatment will be able to define the amount of the cell death mechanisms like apoptosis [53], lytic necrosis, autophagy, and/or mitotic catastrophe [54]. The various metabolisms of the various tumours are increased due to the increased vascular and nutrient supply, causing the hypoxia, central necrosis, and also the important changes in the ADC values. Here, the vascularity and dynamic contrast-enhanced MRI in the tumour volume, can determine the proliferation of the neovascularization of vessels in the tumour. VEGFs, are commonly used for the process of the angiogenesis [55]. Various changes in the parameters by DCE-MRI are useful to access the response to the treatment by the tumours. Again, based on the various measurements and various mathematical models in which the paramagnetic tracer perfusion through the vessels can be evaluated. The healthy vessels in normal tissues may vary with the amount of the blood flow, vessel permeability, and tissue volume fractions of the intravascular or extravascular space. Dynamic contrast-enhanced MRI involves the serial acquisition of MR images of a tissue of interest (e.g., a tumour) before, during, and after an intravenous injection of dynamic contrast-enhanced MRI is being used in the various clinical settings for the assessment of the various tumour responses to treatment. The DSC-MRI is important to evaluate the various data related to the blood volume, blood flow, and mean transit time. The simultaneous assessment of morphological and functional features of the tumour circulation by the DSC-MRI for the characterization of the tumour microenvironment by the non-invasive methods can be done more precisely.

The direct molecular imaging by MRI will be used for the evaluation of various molecular processes in tissues; molecular imaging probes by MRI are possible by two different techniques. The direct evaluation of the imaging probe is the most promising aspect of the imaging. The peculiar property of fluorine is the largest gyromagnetic ratio after hydrogen and thus, will be giving higher strengths which will be producing stronger signals. The second approach is the use of the paramagnetic or superparamagnetic agents capable of the changing proton relaxation times T1, T2 or T2 on the basis of the magnitude of the water signal for the radiofrequency irradiation of the protons that in turn transfer the label to the water via magnetization exchange forming the combination of the chemical exchange saturation transfer (CEST) and paramagnetic chemical exchange saturation transfer (PARACEST) agents [56]. Relaxation of the paramagnetic substances will be affecting the other voxels which are free to move. Another alternative to T1-reducing paramagnetic agents is the susceptibility agents, like the superparamagnetic iron oxide particles [57]. Applying the radiofrequency pulses will be changing the magnetization transfer. This will be communicated to the water protons by magnetization transfer. This forms the basis of the CEST and PARACEST agents [58, 59]. The chemical exchange saturation transfer contrast is equally sensitive for this mechanism [60].

Manganese and gadolinium ions are both effective paramagnetic CAs, but their relaxivities may increase markedly when they are bound to large molecules so that they tumble more slowly, and they may decrease when they are contained in a cage that restricts water access [61]. Similarly, CEST and PARACEST agents can be developed in which the number and rate of exchange of labile protons are altered by an environmental factor such as pH or the presence of specific ligands [62]. This has given rise to the development of "smart agents" in which the characteristics of the probe, e.g., relaxivity, vary with the environment and may report on cellular and molecular processes without the need for specific targeting. For example, the agent may distribute in non-specific manner, but the relaxivity may change only where specific enzymes are abundant that appropriately modify the structure. Similar smart agents have been developed that sense pH or specific solutes such as glucose [63, 64].

7.10.4 Magnetic Resonance Spectral Imaging

The various property of the nuclear imaging is to detect the radioactive decays but not sensitive to the various chemical changes. The various aspects of the high-resolution NMR spectra in which distinct chemical species are separately identifiable by their resonance frequencies provide true chemical specificity. Spectral or chemical shift imaging arguably fits the definition of molecular imaging better than any other modality because the measured quantities actually change with molecular chemistry. Chemical shift imaging has long been used at low spectral resolution for providing fat and water images separately [65, 66], and the SNRs of these images are high because water and lipids occur in high abundance in tissues of interest. Phosphorus-31 metabolites such as adenosine triphosphate (ATP) and phosphocreatine (PCr) will be mapped for their lower sensitivity and spatial resolution [67] will be developed to infer molecular changes associated with tumour composition and muscle and liver metabolism.

Hyperpolarized MRI Nuclear magnetic resonance is insensitive type of due to the small fraction of the nuclei signals. The use of the hyperpolarization will reduce the minimum concentration by using direct imaging of helium in the airways [68]. The hyperpolarized imaging in cancer is based on the direct and indirect assays of pyruvate metabolism. One of the important correlations is based on the abnormal metabolism, where tumours are often more acidic than normal tissue.

The use of the various imaging biomarkers like ADC and DCE-derived parameters, will give an important aspect related to the biophysical, physiological, and metabolic properties of various tissues and important component of the various cellular and molecular imaging methods. PET and single photon emission computed tomography imaging are the important aspects of the higher concentrations of CA for the tissues of interest [69]. Magnetic resonance spectroscopy provides the chemical specific information and for the changes in molecular structures.

7.10.5 Nuclear Medicine

Nuclear Medicine is now being established for the various indications. The invention of newer technologies will be leading to the significant increase in diagnostic and therapeutic applications. 99mTc radioisotope is most commonly used in the diagnosis. 18F-FDG is the most important PET radiopharmaceutical used due to the wide range of the clinical applications, and still more is being used for the clinical applications due to significant changes in the hardware and software.

The concept of dual probe is more of the useful for the guidance of high precision and less invasive robotic surgery. Sentinel lymph node detection and improved lymphadenectomy are the important dual probe applications in clinical practice [70, 71]. The pharmaceutical with the γ or positron emitting radionuclide for the SPECT or PET, or a β minus or α radionuclide emitter for therapeutic purposes can be used. Here based on the concept of theranostics and with the availability of the newer radiopharmaceuticals the concept of the personalized medicine can be seen in the neuroendocrine tumour and prostate cancer.

Advances in Nuclear Medicine and Molecular Imaging based on the

1. Advances in PET radiopharmaceuticals.
2. Developments in equipment.
3. Radiopharmaceutical applications in therapy and theranostics.

7.10.5.1 Advances in PET Radiopharmaceuticals

PET radiopharmaceuticals are used to functionally evaluate the various pathologies. Gallium-68 labelled radiopharmaceuticals are being used increasingly used for the theranostics. Thus, these PET radiopharmaceuticals are being impacted more in the oncology. 18F-FDG (Fluorodeoxyglucose) is a glucose analog, which is being phosphorylated by a hexokinase. 18F-FDG is being trapped within the cells as 18F-FDG-6-phosphate. The use of the FDG is to differentiate between the tumour recurrence vs post-treatment fibrosis, like in the colorectal and head and neck cancers after the post chemoradiotherapy [72, 73]. PSMA (prostate-specific membrane antigen) is also the transmembrane protein which is being expressed in the various prostatic tissues. The prostate cancer staging and monitoring, along with the PSMA ligands for PET is being used in 2012 [74]. PSMA expression is significantly increased in both benign and malignant lesions [75]. The PSMA is being seen in the evaluation of the various malignant and benign non-prostatic pathologies due to the increased neovascularisation of endothelial cells in the various tumours [76]. "European Association of Nuclear Medicine (EANM) Guideline/Society of Nuclear Medicine and Molecular Imaging (SNMMI) Procedure Standard on the use of the 18F-Fluciclovine PET/CT for Prostate Cancer Imaging" defines the use of the various clinical indications for the use of the various PSMA ligands PET/CT [77]. The various other solid and haematological malignancies which are the capable of expressing of the somatostatin receptors can be used [78]. FLT is used for the evaluation of the early response to chemo- and radiotherapy, both in solid and haematological neoplasms and also for the progression-free survival and disease-free survival [79, 80]. 68Ga-FAPI (Fibroblast activation protein inhibitor) is a fibroblast activation protein (FAP), which is the more specific enzyme inhibitor targeting the various cancer associated fibroblasts. Theranostic approach is also possible [81, 82]. FAPI imaging is also useful in the non-cancer agents [81]. These 18F-FES (Fluoroestradiol) target oestrogen receptors which will be useful for the early detection of the breast cancer detection and also for the molecular characterization [83, 84]. 8t9Zr-trastuzumab targets the human epidermal growth factor receptor for the breast cancer patients, [85]. Iodine-124 is for the differentiation of the various thyroid cancer and biochemical recurrence [86]. 18F-FDG is important for the evaluation of the various differentiated thyroid cancer recurrence and also for the poorly differentiated thyroid carcinoma [87, 88].

7.11 Neurology and Psychiatry

There is significant development of the evaluation of the various movement disorders along with the various central nervous system diseases. 123I-Ioflupane (DaTscan™ is the important radiotracer for the evaluation of these conditions [89] along with the specific ligand for the pre-synaptic dopamine transporter (DAT). Striatum uptake is directly related with the synaptic dopaminergic degeneration. The evaluation of the classical nigrostriatal degeneration in the idiopathic Parkinson's disease along with the essential tremor, medication-induced Parkinsonism and for the confirmation of the Parkinsonian plus syndromes can be done more precisely. The pre-synaptic PET radioligand is 18F-FDOPA (e.g., 18F-PE2I) [90]. The common indications are the difference between the idiopathic Parkinson's disease and other parkinsonian plus syndromes. In the Parkinsonian plus syndromes, the D2 post-synaptic receptors activity is significantly reduced along with the Parkinson's disease which is the normal or upregulated. 18F-FDG helps in the diagnosis and the differential diagnosis of the various dementias. The pattern of the uptake in the Alzheimer's disease is different from various other forms of the dementia, like the Lewy Body dementia, frontotemporal lobar degeneration, vascular dementia, and pseudodementia [91]. β-Amyloid tracers deposition are the hallmarks of Alzheimer's disease; β-amyloid in the brain first mapping is being done by the 18FFDDNP [92]. The use of the 11C–labelled Pittsburgh compound B (11C-PIB) [93] helped the earlier detection of the brain β-amyloid deposition in vivo. In 2015, the approved fluorides are the three fluoride-18-labelled amyloid PET radiopharmaceuticals for clinical use [94] Diagram 7.2. Amyloid PET tracer accumulation in cerebral white matter is also seen as the important marker of the myelin [95]. Tau-tracers in the PET imaging are the first- and second-generation compounds which are being commonly used for the mild cognitive impairment for the conversion of the Alzheimer disease. With this the tau-tracers will be more specific for the various neurodegenerative markers and other clinical severity of dementia [96, 97]. The various amino-acid tracers are the 11C-MET (methionine), 18F-FET (tyrosine), 18F-FACBC (fluciclovine), and 18F-FDOPA. The important concept is that the amino acids are more widely used for the evaluation of the essential nutrients, involved in metabolism, cell growth, protein synthesis, and gene expression [98]. Perfusion tracers are also being used of the evaluation of the brain perfusion related with the cerebral ischemia, by the cerebral blood flow and cerebral metabolic rate of oxygen consumption evaluation [99] Diagram 7.3.

7.12 Cardiology

18F-FDG is an important radiotracer for the evaluation of the myocardial viability like the myocardial infarction, stunned and hibernating myocardium, endocarditis, infection of cardiac

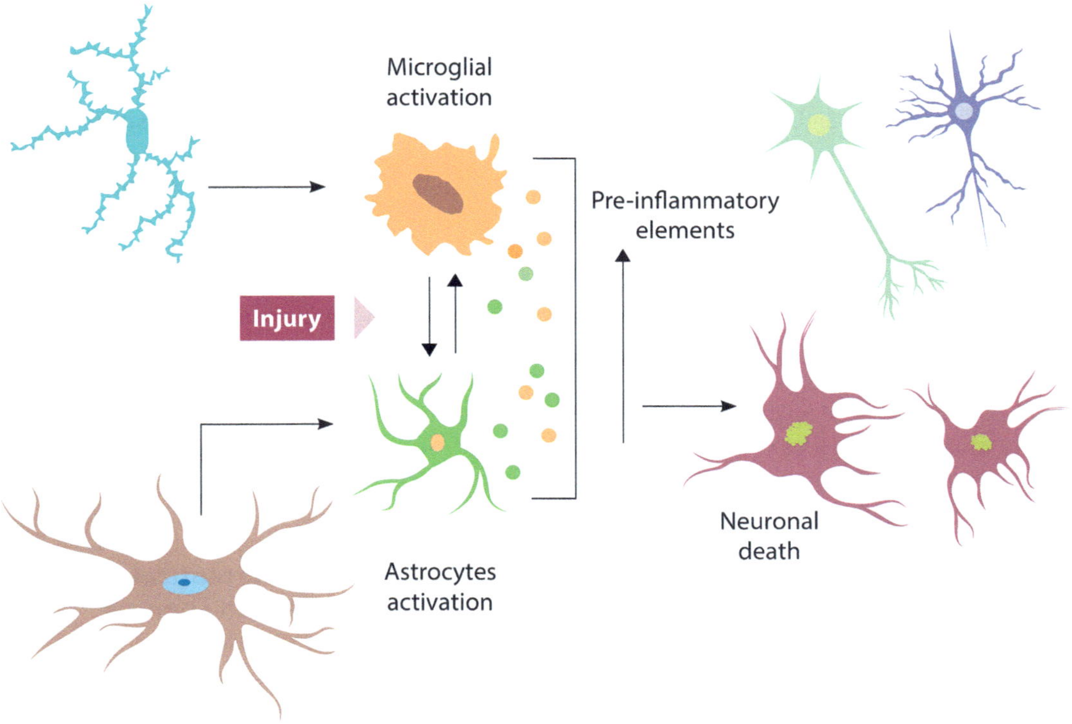

Diagram 7.2 Various interactions and biomarkers which happen in various neurological conditions

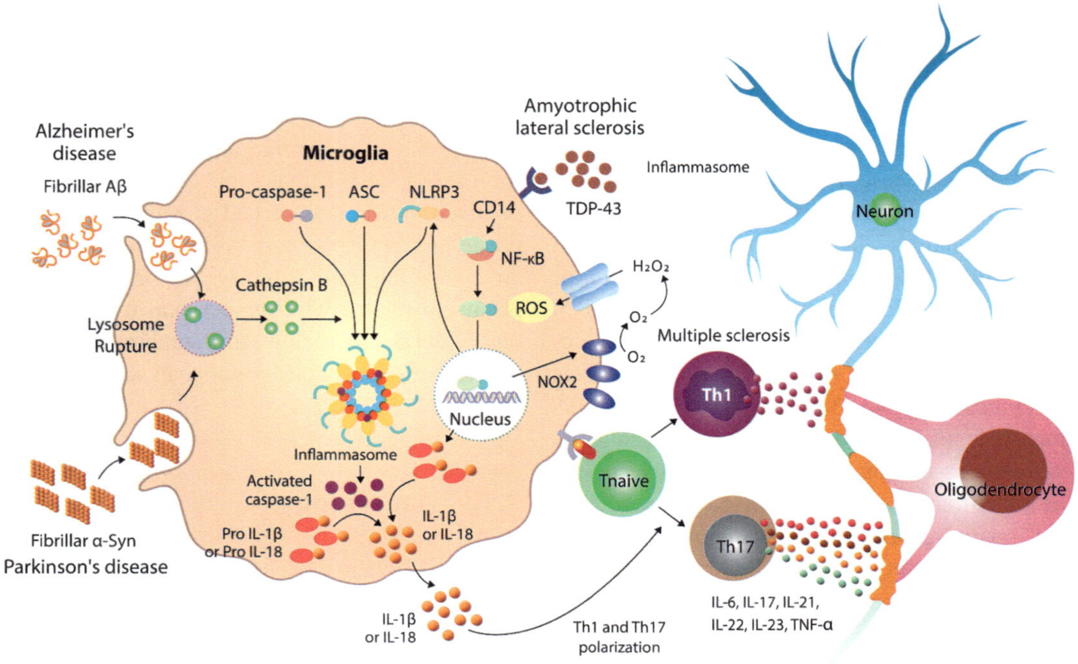

Diagram 7.3 The role of the molecular imaging in the evaluation of the various neuronal cell deaths

devices, metastatic, infectious lesions and endothelial inflammation, and also by the atherosclerosis plaque formation.

7.13 Musculoskeletal System

The use of the 18F-FDG is seen in the arthritis, synovitis, and vasculitis (e.g., polymyalgia rheumatic and large vessel vasculitis) which is mainly due to the various local inflammatory active sites and to monitor response to therapy [100]. 18F-NaF is the newer radiotracer for the evaluation of bone remodelling activity. It is also used for the evaluation of the bone metastases and primary bone malignancies.

7.14 Developments in Equipment

The technical advances in the PET systems are now providing very high spatial resolution. Photomultiplier tubes (analog or digital) are being attached to the single or multiple scintillation crystals. Digital systems use silicon photomultipliers (SiPM) instead of analogs photomultiplier tubes (PMT). Lutetium oxyorthosilicate (LSO) or lutetium yttrium oxyorthosilicate (LYSO) is the most commonly used radiotracer for the scintillator materials [62]. Time of flight (TOF) is used due to the various SiPM for the better performance, LSO, and LYSO [67]. The total body radiopharmaceutical distribution is now possible. Solid-state detectors based on cadmium zinc telluride (CZT) crystals are coupled to PMT.

7.15 Radiopharmaceutical Applications in Therapy and Theranostics

Various dual probes and optical probes are being used more often for the non-invasive molecular imaging and minimally invasive surgery. They are the γ handheld detectors, to locate parathyroid adenomas for sentinel node evaluation by the use of the 99mTc-labelled radio-nano colloids (melanoma, breast, [76] cervical, [77] vulvar, penile, and head and neck cancers [78] and radio guided occult lesion localization procedures using 99mTc-labelled macroaggregates (breast, lung, and thyroid cancers). Higher tissue penetration of γ radiation by this emitter radionuclides and also by the light emitted by the fluorescent probe can be used for the robotic surgery.

Various optical imaging can be done with [82]: (1) fluorescent protein molecules, (2) Cherenkov luminescence imaging, (3) near-infrared light, and (4) quantum dots from Cd/Te or Cd/Se materials. The use of the various substances with the near-infrared and infrared spectrum (700–900 nm) are most useful with very high tissue permeability is there from several millimetres to slightly more than 1 cm [82]. The increasing trends will be giving different aspects of the fluorescence, Cerenkov, optical coherence tomography, and ultrasonography and also along with the various software-based guidance which will lead to the significant changes in various procedures.

7.16 Theranostics

Many newer therapeutic applications of radiopharmaceuticals are available and with the combination of the diagnostic and therapeutic capabilities with radiopharmaceuticals, these are developed. Theranostic applications will be using the same radiolabelled particle with the γ or positron emitter radionuclide for diagnosis and a β minus or α emitter radioisotope for therapy [84, 85]. Radioactive iodine, Iodine-123 (γ emitter)—Iodine-131 (β minus emitter) is being used for many years for the diagnosis of the thyroid disease as well as for therapy. Recently the use of the systemic therapy with peptide receptor radionuclide therapy suggests the important aspect of the metastatic neuroendocrine tumours by using the DOTA-TATE and DOTA-TOC labelled Yttrium-90 or Lutetium-177. The first randomized controlled Phase III study, NETTER-1, [88] revealed disease free for 40 months, and with a response rate of 18%. Due to this the treatment response and also the associated reduced side effects due to the increased research and development in this field and the availability of the new therapeutic agent is being seen now [89–94, 101, 102].

7.17 Conclusion

Many molecular imaging specialties are being impacted by both diagnosis and therapy with the recent innovation of newer radiopharmaceuticals, hardware equipment, regulatory acceptance, and approval. Thus, the PET and SPECT are more evolved as hybrid imaging technologies and along with MRI it is becoming more precise. The multimodality imaging is being more precise and more evolving in the future. The whole-body scanners, use of the dual probes, and also the optical imaging will bring more precise use for the accuracy, radiation exposure, and cost efficiency, thus leading to the personalized imaging. Lastly, the use of the theranostics will be more relevant for the evaluation of the personalized and targeted management. The newer evolving radiolabelled nuclide therapies are a more happening thing in the future management.

References

1. Kircher MF, Hricak H, Larson SM. Molecular imaging for personalized cancer care. Mol Oncol. 2012 Mar 10; 6:182–195. [Epub ahead of print].
2. Gore JC, Yankeelov TE, Peterson TE, Avison MJ. Molecular imaging without radiopharmaceuticals? J Nucl Med. 2009;50(6):999–1007.
3. Pysz MA, Gambhir SS, Willmann JK. Molecular imaging: current status and emerging strategies. Clin Radiol. 2010;65(7):500–16.
4. Willmann JK, van Bruggen N, Dinkelborg LM, Gambhir SS. Molecular imaging in drug development. Nat Rev Drug Discov. 2008;7(7):591–607.
5. Harisinghani MG, Barentsz J, Hahn PF, et al. Noninvasive detection of clinically occult lymph-node metastases in prostate cancer. N Engl J Med. 2003;348(25):2491–9.
6. Saokar A, Braschi M, Harisinghani MG. Lymphotrophic nanoparticle enhanced MR imaging (LNMRI) for lymph node imaging. Abdom Imaging. 2006;31(6):660–7.

7. Wagner S, Schnorr J, Pilgrimm H, Hamm B, Taupitz M. Monomer-coated very small superparamagnetic iron oxide particles as contrast medium for magnetic resonance imaging: preclinical in vivo characterization. Investig Radiol. 2002;37(4):167–77.
8. Weissleder R, Elizondo G, Wittenberg J, Lee AS, Josephson L, Brady TJ. Ultrasmall superparamagnetic iron oxide: an intravenous contrast agent for assessing lymph nodes with MR imaging. Radiology. 1990;175(2):494–8.
9. Weissleder R, Elizondo G, Wittenberg J, Rabito CA, Bengele HH, Josephson L. Ultrasmall superparamagnetic iron oxide: characterization of a new class of contrast agents for MR imaging. Radiology. 1990;175(2):489–93.
10. Clément O, Guimaraes R, de Kerviler E, Frija G. Magnetic resonance lymphography: enhancement patterns using superparamagnetic nanoparticles. Investig Radiol. 1994;29(Suppl 2):S226–8.
11. Guimaraes R, Clément O, Bittoun J, Carnot F, Frija G. MR lymphography with superparamagnetic iron nanoparticles in rats: pathologic basis for contrast enhancement. AJR Am J Roentgenol. 1994;162(1):201–7.
12. Josephson L, Kircher MF, Mahmood U, Tang Y, Weissleder R. Near-infrared fluorescent nanoparticles as combined MR/optical imaging probes. Bioconjug Chem. 2002;13(3):554–60.
13. Kircher MF, Josephson L, Weissleder R. Ratio imaging of enzyme activity using dual wavelength optical reporters. Mol Imaging. 2002;1(2):89–95.
14. Kircher MF, Weissleder R, Josephson L. A dual fluorochrome probe for imaging proteases. Bioconjug Chem. 2004;15(2):242–8.
15. Su SL, Huang IP, Fair WR, Powell CT, Heston WD. Alternatively spliced variants of prostate-specific membrane antigen RNA: ratio of expression as a potential measurement of progression. Cancer Res. 1995;55(7):1441–3.
16. Serda RE, Adolphi NL, Bisoffi M, Sillerud LO. Targeting and cellular trafficking of magnetic nanoparticles for prostate cancer imaging. Mol Imaging. 2007;6(4):277–88.
17. Choi H, Choi SR, Zhou R, Kung HF, Chen IW. Iron oxide nanoparticles as magnetic resonance contrast agent for tumor imaging via folate receptor-targeted delivery. Acad Radiol. 2004;11(9):996–1004.
18. Corot C, Robert P, Lancelot E, et al. Tumor imaging using P866, a high-relaxivity gadolinium chelate designed for folate receptor targeting. Magn Reson Med. 2008;60(6):1337–46.
19. Konda SD, Aref M, Brechbiel M, Wiener EC. Development of a tumor-targeting MR contrast agent using the high-affinity folate receptor: work in progress. Investig Radiol. 2000;35(1):50–7.
20. Meier R, Henning TD, Boddington S, et al. Breast cancers: MR imaging of folatereceptor expression with the folate-specific nanoparticle P1133. Radiology. 2010;255(2):527–35.
21. Swanson SD, Kukowska-Latallo JF, Patri AK, et al. Targeted gadolinium-loaded dendrimer nanoparticles for tumor-specific magnetic resonance contrast enhancement. Int J Nanomedicine. 2008;3(2):201–10.
22. Wang ZJ, Boddington S, Wendland M, Meier R, Corot C, Daldrup-Link H. MR imaging of ovarian tumors using folatereceptor-targeted contrast agents. Pediatr Radiol. 2008;38(5):529–37.
23. Libby P. Inflammation in atherosclerosis. Nature. 2002;420(6917):868–74.
24. Libby P, Ridker PM, Hansson GK. Leducq transatlantic network on Atherothrombosis. Inflammation in atherosclerosis: from pathophysiology to practice. J Am Coll Cardiol. 2009;54(23):2129–38.
25. Libby P, Ridker PM, Maseri A. Inflammation and atherosclerosis. Circulation. 2002;105(9):1135–43.
26. Amirbekian V, Lipinski MJ, Briley-Saebo KC, et al. Detecting and assessing macrophages in vivo to evaluate atherosclerosis noninvasively using molecular MRI. Proc Natl Acad Sci U S A. 2007;104(3):961–6.
27. Amirbekian V, Aguinaldo JG, Amirbekian S, et al. Atherosclerosis and matrix metalloproteinases: experimental molecular MR imaging in vivo. Radiology. 2009;251(2):429–38.
28. Nahrendorf M, Jaffer FA, Kelly KA, et al. Noninvasive vascular cell adhesion molecule-1 imaging identifies inflammatory activation of cells in atherosclerosis. Circulation. 2006;114(14):1504–11.
29. Nahrendorf M, Zhang H, Hembrador S, et al. Nanoparticle PET-CT imaging of macrophages in inflammatory atherosclerosis. Circulation. 2008;117(3):379–87.
30. Skajaa T, Cormode DP, Falk E, Mulder WJ, Fisher EA, Fayad ZA. High-density lipoprotein-based contrast agents for multimodal imaging of atherosclerosis. Arterioscler Thromb Vasc Biol. 2010;30(2):169–76.
31. Cunningham CH, Chen AP, Albers MJ, et al. Double spin-echo sequence for rapid spectroscopic imaging of hyperpolarized 13C. J Magn Reson. 2007;187(2):357–62.
32. Larson PE, Kerr AB, Chen AP, et al. Multiband excitation pulses for hyperpolarized 13C dynamic chemical-shift imaging. J Magn Reson. 2008;194(1):121–7.
33. Levin YS, Mayer D, Yen YF, Hurd RE, Spielman DM. Optimization of fast spiral chemical shift imaging using least squares reconstruction: application for hyperpolarized (13)C metabolic imaging. Magn Reson Med. 2007;58(2):245–52.
34. Reeder SB, Brittain JH, Grist TM, Yen YF. Least-squares chemical shift separation for (13) C metabolic imaging. J Magn Reson Imaging. 2007;26(4):1145–52.
35. Day SE, Kettunen MI, Gallagher FA, et al. Detecting tumor response to treatment using hyperpolarized 13C magnetic resonance imaging and spectroscopy. Nat Med. 2007;13(11):1382–7.

36. Kircher MF, Gambhir SS, Grimm J. Noninvasive cell-tracking methods. Nat Rev Clin Oncol. 2011;8(11):677–88.
37. Grimm J, Kircher MF, Weissleder R. Cell tracking: principles and applications [in German]. Radiologe. 2007;47(1):25–33.
38. Frank JA, Miller BR, Arbab AS, et al. Clinically applicable labeling of mammalian and stem cells by combining superparamagnetic iron oxides and transfection agents. Radiology. 2003;228(2):480–7.
39. Moore A, Weissleder R, Bogdanov A Jr. Uptake of dextran-coated monocrystalline iron oxides in tumor cells and macrophages. J Magn Reson Imaging. 1997;7(6):1140–5.
40. Ahrens ET, Feili-Hariri M, Xu H, Genove G, Morel PA. Receptor-mediated endocytosis of iron-oxide particles provides efficient labeling of dendritic cells for in vivo MR imaging. Magn Reson Med. 2003;49(6):1006–13.
41. Bulte JW, Zhang S, van Gelderen P, et al. Neurotransplantation of magnetically labeled oligodendrocyte progenitors: magnetic resonance tracking of cell migration and myelination. Proc Natl Acad Sci U S A. 1999;96(26):15256–61.
42. Kircher MF, Allport JR, Graves EE, et al. In vivo high resolution three-dimensional imaging of antigen-specific cytotoxic Tlymphocyte trafficking to tumors. Cancer Res. 2003;63(20):6838–46.
43. Kircher MF, Allport JR, Zhao M, Josephson L, Lichtman AH, Weissleder R. Intracellular magnetic labeling with CLIO-tat for efficient in vivo tracking of cytotoxic T cells by MR imaging [abstr]. Radiology. 2002;225(P):453.
44. Bulte JW, Douglas T, Witwer B, et al. Magnetodendrimers allow endosomal magnetic labeling and in vivo tracking of stem cells. Nat Biotechnol. 2001;19(12):1141–7.
45. Deshpande N, Needles A, Willmann JK. Molecular ultrasound imaging: current status and future directions. Clin Radiol. 2010;65(7):567–81.
46. Pysz MA, Willmann JK. Targeted contrastenhanced ultrasound: an emerging technology in abdominal and pelvic imaging. Gastroenterology. 2011;140(3):785–90.
47. Pysz MA, Guracar I, Foygel K, Tian L, Willmann JK. Quantitative assessment of tumor angiogenesis using real-time motion-compensated contrast-enhanced ultrasound imaging. Angiogenesis. 2012 Apr 26;15(3):433–442. [Epub ahead of print].
48. Willmann JK, Lutz AM, Paulmurugan R, et al. Dual-targeted contrast agent for US assessment of tumor angiogenesis in vivo. Radiology. 2008;248(3):936–44.
49. Frangioni JV, Hajjar RJ. In vivo tracking of stem cells for clinical trials in cardiovascular disease. Circulation. 2004;110(21):3378–83.
50. Zhong JH, Gore JC. Studies of restricted diffusion in heterogeneous media containing variations in susceptibility. Magn Reson Med. 1991;19:276–84.
51. Sugahara T, Korogi Y, Kochi M, Ikushima I, Shigematu Y, Hirai T, et al. Usefulness of diffusion-weighted MRI with echo-planar technique in the evaluation of cellularity in gliomas. J Magn Reson Imaging. 1999;9:53–60.
52. Lyng H, Haraldseth O, Rofstad EK. Measurement of cell density and necrotic fraction in human melanoma xenografts by diffusion weighted magnetic resonance imaging. Magn Reson Med. 2000;43:828–36.
53. Kim H, Morgan DE, Zeng H, Grizzle WE, Warram JM, Stockard CR, et al. Breast tumor xenografts: diffusion-weighted MR imaging to assess early therapy with novel apoptosis-inducing anti-DR5 antibody. Radiology. 2008;248(3):844–51.
54. Morse DL, Galons JP, Payne CM, Jennings DL, Day S, Xia G, et al. MRI-measured water mobility increases in response to chemotherapy via multiple cell-death mechanisms. NMR Biomed. 2007;20(6):602–14.
55. Folkman J. Angiogenesis in cancer, vascular, rheumatoid and other disease. Nat Med. 1995;1:27–31.
56. Sherry AD, Woods M. Chemical exchange saturation transfer contrast agents for magnetic resonance imaging. Annu Rev Biomed Eng. 2008;10:391–411.
57. Majumdar S, Zoghbi SS, Pope CF, Gore JCA. Quantitative study of relaxation rate enhancement produced by iron-oxide particles in polyacrylamide gels and tissue. Magn Reson Med. 1989;9:185–202.
58. Zhang S, Merritt M, Woessner DE, Lenkinski RE, Sherry AD. PARACEST agents: modulating MRI contrast via water proton exchange. Acc Chem Res. 2003;36:783–90.
59. Woods M, Woessner DE, Sherry AD. Paramagnetic lanthanide complexes as PARACEST agents for medical imaging. Chem Soc Rev. 2006;5(6):500–11.
60. van Zijl PC, Jones CK, Ren J, Malloy CR, Sherry AD. MRI detection of glycogen in vivo by using chemical exchange saturation transfer imaging (glycoCEST). Proc Natl Acad Sci U S A. 2007;104(11):4359–64.
61. Gore JC, Joers JM, Kennan RP. Contrast agents and relaxation effects. In: Scott A, editor. Magnetic resonance imaging of the brain and spine. 3rd ed. Lippincott: Williams and Wilkins; 2002. p. 79–99. Chapter 4.
62. Ren J, Trokowski R, Zhang S, Malloy CR, Sherry AD. Imaging the tissue distribution of glucose in livers using a PARACEST sensor. Magn Reson Med. 2008;60(5):1047–55.
63. Wu Y, Soesbe TC, Kiefer GE, Zhao P, Sherry AD. A responsive europium(III) chelate that provides a direct readout of pH by MRI. J Am Chem Soc. 2010;132(40):14002–3.
64. Ren J, Trokowski R, Zhang S, Malloy CR, Sherry AD. Imaging the tissue distribution of glucose in livers using a PARACEST sensor. Magn Reson Med. 2008;60(5):1047–55.

65. Dixon WT. Simple proton spectroscopic imaging. Radiology. 1984;153(1):189–94.
66. Gore JC, et al. Magnetic resonance in the era of molecular imaging of cancer. Magn Reson Imaging. 2011;29(5):587–600.
67. Vigneron DB, Nelson SJ, Murphy-Boesch J, Kelley DA, Kessler HB, Brown TR, et al. Chemical shift imaging of human brain: axial, sagittal, and coronal P-31 metabolite images. Radiology. 1990;177(3):643–9.
68. Middleton H, Black RD, Saam B, Cates GD, Cofer GP, Guenther R, et al. MR imaging with hyperpolarized 3He gas. Magn Reson Med. 1995;33(2):271–5.
69. Gore JC, Yankeelov TE, Peterson TE, Avison MJ. Molecular imaging without radiopharmaceuticals? J Nucl Med. 2009;50(6):999–1007.
70. Van Oosterom MN, Rietbergen DDD, Welling MM, Van Der Poel HG, Maurer T, Van Leeuwen FWB. Recent advances in nuclear and hybrid detection modalities for image-guided surgery. Expert Rev Med Devices. 2019;16:711–34. https://doi.org/10.1080/17434440.2019.1642104.
71. van Leeuwen FWB, de Jong M, Committee E. EANM Translational Molecular Imaging Committee. Molecular imaging: the emerging role of optical imaging in nuclear medicine. Eur J Nucl Med Mol Imaging. 2014;41:2150–3. https://doi.org/10.1007/s00259-014-2845-0.
72. Mehanna H, Wong WL, McConkey CC, Rahman JK, Robinson M, Hartley AG, et al. PET-CT surveillance versus neck dissection in advanced head and neck cancer. N Engl J Med. 2016;374(15):1444–54.
73. Jadvar H, Colletti PM, Delgado-Bolton R, Esposito G, Krause BJ, Iagaru AH, et al. Appropriate use criteria for (18)F-FDG PET/CT in restaging and treatment response assessment of malignant disease. J Nucl Med. 2017;58(12):2026–37.
74. Eder M, Schäfer M, Bauder-Wüst U, Hull W-E, Wängler C, Mier W, et al. 68Gacomplex lipophilicity and the targeting property of a urea-based PSMA inhibitor for PET imaging. Bioconjug Chem. 2012;23:688–97. https://doi.org/10.1021/bc200279b.
75. Backhaus P, Noto B, Avramovic N, Grubert LS, Huss S, Bögemann M, et al. Targeting PSMA by radioligands in nonprostate disease-current status and future perspectives. Eur J Nucl Med Mol Imaging. 2018;45:860–77. https://doi.org/10.1007/s00259-017-3922-y.
76. Salas Fragomeni RA, Amir T, Sheikhbahaei S, Harvey SC, Javadi MS, Solnes LB, et al. Imaging of nonprostate cancers using PSMA-targeted radiotracers: rationale, current state of the field, and a call to arms. J Nucl Med. 2018;59:871–7. https://doi.org/10.2967/jnumed.117.203570.
77. Virgolini I, Ambrosini V, Bomanji JB, Baum RP, Fanti S, Gabriel M, et al. Procedure guidelines for PET/CT tumour imaging with 68Ga-DOTA-conjugated peptides: 68GaDOTA-TOC, 68Ga-DOTA-NOC, 68GaDOTA-TATE. Eur J Nucl Med Mol Imaging. 2010;37:2004–10. https://doi.org/10.1007/s00259-010-1512-3.
78. Pauwels E, Cleeren F, Bormans G, Deroose CM. Somatostatin receptor PET ligands - the next generation for clinical practice. Am J Nucl Med Mol Imaging. 2018;8:311–31.
79. Bollineni VR, Kramer GM, Jansma EP, Liu Y, Oyen WJG. A systematic review on [(18) F]FLT-PET uptake as a measure of treatment response in cancer patients. Eur J Cancer. 2016;55:81–97. https://doi.org/10.1016/j.ejca.2015.11.018.
80. Been LB, Suurmeijer AJH, Cobben DCP, Jager PL, Hoekstra HJ, Elsinga PH. [18F] FLT-PET in oncology: current status and opportunities. Eur J Nucl Med Mol Imaging. 2004;31:1659–72. https://doi.org/10.1007/s00259-004-1687-6.
81. Loktev A, Lindner T, Mier W, Debus J, Altmann A, Jäger D, et al. A tumor-imaging method targeting cancer-associated fibroblasts. J Nucl Med. 2018;59:1423–9. https://doi.org/10.2967/jnumed.118.210435.
82. Kratochwil C, Flechsig P, Lindner T, Abderrahim L, Altmann A, Mier W, et al. 68Ga-FAPI PET/CT: tracer uptake in 28 different kinds of cancer. J Nucl Med. 2019;60:801–5. https://doi.org/10.2967/jnumed.119.227967.
83. Chae SY, Ahn SH, Kim S-B, Han S, Lee SH, Oh SJ, et al. Diagnostic accuracy and safety of 16α-[18 F] fluoro-17β-oestradiol PET-CT for the assessment of oestrogen receptor status in recurrent or metastatic lesions in patients with breast cancer: a prospective cohort study. Lancet Oncol. 2019;20:546–55. https://doi.org/10.1016/S1470-2045(18)30936-7.
84. van Kruchten M, de Vries EGE, Brown M, de Vries EFJ, Glaudemans AWJM, Dierckx RAJO, et al. Pet imaging of oestrogen receptors in patients with breast cancer. Lancet Oncol. 2013;14:e465–75. https://doi.org/10.1016/S1470-2045(13)70292-4.
85. Bensch F, Brouwers AH, Lub-de Hooge MN, de Jong JR, van der Vegt B, Sleijfer S, et al. 89Zr-trastuzumab PET supports clinical decision making in breast cancer patients, when HER2 status cannot be determined by standard work up. Eur J Nucl Med Mol Imaging. 2018;45:2300–6. https://doi.org/10.1007/s00259-018-4099-8.
86. Santhanam P, Taieb D, Solnes L, Marashdeh W, Ladenson PW. Utility of I-124 PET/CT in identifying radioiodine avid lesions in differentiated thyroid cancer: a systematic review and meta-analysis. Clin Endocrinol. 2017;86:645–51. https://doi.org/10.1111/cen.13306.
87. Marcus C, Whitworth PW, Surasi DS, Pai SI, Subramaniam RM. Pet/Ct in the management of thyroid cancers. AJR Am J Roentgenol. 2014;202:1316–29. https://doi.org/10.2214/AJR.13.11673.
88. Liu M, Cheng L, Jin Y, Ruan M, Sheng S, Chen L. Predicting 131I-avidity of metastases from differentiated thyroid cancer using 18FFDG PET/CT in postoperative patients with elevated thyroglobu-

lin. Sci Rep. 2018;8:4352. https://doi.org/10.1038/s41598-018-22656-4.

89. Van Laere K, Varrone A, Booij J, Vander Borght T, Nobili F, Kapucu OL, et al. EANM procedure guidelines for brain neurotransmission SPECT/PET using dopamine D2 receptor ligands, version 2. Eur J Nucl Med Mol Imaging. 2010;37:434–42. https://doi.org/10.1007/s00259-009-1265-z.
90. Delva A, Van Weehaeghe D, van Aalst J, Ceccarini J, Koole M, Baete K, et al. Quantification and discriminative power of 18F-FE-PE2I PET in patients with Parkinson's disease. Eur J Nucl Med Mol Imaging 2020; 47(8):1913-1926. https://doi.org/10.1007/s00259-019-04587-y. Epub 27 Nov 2019.
91. Nestor PJ, Altomare D, Festari C, Drzezga A, Rivolta J, Walker Z, et al. Clinical utility of FDG-PET for the differential diagnosis among the main forms of dementia. Eur J Nucl Med Mol Imaging. 2018;45:1509–25. https://doi.org/10.1007/s00259-018-4035-y.
92. Small GW, Kepe V, Ercoli LM, Siddarth P, Bookheimer SY, Miller KJ, et al. Pet of brain amyloid and tau in mild cognitive impairment. N Engl J Med. 2006;355:2652–63. https://doi.org/10.1056/NEJMoa054625.
93. Klunk WE, Engler H, Nordberg A, Wang Y, Blomqvist G, Holt DP, et al. Imaging brain amyloid in Alzheimer's disease with Pittsburgh compound-B. Ann Neurol. 2004;55:306–19. https://doi.org/10.1002/ana.20009.
94. de Wilde A, van der Flier WM, Pelkmans W, Bouwman F, Verwer J, Groot C, et al. Association of amyloid positron emission tomography with changes in diagnosis and patient treatment in an unselected memory clinic cohort: the ABIDE project. JAMA Neurol. 2018;75:1062–70. https://doi.org/10.1001/jamaneurol.2018.1346.
95. Catafau AM, Bullich S. Amyloid PET imaging: applications beyond Alzheimer's disease. Clin Transl Imaging. 2015;3:39–55. https://doi.org/10.1007/s40336-014-0098-3.
96. Okamura N, Harada R, Ishiki A, Kikuchi A, Nakamura T, Kudo Y. The development and validation of tau PET tracers: current status and future directions. Clin Transl Imaging. 2018;6:305–16. https://doi.org/10.1007/s40336-018-0290-y.
97. Ossenkoppele R, Rabinovici GD, Smith R, Cho H, Schöll M, Strandberg O, et al. Discriminative accuracy of [18F] flortaucipir positron emission tomography for Alzheimer disease vs other neurodegenerative disorders. JAMA. 2018;320:1151–62. https://doi.org/10.1001/jama.2018.12917.
98. Sun A, Liu X, Tang G. Carbon-11 and fluorine-18 labeled amino acid tracers for positron emission tomography imaging of tumors. Front Chem. 2017;5:124. https://doi.org/10.3389/fchem.2017.00124.
99. Evans NR, Tarkin JM, Buscombe JR, Markus HS, Rudd JHF, Warburton EA. Pet imaging of the neurovascular interface in cerebrovascular disease. Nat Rev Neurol. 2017;13:676–88. https://doi.org/10.1038/nrneurol.2017.129.
100. Slart R, Writing G, Reviewer G, Members of EC, Members of EI, Inflammation, et al. FDG-PET/CT(A) imaging in large vessel vasculitis and polymyalgia rheumatica: joint procedural recommendation of the EANM, SNMMI, and the PET interest group (PIG), and endorsed by the ASNC. Eur J Nucl Med Mol Imaging. 2018;45(7):1250–69.
101. Yordanova A, Eppard E, Kürpig S, Bundschuh RA, Schönberger S, Gonzalez-Carmona M, et al. Theranostics in nuclear medicine practice. Onco Targets Ther. 2017;10:4821–8. https://doi.org/10.2147/OTT.S140671.
102. Langbein T, Weber WA, Eiber M. Future of theranostics: an outlook on precision oncology in nuclear medicine. J Nucl Med. 2019;60(Suppl 2):13S–9S. https://doi.org/10.2967/jnumed.118.220566.

8 Molecular Imaging Precision Medicine

Key Points (Abstract)

Precision Medicine is the focussed part of the imaging, which is evolving in a very fast way and here the concept is that the right therapy for the right patient, at right time, which is very specific as per the molecular targets which will be expressed in various diseases or tumours which are pertaining to the context of patient's environment and lifestyle. Being the newer concept, it is challenging with the focussed tailor-made diagnostic and treatment options. But there are some limitations related to this modality where the specific biomarkers will be focussed for a particular patient for the diagnostic, mapping of the heterogeneity or homogeneity of particular tissues that are involved, this also includes the various therapy failures and early response to the therapy.

PET is essential to accurately stage patients with potentially curable lung cancer. PET plays a central role in precision medicine by helping to noninvasively assess molecular pathobiology and genetic make-up of disease so that appropriate therapy is selected and started. PET is key for subsequent treatment strategy of patients with lung cancer, including monitoring of therapy response, detection of recurrence, and prediction of patient outcomes.

Keywords

Lung cancer · Positron emission tomography
Solitary pulmonary nodule · Cancer staging
Precision medicine · Targeted cancer therapy

8.1 Introduction

The National Institutes of Health (NIH) is defining the various aspects of Precision Medicine as "an emerging approach for disease treatment and prevention that takes into account individual variability in genes, environment, and lifestyle for each person" [1]. By this approach, the researchers will be able to diagnose the various aspects for accurate treatment, and prevention of these aspects. In 2015, President Obama, as part of his State of the Union address, announced the Precision Medicine initiative—a research effort that focuses on bringing precision medicine to many aspects of health care.

8.2 Precision Medicine in Dementia

Precision medicine is the newer concept of the patient management which has both the components for the prevention and treatment

S. Shaikh, *Advances in Imaging*, https://doi.org/10.1007/978-981-16-9535-3_8

aspects which are tailor made for the individual capacity Diagram 8.1. The important aspect of this is the across the patients for the right management for the right disease and pathologies [2]. The three important aspects of this are the evaluation risk of the risk assessment, early detection of the pathophysiologic processes which are not evident clinically and the management for the individualised concept of the molecular pathophysiology of the focussed disease pattern [3].

8.3 Precision Medicine in Alzheimer Disease

AD is an important condition of the old age which has many diverse disorders having many genetic locations which is the indicator for the increased risk with the higher mutations for the full expression of the disease expression [4, 5]. Traumatic encephalopathy is a heterogeneous entity with many features in particular patients [6]. This will help in the evaluation of chronic

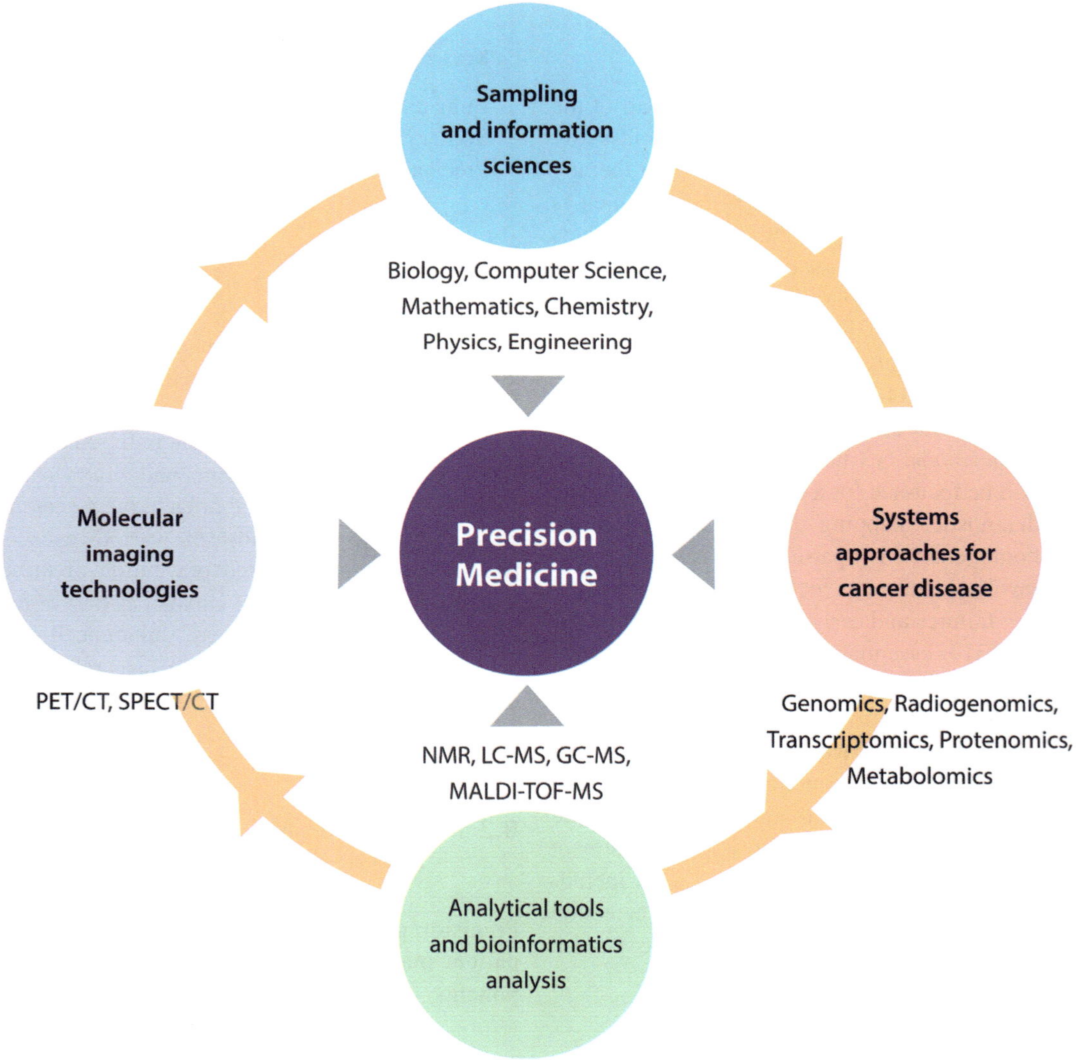

Diagram 8.1 Precision medicine combination of all modalities

traumatic encephalopathy (CTE). There are many biomarkers available for the early diagnosis of AD. The amyloid PET and also the CSF biomarkers are the important biomarkers for the evaluation of cognitive impairment which is always progressive in nature for several years.

High levels of Ab deposition is seen in the cognitively healthy individuals who are having progressive deficits along with the varying degree of the cognitive impairments, which can be seen in the modification of the various lifestyle activities and cognitive functions and also associated with the various genetic markers [7–10]. The use of the MI and CSF biomarkers is for the evaluation of the various stages of AD [11, 12], this helps plan the systematic approach of the various therapies. And unfortunately, there is no permanent cure for this disease. Various types of interventions are involved in reducing acetylcholine degradation or are also associated with ionotropic glutamatergic suppression to improve certain symptoms but cannot completely prevent the disease or slow its progression. The better imaging options are the Amyloid PET, FDG-PET, and tau MI, are also used as the AD biomarkers for evaluating the efficacy of the AD pathophysiology.

8.4 Molecular Imaging and Precision Medicine

8.4.1 Frontotemporal Dementia Syndromes

FTD syndromes are important aspects of varied groups of disorders that are distinct genetically. The majority of the frontotemporal dementias are tauopathies, like the PSP or CBD, and the remaining half are the ubiquitinopathies which are associated various types of the mutations like TDP-43 mutation, and the less entity are comprising of the Fused in Sarcoma RNA binding protein (FUS) inclusions. These FTD syndromes are having specific analytical factors by which they can be easily diagnosed and characterized based on their molecular characteristics and various neuroimaging findings that are crucial in the diagnosis [13]. Precision medicine can be used in these cases by the evaluation of the genetic mappings that are varied and are having different approaches, for example, like PD. We all know that the characteristic feature of PD is heterogeneous in nature having 20 genetic loci having varying risks for PD [14]. The various classical motor symptoms are having many genotypes which can have the clinical based association in relation to the various clinical findings and one of the most common are the cognitive impairment and dementia in PD [15, 16]. With this it can be an established criteria for the genotyping for the various targeted therapies for the evaluation of the various parkinsonian features which are based on the various motor, cognitive, or other atypical parkinsonian symptoms [2, 17] as mentioned the various aspects of the MI, CSF analysis, and peripheral tissue biopsy of the (submandibular gland) is showing the important aspect as a biomarker PD PM. The clinical evaluation of the parkinsonism can be established when there is the approximate loss of the 40–50% of putamen dopamine functional components. By the use of the Quantitative imaging like the PET and SPECT radiotracers which can be able to measure the various striatal DAT binding associated with the various noradrenaline and serotonin transporters systems. Another entity is drug-induced parkinsonism (DIP), which can happen when there are 20% concentrations of the striatal dopamine D2 receptors [18]. DIP is common by the use of the various neuroleptic antipsychotics, sedatives which are being used for the treatment of the vertigo and also the use of the tetra benzamine commonly used for the management of the involuntary movements where there is mismatch of the various components of the striatal DAT function mismatch.

Thus, in this the molecular Imaging. The compensatory downregulation mechanism will be useful for the DAT binding from chronic levodopa exposure as the levodopa medication will be persistent for more than two weeks of the "washout" [19, 20]. The important clinical feature is hyposmia which shows the early synuclein effects in the anterior telencephalon and iRBD will suggest this presence. MI of DAT function will significantly increase the amount of clinical utility. In the suspected PD with normal olfactory discrimination, the negative DAT scan will be demonstrating the various dopaminergic functions. The recent established criterion's for the diagnosis is the dementia occurs before or up to 1 year after the onset of parkinsonism, then it is known as DLB. On the contrary, if dementia is occurring more than a year after the onset of parkinsonism, then it is known as PDD [21]. There is also an association of the DLB with the fluctuating levels of cognitive arousal and visual hallucinations along with parkinsonian motor symptoms.

Thus, here the MI is having an important role in the evaluation of non-invasive, quantitative imaging along with the pathophysiology. The patients with AD and PD are the forms of the atypical MI biomarker which will be benefiting for the identification of the preclinical disease, various risks for the clinical trials and treatments, and also for monitoring new potential interventions.

8.5 Precision Medicine and Cancer

Cancer is the commonest form of malignancy in men and women [22]. As we know the localized disease is treatable, but disseminated disease is the leading cause of death. One of the important aspect is the evaluation of the genetic profiles resulting in the development of resistance. For example, the common form of lung cancer is including various targeted surgery, radiotherapy, chemotherapy, and immunotherapy. With the available modalities, the various aspects of the anatomic and metabolic imaging are important now for the disease evaluation and also for the metabolic evaluation of the various aspects of those cancers, their behaviour, and also in monitoring response to therapy. Positron emission tomography/computed tomography (PET/CT) is important for the evaluation of the tumour heterogeneity.

The 18F-labeled 2-fluoro-2-deoxy-D-glucose (FDG), a glucose analogue is a commonly used radiotracer based on the principle of the increased metabolism of the neoplastic cells to have increased metabolism. And these glucose metabolisms will be depicted before the anatomy and also for the evaluation of the response to the therapy. The amount of uptake is directly proportional to the histology, density of the cancer cells, their aggressiveness, and other various technical parameters also. Thus, the PET/CT can be performed by using standardized technical parameters. The newer various radiotracers like [18F] fluorothymidine (FLT), [18F] fluoromisonidazole (FMISO), [18F] fluoroazomycinarabinofuranoside (FAZA), O-[18F] fluoromethyl-L-tyrosine (FMT), and O-(2- [18F] fluoroethyl)-L-tyrosine (FET) are being used in the lung cancers. By the use of the various PET probes, different regional heterogeneous nature of the disease, are also being studied.

8.6 PET/CT Imaging in Initial Staging of the Patient

FDG-PET/CT is important in various aspects like to (1) characterize an indeterminate solitary pulmonary nodule (SPN), (2) guide biopsy for the most viable tissue in the lesion in the form of the very high uptake of FDG, and (3) for the evaluation of the extent of the disease composed of the primary disease, lymph nodes, and distant metastases. Thus, SPN is an important example for the evaluation of these structures [23]. Here again, many differential diagnoses are various benign and malignant components like infection, inflammation, and lung cancer. Here, the FDG-PET/CT is having a significant increased uptake in the form of the high sensitivity and specificity for the characterization of the lesions whether malignant or benign, especially in the nodules of size that are greater than 8 mm in size [24–27]. Various benign entities like pneumonia, tuberculosis, fungal infections, and sarcoidosis, can also show this FDG avidity. The Society of Nuclear Medicine and Molecular Imaging criteria for the evaluation of FDG-PET/CT with the SPN to (1) for the detection of potentially malignant lesions early in the course of disease, (2) to exclude malignancy in indeterminate grade lesions, and (3) ultimately to increase the sensitivity in the high-risk patients for the curative surgery [28]. PET/CT is having an important role in lung cancer staging, to determine appropriate therapy and prognosis of patients with lung cancer. The local disease is more favourable for surgical resection. CT for the lesion size, location, and invasion of adjacent structures, while PET gives the metabolic information. PET/CT shows that 60% of adenocarcinoma metastases are CT occult [29], having an 8% incidence for the occult metastases of the stage I disease, and up to 24% for stage III disease [30]. The sensitivity, specificity, and accuracy of PET/CT for evaluating systemic metastases usually exceed 90% [31]. PET/CT is more useful for the early osseous metastases and far superior to CT for the detection of liver metastases [32, 33]. In some cases, the histopathological confirmation is to be done in cases of various false-positive PET/CT cases to prevent untoward effects due to aggressive treatment [34, 35]. For the cerebral metastases MRI is better for the evaluation. One study shows that the hybrid PET/MR imaging versus PET/CT are having the same results for lung cancer staging [36].

8.7 PET-Based Molecular Imaging and Precision Medicine in the Treatment Planning of the Lung Cancer

Precision medicine will be classifying the patients into various subgroups by combining the molecular pathobiology with the genetic make-up of disease along with the various clinical findings for the valuation of the proper diagnosis, staging, for the predict treatment response, and also, for the patient outcome [37]. All these components will be used like tailor-made options for the "preventive or therapeutic interventions" thus preventing further unnecessary management of the disease entities. The molecular imaging will now be a more contributing factor in the precision medicine for the extent of disease, monitoring response to treatment, and ultimately be able to prognosticate the findings based on the various specific image signatures. These are in the form of the various predictive biomarkers for early response, cytotoxic and cytostatic treatments, radiotherapy, and to assist the various image-guided interventions. Thus, ultimately the final biomarker for the prognosis of patients with lung cancer. Thus, the precision medicine is influencing to treat, type and intensity of treatment for the tumoral response and also for the adjusting the various treatment algorithms and also for the second-line management options.

8.8 PET as a Predictive Biomarker of Response to Lung Cancer Therapy

Response Evaluation Criteria in Solid Tumours [RECIST] criteria is one of the important criteria for the evaluation of the tumour response or progression after morphologic response criteria for the evaluation of the cytolytic effect of therapy. The targeted therapy is cytostatic, which is very slow and also for the evaluation of the various tumour cell proliferation. The use of these targeted therapies has completely changed the concept of personalize tumour response assessment to therapy [38]. Wahl and colleagues [39] showed with the newer proposed criteria of PET Response Criteria in Solid Tumours which uses the tumoural morphologic phenotype of response (RECIST) as well as the metabolic appearance (PET) for the evaluation of the monitor response to treatment. Thus, FDG-PET is an important biomarker for accessing various therapeutic responses due to the targeted therapies which will be evaluating the various metabolic and pathophysiologic changes that will come before the lesion morphology [40]. And thus, the PET-based molecular imaging will be useful for the evaluation for the response to the treatment as compared with the conventional imaging modalities CT and MRI. In general, the data show that the earlier the response the better the progression-free and overall survival of the patient with cancer. PET response can be used for the early determination of the post-treatment evaluation after couple of the cycles of radiotherapy and also the neoadjuvant chemotherapy [41, 42].

8.9 Assessment of Response to Cytotoxic Cancer Therapy and Radiotherapy

FDG-PET is an important modality for the evaluation of the response to radiotherapy in patients with cancer. Hicks and coinvestigators showed that the associated radiation-induced inflammation after radical radiotherapy for the post-therapeutic response if acquired within 70 days after completion of treatment [43]. For the assessment of the Response to Cytostatic Cancer Therapy Twelve years ago, Paez and colleagues [44] and Lynch and co-workers [45] concluded that the treatment of lung tumours which will be expressing the various somatic mutations of the epidermal growth factor receptor genes with tyrosine kinase inhibitors (TKI) arrested tumour growth. Agents like erlotinib, gefitinib, afatinib, and crizotinib will become the newer aspect of the biomarker management options for the treatment of the lung cancer. The criteria of the tumour size reduction do not signify the concerned cytostatic treatment based on the RECIST or World Health Organization criteria for monitoring response to the treatment for the assessment of the treatment efficacy [46–56].

8.10 PET as a Biomarker of Prognosis in Lung Cancer

The prognostic value of various PET signatures for the evaluation of lung cancer is reported in the literature. The image signatures signify the amount of tumour metabolic activity by the semi-quantitative method of the SUV, the tumour bulk based on the amount of the metabolic volumes and total lesion glycolysis (TLG), metabolic heterogeneity and prognosis based on the FDG uptake. The various aspects of the progression-free survival from the (I through III) based on the various high and low SUV.

8.11 Metabolically Active Tumour Bulk

The tumour bulk is one of the important indicators for the different tumour types, like the lung and pleural malignancies, and also for the clinical decision-making [57]. Metabolic tumour volume (MTV) is showing the metabolically active tumour mass and is quantified by the tumour contouring software by the SUV. Another aspect is the TLG, based on the tumour's mean SUV by the MTV. Whole-body MTV and TLG can be obtained. These parameters will give three-dimensional evaluation of the various total tumour volume and metabolic activity. The amount of the tumoural Metabolic Heterogeneity will be giving the information based on the tumour aggressiveness, resistance to treatment, and poor progression-free and overall survival.

PET image predictors are the indicators for the survival in their patient cohort [58]. These predictors show the prognostic potential.

8.12 Therapeutic Strategies in Gastroenteropancreatic Neuroendocrine Tumours

The gastroenteropancreatic neuroendocrine tumours can be based on the various anatomic site, size, invasiveness, functionality and also the various hormone secretion, and metastatic potential. Early stages surgery is the first option. Later stages including the inoperable advanced/metastatic disease various multiple therapeutic options can be there like the (1) somatostatin analogues, like the octreotide; (2) somatostatin receptors (3) conventional chemotherapeutic agents like cisplatinum-etoposide combination or other combinations and (4) targeted therapy like the various combinations of the locoregional ablative therapies, such as chemoembolization, or radiofrequency ablation or selective internal radiotherapy of therapy among these multiple options are a clinical need of present-day management.

8.13 Personalized Therapeutic Strategy

The use of the various Somatostatin analogues for the various metastatic GEP-NETs, are being used in the various low and intermediate well-differentiated NETs, having the most of the SSTRs [59]. Dual-tracer PET imaging is also used better option for the evaluation for most of the pathologies in the individual patient.

8.14 Precision Medicine in Prostate

Prostate cancer (PCa) is the most common tumour and the third common cause of death in men in Europe and the United States [60, 61]. With the available data the various primary treated localized PCa are having excellent results making up to the up to 50% of the patients treated with radical prostatectomy or external-beam radiotherapy (EBRT) [62–66]. Various clinical and pathologic indicators like prostate-specific antigen (PSA), PSA doubling time [PSAdt], PSA velocity, Gleason score (GS), lymph node (LN) invasion, and the various distant metastases which will be useful for the evaluation of the various local versus systemic recurrence after radical prostatectomy or EBRT.

PSMA PET/computed tomography (CT) has become the most valuable tool for the evaluation of prostate cancer patients along with the chances of recurrence. This 68Ga-PSMA, also acts as an important theranostics agent, capable of delivering higher doses for the various systemic involvements thus a newer approach can be applied. The newer molecular biomarkers will be having the robust test for the analysis of the future management protocols.

The available modalities computed tomography (CT), bone scintigraphy, and MR imaging, are having very lower sensitivities in detecting the sites of PCa recurrence [67]. Molecular function and metabolic activity are being done by the PET modalities as a single-step examination [68]. The newer radiotracers in PET/CT comprising of the 11C-choline and/or 18F-choline has been having the promising roles in the evaluation of the PCa [67, 69] PET/CT by Choline is being seen as the better alternative for restaging PCa patients [67, 69]. This will help in differentiating between early relapse and recurrence with progression [69] and this is well-established protocol in the management of patients with recurrent PCa [70]. The major limitations are the nodal micrometastases, and this also can be provided along with the evaluation of staging PCa before primary therapies like radical prostatectomy or EBRT [71]. High-risk patients with extra prostatic involvement with high PSA values and/or high GS. PET/CT imaging will be able to evaluate the nodal in less common regions. Thus, the pelvic lymph-node dissection or an EBRT can be performed with increased target volume. The choline-PET/CT will prevent the radical therapy due to the assessment of the systemic metastatic spread–diffusion. Choline-PET/CT is having very low sensitivity, in patients with low PSA levels during imaging [72–74]. Molecular mechanisms related to specific resistance to castration in PCa (CRPC) and also for the active androgen receptor (AR) response as the predictive biomarkers for response to antiandrogen therapy.

8.15 PSMA PET-CT Imaging

The newer imaging molecular probe which is targeting the targeting the prostate specific membrane antigen (PSMA) is being developed [75]. PSMA, is the membrane-bound metallopeptidase, seen in the various organs related to prostate, brain, small intestine, and kidney [76]. The catalytic site of PSMA can localize the extracellular domain which will develop the small, highly specific inhibitors inside the cell after ligand binding [77]. The use of these with the focussed targeting the GCPII by the PET-CT imaging for the PCa imaging is being evolved in coming years [78, 79]. The broad range of GCPII enzyme activities as seen by the biodistribution of gallium 68 (68Ga-PSMA) [80]. A significant amount of the uptake is seen in the 68Ga-PSMA is seen in the renal cortex, duodenum, lacrimal, and salivary glands. Moderate uptake is seen in the liver and spleen. There will be higher median uptake in primary prostate tumours in comparison with the normal prostatic parenchyma. PSA levels of the 0.5 to 2.0 ng/mL, showing the positivity rate of 69% for 68Ga-PSMA PET/CT and 31% for 18F-fluoromethylcholine and when PSA greater than 2.0, the positivity rate was 86% for 68Ga-PSMA versus 57% for 18F-fluoromethylcholine. The diffuse bone marrow uptake due to myelosuppression can be seen on the PSMA.

8.16 Biomarkers in Castration-Resistant Prostate Cancer

A severe form of PCa is mostly due to the resistance to castration. Molecular mechanisms that are showing resistance to various castration and are predictive biomarkers for response to antiandrogens [81, 82]. There will be expression within CRPC tumour cells of the AR gene which will mimic at the cell level along with the clinical syndrome of androgen resistance.

PET/CT imaging targeting is used for guiding the various lesion therapies. PSMA inhibitors can also be seen in the high-energy beta emitter (e.g. 177Lu). The radioactive PSMA ligand is directly related to the effectiveness in delivering high doses for systemic radionuclide therapy, by the various newer therapeutic techniques to the patients. With the availability of the various molecular biomarkers, they are capable of evaluation of the newer second-generation antiandrogen agents in CRPC patients.

8.17 Molecular Imaging Precision Medicine

The role of precision medicine in in vivo imaging is for the diagnosis of various biological events at the molecular level, for the early diagnosis and effective management of various diseases [83]. With the use of sophisticated technology in vivo microimaging of the small animals is seen in a better way for the basic science research [84] (Diagram 8.2).

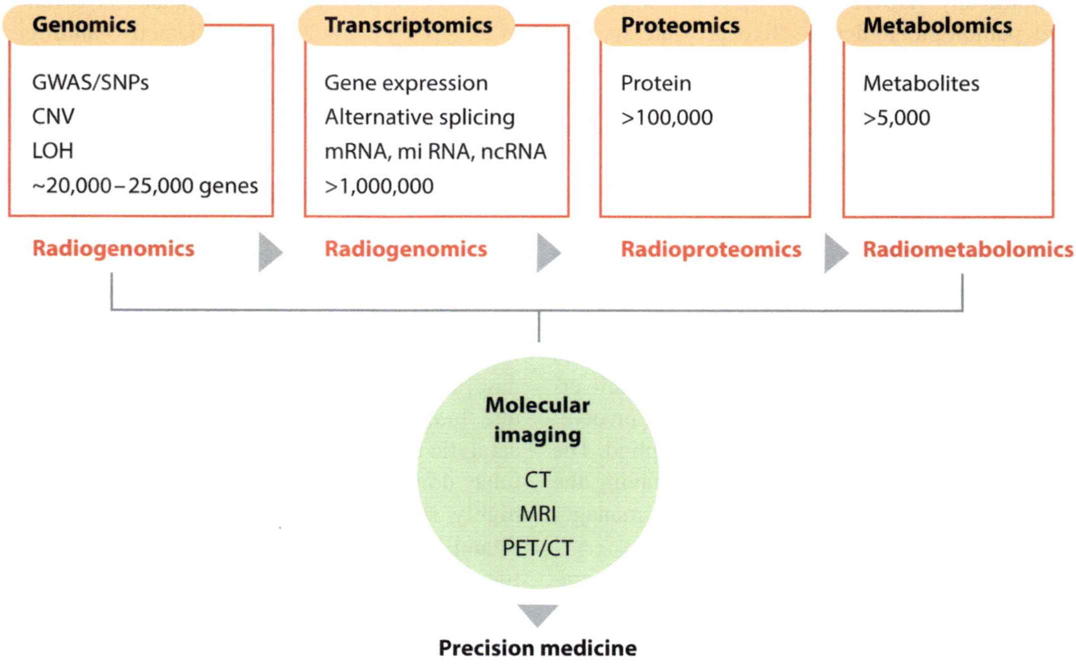

Diagram 8.2 Various genomics involved as the combination for the precision medicine

Molecular imaging is having the limitations like the short light penetration of the molecular optical imaging, non-clear detection, and identification of the various small and deep-seated targets with molecular magnetic resonance (MR) imaging by using surface coils. The use of the physiologic "clearing" of a couple of the various targeted imaging and therapeutic probes in respect to the kidneys and liver in molecular nuclear imaging. Molecular optical imaging is used as a powerful tool for the detection of fluorescence or bioluminescence which will be emitted from the various tissues as well as the small animals. But due to limitations in the penetration of these, it cannot be used as the complete problem-solving tool. The newer concept of interventional molecular imaging where the diagnostic and therapeutic applications can be seen in a single entity. The available interventional radiology can be used for various (a) reach deep-seated targets, (b) which will be enabling the various smaller targets, (c) focussed delivery of non-targeted imaging tracers or therapeutics, and (d) thus offering the supers elective basis of the targeted imaging and treatment. Another advantage of the interventional radiology will be it is the real-time imaging for the use of the minimally invasive diagnostic and therapeutic procedures [85]. Some of the common examples are the use of various percutaneous insertion/guiding of the needles or catheters, deep-seated organs, or targets become accessible to both imaging and intervention. The needle type of optical imager can deliver all deep-seated targets so that the basic point behind the molecular imaging can be done [86, 87]. With this, the use of interventional radiologic will be progressing in the form of the translation molecular imaging for various clinical applications. Optical coherence tomography (OCT) is one of the most emerging biomedical optical imaging techniques which will have the very high spatial resolution, cross-sectional tomographic imaging of microstructure [88]. OCT when modified then will become the endovascular optical imaging tool that can give many small vascular structures, like the wall, vessel wall and the fibrous cap of atherosclerotic plaques. The use of the interventional molecular imaging can is also for the monitoring the delivery of nontargeted imaging tracers or therapeutic agents to their specific targets. Intravascular high spatial resolution MR imaging can also be used for the delivery to vascular walls [89]. These gene vectors when added with the MR contrast agent can be locally infused into the balloon catheter. The gene–contrast material mixture will evaluate the vessel wall intravascular high spatial resolution MR imaging. The molecular imaging guided endovascular gene delivery will also be used for the real-time US [90]. The distribution of various gene carrying echogenic microspheres can also be visualized. The use of the various interventional molecular imaging is more effective for the targeted diagnosis and treatment. One of the important potential clinical applications of molecular imaging is for the monitoring of the systemic delivery of various target-specific imaging and therapeutic probes [91]. The modification for various diagnostic or therapeutic probes in combination with the various monoclonal antibodies can be used for the extracellular domain for PET-CT [92]. These modified probes are cleared by the kidneys and trapped in the liver. With these various interventional radiologic techniques, these probes will be delivered to specific targets such as tumour masses.

8.18 Precision Medicine in Radionuclide Therapy

As there are significant advancements in the field of molecular imaging and cancer therapy, there is also significant advancement happening in radionuclide therapy as a part of precision therapy. The newer concept of the dual-purpose therapeutic and diagnostic use of the various radiopharmaceuticals with the low-dose imaging by the radionuclide for accessing the kinetics for tumour dosimetry, and also for the radionuclide therapy of different patterns. The technological advancements in the PET/computed tomography (CT), PET/MR imaging, and SPECT/CT are more helping in the evaluation and also in the precise localization of radiopharmaceuticals. The exact prediction of the radiation dose before delivery of the therapy is also an important entity of the personalized medicine. The use of various therapies like 131MIBG, 131NaI therapy, peptide radionuclide receptor therapy, and targeted delivery of radionuclides with embolizing 90Y microspheres can be used for personalised medicine.

8.19 Selective Internal Radiation Therapy

The use of selective internal radiation therapy by the use of 90Ylabeled microspheres is the newer concept of nuclear medicine therapeutics. The liver tumours radiation along with the complex procedure, and the use of the multidisciplinary collaboration and coordination, and risk factors can lead to better theranostics. 90Y-labeled glass or resin microspheres are being delivered via intra-arterial route for the treatment of primary hepatocellular carcinoma and metastatic hepatic lesions from colorectal carcinoma primary, respectively [93]. The metastatic liver tumours are also being treated for the "off-label" application. The knowledge of the previous imaging, patient-specific anatomic variants, hepatic function tests, previous chemotherapy, or radiation are important factors for the evaluation of these cancers [93, 94]. In hepatocellular carcinoma, glass microspheres can be delivered based on the volume of liver parenchyma to be treated like lobar or segmental. Hepatic metastatic lesions' resin microspheres are used for the treatment based on the body surface area, hepatic lobe volume, specific tumour load percent on each lobe, and all other factors described previously. Sometimes the preprocedural 99mTc–microaggregated albumin (MAA) imaging and post-procedural 90Y bremsstrahlung SPECT/CT scans will be evaluating the potential of the exact microsphere distribution, and to identify various radiotracer activities in adjacent structures which are outside the tumoural coverage areas [93, 95]. Imaging will follow the step-by-step treatment planning which will be tailor made for the specific patient requirements. After this, the verification of the dose to be delivered to the tumour will be correlated with the treatment dose. Sometimes the use of the 99mTc-MAA SPECT/CT as a predictor of the 90Y radiation dose is not specific [96–98]. The 90Y bremsstrahlung SPECT/CT is semiquantitative but can be used for the estimation of the delivered radiation dose [93, 99]. 90Y has a very low occurrence of positron emission that allows much more accurate post-treatment imaging [100, 101]. Sirtex and theraspheres are also used for targeted therapy of the primary and secondary liver malignancies, by keeping in mind the different patient-specific variables for individualized therapy. Pre- and post-treatment imaging are essential tools for the delivery of precision medicine.

References

1. Collins FS, Varmus H. A new initiative on precision medicine. N Engl J Med. 2015;372(9):793–5.
2. Bu LL, Yang K, Xiong WX, et al. Toward precision medicine in Parkinson's disease. Ann Transl Med. 2016;4(2):26.
3. Montine TJ, Montine KS. Precision medicine: clarity for the clinical and biological complexity of Alzheimer's and Parkinson's diseases. J Exp Med. 2015;212(5):601–5.
4. Lambert JC, Ibrahim-Verbaas CA, Harold D, et al. Meta-analysis of 74,046 individuals identifies 11 new susceptibility loci for Alzheimer's disease. Nat Genet. 2013;45(12):1452–8.
5. Nalls MA, Pankratz N, Lill CM, et al. Large-scale meta-analysis of genome-wide association data identifies six new risk loci for Parkinson's disease. Nat Genet. 2014;46(9):989–93.
6. Armstrong RA, McKee AC, Stein TD, et al. A quantitative study of tau pathology in eleven cases of chronic traumatic encephalopathy. Neuropathol Appl Neurobiol. 2017; 43(2):154–166. https://doi.org/10.1111/nan.12323. [Epub ahead of print]. Molecular Imaging and Precision Medicine 15.
7. Mosconi L, Rinne JO, Tsui WH, et al. Amyloid and metabolic positron emission tomography imaging of cognitively normal adults with Alzheimer's parents. Neurobiol Aging. 2013;34(1):22–34.
8. Vemuri P, Lesnick TG, Przybelski SA, et al. Effect of lifestyle activities on Alzheimer disease biomarkers and cognition. Ann Neurol. 2012;72(5):730–8.
9. Kemppainen NM, Aalto S, Karrasch M, et al. Cognitive reserve hypothesis: Pittsburgh compound B and fluorodeoxyglucose positron emission tomography in relation to education in mild Alzheimer's disease. Ann Neurol. 2008;63(1):112–8.
10. Sperling RA, Aisen PS, Beckett LA, et al. Toward defining the preclinical stages of Alzheimer's disease: recommendations from the National Institute on Aging-Alzheimer's association workgroups

on diagnostic guidelines for Alzheimer's disease. Alzheimers Dement. 2011;7(3):280–92.
11. Albert MS, DeKosky ST, Dickson D, et al. The diagnosis of mild cognitive impairment due to Alzheimer's disease: recommendations from the National Institute on Aging-Alzheimer's association workgroups on diagnostic guidelines for Alzheimer's disease. Alzheimers Dement. 2011;7(3):270–9.
12. McKhann G, Drachman D, Folstein M, et al. Clinical diagnosis of Alzheimer's disease: report of the NINCDS-ADRDA work group under the auspices of Department of Health and Human Services Task Force on Alzheimer's disease. Neurology. 1984;34(7):939–44.
13. Kleinman M, Frank S. Epidemiology and clinical diagnosis of Parkinson disease. PET Clin. 2013;8(4):447–58.
14. Corti O, Lesage S, Brice A. What genetics tells us about the causes and mechanisms of Parkinson's disease. Physiol Rev. 2011;91(4):1161–218.
15. Alcalay RN, Caccappolo E, Mejia-Santana H, et al. Cognitive performance of GBA mutation carriers with early-onset PD: the CORE-PD study. Neurology. 2012;78(18):1434–40.
16. Srivatsal S, Cholerton B, Leverenz JB, et al. Cognitive profile of LRRK2-related Parkinson's disease. Mov Disord. 2015;30(5):728–33.
17. Stamelou M, Bhatia KP. Atypical parkinsonism: diagnosis and treatment. Neurol Clin. 2015;33(1):39–56.
18. Farde L, Nordstrom AL, Wiesel FA, et al. Positron emission tomographic analysis of central D1 and D2 dopamine receptor occupancy in patients treated with classical neuroleptics and clozapine. Relation to extrapyramidal side effects. Arch Gen Psychiatry. 1992;49(7):538–44.
19. Eisensehr I, Linke R, Noachtar S, et al. Reduced striatal dopamine transporters in idiopathic rapid eye movement sleep behaviour disorder. Comparison with Parkinson's disease and controls. Brain. 2000;123(Pt 6):1155–60.
20. Stiasny-Kolster K, Doerr Y, Moller JC, et al. Combination of 'idiopathic' REM sleep behaviour disorder and olfactory dysfunction as possible indicator for alphasynucleinopathy demonstrated by dopamine transporter FP-CIT-SPECT. Brain. 2005;128(Pt 1):126–37.
21. McKeith IG, Dickson DW, Lowe J, et al. Diagnosis and management of dementia with Lewy bodies: third report of the DLB consortium. Neurology. 2005;65(12):1863–72.
22. American Cancer Society. Key statistics for lung cancer. 2016. Available at: http://www.cancer.org/cancer/lungcancer-non-smallcell/detailedguide/non-small-cell-lung-cancer-key-statistics. Accessed July 9, 2016.
23. Gould MK, Tang T, Liu IL, et al. Recent trends in the identification of incidental pulmonary nodules. Am J Respir Crit Care Med. 2015;192(10):1208–14.
24. Gould MK, Maclean CC, Kuschner WG, et al. Accuracy of positron emission tomography for diagnosis of pulmonary nodules and mass lesions: a meta-analysis. JAMA. 2001;287:914–24.
25. Gambhir SS, Czernin J, Schwimmer J, et al. A tabulated summary of the FDG PET literature. J Nucl Med. 2001;42:1S–93S.
26. Cronin P, Dwamena B, Kelly AM, et al. Solitary pulmonary nodules: meta-analytic comparison of cross-sectional imaging modalities for diagnosis of malignancy. Radiology. 2008;246:772–82.
27. Garcia-Velloso MJ, Bastarrika G, de-Torres JP, et al. Assessment of indeterminate pulmonary nodules detected in lung cancer screening: diagnostic accuracy of FDG PET/CT. Lung Cancer. 2016;97:81–6.
28. Fletcher JW, Djulbegovic B, Soares HP, et al. Recommendations on the use of 18F-FDG PET in oncology. J Nucl Med. 2008;49(3):480–508.
29. Sider L, Horejs D. Frequency of extrathoracic metastases from bronchogenic carcinoma in patients with normal-sized hilar and mediastinal lymph nodes on CT. AJR Am J Roentgenol. 1988;151(5):893–5.
30. MacManus MP, Hicks RJ, Matthews JP, et al. High rate of detection of unsuspected distant metastases by PET in apparent stage III non-small-cell lung cancer: implications for radical radiation therapy. Int J Radiat Oncol Biol Phys. 2001;50(2):287–93.
31. Hellwig D, Ukena D, Paulsen F, et al. Onko-PET der Deutschen gesellschaft fur nuklearmedizin. Metaanalysis of the efficacy of positron emission tomography with F-18-fluorodeoxyglucose in lung tumors. Basis for discussion of the German consensus conference on PET in oncology 2000. Pneumologie. 2001;55(8):367–77.
32. Cook GJ, Houston S, Rubens R, et al. Detection of bone metastases in breast cancer by 18FDG PET: differing metabolic activity in osteoblastic and osteolytic lesions. J Clin Oncol. 1998;16(10):3375–9.
33. Hustinx R, Paulus P, Jacquet N, et al. Clinical evaluation of whole-body 18F-fluorodeoxyglucose positron emission tomography in the detection of liver metastases. Ann Oncol. 1998;9(4):397–401.
34. Reed CE, Harpole DH, Posther KE, et al. American College of Surgeons oncology group Z0050 trial. Results of the American College of Surgeons oncology group Z0050 trial: the utility of positron emission tomography in staging potentially operable non-small cell lung cancer. J Thorac Cardiovasc Surg. 2003;126(6):1943–51.
35. Lardinois D, Weder W, Roudas M, et al. Etiology of solitary extrapulmonary positron emission tomography and computed tomography findings in patients with lung cancer. J Clin Oncol. 2005;23:6846–53.
36. Schaarschmidt BM, Grueneisen J, Metzenmacher M, et al. Thoracic staging with 18F-FDG PET/MR in non-small cell lung cancer: does it change therapeutic decisions in comparison to 18F-FDG PET/CT? Eur Radiol. 2017; 27(2):681–688. 10.1007/s00330-016-4397-0. [Epub ahead of print].

37. National Research Council (US) Committee on A Framework for Developing a New Taxonomy of Disease. Toward precision medicine: building a knowledge network for biomedical research and a new taxonomy of disease. Washington, DC: National Academies Press (US); 2011.
38. Erasmus JJ, Gladish GW, Broemeling L, et al. Interobserver and intraobserver variability in measurement of non-small-cell carcinoma lung lesions: implications for assessment of tumor response. J Clin Oncol. 2003;21:2574–82.
39. Wahl RL, Jacene H, Kasamon Y, et al. From RECIST to PERCIST: evolving considerations for PET response criteria in solid tumors. J Nucl Med. 2009;50(Suppl 1):122S–50S.
40. Vansteenkiste J, Fischer BM, Dooms C, et al. Positron-emission tomography in prognostic and therapeutic assessment of lung cancer: systematic review. Lancet Oncol. 2004;5:531–40.
41. Weber WA, Petersen V, Schmidt B, et al. Positron emission tomography in non-small-cell lung cancer: prediction of response to chemotherapy by quantitative assessment of glucose use. J Clin Oncol. 2003;21:2651–7.
42. Cerfolio RJ, Bryant AS, Winokur TS, et al. Repeat 18F-FDG-PET after neoadjuvant therapy is a predictor of pathologic response in patients with non-small cell lung cancer. Ann Thorac Surg. 2004;78:1903–9.
43. Hicks RJ, Mac Manus MP, Matthews JP, et al. Early FDG-PET imaging after radical radiotherapy for non-small-cell lung cancer: inflammatory changes in normal tissues correlate with tumor response and do not confound therapeutic response evaluation. Int J Radiat Oncol Biol Phys. 2004;60(2):412–8.
44. Paez JG, Jänne PA, Lee JC, et al. EGFR mutations in lung cancer: correlation with clinical response to gefitinib therapy. Science. 2004;304(5676):1497–500.
45. Lynch TJ, Bell DW, Sordella R, et al. Activating mutations in the epidermal growth factor receptor underlying responsiveness of non-small-cell lung cancer to gefitinib. N Engl J Med. 2004;350(21):2129–39.
46. Sunaga N, Oriuchi N, Kaira K, et al. Usefulness of FDG-PET for early prediction of the response to gefitinib in non-small cell lung cancer. Lung Cancer. 2008;59(2):203–10.
47. Takahashi R, Hirata H, Tachibana I, et al. Early [18F] fluorodeoxyglucose positron emission tomography at two days of gefitinib treatment predicts clinical outcome in patients with adenocarcinoma of the lung. Clin Cancer Res. 2012;18(1):220–8.
48. van Gool MH, Aukema TS, Schaake EE, et al. NEL study group. Timing of metabolic response monitoring during erlotinib treatment in non-small cell lung cancer. J Nucl Med. 2014;55(7):1081–6.
49. Benz MR, Herrmann K, Walter F, et al. (18)F-FDG PET/CT for monitoring treatment responses to the epidermal growth factor receptor inhibitor erlotinib. J Nucl Med. 2011;52(11):1684–9.
50. Hachemi M, Couturier O, Vervueren L, et al. [18F] FDG positron emission tomography within two weeks of starting erlotinib therapy can predict response in non-small cell lung cancer patients. PLoS One. 2014;9(2):e87629.
51. van Gool MH, Aukema TS, Schaake EE, et al. (18) Ffluorodeoxyglucose positron emission tomography versus computed tomography in predicting histopathological response to epidermal growth factor receptor-tyrosine kinase inhibitor treatment in resectable non-small cell lung cancer. Ann Surg Oncol. 2014;21(9):2831–7.
52. Ullrich RT, Zander T, Neumaier B, et al. Early detection of erlotinib treatment response in NSCLC by 3′- deoxy-3′-[F]-fluoro-L-thymidine ([F]FLT) positron emission tomography (PET). PLoS One. 2008;3(12):e3908.
53. Sohn HJ, Yang YJ, Ryu JS, et al. [18F] Fluorothymidine positron emission tomography before and 7 days after gefitinib treatment predicts response in patients with advanced adenocarcinoma of the lung. Clin Cancer Res. 2008;14(22):7423–9.
54. Kahraman D, Scheffler M, Zander T, et al. Quantitative analysis of response to treatment with erlotinib in advanced non-small cell lung cancer using 18FFDG and 3′-deoxy-3'-18F-fluorothymidine PET. J Nucl Med. 2011;52(12):1871–7.
55. Zander T, Scheffler M, Nogova L, et al. Early prediction of nonprogression in advanced non-small-cell lung cancer treated with erlotinib by using [(18)F]fluorodeoxyglucose and [(18)F]fluorothymidine positron emission tomography. J Clin Oncol. 2011;29(13):1701–8.
56. Bhoil A, Singh B, Singh N, et al. Can 3′-deoxy-3′-(18) F-fluorothymidine or 2′-deoxy-2′-(18) F-fluoro-dglucose PET/CTbetter assess response after 3-weeks treatment by epidermal growth factor receptor kinase inhibitor, in non-small lung cancer patients? Preliminary results. Hell J Nucl Med. 2014;17(2):90–6.
57. Gerbaudo VH, Katz SI, Nowak AK, et al. Multimodality imaging review of malignant pleural mesothelioma diagnosis and staging. PET Clin. 2011;6(3):275–97.
58. Cook GJ, O'Brien ME, Siddique M, et al. Non-small cell lung cancer treated with erlotinib: heterogeneity of (18)F-FDG uptake at PET-association with treatment response and prognosis. Radiology. 2015;276(3):883–93.
59. Oberg K, Kvols L, Caplin M, et al. Consensus report on the use of somatostatin analogs for the management of neuroendocrine tumors of the gastroenteropancreatic system. Ann Oncol. 2004;15(6):966–73.
60. Siegel RL, Miller KD, Jemal A, et al. Cancer statistics. CA Cancer J Clin. 2015;2015(65):5–29.
61. Heidenreich A, Bastian PJ, Bellmunt J, et al. EAU guidelines on prostate cancer. Part 1: screening, diagnosis, and local treatment with curative intentupdate 2013. Eur Urol. 2014;65:124–37.
62. Briganti A, Karnes RJ, Gandaglia G, et al. Natural history of surgically treated high-risk prostate cancer. Urol Oncol. 2015;33(163):e7–13.

63. Punnen S, Cooperberg MR, D'Amico AV, et al. Management of biochemical recurrence after primary treatment of prostate cancer: a systematic review of the literature. Eur Urol. 2013;64:905–15.
64. Freedland SJ, Presti JC Jr, Amling CL, et al. Time trends in biochemical recurrence after radical prostatectomy: results of the SEARCH database. Urology. 2003;61:736–41.
65. Boorjian SA, Eastham JA, Graefen M, et al. A critical analysis of the long-term impact of radical prostatectomy on cancer control and function outcomes. Eur Urol. 2012;61:664–75.
66. Khuntia D, Reddy CA, Mahadevan A, et al. Recurrence-free survival rates after external-beam radiotherapy for patients with clinical T1-T3 prostate carcinoma in the prostate-specific antigen era: what should we expect? Cancer. 2004;100:1283–92.
67. Choueiri TK, Dreicer R, Paciorek A, et al. A model that predicts the probability of positive imaging in prostate cancer cases with biochemical failure after initial definitive local therapy. J Urol. 2008; 179:906–10 [discussion: 10].
68. PhelpsME. Inaugural article: positron emission-tomography provides molecular imaging of biological processes. Proc Natl Acad Sci U S A. 2000;97:9226–33.
69. Castellucci P, Ceci F, Graziani T, et al. Early biochemical relapse after radical prostatectomy: which prostate cancer patients may benefit from a restaging 11C-choline PET/CT scan before salvage radiation therapy? J Nucl Med. 2014;55:1424–9.
70. Ceci F, Herrmann K, Castellucci P, et al. Impact of 11C-choline PET/CT on clinical decision making in recurrent prostate cancer: results from a retrospective two-Centre trial. Eur J Nucl Med Mol Imaging. 2014;41(12):2222–31.
71. Evangelista L, Guttilla A, Zattoni F, et al. Utility of choline positron emission tomography/computed tomography for lymph node involvement identification in intermediate- to high-risk prostate cancer: a systematic literature review and meta-analysis. Eur Urol. 2013;63(6):1040–8.
72. Briganti A, Karnes RJ, Joniau S, et al. Prediction of outcome following early salvage radiotherapy among patients with biochemical recurrence after radical prostatectomy. Eur Urol. 2014;66:479–86.
73. Fossati N, Karnes RJ, Cozzarini C, et al. Assessing the optimal timing for early salvage radiation therapy in patients with prostate-specific antigen rise after radical prostatectomy. Eur Urol. 2015;69(4):728–33.
74. Stephenson AJ, Scardino PT, Kattan MW, et al. Predicting the outcome of salvage radiation therapy for recurrent prostate cancer after radical prostatectomy. J Clin Oncol. 2007;25:2035–41.
75. Ghosh A, Heston WD. Tumor target prostate specific membrane antigen (PSMA) and its regulation in prostate cancer. J Cell Biochem. 2004;91:528–39.
76. Barinka C, Rojas C, Slusher B, et al. Glutamate carboxypeptidase II in diagnosis and treatment of neurologic disorders and prostate cancer. Curr Med Chem. 2012;19:856–70.
77. Foss CA, Mease RC, Fan H, et al. Radiolabeled small-molecule ligands for prostate-specific membrane antigen: in vivo imaging in experimental models of prostate cancer. Clin Cancer Res. 2005;11:4022–8.
78. Afshar-Oromieh A, Avtzi E, Giesel FL, et al. The diagnostic value of PET/CT imaging with the (68) Galabelled PSMA ligand HBED-CC in the diagnosis of recurrent prostate cancer. Eur J Nucl Med Mol Imaging. 2015;42:197–209.
79. Eiber M, Maurer T, Souvatzoglou M, et al. Evaluation of hybrid 68Ga-PSMA ligand PET/CT in 248 patients with biochemical recurrence after radical prostatectomy. J Nucl Med. 2015;56:668–74.
80. Prasad V, Steffen IG, Diederichs G, et al. Biodistribution of [(68)Ga]PSMA-HBED-CC in patients with prostate cancer: characterization of uptake in normal organs and tumour lesions. Mol Imaging Biol. 2016;18(3):428–36.
81. Robinson D, Van Allen EM, Wu YM, et al. Integrative clinical genomics of advanced prostate cancer. Cell. 2015;161(5):1215–28.
82. Nakazawa M, Antonarakis ES, Luo J. Androgen receptor splice variants in the era of enzalutamide and abiraterone. Horm Cancer. 2014;5(5):265–73. Molecular Imaging and Precision Medicine 9
83. Weissleder R, Mahmood U. Molecular imaging. Radiology. 2001;219(2):316–33.
84. Massoud TF, Gambhir SS. Molecular imaging in living subjects: seeing fundamental biological processes in a new light. Genes Dev. 2003;17(5):545–80.
85. Kaufman J, Lee M. Vascular and interventional radiology. Philadelphia, PA: Mosby; 2004. p. xi.
86. Kar S, Kumar A, Gao F, Qiu B, Zhan X, Yang X. Percutaneous optical imaging system to track reporter gene expression from vasculatures in vivo. J Biomed Opt. 2006;11(3):34008.
87. Funovics MA, Weissleder R, Mahmood U. Catheter-based in vivo imaging of enzyme activity and gene expression: feasibility study in mice. Radiology. 2004;231(3):659–66.
88. Fujimoto JG. Optical coherence tomography for ultrahigh resolution in vivo imaging. Nat Biotechnol. 2003;21(11):1361–7.
89. Yang X, Atalar E, Li D, et al. Magnetic resonance imaging permits in vivo monitoring of catheter-based vascular gene delivery. Circulation. 2001;104(14):1588–90.
90. Du X, Yang Y, Le Visage C, et al. In vivo US monitoring of catheter-based vascular delivery of gene microspheres in pigs: feasibility. Radiology. 2003;228(2):555–9.
91. Weissleder R. Molecular imaging in cancer. Science. 2006;312(5777):1168–71.
92. Bouchelouche K, Capala J, Oehr P. Positron emission tomography/computed tomography and radioimmunotherapy of prostate cancer. Curr Opin Oncologia. 2009;21(5):469–74.

93. Camacho JC, Moncayo V, Kokabi N, et al. (90) Y Radioembolization: multimodality imaging pattern approach with angiographic correlation for optimized target therapy delivery. Radiographics. 2015;35(5):1602–18.
94. Murthy R, Nunez R, Szklaruk J, et al. Yttrium-90 microsphere therapy for hepatic malignancy: devices, indications, technical considerations, and potential complications. Radiographics. 2005;25(Suppl 1):S41–55.
95. Ahmadzadehfar H, Sabet A, Muckle M, et al. 99mTc-MAA/90Y-bremsstrahlung SPECT/CT after simultaneous Tc-MAA/90Y-microsphere injection for immediate treatment monitoring and further therapy planning for radioembolization. Eur J Nucl Med Mol Imaging. 2011;38(7):1281–8.
96. Wondergem M, Smits ML, Elschot M, et al. 99mTcmacroaggregated albumin poorly predicts the intrahepatic distribution of 90Y resin microspheres in hepatic radioembolization. J Nucl Med. 2013;54(8):1294–301.
97. Ulrich G, Dudeck O, Furth C, et al. Predictive value of intratumoral 99mTc-macroaggregated albumin uptake in patients with colorectal liver metastases scheduled for radioembolization with 90Y-microspheres. J Nucl Med. 2013;54(4):516–22.
98. Kao YH, Hock Tan AE, Burgmans MC, et al. Imageguided personalized predictive dosimetry by arteryspecific SPECT/CT partition modeling for safe and effective 90Y radioembolization. J Nucl Med. 2012;53(4):559–66.
99. Eaton BR, Kim HS, Schreibmann E, et al. Quantitative dosimetry for yttrium-90 radionuclide therapy: tumor dose predicts fluorodeoxyglucose positron emission tomography response in hepatic metastatic melanoma. J VascInterv Radiol. 2014;25(2):288–95.
100. Willowson KP, Tapner M, Team QI, et al. A multicentre comparison of quantitative (90)Y PET/CT for dosimetric purposes after radioembolization with resin microspheres: the QUEST phantom study. Eur J Nucl Med Mol Imaging. 2015;42(8):1202–22.
101. Lhommel R, van Elmbt L, Goffette P, et al. Feasibility of 90Y TOF PET-based dosimetry in liver metastasis therapy using SIR-spheres. Eur J Nucl Med Mol Imaging. 2010;37(9):1654–62.

9 Positron Emission Tomography/Computed Tomography

Key Points (Abstract)

Total-body PET scans will make immuno-PET imaging and multitracer profiling feasible through delayed imaging and reduced radiation dose. As a result, multidimensional evaluation of disease heterogeneity in vivo will be practical in the clinic. Total-body PET dynamic whole-body imaging allows simultaneous functional and molecular evaluation of multiple organ systems, a concept termed systems biology imaging. Total-body PET systems biology imaging allows the further development and clinical implementation of more robust global disease assessment capabilities.

Keywords

Positron emission tomography/computed tomography · Fluorodeoxyglucose FDG · History · Physics · Instrumentation · Radiochemistry

9.1 Introduction

Medical imaging is revolutionized in recent years and these are being observed in the way medicine is being practiced. Now with this, Molecular imaging has become an important clinical decision-making tree. These modalities are playing an important role in the management of the patients. The routine use of X-ray imaging, ultrasonography, CT, and MR imaging are able to differentiate from the normal tissue and the abnormal tissues which will have the perfusion characteristics based on the enhancement patterns. Again, the normal pattern of the enhancements will be having the different presentations which are based on the post-surgery or radiotherapy changes and can cause significant damage or necrosis of the tissues. There are associated limitations for the evaluation of the anatomic extent of disease, like the radiation treatment or various therapeutic regimens. The anatomic imaging techniques and the functional imaging techniques there will be a significant change in the planar scintigraphy, single-photon emission computed tomography (SPECT), positron emission tomography (PET), and MR spectroscopy which can determine the biochemical and molecular aspect of the disease. The use of the SPECT and PET is done after the injection of radiolabelled isotope which will get accumulated in the region of the interest.

The image registration techniques can produce the "fused" image with the fusion of the SPECT or PET image in colour and CT or MR image of the same anatomic region.

The Society of Nuclear Medicine and Molecular Imaging has defined molecular imag-

S. Shaikh, *Advances in Imaging*, https://doi.org/10.1007/978-981-16-9535-3_9

ing as "the visualization, characterization, and measurement of biological processes at the molecular and cellular levels in humans and other living systems". This molecular imaging is composed of 2-dimensional (2D) or 3-dimensional (3D) imaging [1]. Positron emission tomography (PET) imaging with 2-[18F]fluoro-2-deoxy-D-glucose (FDG) is an important aspect of modern medical imaging in the pretext of personalized medicine. The available PET/computed tomography (PET/CT) is important for various current clinical along with the research applications in neurology, oncology, cardiology, and infection/inflammation.

The concept of the imaging modalities is based on the positron (b1 decay), which can combine with an electron, and these two opposite charges will annihilate to produce the gamma rays annihilation photons of each 511 keV which will be emitting the energy at exact opposite directions at 180 to each other. The positron emission tomography (PET) images are quantitative. Fluorine 18 (^{18}F) is produced by bombarding oxygen 18-enriched water with protons and produced in the cyclotron. Thus, the ^{18}F is the most important aspect of PET radiochemistry. The basic principle is that the tumours will consume more amount of the glucose causing glycolysis (known as the Warburg effect), and this will form the basis of the PET imaging by using the FDG. Again, it is based on the various technical and patient-related factors, normal distribution, physiologic uptake, and common normal variants are pivotal.

9.2 History of PET

Irene and Frederic Joliot-Curie in 1934 demonstrated that the alpha particle irradiation of aluminium, boron, and magnesium will result in the formation of the various radioactive substances which will have a particular half-life which is shorter by emitting positrons and this has formed the basis of the production of the artificial radiation [2]. They produced the first radionuclide nitrogen 13 (^{13}N), which is the important radiotracer for the myocardial PET studies. Ernest O. Lawrence's cyclotron group at Berkeley produced various radionuclides on like the ^{13}N, carbon 11 (^{11}C), oxygen 15 (^{15}O), and fluorine 18 (^{18}F) [3–5]. The detection of annihilation radiation was done by the Wren and co-workers in 1951 and documented the use of the thallium-activated sodium iodide detectors for the localization of the copper 64–phthalocyanine in brain tumours; they also produced the various coincidence detection as compared to the single-photon imaging [6]. Thus, the prototype of the positron-emission trans axial tomography (PET) II was constructed from 1972 to 1973 by the Washington University group headed by Ter-Pogossian [4]. Later, they produced newer generations of PET scanners having the functional whole-body camera, and the newer variant PETT III, having the w48 detectors was presented in 1975 [7–9]. Thus, the evolution in PET instrumentation has coincided with the development of radiochemistry. In the 1970s, Ter-Pogossian and colleagues [10] published an article in the *Scientific American* with 30 new compounds which are labelled with either ^{15}O, ^{13}N, ^{11}C, or ^{18}F. FDG was one of the components which developed in the first half of the 1970s along with the researchers of the Hospital of the University of Pennsylvania (PENN) (including Martin Reivich, David Kuhl, and Abass Alavi), and Brookhaven National Laboratory (BNL) (Alfred Wolf's team including Joanna Fowler and Tatsuo Ito) [11]. The first PET centre was established at PENN in August 1976, with FDG as the radiotracer. These tomographic scanners were of the low-energy gamma photons having the very high-energy collimators for the detection of the positron emission and they performed the first whole-body image having the dual-head rectilinear scanner with high-energy collimators.

9.3 Basic Physics

9.3.1 Positron Emission and Annihilation

PET primarily uses the very short-lived positron-emitting isotopes, which are produced by the cyclotron-produced like the ^{11}C, ^{13}N, ^{15}O, and ^{18}F as well as generator-produced gallium 68 (^{68}Ga) and rubidium 82 (^{82}Rb). By the proton irradiation of natural or enriched targets these radiotracers are being produced. Positron emission is the beta plus decay having an isobaric decay process in which the proton inside the various radionuclide nucleus is converted into a neutron and in this process, the positron and a neutrino (ne) are released. Proton-rich radionuclides are possible in the decay process which will result in the element having an atomic number which is less by one unit. Nuclear transmutation is the process of conversion of one chemical element or isotope into another. This isobaric decay process will be using the mass number of the daughter nuclei which is the same as that of the parent but the atomic number changes. Thus, the protons and neutrons are made up of various particles which are known as quarks. These proton-rich radionuclides can be converted into the stable nucleus by the positron emission or electron capture and these processes are the isobaric decay processes. Electron capture can occur with the isotopes which will have an energy difference which is insufficient. Based on the various energy difference, which is less than 1.022 MeV, then positron emission cannot be possible with the electron capture in the decay mode. Positron emission is more possible in the lower atomic weight nuclei like ^{11}C, ^{13}N, ^{15}O, and ^{18}F, however, the component t of the electron capture is more prominent in the iodine 123. The positron is the electron's antiparticle. The positron decay equation is written as follows1 Y1e11ne X and Y denote the element; A is the mass number; Z is the atomic number; e1 symbolizes the positron; and ne symbolizes an electron neutrino. Here, the positron is highly interactive and can travel for a short distance, which is a function of its energy and is defined by the following equation: Positron energy 1 neutrino energy 5 transition energy -1.022 MeV. The electron when travelling is slowed down by the various materials which will reduce the velocity and there is energy made up of the electron and a positron, which will annihilate to each other in a fraction of a second to produce two various gamma ray photons also known as the annihilation photons having the energy of the 511 keV which is equivalent to the energy equivalent for the combination of the electron and a positron and these are emitted in opposite directions exactly at 180 from each other. These annihilation photons will be emitted at 180 to each other and then these will be detected by PET detectors based on the collimation. TOF is having better contrast PET images with better sensitivity [12], Diagrams 9.1 and 9.2.

9.3.2 PET-Scanner Design

PET scanners are made up of various many small detectors which are being placed with the adjacent rings around the patient port. The modern PET system is having the state-of-the-art detectors which will have the ring diameter of 60–90 cm with the aerial extent of the 10–25 cm totally are made up of the 25,000 detectors. The single PET detector has the scintillator crystal made up of the BGO, lutetium yttrium orthosilicate [LSO], or lutetium yttrium orthosilicate [LYSO], and all these crystals will convert the energy of photons. These scintillators are optically coupled to a device, Basu et al. used the photo multiplier tube (PMT), in this the light is converted into an amplified electric signal. These photons that are being detected and accepted as the coincidence events will be connected to the two detectors. The reconstructed images use the projections, and this imaging is known as the 2D PET. The higher sensitivity can be obtained if inter-ring coincidences are termed 3D PET by the use of 3D. PET images are quantitative in nature and the reconstructed value of each image voxel in vivo for the absolute radioactivity concentration. The inhomogeneity in detector output (normalization) along with the other parameters like the dead-time effects, attenuation of coincidences, and if scattered and random coincidence events are subtracted. The 511-keV photons which are released during the various annihilation events, and they are known as the random coincidences. Fifty percent of all single scattered photons are having emitted energies which are more than 425 keV, scatter fraction is more than 50%. Most modern PET/CT systems models will be scattering the simulation model which was proposed by Watson and colleagues (Figs. 9.1 and 9.2).

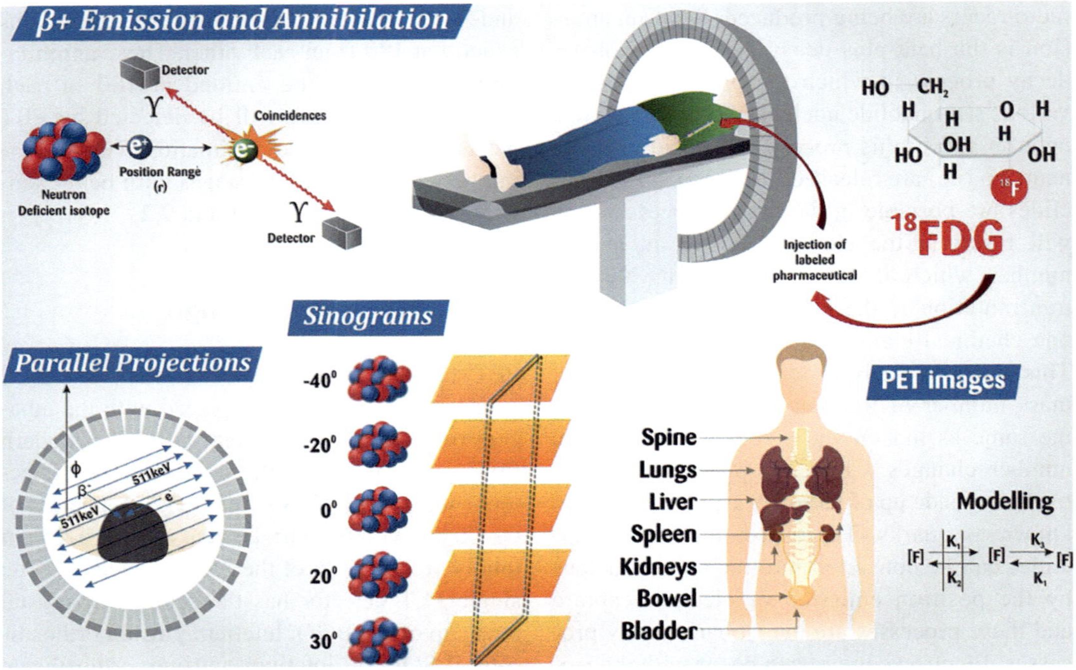

Diagram 9.1 The Emission, annihilation, and image formation of the PET-CT

Diagram 9.2 The smaller PMT blocks

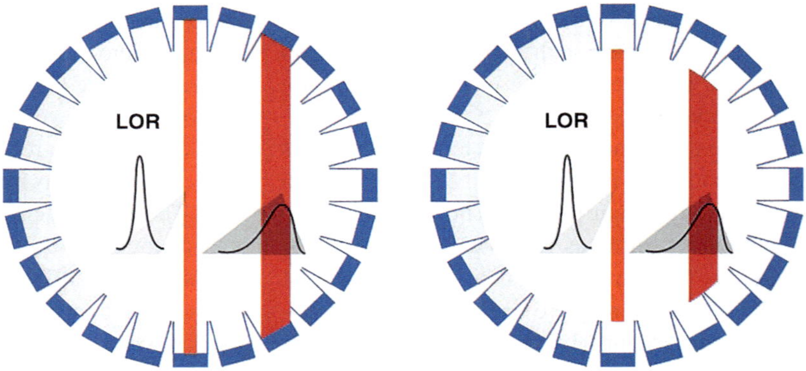

9.3.3 Novel Developments

With the advancements in the PET instrumentation, there is a significant increase in the evaluation and characterization of the small lesions and nodules by increasing the image contrast and also the partial volume effects. The major reason for the limitations of the PET spatial resolution is that there are partial volume effects in the smaller nodules due to the spill-out of the activity. Again, the size of the spatial resolution is based on the size of the detector crystals; for increasing the spatial resolution by adding the smaller crystals. The light output from the particular crystal is shared by several PMTs in our conventional PET. The important way for this PET system is to have the layer of the crystals with the 511-keV photons [13] (Diagram 9.3). Spatial resolution response from the measured response is known as the point-spread function, which is being corrected by the iterative reconstruction algorithm. The newer generation PET systems are having the

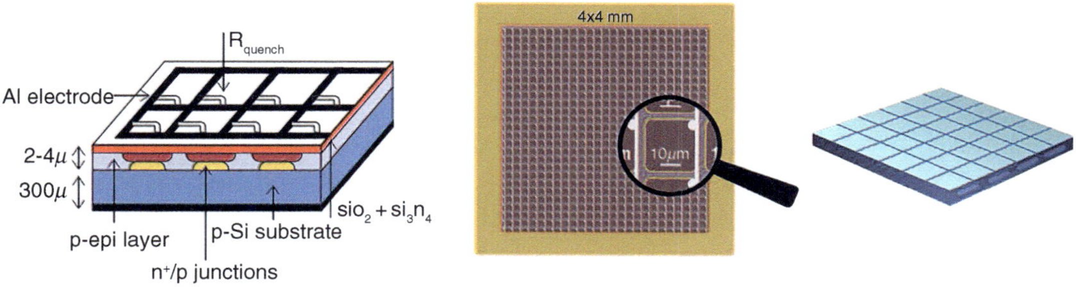

Fig. 9.1 PET-CT machine scintillators

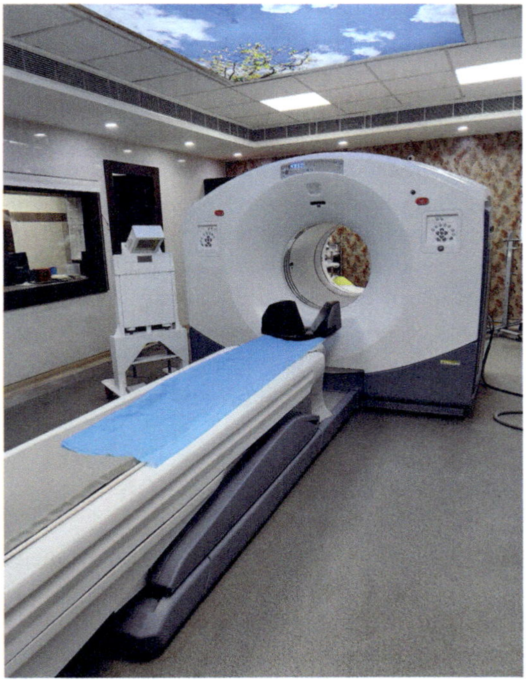

Fig. 9.2 PET-CT machine image (Image courtesy Dr. Madhur Srivastava, Department of Nuclear Medicine and PET-CT, Nizams Institute of Medical Sciences, Hyderabad)

TOF capabilities, and the biggest advantage is the TOF-PET where the image contrast is improved, and noise is reduced by making the annihilation position. Newer designs are also being focused on the reduction in patient radioactive dose and the total scan time by increasing the PET sensitivity by increasing the axial dimensions of the PET detector. Thus, the sensitivity of this is being increased significantly due to the PET and CT

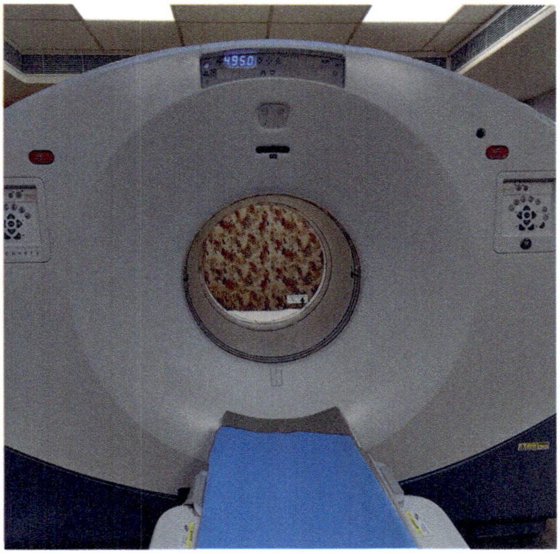

Diagram 9.3 Showing the PET-CT machine with Gantry and patient table

also and also by the PET image quality which is improved and obtained from the CT images after the attenuation correction (Fig. 9.3).

9.4 PET Radionuclides and Production of FDG

^{18}F is the important and most widely used radiotracer in PET radiochemistry. This is produced in a cyclotron by the nuclear reaction between oxygen 18 (^{18}O)-enriched water which is being bombarded with protons thus reducing the production equation. ^{18}F is produced when bombarded with the ^{18}O-enriched water. Hydrogen fluoride (HF) in water is formed by the synthesis module and

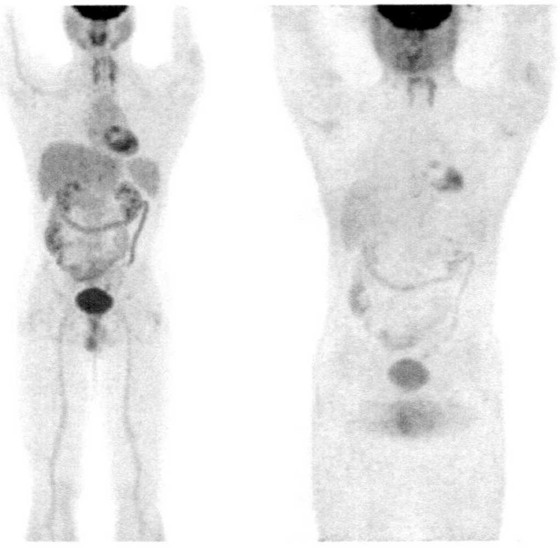

Fig. 9.3 The corrected and uncorrected image differences

Table 9.1 Important PET nuclides and their preparation

Nuclide	Production	Half-life
F-18(F^-)	$^{18}O(p,n)^{18}F$	110 min
F-18(F_2)	$^{20}Ne(d,\alpha)^{18}F$	110 min
C-11	$^{14}N(p,\alpha)^{11}C$	20 min
N-13	$^{16}O(p,\alpha)^{13}N$	10 min
O-15	$^{14}N(d,n)^{15}O$	2 min
Ga-68	$^{68}Ge/^{68}Ga$-generator	68 min
Rb-82	$^{82}Sr/^{82}Rb$-generator	1.3 min

absorbed on the QMA column. Thus, the sodium hydroxide is being purified by the purification cartridges before sterile filtration and formulation into sodium chloride and ethanol (Table 9.1).

9.4.1 The FDG Concept

Tumours have increased glycolysis (known as the Warburg effect) due to consumption of more glucose and this principle is used for the common use of FDG as a tracer in the PET. FDG is a radiolabelled glucose analogue in which the ^{18}F is substituted by the 20-hydroxyl group. The uptake in the tissue is similar to that of the normal glucose. This FDG is passed through the cellular membrane which is mediated by the glucose transporters (GLUTs), and there are 14 different isoforms that are being identified [14]. GLUT1 is the commonest glucose transporter in humans and GLUT3 is more commonly expressed in the tumours [15]. The half-life of 110 minutes is ideal for the synthesis and the low positron energy (640 keV) will be resulting in a short tissue range (2.3 mm) higher resolution and low radiation dose. ^{18}F can be used for dynamic studies also. Final steps in FDG synthesis: (1) Acetylated mannose triflate. (2) Acetylated FDG. (3) FDG.

The Basic Principles of FDG-PET/CT Imaging is showing the most commonly use in the various cancers like (e.g. breast cancer) [16]. The GLUT1 expression will be correlating with the tumour development which is not favourable [17]. FDG inside the cell is phosphorylated by hexokinase resulting in the FDG-6-phosphate, and this cannot be further metabolized. The reduced levels of glucose-6-phosphatase in cancer cells will cause the accumulation of FDG-phosphate in cancer cells [18, 19]. But the biggest disadvantage is that the FDG is not specific for cancer and is accumulated in the infection and inflammation and also in the various normal tissue which is having high glucose turnover.

9.4.2 Factors Influencing FDG

FDG uptake in cancer cells is based on the metabolic activity of tumour. There are other factors that will have an impact are tumour cells, histologic type, tumour grade, proliferative activity, and neovascularization which is important for the delivery of enough quantity of glucose and oxygen [20]. If the vascularization is less, then it will lead to hypoxia, due to the lower partial pressure of oxygen in comparison to the normal tissue. Hypoxia varies in a solid tumour, and these hypoxic states will have hypoxic regions indicating the sign of more malignancy and aggressiveness of tumours which will be having a poor prognosis and also resistance to the therapy [21]. This hypoxic response is based on the hypoxia-inducible factor (HIF) due to accumulation of DNA-binding transcription factors due to rapid degradation [22]. ^{18}F-FDG Accumulation along with the GLUT, HK, HIF, and Glucose6-

Phosphatase causes increased in the glucose metabolism based on the amount of the glycolysis. The amount of FDG uptake is quantified by the standardized uptake value [SUV] with the expression of the GLUTs, hexokinases, glucose-6-phosphatase, and also, the Ki67, a proliferation marker [23]. This expression is done by immunohistochemical staining. One of the studies is showing the correlation between SUV and the glucose-6-phosphatase expression but no significant correlation is being found with the OSCC, along with the GLUT1, HK2, and HIF [24, 25].

9.5 Patient Preparation, Physiologic Uptake, and Pitfalls

FDG is a glucose analogue, and the distribution pattern is based on the physiologic glucose metabolism. For the evaluation of various pathologies by FDG the blood glucose levels should be in the normal range, of the (w150–200 mg/dL). If the glucose levels are higher than this, then the procedure should be postponed rather than doing it with the insulin injection and stabilizing the glucose levels to normal. The basis of insulin-induced hypoglycaemia will cause the reduction in the tumour uptake which will be facilitating the increased physiologic uptake in muscles and fat, causing the reduction in the tumour-to-background ratio. Higher levels can also be accepted in patients with known type 2 diabetes which will cause the hyperglycaemia (>11 mmol/L, w200 mg/dL) impacting least on the FDG uptake [26].

9.6 Normal FDG-PET

The normal concentration of the radiotracer activity will be seen in the brain, heart, and salivary glands. The tracer accumulation is also seen in the urinary bladder due to the excretion in the urinary bladder. If the patient is not properly fasting, then the physiologic uptake will be seen in the muscles (Fig. 9.4). The myocardium uptake will be uniform and intense due to the myocardial activity. This uptake pattern is more prominent in the left ventricle on contrary the right ventricle and atria will not have any FDG uptake. In the cases of prolonged fasting of more than 18 hours, the low-carbohydrate high-fat diet will be causing the substrate to shift from glucose to free fatty acids. The uptake patterns in liver, spleen, and bone marrow are uniformly homogenous and low. There can be a diffuse increase in the bone marrow uptake in various systemic inflammations, prolonged bleeding, or various therapeutic interventions associated with chemotherapy or bone marrow stimulants. Skeletal muscles consume the maximum amount of glucose, and the pattern of uptake is uniform unless it is due to voluntary movements which will be showing increased activity. But sometimes there will be increased activity due to the anxiety and anxiolytic can be given, if necessary, sometimes. Brown fat is also an important cause of increased metabolic activity, especially in children and young adults during the cold months. This brown fat uptake needs to be differentiated from other pathological conditions like lymphoma and various head-and-neck cancers. The concept is that the brown fat is sympathetically innervated, sometimes the beta-blockers can be administered for controlling the temperature. As already mentioned, the physiologic FDG uptake in the genitourinary system is also the bigger challenge This can be partly adjusted by giving proper hydration, sometimes diuretics, and also bladder catheterization but these are not accepted as standard protocols to be practised. Testicles uptake is sometimes moderate and is seen due to age. Similarly is the case with the ovaries and uterine cavity in premenopausal women during ovulation and menstruation. A similar amount of uptake is also seen in glandular tissue of the breast. Another area of the uptake which is seen is the thyroid gland and the gastrointestinal tract. The thyroid uptake patterns can be foal or represent the nodule of thyroiditis, respectively. But these sorts of findings are also seen in the malignancies or premalignant conditions in approximately 33% of patients [27]. Gastrointestinal tract uptake is also a common finding and is variable in locations. Focal uptake seen at the gastroesophageal junction which is mostly physiologic or but sometimes the association can be with the ulcers as well as reflux.

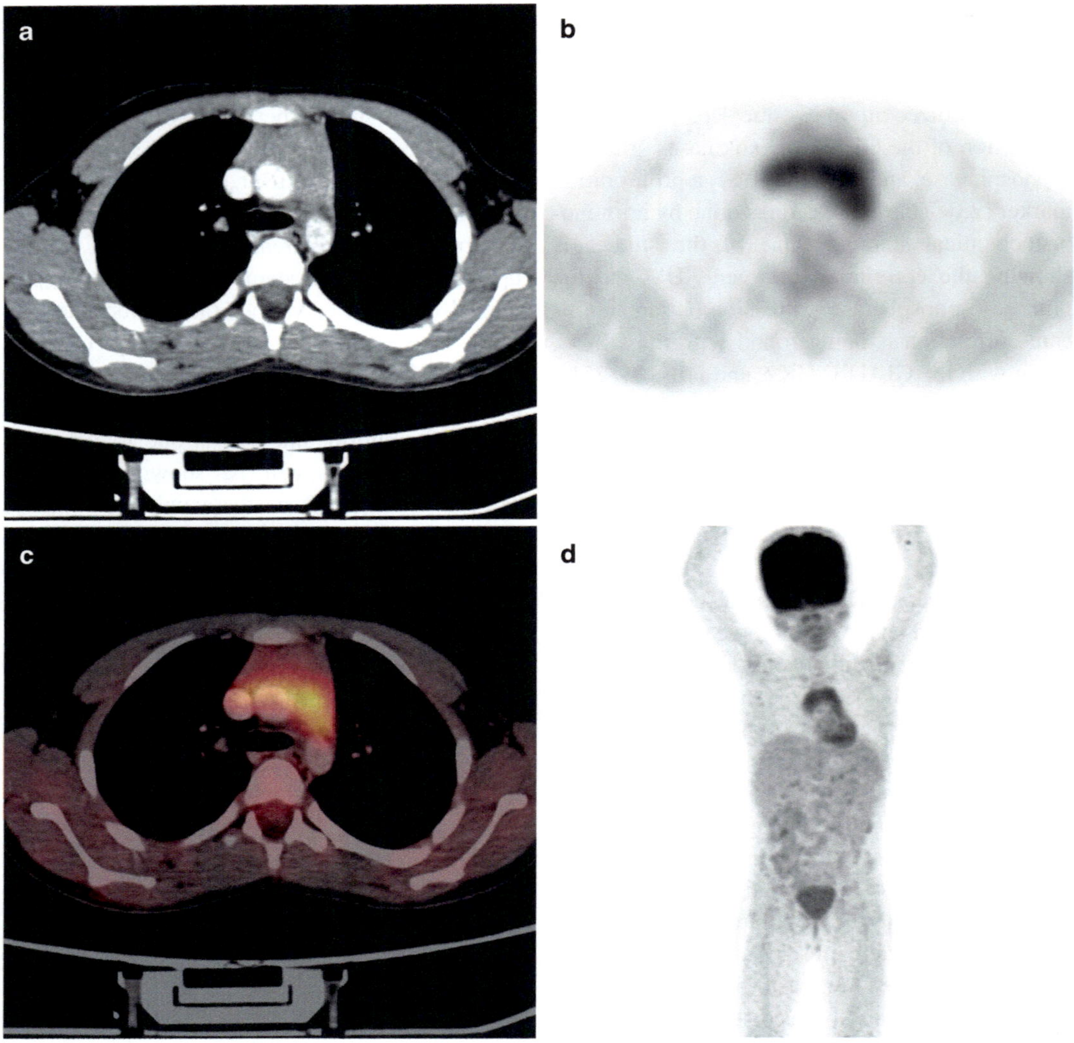

Fig. 9.4 Normal PET-CT image with normal physiological uptake in Brain, Cardiac, and Urinary bladder. (**a–c**) Axial images at the level of mediatinum showing normal physiological uptake. (**d**) Whole body PET image showing normal physiological uptake in brain, cardia and urinary bladder

Also, the normal cerebral cortex has more little uptake (Fig. 9.5).

The physiologic colonic uptake can be faint and diffuse or intense and focal; and can be seen in the entire colon but the caecum and rectosigmoid are common regions of the uptake. The mechanism of this intestinal uptake is probably due to the smooth muscle activity, metabolically active mucosa, luminal contents, or glycolytic bacteria but not clearly established criteria.

The PET/CT imaging with FDG and other radiotracers is based on the various physiologic, pathophysiologic, chemical, radiochemical, physical, radio physical, and various technical concepts and processes, due to which the imaging modalities will be little difficult to understand.

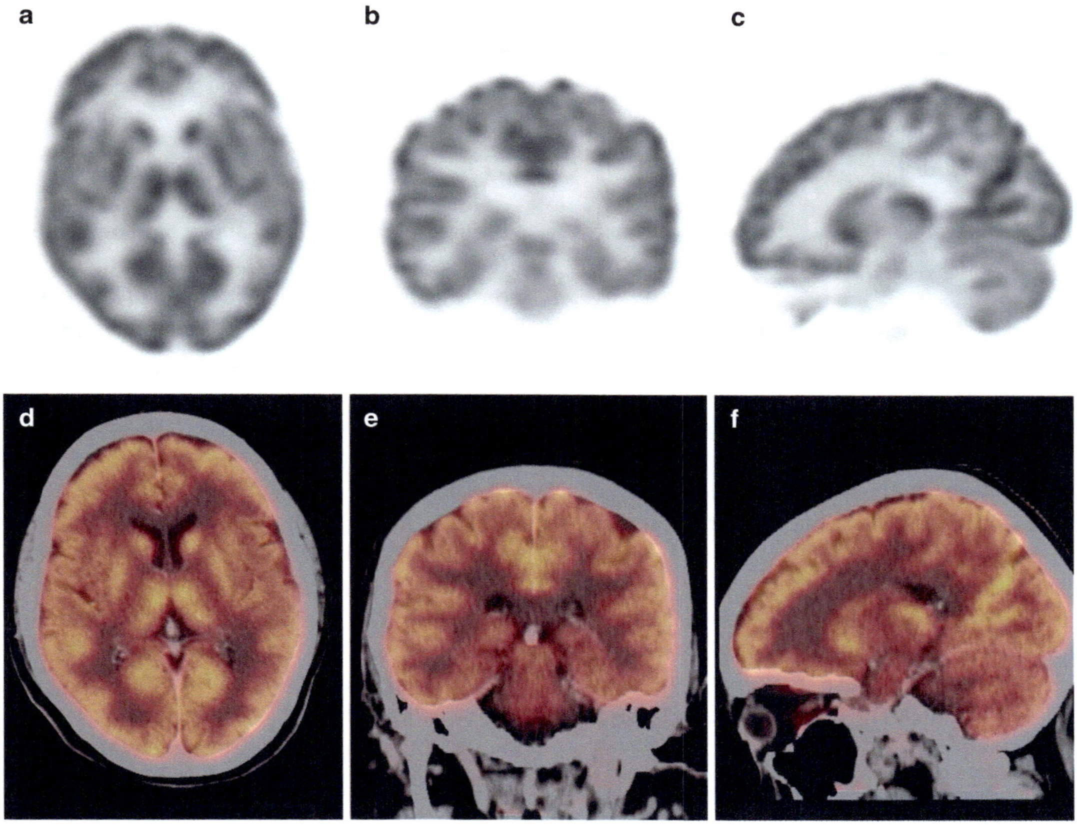

Fig. 9.5 Normal cerebral parenchyma uptake. **a**, **b** and **c** are PET Brain images showing the normal uptake in cerebral parenchyma. **d**, **e** and **f** showing fused PET-CT images with normal cerebral parenchyma

9.7 Whole-Body PET

WB-PET imaging protocol has significantly increased the sensitivity, and this can be used for various strategies like the signal-to-noise ratio, temporal resolution, or less radioactive dose [28, 29].

9.8 Clinical Applications

The conventional PET imaging techniques is having some of limitations in diffuse lesions, which are involving many structures in the body. Limited sensitivity and field of view approximately up to 20–30 cm, for the whole-body imaging is little tedious taking more time for the imaging [30].

Whole-body imaging is the concept used in the various common pathologies like cancer, inflammatory and immunologic disorders, cardiovascular disease, and osteoporosis, where many structures and organs of the body need to be evaluated [31, 32]. Hybrid molecular and structural imaging with PET and computed tomography (CT) scans or MR imaging are the modalities for the diagnosis of these pathologies. More focus is seen on the structures which are to be evaluated in the form of cancer, atherosclerosis, systemic inflammation, and musculoskeletal disorders [33–40]. It can be used for improving the temporal resolution for evaluation of tumour burden, for better management of the serious, disabling, and various fatal diseases and disorders. The use of dynamic whole-body imaging to perform delayed imaging can be evaluated for pathobiology kinetics [41]. Better signal-to-noise ratio (SNR), enhanced temporal resolution (T), or reduction of the required dose of the radiotracer injection can be analyzed. The cardiovascular involvement of autoimmune disorders is the tip of the iceberg.

9.9 Oncology Dose Reduction

Due to the significantly increased sensitivity of PET imaging, reduced dose amount is needed for the imaging [42, 43]. Tumour heterogeneity is an important aspect of the treatment failure in cancer [30].

Molecular imaging for the treatment evaluation can be seen in the personalized management of diseases [30]. The amount of radiation exposure for the immuno-PET imaging is more confirmed by various clinical studies and research and cannot be justified. The whole-body PET-CT to characterize tumour heterogeneity with multiple immuno-PET tracers in series with conventional PET imaging the exposure will be more than 100 mSv.

9.10 Delayed Imaging

Delayed imaging is being done for the evaluation of the varied pathologies like rectal lesions, to differentiate between the infection inflammation and malignancies based on the metabolic activity changes [44–46]. Basu and colleagues [46] demonstrated a significant increase in metabolic activity in lung primary cancer lesions even after 8 hours after the injection. This concept not only clearly signifies the cancer activity in the primary sites, and along with this there will be increased activity and sensitivity for the accurate staging of the tumours. Another aspect of the imaging is the FDG uptake decreases after 1–3 h of the injection in the majority of normal tissues, benign lesions except heart and bone marrow. Thus, enhancing the contrast between tumour activity and the adjacent lesion in surrounding tissues [47]. The disadvantage is that the physiological bone marrow activity needs to be differentiated between the metastatic marrow lesions. Thus, delayed FDG-PET imaging will be helpful in the evaluation of the various stages of the disease.

9.11 Dynamic Imaging

Full field of view and enhanced temporal resolution will be improving the dynamic quantification of radiotracer uptake [48]. This kinetic analysis is being used in FDG PET imaging. The tumours which show increased uptake over the period of time are aggressive lesions as compared to the lesions which will have the decreasing standardized uptake value over time. Dynamic imaging is more helpful in the evaluation of the various effects and the side effects on various body organs and the systems. Atherosclerosis can be seen with the significant morbidity and mortality associated with the various disorders [49, 50]. FDG40 and ^{18}F-sodium fluoride (NaF), [51–53] are being used commonly for the PET imaging of patients having malignancies best suited for the detection of the various atherosclerotic plaques. Early detection and management of venous thromboembolism in malignant diseases can be evaluated. NaF-PET imaging is important for the evaluation of the bone turnover [54] and for these various quantitative methods are being used [55, 56]. This bone turnover evaluation can be helpful for the prevention of disease-related fractures.

9.12 Inflammation

Autoimmune disorders are usually starting in one organ and involving multiple organs in the definition [57]. The assessment of the inflammation in various organs like the musculoskeletal pathologies will be benefitted from the whole-body imaging with PET. The coronal fused images are showing the increased metabolism. Autoimmune disorders and viral infections are multisystemic and the severe acute respiratory syndrome coronavirus-2 coronavirus disease-2019 disease are systemic in nature and will be involving the various organs in the body [58].

Cardiovascular Atherosclerosis is also the commonest cause of morbidity and mortality, especially in the elderly patients with significant involvement of the arteries in the body. The atherosclerotic plaques are showing increased uptake with the increased glycolytic activity and can be diagnosed by FDG-PET. Delayed imaging after the first scans will be better or better results.

9.13 Osteoporosis

Osteoporosis is the commonest cause of morbidity in older age patients and especially in postmenopausal patients in women. The osteoporosis can be due to the changes impacted due to chemotherapeutic agents. More commonly seen in the spine and lower extremities resulting in the pulmonary embolism. NaF-PET imaging is being used in osteoporosis and can be detected in dual-energy X-ray scans. NaF PET scanning has become the modality of choice for osteoporosis.

9.14 Advances in Anatomically Guided Quantification of PET Data

Multimodality imaging is based on the fusion of functional and anatomic imaging data for the anatomic and functional localization. Zaidi et al. showed the various abnormalities in the region-of-interest (ROI). Various factors like attenuation correction, transmission-based modelling, motion detection, and also motion correction and volume correction will be impacting on the image quality [59]. PET Attenuation and Scatter Compensation attenuation has greater advantages seen in the conventional transmission-based scanning [60]. The misregistration between CT and PET images can have respiratory motion, truncation artefacts, various contrast mediums, metallic implants, X-ray scatter in CT images [61]. MR imaging-guided attenuation is still not being as set protocol for the whole-body imaging [62, 63]. Without this, it will be easier for the hybrid PET/MR imaging to be done. The physics of interaction and detection of emitted photons to estimate the scatter magnitude and distribution accurately [64].

Various transmission-based scatter corrections by the various attenuation map for the distribution of scattered events using line integrals will be calculated as part of the attenuation correction options [65–67].

9.14.1 Anatomically Guided PET Image Reconstruction

Maximum likelihood–expectation maximizations (ML-EM) are the newer algorithms in which the number of iterations can be maximum and will significantly increase the noise of the PET images [68].

9.14.2 Anatomically Guided Partial Volume Correction in PET

The low spatial resolution is the basis for the various scanners. The activity concentration is equal to or twice the system's spatial resolutions with the full-width-at-half-maximum (FWHM). PET/CT is helpful for the identification of the gross tumour volume, which can be delineated for radiotherapy treatment planning. Zaidi et al. showed that the reconstruction process for the PVE along with the photon attenuation, scattered radiation, and other physical effects will be directly related to the reconstructed algorithm.

The ongoing advancements will be doing the various developments in software- and hardware-based multimodality imaging which will be combining the PET with PET/CT or PET/MR imaging [69]. The concept of multimodality imaging is being revolutionized in the last two decades last 2 decades [70]. Some doubts are there related to the future role of SPECT in the era of PET [71–74]. The dual-modality imaging systems of the PET are the important key components for the assessment of response to treatment, and also for the delivery of personalized treatments and targeted therapies [75, 76].

References

1. Mankoff DA. A definition of molecular imaging. J Nucl Med 2007;48:18N, 21N.
2. Joliot-Curie F, Curie I. Artificial production of a new kind of radioelement. Nature. 1934;133:201.
3. Ter-Pogossian M. The origins of positron emission tomography. Semin Nucl Med. 1992;22(3):140–9.
4. Rich DA. A brief history of positron emission tomography. J Nucl Med Technol. 1997;25(1):4–11.
5. Wagner HW Jr. A brief history of positron emission tomography (PET). Semin Nucl Med. 1998;28(3):213–20.
6. Kuhl DE, Edwards RQ. Image separation radioisotope scanning. Radiology. 1963;80:653–61.
7. Cho ZH, Chan JK, Eriksson L. Circular ring transverse axial positron camera for three-dimensional reconstruction of radionuclides distribution. IEEE Trans Nucl Sci. 1976;NS-23:613–22.
8. Cho ZH, Farukhi MR. Bismuth germinate as a potential scintillation detector in positron cameras. J Nucl Med. 1977;18:840–4.
9. Ter-Pogossian MM, Mullani NA, Ficke DC, et al. Photon time-of-flight-assisted positron emission tomography. J Comput Assist Tomogr. 1981;5:227–39.
10. Ter-Pogossian MM, Raichle ME, Sobel BE. Positron emission tomography. Sci Am. 1980;243:170–81.
11. Hess S, Høilund-Carlsen PF, Alavi A. Historic images in nuclear medicine 1976: the first issue of clinical nuclear medicine and the first human FDG study. Clin Nucl Med. 2014;39:701–3.
12. Karp JS, Surti S, Daube-Witherspoon ME, et al. Benefit of time-of-flight in PET: experimental and clinical results. J Nucl Med. 2008;49(3):462–70.
13. Sossi V, de Jong HW, Barker WC, et al. The second generation HRRT: a multi-Centre scanner performance investigation. IEEE Nucl Sci Symp Conf Rec. 2005;4:2195–9.
14. Macheda ML, Rogers S, Best JD. Molecular and cellular regulation of glucose transporter (GLUT) proteins in cancer. J Cell Physiol. 2005;202:654–62.
15. Ganapathy V, Thangaraju M, Prasad PD. Nutrient transporters in cancer: relevance to Warburg hypothesis and beyond. Pharmacol Ther. 2009;121:29–40.
16. Moadel RM, Weldon RH, Katz EB, et al. Positherapy: targeted nuclear therapy of breast cancer with 18F-2-deoxy-2-fluoro-D-glucose. Cancer Res. 2005;65:698–702.
17. Szablewski L. Expression of glucose transporters in cancers. Biochim Biophys Acta. 2013;1835:164–9.
18. Nelson CA, Wang JQ, Leav I, et al. The interaction among glucose transport, hexokinase, and glucose-6-phosphatase with respect to 3H-2-deoxyglucose retention in murine tumor models. Nucl Med Biol. 1996;23:533–41.
19. Yamada T, Uchida M, Kwang-Lee K, et al. Correlation of metabolism/hypoxia markers and fluorodeoxyglucose uptake in oral squamous cell carcinomas. Oral Surg Oral Med Oral Pathol Oral Radiol. 2012;113:464–71.
20. Bos R, van Der Hoeven JJ, van Der Wall E, et al. Biologic correlates of (18)fluorodeoxyglucose uptake in human breast cancer measured by positron emission tomography. J Clin Oncol. 2002;20:379–87.
21. Bertout JA, Patel SA, Simon MC. The impact of O2 availability on human cancer. Nat Rev Cancer. 2008;8:967–75.
22. Avril N, Menzel M, Dose J, et al. Glucose metabolism of breast cancer assessed by 18F-FDG PET: histologic and immunohistochemical tissue analysis. J Nucl Med. 2001;42:9–16.
23. Scholzen T, Gerdes J. The Ki-67 protein: from the known and the unknown. J Cell Physiol. 2000;182:311–22.
24. Tixier F, Le Rest CC, Hatt M, et al. Intratumor heterogeneity characterized by textural features on baseline 18F-FDG PET images predicts response to concomitant radio chemotherapy in oesophageal cancer. J Nucl Med. 2011;52:369–78.
25. Tixier F, HattM VC, et al. Visual versus quantitative assessment of intratumor 18F-FDG PET uptake heterogeneity: prognostic value in non-small cell lung cancer. J Nucl Med. 2014:pii:jnumed.113.133389.
26. Hara T, Higashi T, Nakamoto Y, et al. Significance of chronic marked hyperglycaemia on FDG-PET: is it really problematic for clinical oncologic imaging? Ann Nucl Med. 2009;23:657–69.
27. Shie P, Cardarelli R, Sprawls K, et al. Systematic review: prevalence of malignant incidental thyroid nodules identified on fluorine-18 fluorodeoxyglucose positron emission tomography. Nucl Med Commun. 2009;30(9):742–8.
28. Cherry SR, Jones T, Karp JS, et al. Total-body PET: maximizing sensitivity to create new opportunities for clinical research and patient care. J Nucl Med. 2018;59(1):3–12.
29. Badawi RD, Shi H, Hu P, et al. First human imaging studies with the EXPLORER total-body PET scanner. J Nucl Med. 2019;60(3):299–303.
30. Alavi A, Werner TJ, Høilund-Carlsen PF. What can be and what cannot be accomplished with PET: rectifying ongoing misconceptions. Clin Nucl Med. 2017;42(8):603.
31. Raynor WY, Al-Zaghal A, Zadeh MZ, et al. Metastatic seeding attacks bone marrow, not bone: rectifying ongoing misconceptions. PET Clin. 2019;14(1):135–44.
32. Raynor WY, Zadeh MZ, Kothekar E, et al. Evolving role of PET-based novel quantitative techniques in the management of hematological malignancies. PET Clin. 2019;14(3):331–40.
33. Raynor WY, Jonnakuti VS, Zirakchian Zadeh M, et al. Comparison of methods of quantifying global synovial metabolic activity with FDG-PET/CT in rheumatoid arthritis. Int J Rheum Dis. 2019;22(12):2191–8.
34. Khosravi M, Peter J, Wintering NA, et al. 18F-FDG is a superior indicator of cognitive performance compared to 18F-florbetapir in Alzheimer's disease and mild cognitive impairment evaluation: a global quantitative analysis. J Alzheimers Dis. 2019;70(4):1197–207.

35. Saboury B, Parsons MA, Moghbel M, et al. Quantification of aging effects upon global knee inflammation by 18F-FDG-PET. Nucl Med Commun. 2016;37(3):254–8.
36. Peter J, Houshmand S, Werner TJ, et al. Applications of global quantitative 18F-FDG-PET analysis in temporal lobe epilepsy. Nucl Med Commun. 2016;37(3):223–30. https://doi.org/10.1097/MNM.0000000000000440.
37. Fardin S, Gholami S, Samimi S, et al. Global quantitative techniques for positron emission tomographic assessment of disease activity in cutaneous T-cell lymphoma and response to treatment. JAMA Dermatol. 2016;152(1):103–5.
38. Marin-Oyaga VA, Salavati A, Houshmand S, et al. Feasibility and performance of an adaptive contrast-oriented FDG PET/CT quantification technique for global disease assessment of malignant pleural mesothelioma and a brief review of the literature. Hell J Nucl Med. 2015;18(1):11–8.
39. Basu S, Zaidi H, Salavati A, et al. FDG PET/CT methodology for evaluation of treatment response in lymphoma: from "graded visual analysis" and "semiquantitative SUVmax" to global disease burden assessment. Eur J Nucl Med Mol Imaging. 2014;41(11):2158–60.
40. Seraj SM, Ayubcha C, Zadeh MZ, et al. The evolving role of PET-based novel quantitative techniques in the interventional radiology procedures of the liver. PET Clin. 2019;14(4):419–25.
41. Høilund-Carlsen PF, Edenbrandt L, Alavi A. Global disease score (GDS) is the name of the game! Eur J Nucl Med Mol Imaging. 2019;46(9):1768–72.
42. Pinu FR, Beale DJ, Paten AM, et al. Systems biology and multi-omics integration: viewpoints from the metabolomics research community. Meta. 2019;9(4):76.
43. Mardinoglu A, Boren J, Smith U, et al. Systems biology in hepatology: approaches and applications. Nat Rev Gastroenterol Hepatol. 2018;15(6):365–77.
44. Pauwels EK, Ribeiro MJ, Stoot JH, et al. FDG accumulation and tumor biology. Nucl Med Biol. 1998;25(4):317–22.
45. Zhuang H, Pourdehnad M, Lambright ES, et al. Dual time point 18F-FDG PET imaging for differentiating malignant from inflammatory processes. J Nucl Med. 2001;42(9):1412–7.
46. Basu S, Kung J, Houseni M, et al. Temporal profile of fluorodeoxyglucose uptake in malignant lesions and normal organs over extended time periods in patients with lung carcinoma: implications for its utilization in assessing malignant lesions. Q J Nucl Med Mol Imaging. 2009;53(1):9.
47. Cheng G, Alavi A, Lim E, et al. Dynamic changes of FDG uptake and clearance in normal tissues. Mol Imaging Biol. 2013;15(3):345–52.
48. Cherry SR, Badawi RD, Karp JS, et al. Total-body imaging: transforming the role of positron emission tomography. Sci Transl Med. 2017;9(381):eaaf6169.
49. Ogawa A, Kanda T, Sugihara S, et al. Risk factors for myocardial infarction in cancer patients. J Med. 1995;26(5–6):221–33.
50. Dardiotis E, Aloizou A-M, Markoula S, et al. Cancer associated stroke: pathophysiology, detection and management. Int J Oncol. 2019;54(3):779–96.
51. Beheshti M, Saboury B, Mehta NN, et al. Detection and global quantification of cardiovascular molecular calcification by fluoro18-fluoride positron emission tomography/computed tomography–a novel concept. Hell J Nucl Med. 2011;14(2):114–20.
52. Moghbel M, Al-Zaghal A, Werner TJ, et al. The role of PET in evaluating atherosclerosis: a critical review. Semin Nucl Med. 2018;48(6):488–97.
53. Høilund-Carlsen PF, Sturek M, Alavi A, et al. Atherosclerosis imaging with 18F-sodium fluoride PET: state-of-the-art review. Eur J Nucl Med Mol Imaging. 2020;47(6):1538–51.
54. Blake GM, Siddique M, Frost ML, et al. Imaging of site-specific bone turnover in osteoporosis using positron emission tomography. Curr Osteoporosis Rep. 2014;12(4):475–85.
55. Raijmakers P, Temmerman OPP, Saridin CP, et al. Quantification of F-18-fluoride kinetics: evaluation of simplified methods. J Nucl Med. 2014;55(7):1122–7.
56. Al-beyatti Y, Siddique M, Frost ML, et al. Precision of F-18-fluoride PET skeletal kinetic studies in the assessment of bone metabolism. Osteoporosis Int. 2012;23(10):2535–41.
57. Rankin LC, Artis D. Beyond host defence: emerging functions of the immune system in regulating complex tissue physiology. Cell. 2018;173(3):554–67.
58. Henrich TJ, Hsue PY, VanBrocklin H. Seeing is believing: nuclear imaging of HIV persistence. Front Immunol. 2019;10:2077.
59. Basu S, Zaidi H, Houseni M, et al. Novel quantitative techniques for assessing regional and global function and structure based on modern imaging modalities: implications for normal variation, aging and diseased states. Semin Nucl Med. 2007;37:223–39.
60. Zaidi H. Is radionuclide transmission scanning obsolete for dual-modality PET/CT systems? Eur J Nucl Med Mol Imaging. 2007;34:815–8.
61. Zaidi H, Montandon M-L, Alavi A. Advances in attenuation correction techniques in PET. PET Clinics. 2007;2:191–217.
62. Zaidi H. Is MRI-guided attenuation correction a viable option for dual-modality PET/MR imaging? Radiology. 2007;244:639–42.
63. Hofmann M, Pichler B, Scholkopf B, et al. Towards quantitative PET/MRI: a review of MR-based attenuation correction techniques. Eur J Nucl Med Mol Imaging. 2009;36:93–104.
64. Zaidi H, Montandon M-L. Scatter compensation techniques in PET. PET clinics 2007;2:219–34. 102. Watson CC. New, faster, image-based scatter correction for 3D PET. IEEE Trans Nucl Sci. 2000;47:1587–94.

65. Levin CS, Dahlbom M, Hoffman EJ. A Monte Carlo correction for the effect of Compton scattering in 3-D PET brain imaging. IEEE Trans Nucl Sci. 1995;42:1181–8.
66. Zaidi H. Comparative evaluation of scatter correction techniques in 3D positron emission tomography. Eur J Nucl Med. 2000;27:1813–26.
67. Holdsworth CH, Levin CS, Janecek M, et al. Performance analysis of an improved 3-D PET Monte Carlo simulation and scatter correction. IEEE Trans Nucl Sci. 2002;49:83–9.
68. Reader AJ, Zaidi H. Advances in PET image reconstruction. PET Clinics. 2007;2:173–90.
69. Baete K, Nuyts J, Laere KV, et al. Evaluation of anatomy-based reconstruction for partial volume correction in brain FDG-PET. NeuroImage. 2004;23:305–17.
70. Zaidi H. Navigating beyond the 6th dimension: a challenge in the era of multi-parametric molecular imaging. Eur J Nucl Med Mol Imaging. in press
71. Rahmim A, Zaidi H. PET versus SPECT: strengths, limitations, and challenges. Nucl Med Commun. 2008;29:193–207.
72. Alavi A, Basu S. Planar and SPECT imaging in the era of PET and PET–CT: can it survive the test of time? Eur J Nucl Med Mol Imaging. 2008;35:1554–9.
73. Mariani G, Bruselli L, Duatti A. Is PET always an advantage versus planar and SPECT imaging? Eur J Nucl Med Mol Imaging. 2008;35:1560–5.
74. Seret A. Will high-resolution/high-sensitivity SPECT ensure that PET is not the only survivor in nuclear medicine during the next decade? Eur J Nucl Med Mol Imaging. 2009;36:533–5.
75. Hess S, Blomberg BA, Zhu H, et al. The pivotal role of FDG-PET/CT in modern medicine. Acad Radiol. 2014;21:232–49.
76. Kinahan PE, Hasegawa BH, Beyer T. X-ray–based attenuation correction for positron emission tomography/computed tomography scanners. Semin Nucl Med. 2003;33:166–79.

PET-MRI

10

Key Points (Abstracts)

PET/MR is the recent and one of the key available imagings. The biggest advantage is the non-invasive nature used for the characterization and quantitative evaluation of various molecular and physiologic processes by the biomarkers in vivo at the cellular level in healthy as well as the various disease states, including neurology, psychiatry, cardiology, and oncology. Thus, hybrid imaging is the combination of PET with CT and MRI which are the anatomical imaging modalities which have revolutionized the concept of molecular imaging.

Keywords

PET-MR · Annihilation · Attenuation correction · DWI

10.1 Introduction

10.1.1 Instrumentation and Design of PET/MR

The available PET/MR imaging scanners are of two prototypes: sequential and simultaneous systems [1]. In the sequential PET/MR systems, there are two separate PET and MR imaging systems which are physically separated by a rotating table. This is rather simple in the construction and only minor modifications can make this system viable. This will be more prone to image misregistration due to the separation of the PET and MR imaging data and need more space [2–4]. Integrated PET/MR imaging is a little complex modality where the PET detectors are inserted between the gradient and radiofrequency body coils of the scanner. The electromagnetic interactions between magnetic field-insensitive avalanche photodiodes and silicon photomultiplier detectors need to be avoided to a larger extent. The simultaneous acquisition of the data has shorter scan times and misregistration is less. But the respiratory motion artefacts are more common in the upper abdomen [5–7] (Fig. 10.1).

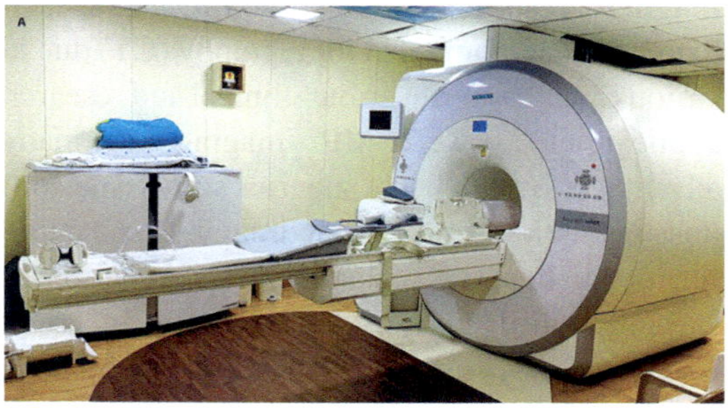

Fig. 10.1 PET-MR Machine

S. Shaikh, *Advances in Imaging*, https://doi.org/10.1007/978-981-16-9535-3_10

10.2 PET/MR Imaging Protocol

Integrated whole-body PET/MR is made up of two parts: whole-body PET/MR imaging and dedicated regional MR imaging. The whole-body imaging protocol is same while the regional analysis of the area or region of interest is variable. PET/MR imaging efficiency will be based on the timing of the scans which should not extend beyond too much time [8, 9]. Again, the use of the focussed dedicated MR imaging can also have an impact on the MR imaging sequences based on the various clinical indications. This is very important in oncologic patients [10].

10.3 Whole-Body PET/MR Imaging Protocol

Commonly used whole-body MR imaging sequences will include DWI and short tau inversion recovery (STIR) imaging sequences. Whole-body DWI is more preferred in the lymphoma, [11, 12] and whole-body coronal STIR imaging for the detection of bony lesions. DWI with apparent diffusion coefficient (ADC) maps will be more useful to evaluate the primary tumour and also to differentiate the posttreatment inflammation versus fibrosis from viable neoplasm [13–15]. DWI is also having a very high sensitivity for the detection of lymph node and peritoneal metastases [16, 17].

Positron emission tomography (PET) and magnetic resonance (MR) imaging are superior to that of PET/computed tomography (CT) due to various applications, various clinical and research applications as well. MR imaging has many advantages over CT like superior soft-tissue contrast resolution, multiplanar imaging, and other functional imaging techniques, diffusion-tensor imaging, diffusion-weighted (DW) imaging, functional MR imaging, MR elastography, MR spectroscopy, perfusion-weighted imaging, MR imaging with very short echo times, and the availability of some targeted MR imaging contrast agents. No ionizing radiation from MR imaging is the biggest advantage, especially in the paediatric, young adult, or pregnant patients for scanning. The safety profile of MR contrast agents is more favourable as compared with the iodinated CT contrast agents. Now the MR imaging is being used for the PET image reconstruction, partial volume correction, and motion with more accurate disease quantification and also for the anatomic localization of radiotracer uptake, improving diagnostic performance, and also for evaluation of the regional and global structural, functional, and molecular assessment of various clinical disorders. The different aspects of the development, related with the software-based registration, with the various instrumentation and designs, the quantification issues, various clinical applications, with the excellent potential clinical roles of image segmentation and global disease assessment, and also the challenges which are related to PET/MR imaging.

10.4 Image Registration Techniques

Image registration techniques are the techniques where the images can be fused or combined, and in the PET, the images will be displayed in various colour codings along with the MR image of the same anatomical region [18, 19]. The combined use of the PET and MR imaging systems will be better for more flexibility and also will be more complementary based on the different approaches [20, 21]. The other parameters which will have an impact on these are the noise, limited spatial resolution, attenuation correction, scatter, and partial volume effect along with various other factors like the blood pool activity radiotracer uptake along with the landmark localization. The various aspects of the MR images are during to the various breath-hold techniques along with the reconstructed images in all the phases of respiration [22]. This will cause the inconsistency of the images between the PET and MR. To avoid this various short dual-modality, imaging protocols are being used to avoid the various breath-holding problems [23].

10.5 PET-MR Imaging

MR is an important imaging modality which has very excellent resolution and many advanced functional MR imaging options are available to complement the molecular information PET that provides. PET/MR imaging should be done end to end in a single gantry. PET spatial resolution is based on the design of the PET systems, and this will be the same even in the various hybrid imaging systems. These photodetector technologies are insensitive to magnetic fields where various heat radiations are required [24]. MR imaging unit will not have any impact due to the various electronic interactions due to the various radiofrequency and gradient coils on the PET systems. The photomultiplier tubes are now being replaced by the avalanche photodiodes [25]. The scintillation light which is not in the range of the various magnetic fields will have very much restriction due to the PET [26]. Scintillation light loss will have an impact degrading the various energy resolution of PET detectors. There were three PET/MR imaging systems: PET insert, fully integrated PET/MR imaging, and the split-field magnet [24, 27]. Photomultiplier tube-based designs having the s split-magnet low-field-strength MR imaging systems along with the various PET detectors can be seen in the various fibre length [27] MicroPET Focus 120 preclinical system (Siemens Molecular Imaging Preclinical Solutions, Knoxville, Tenn) [28], with the 1-T actively-shielded superconducting magnet. Newer state-of-art solid-state detectors, like the avalanche photodiodes, can be used for the detection of the PET detector which are not sensitive in the magnetic field, and which can be placed in the MR imaging unit [25, 29–43] and in research this is focussed on the small animal imaging [44]. The various challenges are for the poor timing resolution of these various avalanche photodiode-based detectors preventing the time-of-flight technology [45]. Sometimes the use of MR and PET electronics will have an impact on PET performance [44]. PET and MR imaging as a single unit and as a single device will be more helpful for this evaluation. The optimal system performance can also be compromised if the shims, gradients, and radiofrequency transmitters are not integrated together [24]. Biograph mMR whole-body PET/MR imaging is an example of the integrated compact hybrid system. In the Biograph mMR MR is fully integrated with the PET system [24]. The various hybrid PET/MR imaging technologies are more focussed on dedicated high-performance specific integrated circuits. Multicell Geiger-mode avalanche photodiodes for light detection are important for the future design of integrated PET/MR imaging systems which will not have any interference between them. In comparison with the various solid-state photodetectors the avalanche photodiodes, silicon photomultiplier tubes are having more gain, signal-to-noise ratio, timing, and are very good technical time-of-flight PET [46] and also for the time-of-flight PET/MR imaging systems. The digital solid-state detectors will have very dedicated components like amplifiers, like the integrated circuits, and the various digital analogue-to-digital converters. The future of PET detectors is capable of three-dimensional spatial information with very high efficiency. MR imaging-guided motion correction is rarely applied to the PET along with the MR images which will have a significant measurement pattern for the quantitative measurement of tissue motion [47]. The simple dictum is that there will be less time of acquisition in the neurologic, cardiovascular, and musculoskeletal disease based on the area of the coverage. In the oncological settings the MR imaging will be more useful for the structural and functional information, and this is also complimentary to the PET [48–54]. MR imaging will be providing very high spatial resolution of tumour volume the local extent based on the superior soft tissue contrast and this is based on the primary tumour locations like the brain, head and neck, spinal cord, liver, pelvic organs, breasts, and musculoskeletal system.

PET and MR imaging are complementary to each other in most cases which is again based on the various tumour characteristics like the amount of the metabolism, cell proliferation, and hypoxia, the size of metastases, and the regions involved. The MR imaging will be superior to the CT on the early detection and characterization of metastases in bone marrow, liver, and brain; otherwise, the CT is superior for the evaluation of small lung metastases [55–59].

PET/MR imaging is having a very important modality for the assessment of the various types of cancer before, during, and after therapeutic intervention. It is also useful for optimizing drug development like pharmacokinetics which is based on the absorption, biodistribution, metabolism, and elimination and various pharmacodynamics of novel therapeutic agents of interest [60, 61].

10.6 Neurologic Disease

PET/MR imaging is very important for the various integrated multidimensional and multiparametric structural and functional assessment of the central nervous system in various pathologies like neurodegenerative, ischemic, vascular, neurologic-oncologic, traumatic, psychiatric, behavioural, seizure-related, and age-related conditions and useful for the assessment of various cellular and gene therapies [54, 62, 63]. Various degrees of spatial and temporal coregistration of PET and MR imaging are also based on the various aspects of the metabolism, perfusion, oxygen consumption, receptor expression, and function in even the smallest neurologic-anatomic structures [64, 65] (Fig. 10.2a, b, and c).

PET/MR imaging is useful for the evaluation of the various metabolic activities, various neurotransmitter concentrations, and enzyme expression in small structures of the brain [66, 67]. Normal MR imaging examinations can be there with mild type I cortical dysplasia [68]. DWI along with the PET parameters of the oxygen consumption and the perfusion. The immediate planning of brain tumours will be useful for the various peritumoural oedema like the infiltrative tumour, various pre-treatment assessments of white matter tract involvement by tumour, and also for the various intraoperative visualization and localization of major white matter tracts preventing the chances of the injury [69, 70]. DW imaging with PET can also be used for the detection, characterization, and monitoring the various changes in brain tumours after various therapeutic interventions [52]. Diffusion tensor imaging will be due to the various white matter bundles, which can be useful for the planning of various brain tumours differentiating from the perilesional oedema, white matter tract involvement, and also the various intraoperative visualization and localization of major white matter tracts preventing the chances of the injury to the surrounding normal tissues [69, 70].

10.7 Perfusion-Weighted Imaging Along with the PET

Is very crucial for the evaluation of the various pathologies like the ischemic or vascular, neurodegenerative, and neoplastic brain disorders. The functional MR imaging is also useful for the evaluation of the cerebral cortex and also to evaluate the reduced timing of the surgery and also for minimizing the intraoperative cortical stimulation during surgical resection [71, 72]. Some studies were there for the assessment of the activation of the various transmitter release or receptor binding, and also, for the drug usage and withdrawal [64]. PET/MR is also useful for the evaluation of the various spinal cord and peripheral nerve disease abnormalities. Behera et al. [73] showed the importance of neuropathic pain with significant increased FDG uptake in the affected nerve and can be used to the localization of the FDG uptake in peripheral nerves.

10.8 Cardiovascular Disease PET/MR Imaging

It is having an important role in the evaluation of myocardial viability and infarction, ventricular function, cardiomyopathy, myocarditis, pericarditis, atherosclerosis, vasculitis, and other cardiovascular pathologies. As MR imaging is already well established by virtue of the various pulse sequences for the imaging of cardiovascular structure and function, where multiple PET radiotracers along with the probe molecular processes will be involved. MR imaging is also more

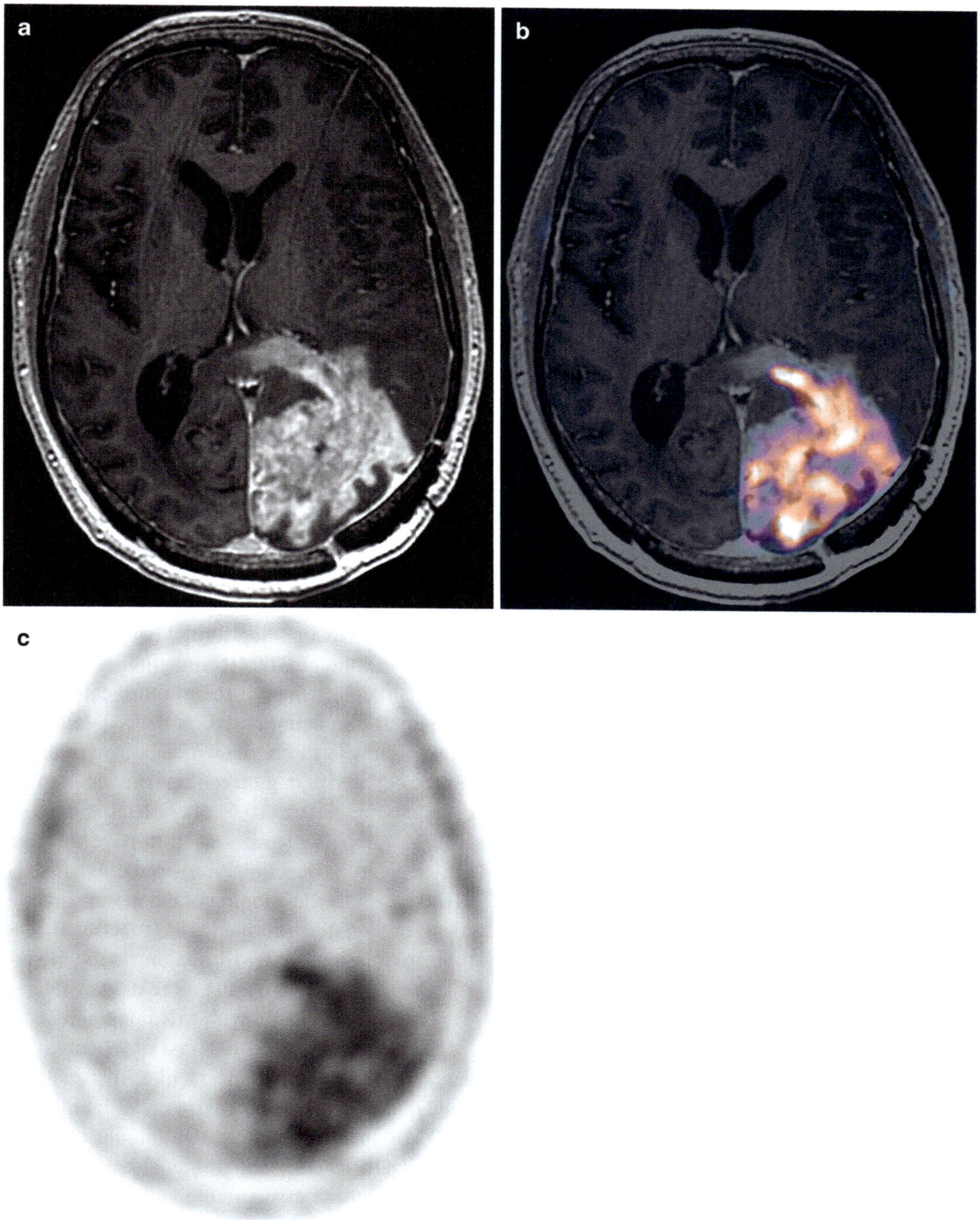

Fig. 10.2 (**a**) MR post-contrast image showing densely enhancing lesion in the left parieto-occipital region with local infiltrations. (**b**) is the fused PET-MR image showing significant uptake corresponding to the area of the enhancement on MR. (**c**) is the PET image showing significantly increased uptake in these regions

useful for the measurement of various cardiac chambers, wall thickness, wall motion, and vessel diameters; provides quantitative measures of flow; is useful to assess myocardial perfusion with pharmacological stress testing; and can allow detection and quantification of myocardial fibrosis. MR imaging is also useful to show the precise anatomic extent and location of cardiac and pericardiac tumours and is also complimentary to the FDG PET for response assessment purposes [74–76]. This imaging will allow the assessment of cellular and gene therapies like cardiac stem cell transplantation [77]. Vascular system is also being evaluated with the regional and global detection, characterization, and also for the quantification of atherosclerotic disease to quantify the risk assessment and various drug response as it can provide the assessment of the vascular wall thickness, wall inflammation, plaque vulnerability, and degree of luminal narrowing [74, 78–80].

10.9 Musculoskeletal Disease PET/MR Imaging

In many conditions because MR imaging will provide excellent soft tissue contrast in evaluating the bone marrow, muscles, tendons, ligaments, cartilaginous structures, and fat thus it will have very high sensitivity [52]. The FDG PET and MR imaging are complimentary for the detection and characterization of various complications in diabetes, like Charcot neuroarthropathy, osteomyelitis, and soft-tissue infection. The total evaluation of the various molecular and volumetric measurements will be able to quantify for pretreatment planning, prognosis, and prediction and assessment of treatment response [57]. Image segmentation and global disease assessment can also be done along with the PET and MR imaging which are as follows. Nawaz et al. [81] studied 27 patients with diabetes who underwent lower-extremity FDG PET and MR imaging. Evaluation of the popliteal artery-to-background ratio and whole-foot metabolic volumetric product . The various standardized criteria, image acquisition parameters, and radiotracer and contrast material-injection protocols for PET/MR imaging can be used for the evaluation of the specific patients, disease conditions, and various body parts of interest, with the newer procedural, safety, and quality control guidelines (Fig. 10.3).

In gynaecologic cancers, the role of the PET is well established along with the superior soft-tissue contrast and various anatomical resolution, lack of ionizing radiation, assess cellular density based on the diffusion-weighted imaging (DWI), and tissue perfusion and oxygenation by dynamic contrast-enhanced (DCE) MR imaging [82–84] (Fig. 10.4).

An increasing number of PET/MR whole-body for the evaluation of the gynaecologic cancers is based on the excellent soft-tissue contrast and the various application techniques like the DWI, DCE MR imaging for the better evaluation of the lesions. PET/MR imaging is also the important component of the multimodality, multiparametric imaging based on the SUVmax and ADC values in the tumour metabolism and also for the cellularity in gynaecologic and abdominal cancers (Figs. 10.5, 10.6, 10.7, 10.8 and 10.9). PET/MR imaging studies need to have the various standardized acquisition protocols; for the MR-AC; for the developing of the newer imaging focussing on the morphologic, functional, and molecular levels, PET/MR imaging is the modality which will be having the more diagnostic values for the comparison with MR imaging.

Excellent soft-tissue contrast of MR imaging can evaluate various cancers like lung cancers, renal cell carcinoma, and extra nodal lymphoma. PET/MR imaging reduces the amount of radiation. FDG PET/MR imaging is also feasible for therapy response assessment in all these tumours more focussed for lymphoma but has not been compared with other modalities for this purpose (Figs. 10.10, 10.11 and 10.12a and b).

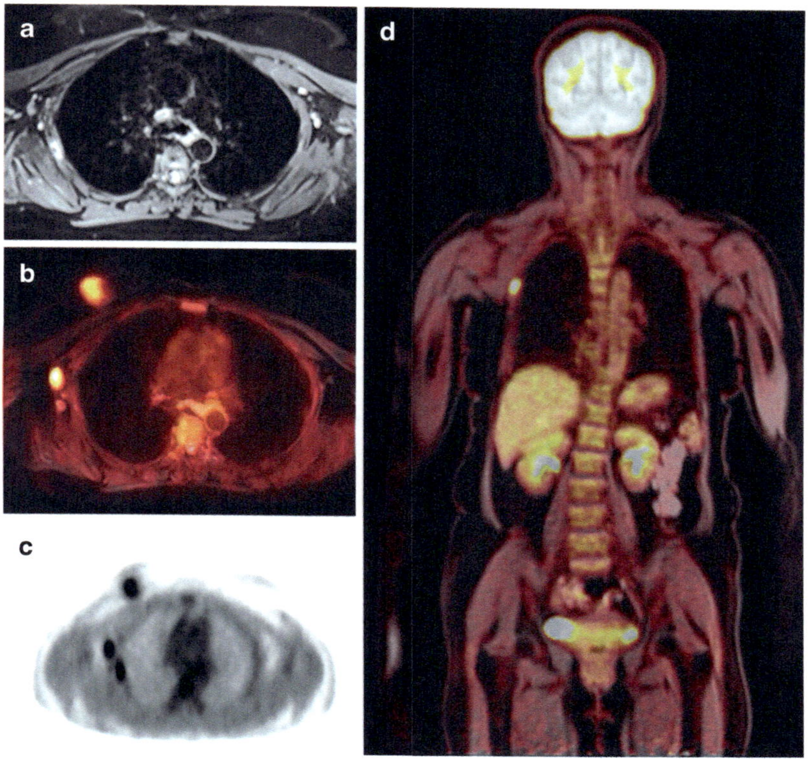

Fig. 10.3 Carcinoma Right Breast showing (**a**) MRI image showing the small right breast nodule with the small axillary nodes with right rib lesion. (**b** and **d**) PET-MRI fused image showing significant uptake in the right breast parenchyma, right axillary nodes, and in the right rib lesion. (**c**) is the PET image corresponding to the lesions seen in the MRI

10.10 Potential of Hyperpolarized MR Imaging

PET/MR imaging along with the component of the hyperpolarized MR imaging. The various imaging techniques are there for the evaluation of the various cancers and also the other pathologies which will give the metabolic information like that of the PET [85, 86]. The hyperpolarized 13C MR imaging uses a recently developed technique, solution dynamic nuclear polarization (DNP), to dramatically increase the signal of 13C-enriched metabolic agents. Metabolism is based on the various new resonances of the hyperpolarized 13C spectrum, resulting in the difference of the 13C small molecules in vivo. The hyperpolarized 13C MR imaging will be required in chemistry, biochemistry, engineering, pulse sequence design, pharmaceutical sciences, and data processing. Thus, the PET is typically limited to 1 targeted probe: in combination with the hyperpolarized MR imaging and PET.

10.11 Nontargeted Molecular Probes

PET/MR imaging is now being used for the various nontargeted molecular imaging agents. Imaging of the cell processes, and nontargeted molecular imaging for the abnormal cell physiology and monitor cellular changes over time. The radiolabelled versions of compounds are the nontargeted probes used for the various targeted pathologic process when compared with normal physiologic ones. The most common cellular processes are the use of the glucose metabolism (18F-FDG), lipogenesis (11C-choline,

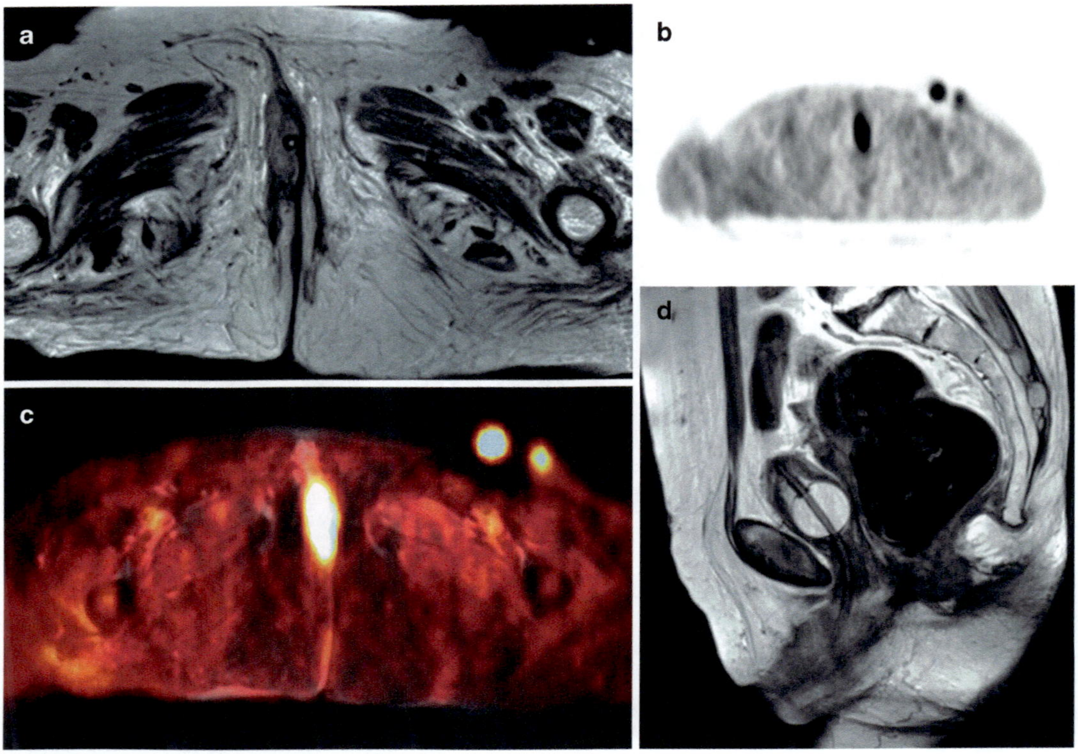

Fig. 10.4 (**a** and **d**) MRI images showing the Bulky uterus with perianal lesion with left inguinal lymph nodes. (**c**) corresponding PET-MR fused image showing the perineal lesion with left inguinal node with significant amount of metabolic activity. (**b**) Invert grey PET image showing the perianal lesion and left inguinal nodes which shows a significant amount of the uptake in these areas

11C-acetate), cellular proliferation or DNA synthesis (18F-fluorothymidine, 18F-FMAU), and cellular hypoxia (18F-fluoromisonidazole, nitroimidazole compounds). As glucose metabolism is a very common metabolism that is not specific to tumours, areas of naturally high or increased metabolism also demonstrate increased uptake, such as the brain, heart, or bowel, in addition to inflammatory or infectious processes.

18F-choline also shows the increased uptake in prostate and parathyroid cancers as there will be significantly increased choline kinase activity and also increased choline transport [87, 88]. The PET/MR imaging with 18F-choline shows very high prediction rate of prostate cancer in targeted biopsies as compared with MR imaging alone [89]. It also shows the increased detection of both androgen-dependent and independent prostate cancers in vitro [90]. Incidental parathyroid adenomas on18F-choline PET/MR imaging are used for prostate cancer staging [91]. PET/MR imaging also provides detailed anatomic information to the surgeons [92].

10.12 Targeted Molecular Imaging

Targeted molecular imaging agents are specific targets such as transporters or enzymes, are capable of the very highly sensitive biomarkers of therapeutic efficacy. The various targeted molecular imaging probes are divided into the various different targeted ligands, monoclonal antibodies, fragments, natural peptide ligands or their analogues, tyrosine kinase inhibitors or their analogues, and high-affinity peptides. In the concept

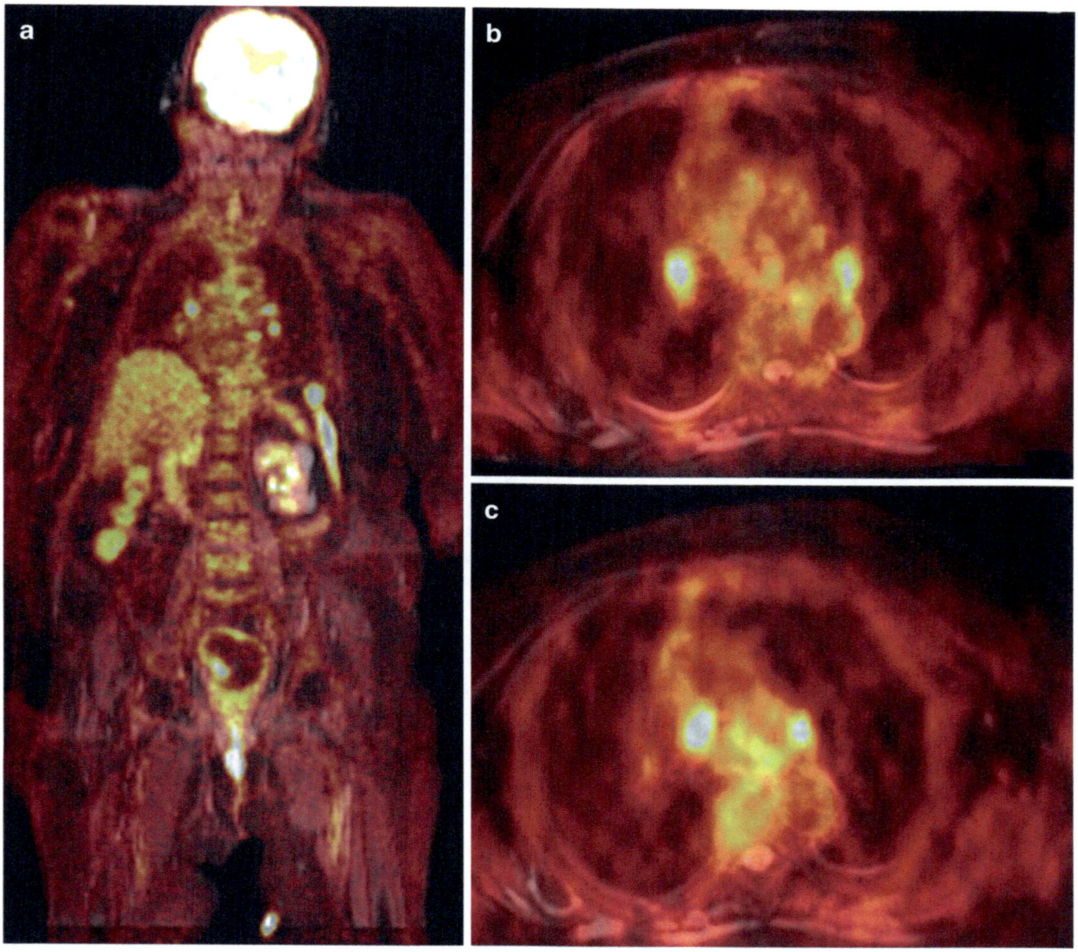

Fig. 10.5 (**a**) PET-MR fused images showing the focal area of the wall thickening in the rectum and also left sub-diaphragmatic peritoneal thickening which is corresponding to the uptake on this image. (**b** and **c**) fused images showing the mediastinal nodes and uptake in these regions suggestive of the metastases

of precision medicine PET/MR imaging can be applied in different ways, most commonly in prostate and neuroendocrine tumour (NET).

10.13 Paediatric PET/MR

Paediatric imaging is important by the PET/MRI. Paediatric oncologic imaging is most commonly used by the 18F-FDG-PET/MRI for the precise assessment of the tumour spread and also for the monitoring response to the therapy [93–95]. Lower radiation exposure in comparison to the CT or PET/CT is the biggest advantage. Already along with the whole-body MRI, PET inclusion will improve significant diagnostic specificity in the post-therapy evaluation situation [93, 94, 96]. Paediatric oncologic PET/MRI is used for the primary staging, therapy monitoring, and follow-up imaging of paediatric patients and in solid malignancies like lymphoma, sarcoma, and neuroblastoma [97–101]. Non-oncologic imaging is not clearly defined in paediatric applications. Many PET/MRI is being used for various targeting inflammatory condition like PET-CT [102, 103]. MRI also useful for the imaging of disease spread and various conditions like chronic inflammatory bowel disease,

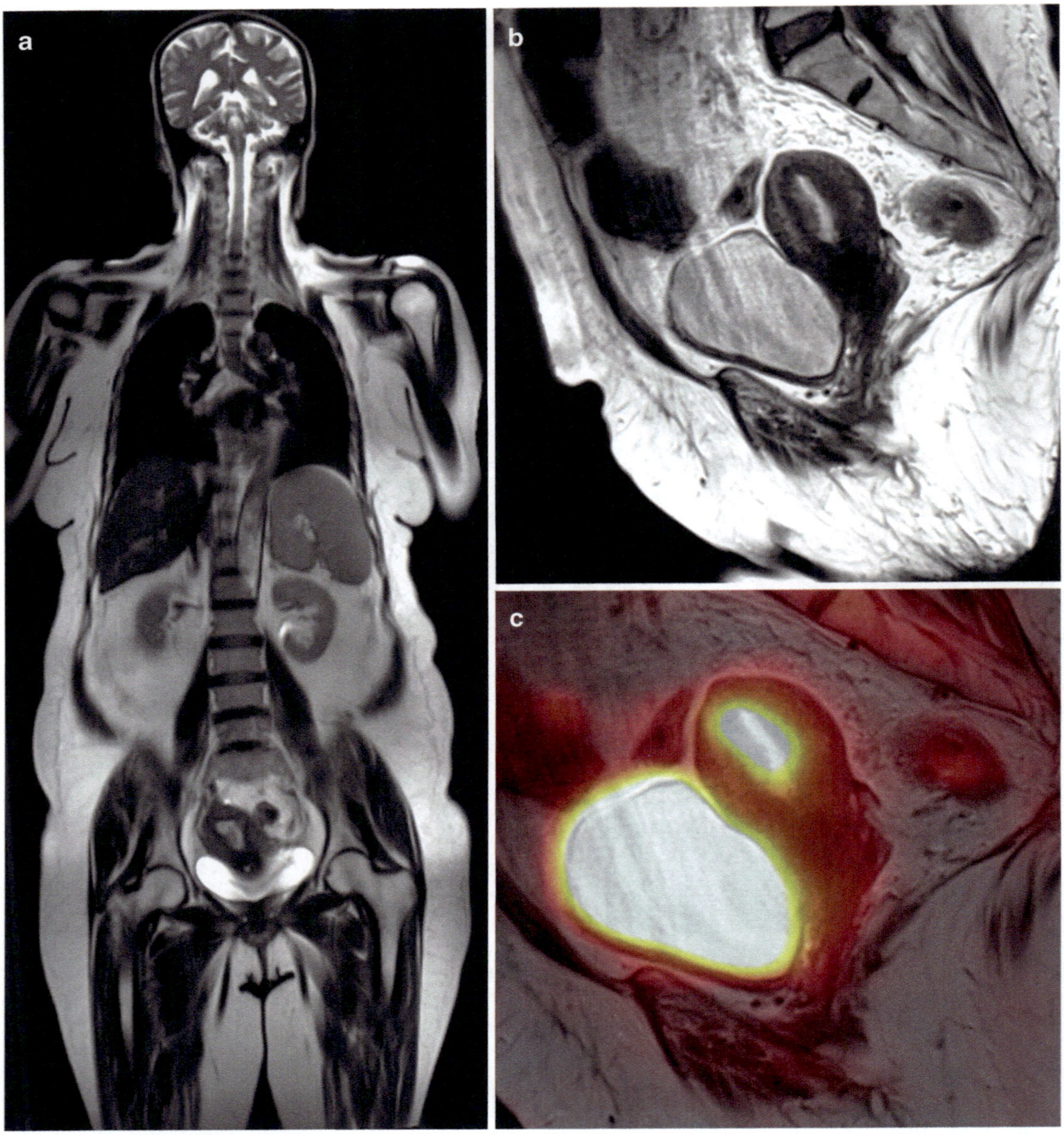

Fig. 10.6 (**a** and **b**) MRI images showing subtle irregularity involving the endometrial cavity. (**c**) fused PET-MR image showing the corresponding increased uptake in the endometrium

rheumatoid disorders, or chronic infectious disease. It is important to point out that the availability of combined PET/MRI is still limited. Multiparametric imaging in PET/MRI will be more useful for the precise location of the biological effects of novel therapeutic agents.

PET/MRI imaging is the modality of choice in paediatric lymphoma patients. FDG-PET has been also for the various amount of the metabolic tumour volume of sarcoma, thus offering prognostic information [103, 104]. FDG-PET/MRI will also provide important diagnostic information in a post-therapeutic setting [105]. MRI alone is less sensitive for the use to distinguish between the post-therapeutic changes and possible tumour recurrence [96]. The specific PET tracers for the imaging of neuroendocrine tumours is 68Ga-DOTATATE. 18F-FDG-PET is

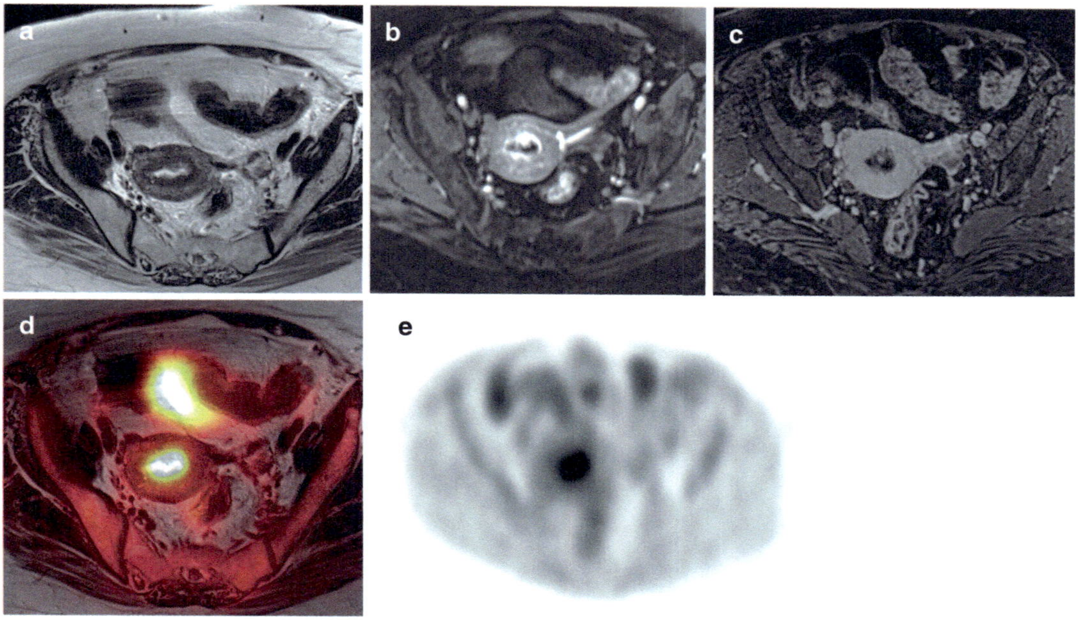

Fig. 10.7 (**a**, **b** and **c**) MR images showing the diffuse circumferential and irregular wall thickening involving the Sigmoid colon. Small endometrial polypoidal lesion also noted. (**d**) fused PET-MR image showing the corresponding uptake in the Sigmoid colon and in the endometrial lesion. (**e**) PET image showing the significantly increased uptake in the areas mentioned in the fused PET-MR images

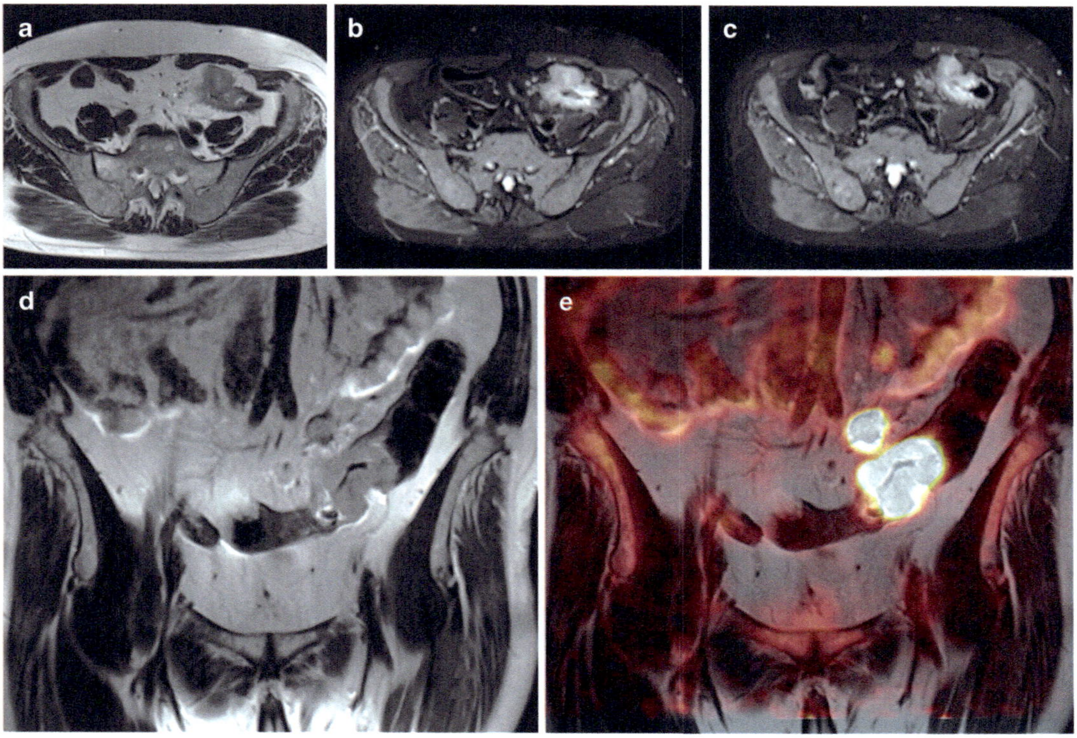

Fig. 10.8 MR, axial images (**a**–**c**) showing diffuse irregular circumferential wall thickening, (**d**) axial MR image showing thickening with adjacent perilesional node, (**e**) fused PET-MR significant amount of the uptake on PET in sigmoid colon and adjacent perilesional node

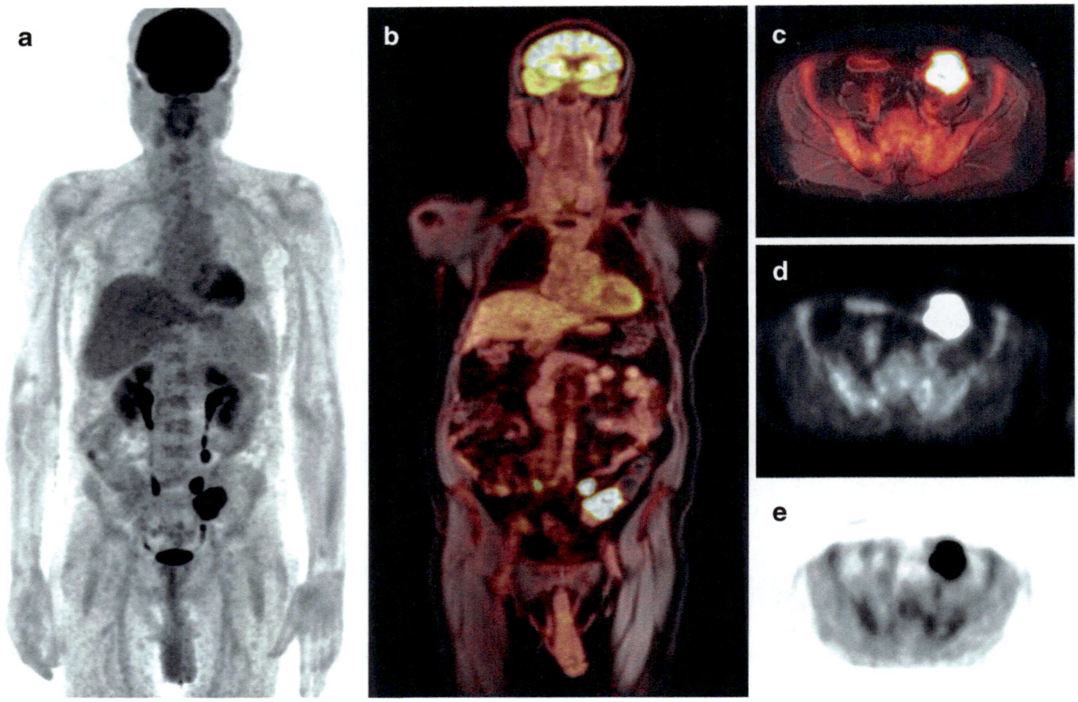

Fig. 10.9 PET-MR, (**a**) PET image and (**b**) fused PET-MR image showing diffuse increased sigmoid colon lesion uptake with local node and no distant metastases. (**c–e**) axial fused PET-MR, MR and PET images showing diffuse sigmoid colon wall thickening with peri colonic node with significant metabolic activity

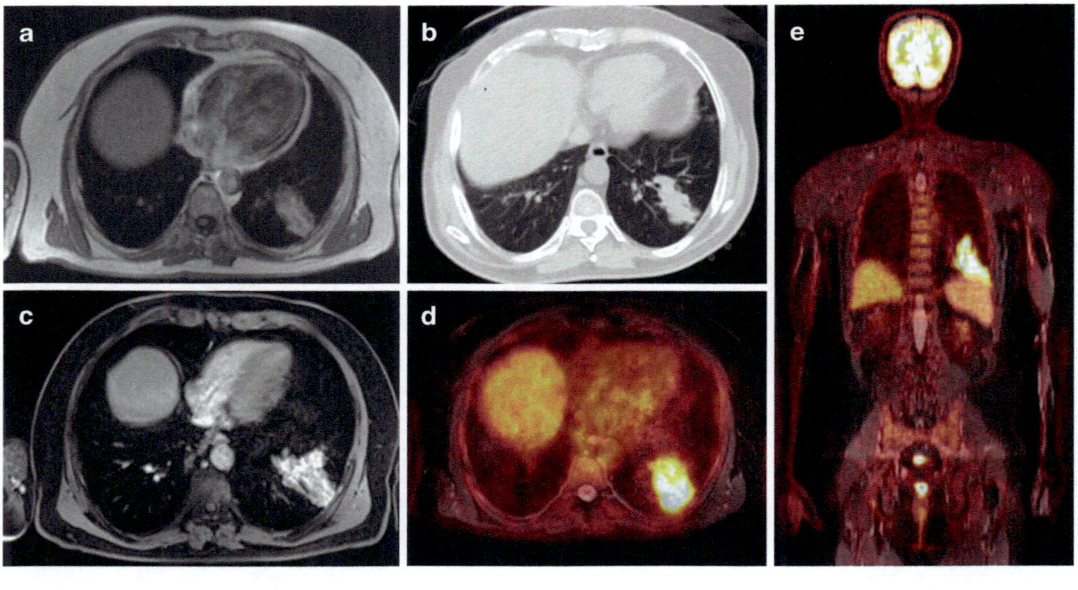

Fig. 10.10 (**a** and **c**) MR images showing the left lower lobe lesion, which corresponding to the Image (**b**) CT lung window. (**d** and **e**) showing significant uptake on the fused PET-MR images. Rest of the body is normal

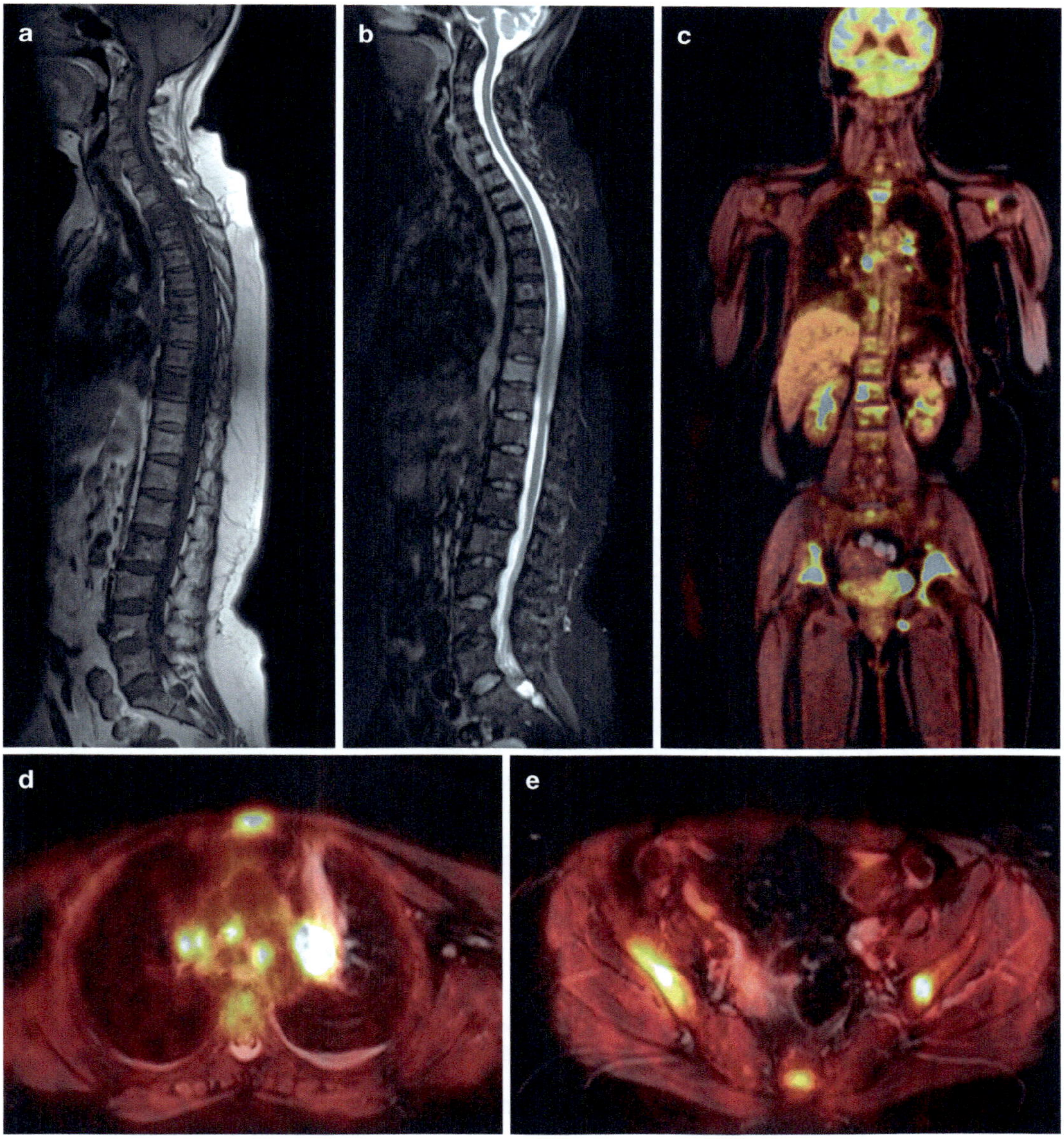

Fig. 10.11 Multiple Myeloma case, (**a** and **b**) MR whole-body images showing disseminated skeletal lesions with mediastinal nodes. (**c**, **d**, and **e**) fused images showing the significant amount of the uptake in the skeletal lesions and in the mediastinal nodes

used to monitor and track the malignant transformation of plexiform neurofibromas to malignant peripheral nerve sheath tumours. Elevated FDG-uptake correlates with the malignant transformation based on the higher standardized uptake values (SUV) [106, 107]. MRI can delineate the better progression of the widespread tumours also in relation to the biological evaluation by diffusion-weighted imaging (DWI) [108]. PET/MRI in primary CNS tumours imaging is already commonly done by the MRI. Higher soft tissue contrast along with the various functional imaging will be more characterized for the CNS anatomy and pathologies. And along with PET, it

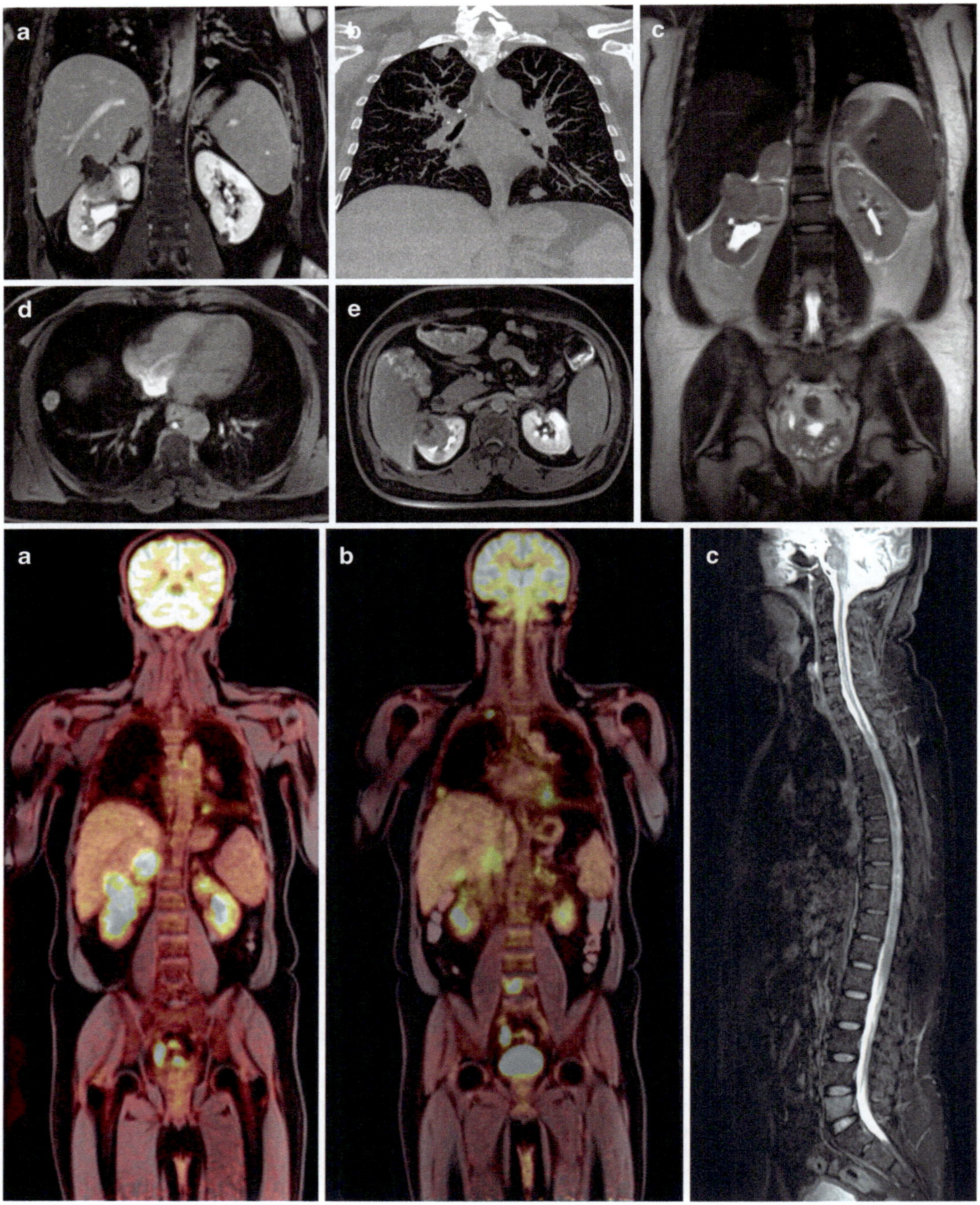

Fig. 10.12 (**A** and **B**): **Image A**, (**a**, **c** and **e**) MR image showing the right renal lesion diagnosed as Renal cell carcinoma, (**d**) MR image showing right lung nodule and (**e**) CT lung window shows the right lung nodular lesion suggestive of the metastases. **Image B**, (**a** and **b**) are fused PET-MR images showing significant uptake in the primary right renal lesion with lumbar vertebral metastases corresponding to the (**c**) MR image. **Image Courtesy**: Dr. Nidhi Goyal Senior Consultant Radiologist, Apollo Indraprastha Hospitals New Delhi. Dr. Amit Chaudhari Assistant Professor, Department of Radiology. Tata Memorial Hospital. Mumbai

gives more information on the metabolism of the tumour [109]. 18F-FET or 11C-Methionine is more commonly used in the primary CNS tumours evaluation [110]. Non-oncologic applications of FDG-PET/MRI for the functional assessment of various inflammatory changes, for the diagnosis and therapy assessment of various acute and chronic inflammatory diseases like fever of unknown origin, chronic inflammatory bowel disease, vasculitis, and rheumatoid disease [111]. Here the role of the MRI can also be important for the morphological and functional changes of inflammation like perfusion, oedema, or wall thickening, etc. [112, 113].

MRI is already the established modality of choice for the detection of morphological which will be correlating with the epileptic foci in cases of the various primary CNS tumours or focal cortical dysplasia. FDG-PET can also evaluate the various functional extent based on the asymmetric cortical hypometabolism [114, 115]. The diagnostic radiation exposure is also being associated with PET. Whole-body MRI sequences are T1-weighted gradient-echo sequences, inversion recovery (STIR) sequences in coronal, and diffusion-weighted MRI (DWI).

The biggest advantage of PET/MRI over PET/CT is the various paediatric applications based on the significant reduction in diagnostic radiation exposure. The implementation of paediatric PET/MR imaging is based on the different sites and also in the cardiac MR imaging.

10.14 PET/MR Imaging Musculoskeletal Tumours

Characterization of bony as well as soft tissue tumours, the contrast-enhanced MRI is the commonest protocol, having excellent superior soft-tissue contrast, the associated tumour involvement of soft tissue and neurovascular structures, and marrow changes on MRI. MRI for the identification, treatment planning,follow-up in patients with sarcoma is unique for them. This will give the rough estimation of metabolism, along with the information of the tumour nature, histopathologic findings, response to neoadjuvant therapy, and musculoskeletal tumours outcomes. Bone scintigraphy is the modality of choice for the diagnosis of the bony metastases, along with the increased local bone turnover. But low spatial resolution, bone marrow infiltration, or osteolytic metastases can be there with normal bone turnover [116, 117]. MRI high spatial and soft-tissue resolution intramedullary metastases before further cortical destruction occurs (Fig. 10.5).

10.14.1 PET/MR Imaging in Inflammatory and Infectious Musculoskeletal Disorders

The contrast-enhanced MRI is more commonly used for the early diagnosis and follow-up of various inflammatory and infectious musculoskeletal disease conditions. High resolution of the MRI will be delineating the extent of tissue inflammation. PET and MRI in the evaluation of patients with rheumatoid arthritis will be able to quantify the amount of the synovial joint inflammation to quantify the amount of the disease activity [118, 119]. The common soft tissue infections are hematogenous cellulitis/myositis or a wound infection and all these are nonspecific. PET/MRI is also able to differentiate between the non-necrotizing soft tissue infections and inflammatory conditions, and also the necrotizing fasciitis. PET/MRI protocols are more useful for high-resolution imaging device.

The musculoskeletal system, because combining PET molecular and functional information with MRI structural information and multiparametric lesion evaluation is possible in a single device with a one-stop shop. The PET/MRI protocol is convenient and would solve the major problem faced during musculoskeletal system evaluation. In addition, the use of a specific radiotracer other PET/CT & PET/MRI for Musculoskeletal Applications 473 than FDG can potentially provide molecular information that is complementary to MRI in hybrid PET/MRI.

10.15 PET/MR Imaging for Atherosclerosis

MR imaging due to its very high soft tissue resolution and excellent tissue contrast tissue the plaques can eb quantified and this can also be done for the various molecular imaging targets. MR imaging is used for the evaluation of the vessel wall and plaque quantification. MR imaging is best for the evaluation of the regional information for atherosclerotic imaging, for the carotid or coronary arteries. Whole-body imaging is advisable if the use is there for the systemic disease. The PET/MR systems are newer imaging techniques; these will be more challenging for the evaluation and also showing the inability to get PET quantification right as CT-based attenuation is not there [120].

Hybrid PET/MR Imaging for Vascular Imaging of Atherosclerosis will use PET and MR for imaging of vessels based on the simultaneous hybrid PET/MR imaging for arterial wall imaging [121]. FDG-PET uptake in carotid arteries wall was there along with the human immunodeficiency virus without any cardiac disease. A comparison was done on ahead-to-head basis with PET/CT and found no difference in FDG quantification [122]. 64Cu-DOTATATE-PET/MR imaging was done before operation; these plaques were evaluated for molecular analyses. These molecular analyses showed that the 64Cu-DOTATATE uptake is also associated with the haemorrhage-associated macrophage load. Here there is great potential for the specific PET tracers to be combined for the various morphologic and functional information.

MR and PET have been important imaging tools to evaluate atherosclerosis and various plaque vulnerability. Fast MR sequences along with the specific PET tracers are the key markers of atherosclerosis and plaque vulnerability. Thus, the PET-MR is the one-stop shop for the hybrid PET/MR imaging scanners for the evaluation of atherosclerosis and also for the characterization of atherosclerotic plaques.

References

1. Delso G, Ziegler S. PET/MRI system design. Eur J Nucl Med Mol Imaging. 2009;36(suppl 1):S86–92.
2. Herzog H, Van Den Hoff J. Combined PET/MR systems: an overview and comparison of currently available options. Q J Nucl Med Mol Imaging. 2012;56:247–67.
3. Torigian DA, Zaidi H, Kwee TC, et al. PET/MR imaging: technical aspects and potential clinical applications. Radiology. 2013;267:26–44.
4. Vaska P, Cao T. The state of instrumentation for combined positron emission tomography and magnetic resonance imaging. Semin Nucl Med. 2013;43:11–8.
5. Lecomte R, Cadorette J, Rodrigue S, et al. Initial results from the Sherbrooke avalanche photodiode positron tomograph. IEEE Trans Nucl Sci. 1996;43:1952–7.
6. Yoon HS, Ko GB, Kwon S, et al. Initial results of simultaneous PET/MRI experiments with an MRI compatible silicon photomultiplier PET scanner. J Nucl Med. 2012;53:608–14.
7. Yankeelov TE, Peterson TE, Abramson RG, et al. Simultaneous PET-MRI in oncology: a solution looking for a problem? Magn Reson Imaging. 2012;30:1342–56.
8. Yoo HJ, Lee JS, Lee JM. Integrated whole body MR/PET: where are we? Korean J Radiol. 2015;16(1):32–49.
9. Werner M, Schmidt H, Schwenzer N. MR/PET: a new challenge in hybrid imaging. Am J Roentgenol. 2012;199:272.
10. Bagade S, Fowler KJ, Schwarz JK, et al. PET/MRI evaluation of gynaecologic malignancies and prostate cancer. Semin Nucl Med. 2015 Jul;45(4):293–303.
11. Gu J, Chan T, Zhang J, et al. Whole-body diffusion weighted imaging: the added value to whole-body MRI at initial diagnosis of lymphoma. AJR Am J Roentgenol. 2011;197(3):W384–91.
12. Abdulqadhr G, Molin D, Aström G, et al. Whole body diffusion-weighted imaging compared with FDG-PET/CT in staging of lymphoma patients. Acta Radiol. 2011;52:173–80.
13. Partovi S, Kohan A, Rubbert C, et al. Clinical oncologic applications of PET/MRI: a new horizon. Am J Nucl Med Mol Imaging. 2014;4(2):202–12.
14. Fraum TJ, Fowler KJ, McConathy J, et al. PET/MRI for the body imager: abdominal and pelvic oncologic applications. Abdom Imaging. 2015;40(6):1387–404. PET/MR Imaging in Cancers of the Gastrointestinal Tract 17
15. Sugita R, Ito K, Fujita N, et al. Diffusion-weighted MRI in abdominal oncology: clinical applications. World J Gastroenterol. 2010;16(7):832–6.
16. Vandecaveye V, De Keyzer F, Vander Poorten V, et al. Head and neck squamous cell carcinoma: value

of diffusion-weighted MR imaging for nodal staging. Radiology. 2009;251:134–46.
17. Fujii S, Matsusue E, Kanasaki Y, et al. Detection of peritoneal dissemination in gynecological malignancy: evaluation by diffusion-weighted MR imaging. Eur Radiol. 2008;18(1):18–23.
18. Zaidi H, Mawlawi O, Orton CG. Point/counterpoint. Simultaneous PET/MR will replace PET/CT as the molecular multimodality imaging platform of choice. Med Phys. 2007;34(5):1525–8.
19. Zaidi H, Montandon ML, Alavi A. The clinical role of fusion imaging using PET, CT, and MR imaging. Magn Reson Imaging Clin N Am. 2010;18(1):133–49.
20. Pietrzyk U. Does PET/CT render software fusion obsolete? Nuklearmedizin. 2005;44(Suppl 1):S13–7.
21. Weigert M, Pietrzyk U, Müller S, Palm C, Beyer T. Whole-body PET/CT imaging: combining software- and hardware-based co-registration. Z Med Phys. 2008;18(1):59–66.
22. Nehmeh SA, Erdi YE. Respiratory motion in positron emission tomography/computed tomography: a review. Semin Nucl Med. 2008;38(3):167–76.
23. Slomka PJ, Baum RP. Multimodality image registration with software: state-of-the-art. Eur J Nucl Med Mol Imaging. 2009;36(Suppl 1):S44–55.
24. Zaidi H, Del Guerra A. An outlook on future design of hybrid PET/MRI systems. Med Phys. 2011;38(10):5667–89.
25. Catana C, Wu Y, Judenhofer MS, Qi J, Pichler BJ, Cherry SR. Simultaneous acquisition of multislice PET and MR images: initial results with a MR-compatible PET scanner. J Nucl Med. 2006;47(12):1968–76.
26. Frach T, Prescher G, Degenhardt C, et al. The digital silicon photomultiplier – system architecture and performance evaluation. In IEEE NSS-MIC Conference Record, October 30–November 6, 2010, Knoxville, TN, pp. 1722–7.
27. Lucas AJ, Hawkes RC, Ansorge RE, et al. Development of a combined microPET-MR system. Technol Cancer Res Treat. 2006;5(4):337–41.
28. Kim JS, Lee JS, Im KC, et al. Performance measurement of the microPET focus 120 scanner. J Nucl Med. 2007;48(9):1527–35.
29. Pichler B, Lorenz E, Mirzoyan R, Pimpl W, Roder F, Schwaiger M. Performance tests of a LSO-APD PET module in a 9.4 tesla magnet. In: IEEE Nuclear Science Symposium and Medical Imaging Conference Record. Albuquerque, NM: IEEE; 1997. p. 1237–9.
30. Marsden PK, Strul D, Keevil SF, Williams SC, Cash D. Simultaneous PET and NMR. Br J Radiol 2002;75(Spec No):S53–S59.
31. Cherry SR. Multimodality in vivo imaging systems: twice the power or double the trouble? Annu Rev Biomed Eng. 2006;8:35–62.
32. Cherry SR, Louie AY, Jacobs RE. The integration of positron emission tomography with magnetic resonance imaging. Proc IEEE. 2008;96(3):416–38.
33. Pichler BJ, Judenhofer MS, Catana C, et al. Performance test of an LSO-APD detector in a 7-T MRI scanner for simultaneous PET/MRI. J Nucl Med. 2006;47(4):639–47.
34. Schlyer D, Vaska P, Tomasi D, et al. A simultaneous PET/MRI scanner based on the RatCAP in small animals. IEEE Nucl Sci Symp Conf Rec. 2007;5:3256–9.
35. Woody C, Schlyer D, Vaska P, et al. Preliminary studies of a simultaneous PET/MRI scanner based on the RatCAP small animal tomograph. NuclInstr Meth A. 2007;571(1–2):102–5.
36. Judenhofer MS, Catana C, Swann BK, et al. PET/MR images acquired with a compact MR-compatible PET detector in a 7-T magnet. Radiology. 2007;244(3):807–14.
37. Judenhofer MS, Wehrl HF, Newport DF, et al. Simultaneous PET-MRI: a new approach for functional and morphological imaging. Nat Med. 2008;14(4):459–65.
38. Ravindranath B, Junnarkar SS, Purschke ML, et al. Results from prototype II of the BNL simultaneous PET-MRI dedicated breast scanner. IEEE Nucl Sci Symp Conf Rec. 2009: 3315–3317.
39. Pichler BJ, Kolb A, Nägele T, Schlemmer HP. PET/MRI: paving the way for the next generation of clinical multimodality imaging applications. J Nucl Med. 2010;51(3):333–6.
40. Kang J, Choi Y, Hong KJ, et al. A feasibility study of photosensor charge signal transmission to preamplifier using long cable for development of hybrid PET-MRI. Med Phys. 2010;37(11):5655–64.
41. Wu Y, Catana C, Farrell R, et al. PET performance evaluation of an MR-compatible PET insert. IEEE Trans Nucl Sci. 2009;56(3):574–80.
42. Schlemmer HP, Pichler BJ, Schmand M, et al. Simultaneous MR/PET imaging of the human brain: feasibility study. Radiology. 2008;248(3):1028–35.
43. Wehrl HF, Judenhofer MS, Thielscher A, Martirosian P, Schick F, Pichler BJ. Assessment of MR compatibility of a PET insert developed for simultaneous multiparametric PET/MR imaging on an animal system operating at 7 T. Magn Reson Med. 2011;65(1):269–79.
44. Wehrl HF, Judenhofer MS, Wiehr S, Pichler BJ. Pre-clinical PET/MR: technological advances and new perspectives in biomedical research. Eur J Nucl Med Mol Imaging. 2009;36(Suppl 1):S56–68.
45. Fontaine R, Belanger F, Viscogliosi N, et al. The hardware and signal processing architecture of LabPET, a small animal APDbased digital PET scanner. IEEE Trans Nucl Sci. 2009;56(1):3–9.
46. Conti M. Focus on time-of-flight PET: the benefits of improved time resolution. Eur J Nucl Med Mol Imaging. 2011;38(6):1147–57.

47. Chun SY, Reese TG, Ouyang J, et al. MRIbased nonrigid motion correction in simultaneous PET/MRI. J Nucl Med. 2012;53(8):1284–91.
48. Kwee TC, Basu S, Saboury B, Alavi A, Torigian DA. Functional oncoimaging techniques with potential clinical applications. Front Biosci (Elite Ed). 2012;4:1081–96.
49. Shamim SA, Torigian DA, Kumar R. PET, PET/CT, and PET/MRI assessment of breast cancer. PET Clin. 2008;3(3):381–93.
50. Hustinx R, Torigian DA, Namur G. Complementary assessment of abdominopelvic disorders with PET/CT and MRI. PET Clin. 2008;3(3):435–49.
51. Katz S, Ferrara T, Alavi A, Torigian DA. PET, CT, and MRI for assessment of thoracic malignancy: structure meets function. PET Clin. 2008;3(3):395–410.
52. Chen K, Blebea J, Laredo JD, Chen W, Alavi A, Torigian DA. Evaluation of musculoskeletal disorders with PET, PET/CT, and PET/MRI. PET Clin. 2008;3(3):451–65.
53. Goldberg MF, Chawla S, Alavi A, Torigian DA, Melhem ER. PET and MRI of brain tumours. PET Clin. 2008;3(3):293–315.
54. Antoch G, Bockisch A. Combined PET/MRI: a new dimension in whole-body oncology imaging? Eur J Nucl Med Mol Imaging. 2009;36(Suppl 1):S113–20.
55. Donati OF, Hany TF, Reiner CS, et al. Value of retrospective fusion of PET and MR images in detection of hepatic metastases: comparison with 18F-FDG PET/CT and Gd-EOB-DTPA-enhanced MRI. J Nucl Med. 2010;51(5):692–9.
56. Antoch G, Vogt FM, Freudenberg LS, et al. Whole-body dual-modality PET/CT and whole-body MRI for tumor staging in oncology. JAMA. 2003;290(24):3199–206.
57. Torigian DA, Lopez RF, Alapati S, et al. Feasibility and performance of novel software to quantify metabolically active volumes and 3D partial volumes corrected SUV and metabolic volumetric products of spinal bone marrow metastases on 18F-FDGPET/CT. Hell J Nucl Med. 2011;14(1):8–14.
58. Kwee TC, Basu S, Saboury B, Ambrosini V, Torigian DA, Alavi A. A new dimension of FDG-PET interpretation: assessment of tumor biology. Eur J Nucl Med Mol Imaging. 2011;38(6):1158–70.
59. Kwee TC, Takahara T, Ochiai R, et al. Whole-body diffusion-weighted magnetic resonance imaging. Eur J Radiol. 2009;70(3):409–17.
60. Wolf W. The unique potential for non-invasive imaging in modernizing drug development and in transforming therapeutics: PET/MRI/MRS. Pharm Res. 2011;28(3):490–3.
61. Benveniste H, Fowler JS, Rooney WD, et al. Maternal-fetal in vivo imaging: a combined PET and MRI study. J Nucl Med. 2003;44(9):1522–30.
62. Musiek ES, Torigian DA, Newberg AB. Investigation of non-neoplastic neurologic disorders with PET and MRI. PET Clin. 2008;3(3):317–34.
63. Heiss WD. The potential of PET/MR for brain imaging. Eur J Nucl Med Mol Imaging. 2009;36(Suppl 1):S105–12.
64. Boss A, Bisdas S, Kolb A, et al. Hybrid PET/MRI of intracranial masses: initial experiences and comparison to PET/CT. J Nucl Med. 2010;51(8):1198–205.
65. Cho ZH, Son YD, Kim HK, et al. Substructural hippocampal glucose metabolism observed on PET/MRI. J Nucl Med. 2010;51(10):1545–8.
66. Eggers C, Szelies B, Bauer B, et al. Imaging of acetylcholine esterase activity in brainstem nuclei involved in regulation of sleep and wakefulness. Eur J Neurol. 2007;14(6):690–3.
67. Lee KK, Salamon N. [18F] fluorodeoxyglucose-positron-emission tomography and MR imaging coregistration for presurgical evaluation of medically refractory epilepsy. AJNR Am J Neuroradiol. 2009;30(10):1811–6.
68. Salamon N, Kung J, Shaw SJ, et al. FDGPET/MRI coregistration improves detection of cortical dysplasia in patients with epilepsy. Neurology. 2008;71(20):1594–601.
69. Cruz LC Jr, Sorensen AG. Diffusion tensor magnetic resonance imaging of brain tumors. Magn Reson Imaging Clin N Am. 2006;14(2):183–202.
70. Boss A, Kolb A, Hofmann M, et al. Diffusion tensor imaging in a human PET/MR hybrid system. Investig Radiol. 2010;45(5):270–4.
71. Vlieger EJ, Majoie CB, Leenstra S, Den Heeten GJ. Functional magnetic resonance imaging for neurosurgical planning in Neurooncology. Eur Radiol. 2004;14(7):1143–53.
72. Ogawa S, Lee TM, Kay AR, Tank DW. Brain magnetic resonance imaging with contrast dependent on blood oxygenation. Proc Natl Acad Sci U S A. 1990;87(24):9868–72.
73. Behera D, Jacobs KE, Behera S, Rosenberg J, Biswal S. (18)F-FDG PET/MRI can be used to identify injured peripheral nerves in a model of neuropathic pain. J Nucl Med. 2011;52(8):1308–12.
74. Takalkar A, Chen W, Desjardins B, Alavi A, Torigian DA. Cardiovascular imaging with PET, CT, and MRI. PET Clin. 2008;3(3):411–34.
75. Syed IS, Feng D, Harris SR, et al. MR imaging of cardiac masses. Magn Reson Imaging Clin N Am. 2008;16(2):137–64. vii
76. Probst S, Seltzer A, Spieler B, Chachoua A, Friedman K. The appearance of cardiac metastasis from squamous cell carcinoma of the lung on F-18 FDG PET/CT and post hoc PET/MRI. Clin Nucl Med. 2011;36(4):311–2.
77. Higuchi T, Anton M, Dumler K, et al. Combined reporter gene PET and iron oxide MRI for monitoring survival and localization of transplanted cells in the rat heart. J Nucl Med. 2009;50(7):1088–94.
78. Bural GG, Torigian DA, Chamroonrat W, et al. Quantitative assessment of the atherosclerotic burden of the aorta by combined FDG-PET and CT image analysis: a new concept. Nucl Med Biol. 2006;33(8):1037–43.

79. Tahara N, Kai H, Ishibashi M, et al. Simvastatin attenuates plaque inflammation: evaluation by fluorodeoxyglucose positron emission tomography. J Am Coll Cardiol. 2006;48(9):1825–31.
80. Fayad ZA, Mani V, Woodward M, et al. Safety and efficacy of dalcetrapib on atherosclerotic disease using novel non-invasive multimodality imaging (dal-PLAQUE): a randomised clinical trial. Lancet. 2011;378(9802):1547–59.
81. Nawaz A, Torigian D, Zhuang H, Alavi A. Study on the correlation of atherosclerosis in the popliteal artery with metabolic activity and metabolic volumetric product of the diabetic foot. J Nucl Med. 2008;49(Suppl 1):197P.
82. von Schulthess GK, Schlemmer HP. A look ahead: PET/MR versus PET/CT. Eur J Nucl Med Mol Imaging. 2009;36(Suppl 1):S3–9.
83. Drzezga A, Souvatzoglou M, Eiber M, et al. First clinical experience with integrated whole-body PET/MR: comparison to PET/CT in patients with oncologic diagnoses. J Nucl Med. 2012;53(6):845–55.
84. Al-Nabhani KZ, Syed R, Michopoulou S, et al. Qualitative and quantitative comparison of PET/CT and PET/MR imaging in clinical practice. J Nucl Med. 2014;55(1):88–94.
85. Di Gialleonardo V, Wilson DM, Keshari KR. The potential of metabolic imaging. Semin Nucl Med. 2016;46(1):28–39.
86. Kurhanewicz J, Bok R, Nelson SJ, et al. Current and potential applications of clinical 13C MR spectroscopy. J Nucl Med. 2008;49(3):341–4.
87. Ramirez de Molina A, Rodriguez-Gonzalez A, Gutierrez R, et al. Overexpression of choline kinase is a frequent feature in human tumor-derived cell lines and in lung, prostate, and colorectal human cancers. Biochem Biophys Res Commun. 2002;296(3):580–3.
88. Awwad HM, Geisel J, Obeid R. The role of choline in prostate cancer. Clin Biochem. 2012;45(18):1548–53.
89. Piert M, Montgomery J, Kunju LP, et al. 18F-choline PET/MRI: the additional value of PET for MRI-guided transrectal prostate biopsies. J Nucl Med. 2016;57(7):1065–70.
90. Price DT, Coleman RE, Liao RP, et al. Comparison of [18F]Fluorocholine and [18F]Fluorodeoxyglucose for positron emission tomography of androgen dependent and androgen independent prostate cancer. J Urol. 2002;168(1):273–80.
91. Cazaentre T, Clivaz F, Triponez F. False-positive result in 18F-fluorocholine PET/CT due to incidental and ectopic parathyroid hyperplasia. Clin Nucl Med. 2014;39(6):e328–30.
92. Bouchelouche K, Turkbey B, Choyke PL. PSMA PET and radionuclide therapy in prostate cancer. Semin Nucl Med. 2016;46(6):522–35.
93. Gatidis S, Schmidt H, Gucke B, Bezrukov I, Seitz G, Ebinger M, et al. Comprehensive oncologic imaging in infants and preschool children with substantially reduced radiation exposure using combined simultaneous (1)(8)F-Fluorodeoxyglucose positron emission tomography/magnetic resonance imaging: a direct comparison to (1)(8)FFluorodeoxyglucose positron emission tomography/computed tomography. Investig Radiol. 2016;51(1):7–14.
94. Schafer JF, Gatidis S, Schmidt H, Guckel B, Bezrukov I, Pfannenberg CA, et al. Simultaneous whole-body PET/MR imaging in comparison to PET/CT in pediatric oncology: initial results. Radiology. 2014;273(1):220–31.
95. Hirsch FW, Sattler B, Sorge I, Kurch L, Viehweger A, Ritter L, et al. PET/MR in children. Initial clinical experience in paediatric oncology using an integrated PET/MR scanner. Pediatr Radiol. 2013;43(7):860–75.
96. Pfluger T, Melzer HI, Mueller WP, Coppenrath E, Bartenstein P, Albert MH, et al. Diagnostic value of combined (1)(8)F-FDG PET/MRI for staging and restaging in paediatric oncology. Eur J Nucl Med Mol Imaging. 2012;39(11):1745–55.
97. Stauss J, Franzius C, Pfluger T, Juergens KU, Biassoni L, Begent J, et al. Guidelines for 18F-FDG PET and PET-CT imaging in paediatric oncology. Eur J Nucl Med Mol Imaging. 2008;35(8):1581–8.
98. Goo HW. Whole-body MRI of neuroblastoma. Eur J Radiol. 2010;75(3):306–14.
99. Krohmer S, Sorge I, Krausse A, Kluge R, Bierbach U, Marwede D, et al. Whole-body MRI for primary evaluation of malignant disease in children. Eur J Radiol. 2010;74(1):256–61.
100. Riad R, Omar W, Kotb M, Hafez M, Sidhom I, Zamzam M, et al. Role of PET/CT in malignant pediatric lymphoma. Eur J Nucl Med Mol Imaging. 2010;37(2):319–29.
101. Volker T, Denecke T, Steffen I, Misch D, Schonberger S, Plotkin M, et al. Positron emission tomography for staging of pediatric sarcoma patients: results of a prospective multicenter trial. J Clin Oncol. 2007;25(34):5435–41.
102. Kaste SC. PET-CT in children: where is it appropriate? Pediatr Radiol. 2011;41(Suppl 2):509–13.
103. Love C, Tomas MB, Tronco GG, Palestro CJ. FDG PET of infection and inflammation. Radiographics : a review publication of the Radiological Society of North America. Inc. 2005;25(5):1357–68.
104. Byun BH, Kong CB, Park J, Seo Y, Lim I, Choi CW, et al. Initial metabolic tumor volume measured by 18F-FDG PET/CT can predict the outcome of osteosarcoma of the extremities. J Nuclear Med: Official Publication, Society of Nuclear Medicine. 2013;54(10):1725–32.
105. Andersen KF, Fuglo HM, Rasmussen SH, Petersen MM, Loft A. Volume-based F-18 FDG PET/CT imaging markers provide supplemental prognostic information to histologic grading in patients with high-grade bone or soft tissue sarcoma. Medicine. 2015;94(51):e2319.
106. Warbey VS, Ferner RE, Dunn JT, Calonje E, O'Doherty MJ. [18F]FDG PET/CT in the diagnosis of malignant peripheral nerve sheath tumours in neu-

rofibromatosis type-1. Eur J Nucl Med Mol Imaging. 2009;36(5):751–7.
107. Bredella MA, Torriani M, Hornicek F, Ouellette HA, Plamer WE, Williams Z, et al. Value of PET in the assessment of patients with neurofibromatosis type 1. AJR Am J Roentgenol. 2007;189(4):928–35.
108. Wasa J, Nishida Y, Tsukushi S, Shido Y, Sugiura H, Nakashima H, et al. MRI features in the differentiation of malignant peripheral nerve sheath tumors and neurofibromas. AJR Am J Roentgenol. 2010;194(6):1568–74.
109. Bisdas S, Ritz R, Bender B, Braun C, Pfannenberg C, Reimold M, et al. Metabolic mapping of gliomas using hybrid MR-PET imaging: feasibility of the method and spatial distribution of metabolic changes. Investig Radiol. 2013;48(5):295–301.
110. la Fougere C, Suchorska B, Bartenstein P, Kreth FW, Tonn JC. Molecular imaging of gliomas with PET: opportunities and limitations. Neuro-Oncology. 2011;13(8):806–19.
111. Vaidyanathan S, Patel CN, Scarsbrook AF, Chowdhury FU. FDG PET/CT in infection and inflammation--current and emerging clinical applications. Clin Radiol. 2015;70(7):787–800.
112. Chalian M, Ozturk A, Oliva-Hemker M, Pryde S, Huisman TA. MR enterography findings of inflammatory bowel disease in pediatric patients. AJR Am J Roentgenol. 2011;196(6):W810–6.
113. Narvaez JA, Narvaez J, De Lama E, De Albert M. MR imaging of early rheumatoid arthritis. Radiographics : a review publication of the Radiological Society of North America. Inc. 2010;30(1):143–63. discussion 163–145
114. Gok B, Jallo G, Hayeri R, Wahl R, Aygun N. The evaluation of FDG-PET imaging for epileptogenic focus localization in patients with MRI positive and MRI negative temporal lobe epilepsy. Neuroradiology. 2013;55(5):541–50.
115. Rastogi S, Lee C, Salamon N. Neuroimaging in pediatric epilepsy: a multimodality approach. Radiographics : a review publication of the Radiological Society of North America. Inc. 2008;28(4):1079–95.
116. Talbot JN, Paycha F, Balogova S. Diagnosis of bone metastasis: recent comparative studies of imaging modalities. Q J Nucl Med Mol Imaging. 2011;55:374–410.
117. Yang HL, Liu T, Wang XM, et al. Diagnosis of bone metastases: a meta-analysis comparing 18FDG PET, CT, MRI and bone scintigraphy. Eur Radiol. 2011;21:2604–17.
118. Goerres GW, Forster A, Uebelhart D, et al. F-18 FDG whole-body PET for the assessment of disease activity in patients with rheumatoid arthritis. Clin Nucl Med. 2006;31:386–90.
119. Palmer WE, Rosenthal DI, Schoenberg OI, et al. Quantification of inflammation in the wrist with gadolinium-enhanced MR imaging and PET with 2- [F-18]-fluoro-2-deoxy-D-glucose. Radiology. 1995;196:647–55.
120. Andersen FL, Ladefoged CN, Beyer T, et al. Combined PET/MR imaging in neurology: MR-based attenuation correction implies a strong spatial bias when ignoring bone. NeuroImage. 2014;84:206–16.
121. Ripa RS, Knudsen A, Hag AMF, et al. Feasibility of simultaneous PET/MR of the carotid artery: first clinical experience and comparison to PET/CT. Am J Nucl Med Mol Imaging. 2013;3(4):361–71.
122. Pedersen SF, Graebe M, Fisker Hag AM, Hojgaard L, Sillesen H, Kjaer A. Gene expression and 18FDG uptake in atherosclerotic carotid plaques. Nucl Med Commun. 2010;31(5):423–9.

11 Nanoimaging I

Key Points (Abstract)

Nanotechnology refers to the design, creation, and manipulation of structures on the nanometre scale. The recent research and development of nanotechnology are based and focused for the development of the novel methods of imaging and delivery of therapeutics through easiest ways. Multifunctional nanoparticles play an important role in the molecular imaging for therapeutics to molecular targets. Nanoparticle-based contrast agents have been developed for all imaging modalities.

Keywords

SPECT · PET · USPIO · Nanoparticles

11.1 Introduction

The term nanotechnology refers to the creation of objects with dimensions between 1.0 and 100.0 nm, or between one and 100 billionths of a meter. The difference between the nanoparticles and microparticles is based on the size, and nanoparticle size is ranging from the 5 to 700 nm in diameter, while the microparticles 3 μm in diameter (Diagram 11.1). Nanomaterials have similarities in scale to molecules and cellular structures affected by disease processes, and nanomaterials can be engineered in different ways to serve various functions. Due to the very small size of the nanoparticles, they can enter the cells easily to create various functions like intracellular imaging, targeting of various molecules, and also for the delivery of drugs or genes into the cells [1]. The goal of the field of nanomedicine is to use the properties and physical characteristics of nanotechnologies to diagnose and treat diseases at the molecular level [1]. Recent advances in the nanotechnologies are allowing the targeted and molecular imaging of tumours and other conditions in a better way. Nanoparticle-based contrast agents have been developed for single-photon emission computed tomography (SPECT) and positron emission tomography (PET), magnetic resonance (MR) imaging, ultrasonography (US), computed tomography (CT), and optical imaging. Nanotechnologies cover all aspects of radiology and also allow targeted drug delivery to novel molecular targets. Tumour biology and the barriers of the tumour microvasculature and microenvironment need to be studied for understanding the potential and limitations of nanotechnology-based targeted imaging and therapeutics. The newer development in properties of nanotechnologies has newer concepts of the drug delivery agents, contrast agents, and diagnostic devices. Nanomaterials are their large surface area-to-volume ratio, which may be orders of magnitude greater than that of current materials, a feature that allows the surface of the nanoparticle to be coated with a large amount of imaging or therapeutic moieties.

S. Shaikh, *Advances in Imaging*, https://doi.org/10.1007/978-981-16-9535-3_11

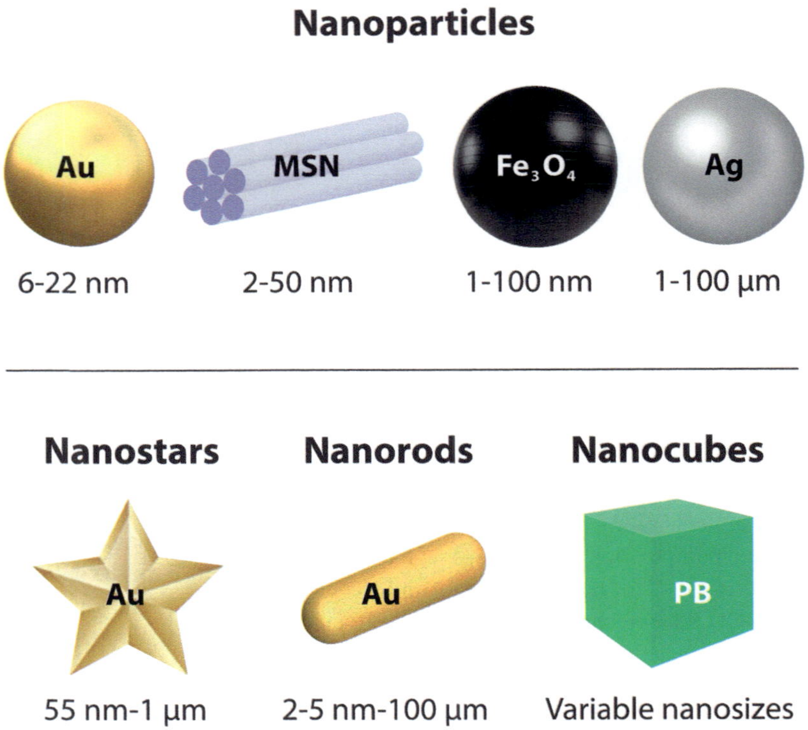

Diagram 11.1 The various sizes of the nanoparticles

11.2 History and Development of Nanotechnology

Richard Feynman is credited for inspiring the development of the field of nanotechnology when he delivered a lecture at the California Institute of Technology on December 29, 1959, entitled "There's Plenty of Room at the Bottom: An Invitation to Enter a New Field of Physics". In the 1970s, Eric Drexler initiated investigations into molecular manufacturing, and in 1986 he introduced the term nanotechnology in his book *Engines of Creation* [2]. In 1992, Drexler expanded on this work and published nanosystems [3], a technical work that outlines how to manufacture extremely high-performance machines out of molecular carbon lattices. Nanosystems were the first nanotechnology textbook in the world.

"Nano" means one-billionth; thus, a nanometre is one-billionth of a meter. The term nanotechnology refers to the creation of objects with nanoscale dimensions between 1.0 and 100.0 nm [4]. Nanoparticles are approximately 1/1000 the diameter of a hair, approximately the size of a cellular organelle [5]. Due to the very small size, which is on the order of molecules and organelles, nanoparticles may be used for molecular imaging and to deliver therapeutics to molecular targets [1]. One of the biggest advantages of the use of nanoparticles includes a high signal-to-noise ratio, ease of integrating multiple properties, lengthy circulation times, and the possibility of delivering high concentrations of contrast or therapeutic agents.

The use of the nanoimaging can be in varied presentations like the specific probe or tracer which can be used for the various functions and various physical and chemical properties of nanoparticles based on these they can be attached to the ligands. These ligands are various monoclonal antibodies, peptides, small protein like having both natural and non-natural amino acids, vitamins, or the aptamers which are the various small molecules binding to another molecule [6]. These nanoparticles also can be used as the therapeutic carrier which can carry the various nanoparticles for carrying the various drugs, genes, or proteins.

These various therapeutic agents will be attached to the target-specific imaging particle [7].

11.3 Nanotechnologies Interventional Radiologists Role

Many therapeutic options are available which may directly or indirectly affect the practice of interventional radiology. This can be used for the pain control with transdermal local anaesthetics, sustained-release antimicrobials for treatment of infection, and the use of nanocapsules and liposomes as haemoglobin carriers in the development of blood substitutes [8]. Nanoparticles that contain streptokinase and that are targeted to fibrin have been described as yielding the same degree of thrombolysis as a 1000-fold greater dose of free enzyme [9]. Liposomes both with and without encapsulated thrombolytics have been used for clot lysis in applying US energy to rupture the liposomes and disrupt the clot [10, 11]. Drug-eluting stents that release agents such as sirolimus and paclitaxel have the potential to reduce intimal hyperplasia, leading to in-stent restenosis [12, 13]. The use of novel nanoparticles to coat stents with a thin and uniform layer of biodegradable polymeric nanoparticles that carry a number of therapeutic agents and paclitaxel eluting porous carbon-carbon nanoparticle coated stents has been described as a potential strategy [13, 14]. Injuring the vascular wall with angioplasty or stent placement leads to increased localized uptake of nanoparticles, including dexamethasone-loaded nanoparticles and nanoparticle formulation of paclitaxel within the vessel wall [15]. Antibodies and ligands for av. b3 integrin have also been used to target drug-carrying nanoparticles to the vessel wall [16]. Finally, novel nanoparticle-based haemostatic agents are being developed for percutaneous arterial puncture [17]. Interventional molecular imaging entails minimally invasive (e.g. percutaneous, catheter-directed intravascular, and endoluminal) placement of imaging tools, such as optical imaging probes. The aim of this approach is to extend the capabilities of currently available molecular imaging techniques to (a) reach deep-seated targets, (b) enable a close look at small targets, (c) precisely guide delivery of nontargeted imaging tracers or therapeutic agents, and (d) super selectively enhance the effectiveness of targeted imaging [18].

11.4 Nanotechnologies for Cancer Therapy

Multifunctional nanoparticles may be used to target therapeutics to the tumour (Diagram 11.2). Many newer therapeutic strategies are being developed and also an ever-increasing number of potential tumour-specific targets which can be active as well as passive targets which are being identified (Diagram 11.3). Promising targets that are expressed exclusively or preferentially within the tumour, tumour vasculature, and neoplastic cells have been targeted. For example, angiogenic tumour vessels are rich in av. b3 integrin and vascular endothelial growth factor or platelet-derived growth factor kinase receptors, whereas tumour cells may demonstrate unique, increased expression of surface proteins such as endothelial growth factor receptors, oestrogen receptor, proteases, folate and transferrin receptors, prostate-specific antigen, and carcinoembryonic antigen. Nanoparticle-based therapeutics may vary with respect to the component materials, size, shape, therapeutic agent, and drug or therapeutic incorporation method. Nanoparticle-based therapeutics has different characteristics in terms of drug-loading capacity, drug release rates, and potential for targeted drug delivery [19]. The use of radiofrequency ablation to increase vascular permeability is feasible, with resultant enhanced intratumoral accumulation of liposomal doxorubicin and tumouricidal activity in areas of sublethal hyperthermia, leading to improved clinical efficacy [20]. Sublethal heat at the periphery of the tumour and between spheres of ablative heat may also destabilize tumour cell membranes and deactivate multidrug-resistant pumps, leading to neoplastic cells that are more susceptible to the effects of chemotherapeutics. The size of the nanoparticles was found to significantly influ-

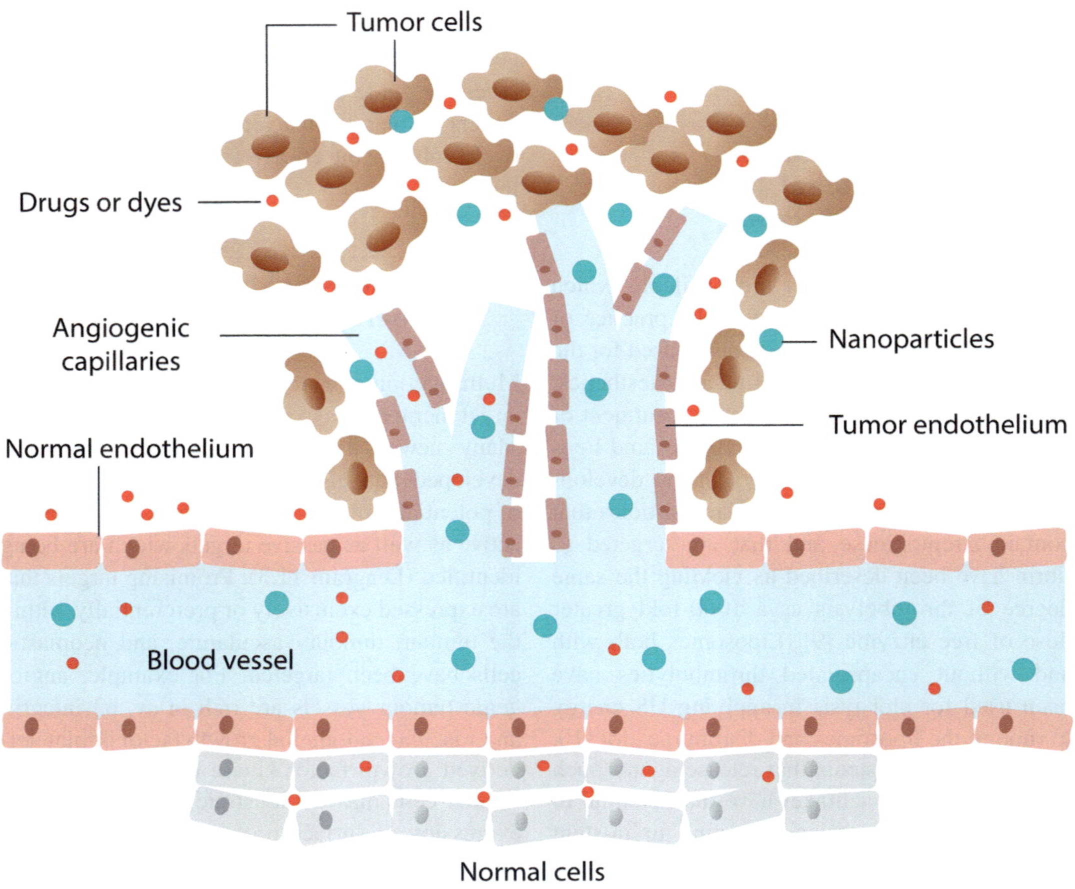

Diagram 11.2 Showing the difference between the normal and tumour endothelium and also the movement of the nanoparticles through the tumour endothelium

ence the extent of tumour destruction; liposomes with a diameter of 100 nm produced a greater effect than those with larger diameters [21], a finding that likely is related to the size of endothelial gaps available for transvascular transport, which imposes barriers to the delivery of larger particles [22]. Another common approach is the use of tumour-targeted nanoparticles to generate lethal ablative thermal energy. Nanoparticles may be light or laser-activated for photodynamic therapy [23]. Magnetic nanoparticles may absorb energy from an alternating magnetic field and convert it into heat, a process described by Hilger et al. [24]. Magnetic nanoparticles may be infused intravenously. Furthermore, percutaneous intratumoral and catheter-directed intraarterial delivery of these agents has been described [25, 26]. Gold nanoshells, or quantum dots, absorb near-infrared light and are capable of producing lethal heat [27]. Although there is great potential for nanoparticle-based imaging and treatment, there is considerable concern regarding potential toxicities [28, 29]. The toxicity of a nanoparticle has been shown to depend on its size, morphologic characteristics, and chemical composition. Active targeting implies incorporation of a ligand or antibody that is specific to cell or vessel molecules, enabling the nanoparticle to bind to a target and enhance accumulation of the therapeutic at the desired site. Passive targeting relies on the concept of enhanced permeability and retention of the tumour microvasculature, a result of the small size of the nanoparticle. Circulating agents are cleared from the blood-

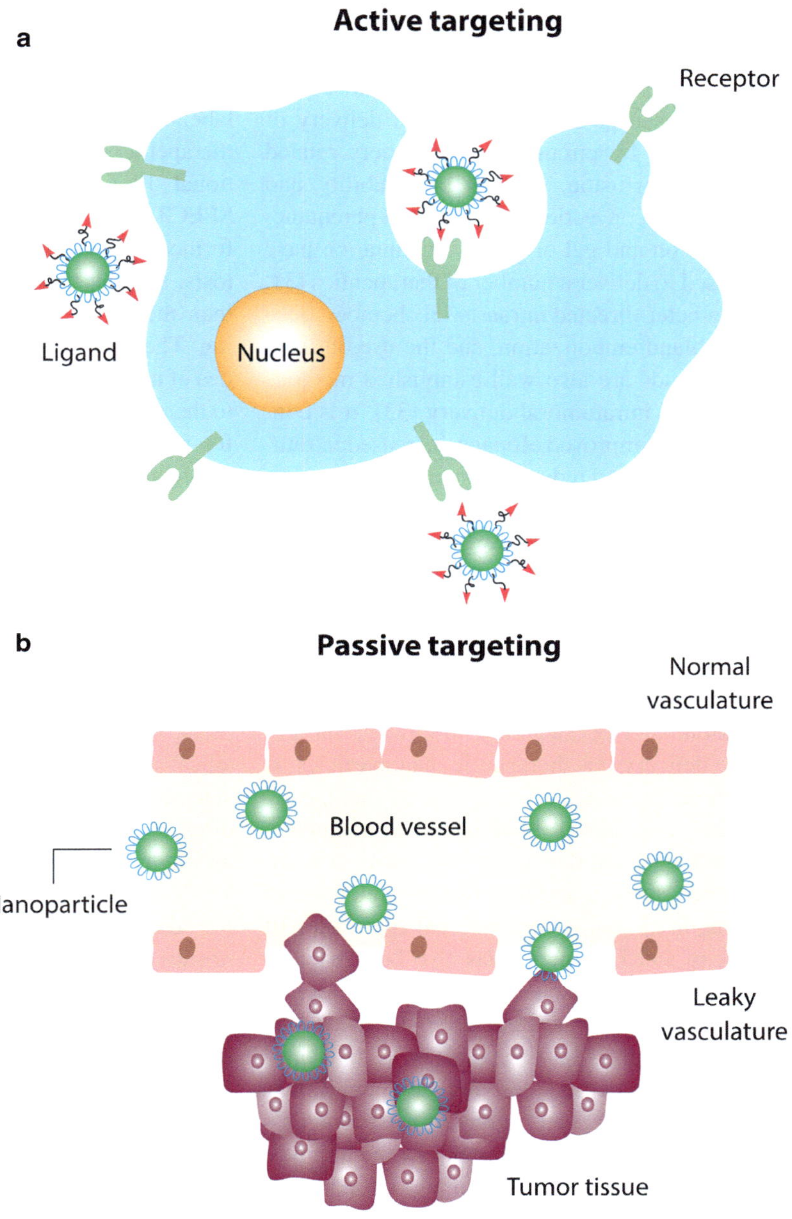

Diagram 11.3 Two different types of the targeting of the nanoparticles active and passive. (**a**) is active targeting and (**b**) is passive targeting due to leaky vasculature

stream by the reticuloendothelial system in the spleen and liver. Tumours may be thought of as comprising three compartments: the vasculature, interstitium, and the neoplastic cells themselves. Each of these compartments has intrinsic barriers. For instance, blood vessels in tumours are heterogeneously distributed. Furthermore, temporal and spatial heterogeneity of tumour perfusion has been demonstrated [30]. Extravasation of therapeutic agents from blood vessels into the interstitium is limited by the permeability of blood vessels. Elevated interstitial pressure limits intratumoral convection of therapeutic agents so they are unable to move from the blood vessel, across the interstitium, and into the tumour cells. Once they arrive at the tumour cell, therapeutic agents must cross the cellular or nuclear membranes. When administered intravenously, intratumoral deposition of therapeutic agents is augmented by active and passive targeted delivery of these agents. There is great potential for the use of imaging-based guidance to augment delivery of these agents by circumventing barriers related to tumour perfusion, vascular permeability, and intratumoral convection. Intratumoral percutaneous infusion and gel or wafer implantation have been used to deliver a number of therapeutics [31, 32]. Catheter-directed intraarterial chemoembolization, bland embolization, and the use of drug-eluting beads are also well-established methods of localized intratumoral delivery [33]. It is conceivable that improved efficacy, increased intratumoral dosage, and reduced systemic toxicity may result from the use of these strategies. US-assisted delivery has been described for liposomal carriers and may be used to target circulating multi-functional nanotherapeutics to the tumour [34]. Greater homogeneity of intratumoral distribution of therapeutic agents may be possible and may not depend on microvascular distribution, perfusion, and permeability. Improved intratumoral delivery of therapeutic nanoparticles is hypothesized to result in optimized therapeutic efficacy. Intratumoral injection of a therapeutic agent allows local delivery of high drug concentration to a tumour and may increase retention of the drug in tumour tissue. External application of magnetic and US energy has also been used to help iron-containing nanoparticles and liposomal agents, respectively, accumulate [34]. The use of US-activated drug delivery vehicles such as liposomes, polymeric micelles, and nanobubbles has been reported. US energy may drive such agents against the vessel wall, through cell membranes, and into tumour cells. Imaging of patients' response to targeted therapeutic agents may focus on the expected physiologic effect of the therapy rather than on anatomic imaging, such as the linear tumour measurements described in the response evaluation criteria in solid tumours (RECIST). However, these novel approaches to functional imaging, such as dynamic contrast-enhanced MR imaging, must first be validated with appropriate clinical studies and then sufficiently standardized [35]. For example, if a therapeutic agent targets the endothelium, assessment of the patient's response may be determined at dynamic contrast-enhanced MR imaging or by measuring tumour hypoxia with fluorine18-labelled fluoromisonidazole and copper-64. If a therapeutic agent targets neoplastic cells, functional PET with 18F fluorodeoxyglucose or SPECT with 18F-fluorothymidine may be performed to evaluate glucose metabolism or apoptosis, and the findings may be more meaningful than those obtained with usual anatomic imaging. There is substantial interest in the capabilities of molecular imaging for measuring response to therapy. Targeted nanoparticles have been used for molecular imaging, which may represent a future approach to response assessment [36, 37]. Multivalent nanoparticles that contain therapeutic and imaging moieties also may allow imaging of intratumoral accumulation and trafficking of therapeutic agents, which in turn would allow assessment of drug distribution and its association with efficacy, local failure, and recurrence.

Nano- and microparticles based on polymers, proteins, lipids, lipoproteins, metals, and silica, as well as fullerenes, carbon nanotubes, selenium-cadmium nanocrystals (i.e. quantum dots), and microbubbles, are frequently suggested as diagnostic and theranostic agents (Diagram 11.4). In general, one can distinguish between nanodiagnostics (1 nm to, 1 μm) and microdiagnostics (1 μm to, 1 mm; however, most microdiagnostics are 1–5 μm) on the basis of their size. Theranostics nanomedicines are nanoparticles that act as both diagnostic and therapeutic agents. In this context, depending on the particle design, the obtained diagnostic information can be different, for example, providing insights into the availability of a molecular target in the tissue, the vascular permeability and retention of the molecule, the drug release from the particle, and the response of the target tissue.

The intrinsic properties of nanoparticles do not always correlate with the pharmacokinetic and pharmacodynamic requirements. As per their size, which is ranging from a few nanometres for small polymers and dendrimers to more than 1000 nm for microbubbles, the biodistribution of nanoparticles is restricted to the compartment in which they are injected. If they are administered

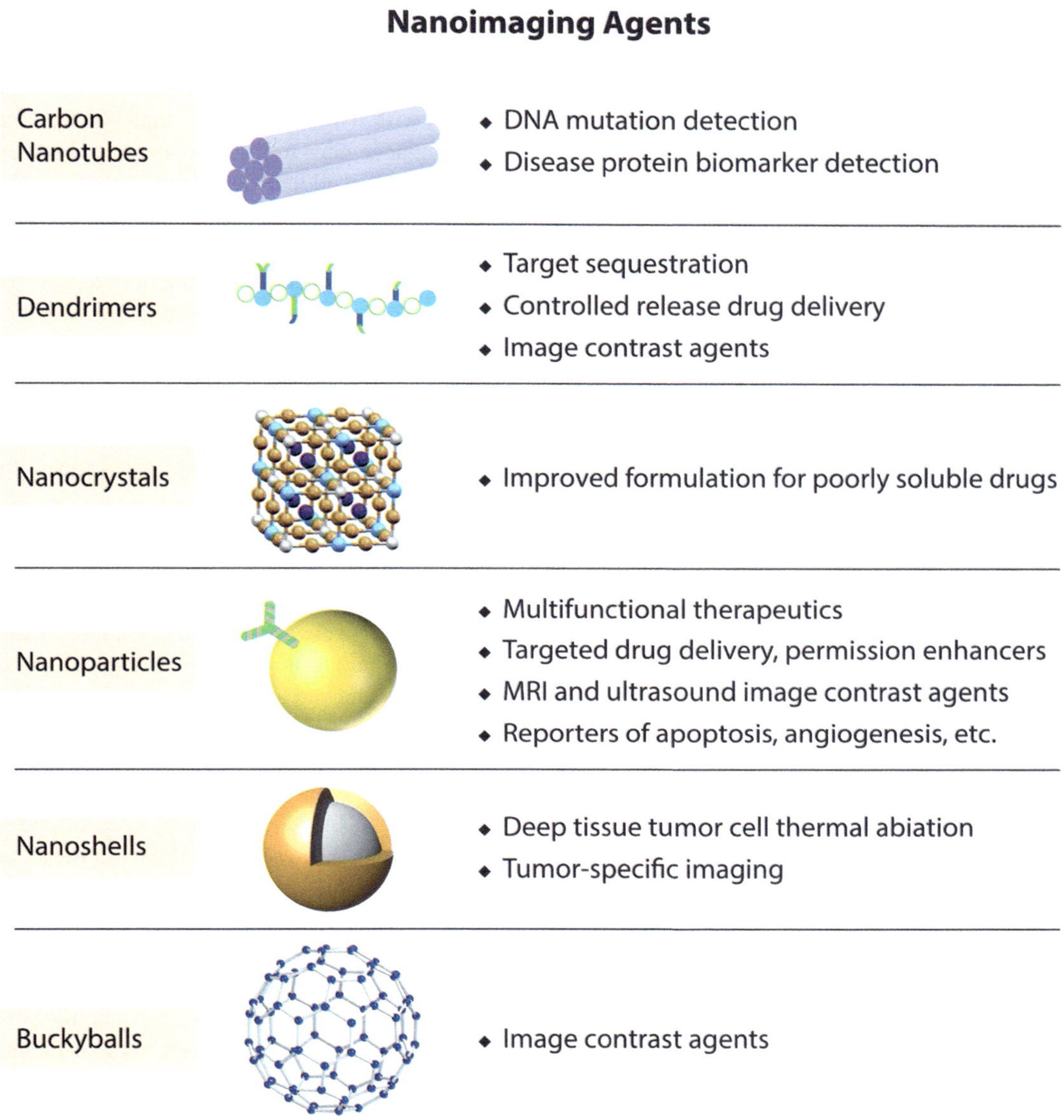

Diagram 11.4 Different types of the nanoimaging materials

locally, then they will be located around the site of injection, and the clearance is very slow and cleared by the lymphatic drainage. When these nanoparticles are given orally, they are confined to the gastrointestinal tract and are excreted via the faces. When administered intravenously, then based on their size, charge, and surface properties, their biodistribution will be restricted to the vascular system and liver and spleen, tumours and inflammation sites; these are characterized by fenestrated endothelium and enhanced vascular leakiness. The larger the size of nanoparticles, then these nanoparticles spent more time in the circulation system, and intact vascular endothelium normally will prevent them to get accumulated in the majority of normal tissues, thus reducing the side effects. In the abnormal and leaky neovasculature of tumours and inflammation, there will be extravasation due to the increased permeability and retention (EPR) effect, thus reducing the therapeutic efficacy [38–43]. EPR is due to the long-circulating properties of nanoparticles which is gradually increasing over the time and peaking approximately between 12 and 48 h. The systemically administered nanoparticles for diagnostic purposes are relating to the (a) poor penetration in the tissues (due to their large size, thereby constraining their access to target cells which are located away from blood vessels), (b) their prolonged staying in certain organs like the liver and spleen will give rise to the long-term side effects when administered repeatedly, and (c) their composition like heavy metal-based quantum dots is having concerns with the biocompatibility. The use of the blood pool contrast agents when used for MPS, labelling, and tracking of stem cells, monitoring of implant materials by the tissue engineering, vascular targets, facilitating interventional radiologic management options, and various theranostic approaches this will lead to the concept of the personalize nanomedicine treatments by combination of drug targeting and imaging.

11.5 Nanoparticles as Blood Pool Contrast Agents

The imaging of the various small and larger blood vessels is of significance for many diseases, which includes the atherosclerosis, thrombosis, venous insufficiency, vascular inflammation, and cancer. There are two major concepts for the achievement of the good contrast of vessels with background by administering the contrast agents. For this the contrast agents with long blood half-lives are usually preferred contrast agents. In magnetic resonance (MR) imaging, various positive (T1) and negative (T2) nanosized contrast agents are being developed, and a couple of them are being used for the clinical evaluation. As positive MR contrast agents which are bright in T1-weighted imaging, gadolinium-loaded polymers [44], paramagnetic liposomes [45], and very small superparamagnetic iron oxide (SPIO) nanoparticles like the citrate-coated very small SPIO nanoparticles [46] are being used successfully in preclinical and/or clinical trials, as the macromolecular MR contrast agents are not being commonly used in the preclinical studies, like the assessment of the functional vascular information status in tumours with dynamic contrast material leading to the enhancement in the MR imaging. Further these agents had added value due to the clinically available low-molecular-weight agents as they are lower and more “tumour-specific” extravasation, further decreasing the temporal resolution on dynamic images, and further facilitating the differentiation of the perfusion and permeability effects [44, 47]. This is possible due to the very slower extravasation and also the stable relaxivities. Small protein-binding gadolinium chelates like gadofosveset and gadocoletic acid [44] will be changing their relaxivity while interacting with their proteins causing less concentration in the tissues of the interest. The clinical CT scanners’ image acquisition is very short due to the low-molecular-weight contrast agents having the iodine concentrations of 300–400 mg of iodine per millilitre and can easily be scanned including the large parts of the body, which will be rendering the various blood pool CT contrast agents for most clinical applications. Microbubbles are the established blood pool contrast agents used in the ultrasonography (US) and having the 1- to 3-mm large gas bubbles which will be stabilizing the various phospholipids, polymers, sugars, or denaturized proteins. US can detect the microbubbles with high sensitivity and specificity and thus the microvessel evaluation to quantify perfusion along with the destruction replenishment techniques [48].

11.6 Imaging the MPS

Most nanoparticles are ideal for imaging of the MPS (formerly reticuloendothelial system), comprising of the liver, spleen, and the lymphatics, and these are being taken in the various tissues where most of the particles are taken up. The basis for this targeting of particles to the MPS is due to the high content of macrophages (Kupffer cells in the liver) in these organs. Majority of the particles end up in the MPS, and thus the nanoparticle-based MPS imaging agents are being used for the various modalities, like MR imaging [49–55], CT [56–62], single-photon emission CT (SPECT) [63], optical imaging [64], photoacoustic imaging [65], and even US [66, 67]. Iron oxide nanoparticles (MR imaging [55]), quantum dots (optical imaging [64]), gold nanocages (photoacoustic imaging [65]), and microbubbles (US are being used [66, 67]).

MR imaging is possible due to their superparamagnetic nature. Their coating like the polymer-coated iron cores will be inducing the proton dephasing and decreasing the signal intensity on T2-weighted images thus creating local heterogeneities in the magnetic field, which are causing the local susceptibility changes further decreasing the T2 signal, thus allowing the MPS-specific MR imaging contrast agent [68]. The nanoparticles which are larger than approximately 5–10 nm, SPIO and USPIO nanoparticles are usually cleared from the blood due to the phagocytosis through macrophages (e.g. Kupffer cells), which will result in the uptake in the liver, spleen, and lymph nodes [69]. The uptake in liver is seen in the normal liver tissue having Kupffer cells. Majority of the abnormalities like scarring, regeneration, and shunting in cirrhotic liver and inflammatory or infectious processes all these will reduce uptake of SPIO causing the bright focal area in the signal reduced liver parenchyma on T2-weighted images. In malignant liver tumours, Kupffer cells are displaced by tumour cells and due to this these lesions will be not having the T2-reduced signal on the MR images, and this can differentiate them from the surrounding normal liver with reduced T2 signal [49, 70]. For the diagnosis of the liver metastasis SPIO-enhanced liver MR imaging is very sensitive [71, 72]. Kupffer cells still present in early stages of hepatocellular carcinoma can sometimes cause particle uptake similar to that seen in hepatic adenomas [73]. Positive contrast of SPIO during its blood pool phase can support diagnosis finding by depicting, for example, early arterial feeding in small hepatomas or a gradual centripetal fill-in pattern in haemangiomas. The presence of the iron oxide particles causes a decrease in signal intensity on T2- and T2-weighted MR images. Contrast-enhanced MR lymphography with these agents has been shown to improve the detection of lymph node metastasis and the differentiation between reactive and metastatically infiltrated lymph nodes in patients with prostate cancer [52, 74], breast cancer [75], head and neck tumours [50], and renal cancer [76].

Imaging inflammation, plaques) it is important to know that various monocyte subsets will internalize not all particles with the same avidity, resulting in variable loading efficacy and thus causing a signal intensity change at MR imaging, which possibly reflecting different biologic properties [77]. Successful preclinical imaging with iron oxide nanoparticles has also been achieved to image transplant rejection [78] and tissue repair processes such as postischemic lesions in the brain [53] and heart [79]. MR imaging with iron oxide nanoparticles has been used in animals and ultimately in patients to visualize insulitis as early manifestation of type I diabetes, where an autoimmune process leads to an inflammatory destruction of the islet cells.

11.7 Cell Labelling and Tracking

Cell tracking can be performed by means of either direct or indirect cell labelling [80–82]. In direct cell-labelling approaches, the cells are labelled ex vivo with the imaging markers and then transplanted. Indirect cell-labelling methods take advantage of reporter genes that make the cells produce or accumulate imaging markers after their transplantation in vivo [80]. However, direct cell labelling is simply achieved by incubating the cells with the labelling nanoparticle [80]. In phagocytosing cells, these are then usually labelled relatively quickly [83, 84]. With direct labelling methods, the nanoparticles become diluted in an 1expanding cell population through distribution over daughter cells, who then carry approximately 50% of the original labelling density if distributed symmetrically, or the label can be lost by the cells, as has been shown, for example, for indium 111 (111In) oxine [85, 86]. Importantly, direct labelling methods also do not allow for the evaluation of the viability, proliferation, activation, or death of the cells, and, in the worst case, the label can be incorporated by other cells (e.g. macrophages) that metabolize the remnants of the dead cellular transplants, which can lead to severe misinterpretation of the imaging findings. For cell labelling, primarily nanoparticles suitable for MR imaging have been used. The iron oxide core usually contains several thousands of iron atoms, significantly increasing the local iron concentration and enabling the detection of lower concentrations of particles. The relatively small intracellular particle concentration results in a relaxivity change sufficient for the detection of locally concentrated cells in vitro. Cells that are more actively phagocytosing, such as dendritic cells [87] or pancreatic islet cells [88], can accumulate sufficient amounts of nanoparticles to allow for in vivo detection. The development of new MR pulse sequences such as off-resonance MR imaging, which generates positive contrast through suppression of background tissue, may help increase the robustness of cell detection. Cell labelling was achieved by using an additional transfection agent, and the cells were stereotactically injected near the side of the brain injury. Dynamic changes in the observed hypointensities were attributed to assumed movement of the cells towards the lesion [89]. The accurate MR assessment enabled the determination of the proper operation of the implants and revealed related complications such as shrinkage or adhesions without additional invasive surgical revision [90]. Beyond that, gold and silver nanoparticles have also been incorporated into approaches that combine tailored mechanical properties' biodegradable polymeric blend of poly(lactide)/poly/(4-hydroxybutryrate) to improve image enhancement in X-ray and near-infrared imaging of an absorbable vascular graft [91]. Diagnostic particles have also been used to label biohybrid tissue-engineered implants and cellular transplants. MR imaging is to monitor tissue-engineered vascular grafts in vivo with the use of human aortic smooth muscle cells labelled with iron oxide nanoparticles. MR imaging was used to evaluate the structure and function of the human tissue-engineered vascular grafts in addition to investigating the fate of the cells in vivo during a 3-week time course [92]. Especially important is gathering information about the fate of tissue-engineered endothelium in a vascular graft, as this cell layer provides an anticoagulant and antithrombotic barrier and modulates vascular tone, growth, inflammation, and haemostasis by secreting biologically active mediators. Labelling of the endothelial cells with superparamagnetic nanoparticles provided a valuable tool for monitorable seeding procedures and offered details about the intactness of the endothelial monolayer after implantation [93]. In the field of cellular transplants, islet cell transplantation has received considerable attention as an effective therapy for type I diabetes mellitus. However, the therapeutic effect is often limited owing to immunologic reactions and graft rejection. To protect pancreatic islet cells from immune reactions leading to rejection of the graft, encapsulation into hydrogel structures has effectively prolonged islet cell viability and improved their insulin secretion. Capsules labelled with gadolinium-containing or gold nanoparticles could be further visualized with MR imaging, CT, and US [94, 95]. Immunoprotected alginate microcapsule formulations with coembedded perfluorocarbons also enabled multimodality imaging with CT, US, and 19F MR imaging. In addition, perfluorocarbons increased oxygen tension in the immediate proximity of the cells owing to their high oxygen solubility [96]. This probe allowed the local sensing of pH changes in the microenvironment associated with cell death and provided conclusive information about the time period of cell survival and the reasons for incomplete immune protection. In conclusion, it has been demonstrated that the labelling of implant material and cells with nanoparticles is an efficient method for visualizing the location and fate of implanted devices.

In nano- and microparticles for molecular imaging from a pharmacologic and imaging point of view, molecular imaging probes should fulfil several demands: good delivery to the target, highly specific binding (and internalization), low non-specific accumulation, rapid elimination of the unbound probe, and highly sensitive detection (optimally enabling micro dosing). Until now, most clinically applied molecular imaging agents have been small molecules with fast renal clearance for imaging with PET or SPECT—the modalities with the highest sensitivity for probes (pico- and nanomolar concentrations can be detected). For other imaging modalities with lower contrast agent sensitivity, such as MR imaging (sensitivity up to nanomolar range) or CT (sensitivity in the millimolar range), nanoparticles can be designed as highly potent signal-altering molecules. Examples are targeted SPIO nanoparticles such as USPIO and crossed-linked iron oxide [97–100], as well as paramagnetic liposomes [101] for MR imaging and different functionalized gold nanoparticles for CT (Table) [102–105]. Targeted nanoparticles for PET and SPECT, the most widely used molecular imaging modalities in clinical applications, are rarely used. In addition, injected amounts of targeted nanoparticles in many preclinical studies are much higher than would ever be acceptable for humans. On one hand, the expected key market for molecular imaging probes that target angiogenesis and inflammation is large because both processes play a pivotal role in a multitude of diseases, including cancer, atherosclerosis, and cardiac and cerebral infarction. Many related target structures are located at the surface of endothelial cells, extravasation of the diagnostic probes is not required, and the low extravasation can even be beneficial to keep the non-specific background signal low. Thus, nano- and microparticles are well suited for these targets. Molecular US contrast agents are the only ligand-targeted diagnostic microparticles that are being clinically evaluated at the moment. Depending on the shell composition, soft- and hard-shell microbubbles can be distinguished, as reviewed by Kiessling et al. [106]. After preclinical testing in models of breast [107] and prostate [108] cancer in addition to their use for monitoring antiangiogenic tumour therapies [109], the diagnostic potential of vascular endothelial growth factor receptor 2-targeted soft-shell microbubbles with a perfluorobutane core and a PEGylated phospholipid shell [110] is now being evaluated in patients suspected of having prostate carcinoma. Advantages of this class of contrast agents are as follows: (a) highly sensitive detection with US, (b) rapid binding (short time between injection and imaging), (c) no extravasation (low non-specific background), and (d) rapid elimination from the body (after microbubble disintegration, by means of exhalation of the core gas and metabolization of the phospholipids).

11.8 Nanoparticles for Imaging-Guided Interventions

Nano- and microparticles have been used for tumour embolization in the kidney, liver, and brain. During the past several years, nano- and microparticles for embolization therapies have been developed that can be imaged with CT and MR imaging (Diagram 11.5). Trans-arterial chemoembolization is another procedure that may benefit from the use of novel theranostic nano- and/or microparticle agents, which have been excellently reviewed by Lewis and Dreher [111]. Here, chemotherapeutic drugs can be encapsulated in degradable and nondegradable carrier materials based, for example, on polymers of poly(lactic/glycolic) acid, polyvinyl acetate, and natural substances like plasma proteins, alginate, and chitosan. The properties of theranostic microparticles with variable constitution and radiolabels that are used for selective internal radiation therapy treatment of liver tumours are reviewed by Van de Wiele et al. [112].

Because of the local administration and the use of high doses, however, PET-based distribution measurements of 90Y microspheres are feasible during selective internal radiation therapy treatment.

11.9 Nano- or Microparticles for Imaging-Guided Hyperthermia Treatment

The basic principle of nano- or microparticle-based hyperthermia is to use particles that absorb energy and transform it into heat. This can be achieved by means of irradiation with acoustic [113, 114] and electromagnetic [115] waves, as well as with light [116–119]. The major prob-

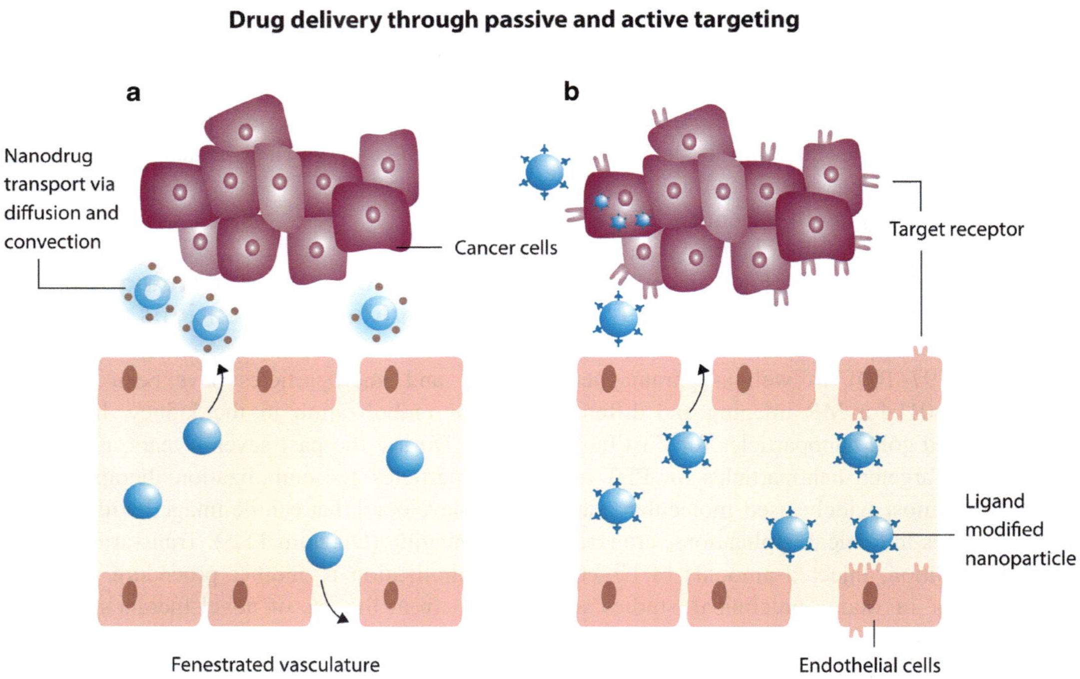

Diagram 11.5 A showing the passive targeting due to the diffusion and active targeting by using the specific target receptor. (**a**) showing the passive targeting due to fenestrated vasculature (**b**), by direct target receptors

lem and the motivation for choosing a theranostic approach is the control of the homogeneous and quantitatively sufficient accumulation of the nanoparticles in the target tissue which is the major problem for most of these approaches and limits the therapeutic outcome. In this context, injections of particles into the target tissue, catheter-based local arterial injections, and systemic intravenous injections have been evaluated [120, 121]. Account the available alternative treatments, which include high-intensity focused ultrasound, radiofrequency ablation, cryoablation, and embolization, as well as radiation therapy, trans-arterial chemoembolization, and selective internal radiation therapy treatment. Malignant brain tumours are suited for nanoparticle-based magnetic fluid hyperthermia because after surgery, radiation therapy, and chemotherapy, further therapeutic options for malignant brain tumours are limited. Imaging-guided drug delivery final interesting and increasingly recognized application of nanoparticles is for imaging-guided drug delivery. By developing nanomedicine formulations containing both diagnostic and therapeutic properties, their biodistribution and target site accumulation can be visualized and quantified, their local activation can be monitored (in case of triggered drug release), and their therapeutic efficacy can be assessed non-invasively and longitudinally [122–124]. The latter strategy could, for example, be relevant in case of long-circulating blood pool contrast agents that contain antiangiogenic drugs or vascular disrupting agents, which would enable targeted reduction of blood vessels in tumours as well as simultaneous monitoring of therapeutic efficacy [125, 126]. The use of nanoparticles that contain both drugs and imaging agents for visualizing their biodistribution and target site accumulation is arguably the most relevant application of imaging-guided drug delivery. Convincing clinical proof of principle is available showing that tumours associated with a strong EPR effect, such as Kaposi sarcomas and head and neck tumours, respond relatively well to liposome-based nanotherapeutics, whereas tumours that generally have poor EPR, such as breast carcinomas, do not seem to benefit too much from such targeted interventions—at least not when it comes to increasing response rates and prolonging progression-free and overall survival times [39, 127, 128]. Hybrid imaging approaches that aim to non-invasively monitor therapeutic efficacy can be implemented to further refine and personalize nanomedicine treatments. Conclusion diagnostic nanoparticles are favourably suited for labelling the MPS (e.g. liver, spleen, lymph nodes), and the use of diagnostic nanoparticles is indicated for ex vivo labelling of cells, scaffolds, and other kinds of tissue-engineered implants that are to be because of the local administration and the use of high doses, however, PET-based distribution measurements of 90Y microspheres are feasible during selective internal radiation therapy treatment.

11.10 Imaging-Guided Drug Delivery

A final interesting and increasingly recognized application of nanoparticles is for imaging-guided drug delivery. By developing nanomedicine formulations containing both diagnostic and therapeutic properties, their biodistribution and target site accumulation can be visualized and quantified, their local activation can be monitored (in case of triggered drug release), and their therapeutic efficacy can be assessed non-invasively and longitudinally [122–124] (Diagram 11.6). The latter strategy could, for example, be relevant in case of long-circulating blood pool contrast agents that contain antiangiogenic drugs or vascular disrupting agents, which would enable targeted reduction of blood vessels in tumours as well as simultaneous monitoring of therapeutic efficacy [125, 126]. The potential value of monitoring triggered drug release has, on several occasions, been elegantly demonstrated by using temperature-sensitive liposomes containing chemotherapeutic drugs and T1-weighted MR imaging contrast agents [129]. When used in combination with local radiofrequency ablation or MR imaging-guided high-intensity-focused ultrasound-mediated hyperthermia, such

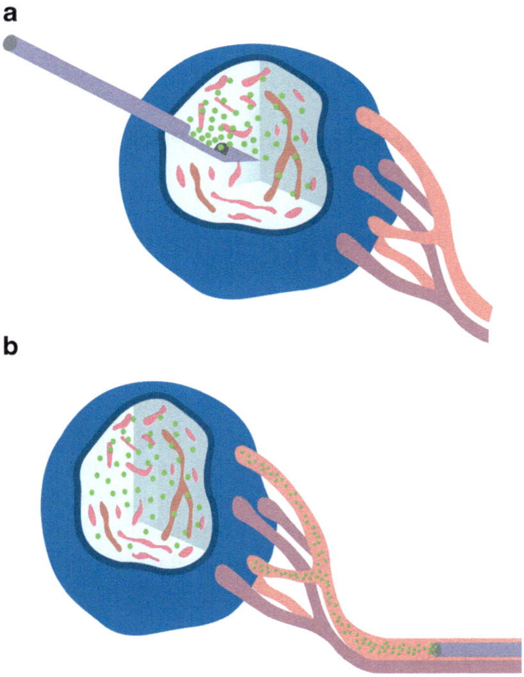

Diagram 11.6 (**a**) is direct drug delivery and (**b**) is passive drug delivery in the tumour regions

stimuli-sensitive nanotheranostics, they provide real-time feedback on the efficacy of temperature-induced drug release [130–132]. Convincing clinical proof of principle is available showing that tumours associated with a strong EPR effect, such as Kaposi sarcomas and head and neck tumours, respond relatively well to liposome-based nanotherapeutics, whereas tumours that generally have poor EPR, such as breast carcinomas, do not seem to benefit too much from such targeted interventions at least not when it comes to increasing response rates and prolonging progression-free and overall survival times [39, 127, 128]. On the basis of the above notion that a substantial target site accumulation of nanomedicines, as observed in Kaposi sarcomas and head and neck cancers, also leads to significant therapeutic efficacy, it seems reasonable to incorporate imaging much more strongly into nanomedicine-based chemotherapeutic interventions [128, 133]. Hybrid imaging approaches that aim to non-invasively monitor therapeutic efficacy can be implemented to further refine and personalize nanomedicine treatments.

11.11 Nanoimaging for Prion Diseases

Misfolding and aggregation of prion proteins is linked to a number of neurodegenerative disorders such as Creutzfeldt-Jakob disease (CJD) and its variants: Kuru, Gerstmann-Straussler-Scheinker syndrome, and fatal familial insomnia. In prion diseases, infectious particles are proteins that propagate by transmitting a misfolded state of a protein, leading to the formation of aggregates and ultimately to neurodegeneration. Prion phenomenon is not restricted to humans. There are a number of prion-related diseases in a variety of mammals, including bovine spongiform encephalopathy (BSE, also known as "mad cow disease") in cattle. All known prion diseases, collectively called transmissible spongiform encephalopathies (TSEs), are untreatable and fatal. Prion proteins were also found in some fungi where they are responsible for heritable traits. Prion proteins in fungi are easily accessible and provide a powerful model for understanding the general principles of prion phenomenon and molecular mechanisms of mammalian prion diseases. Presently, several fundamental questions related to prions remain unanswered. For example, it is not clear how prions cause the disease. Other unknowns include the nature and structure of infectious agent and how prions replicate. Generally, the phenomenon of misfolding of the prion protein into infectious conformations that have the ability to propagate their properties via aggregation is of significant interest. Despite the crucial importance of misfolding and aggregation, very little is currently known about the molecular mechanisms of these processes. While there is an apparent critical need to study molecular mechanisms underlying misfolding and aggregation, the detailed characterization of these single molecule processes is hindered by the limitation of conventional methods. Although some issues remain unresolved, much progress has been recently made primarily due to the application of nanoimaging tools. The use of nanoimaging methods shows great promise for understanding the molecular mechanisms of prion phenomenon, possibly leading towards early diagnosis and effective treatment of these devastating diseases. This review article summarizes recent reports which advanced our understanding of the prion phenomenon through the use of nanoimaging methods.

Significant progress has been made in understanding the structure of aggregated species at the atomic level using both computational modelling and experimental studies such as X-ray crystallography and solid-state NMR. It is widely accepted that the infectious form of prions is self-propagating fibrillar or amyloid PrP. The formation of amyloid has been tightly linked to the development of the disease. Amyloids share common structural features and biophysical properties, including binding of specific dyes, elongated morphology, and nucleation-dependent kinetics of aggregation. Based on solid-state NMR and X-ray crystallography data, the underlying structure of prion amyloids was found to share common structural features. Differences in the packing of these beta-sheets, originating from side chain packing, and register or topology of beta-sheets may explain morphological variants of fibrillar structure.

The mechanical properties of fibrillar structures were characterized by AFM topographic data which enabled the analysis of the decay of tangent along the fibril [134]. The above-described finding only reinforces the hypothesis that the ability to form amyloid fibril is a generic property because these structures are stabilized by main chain interactions of the polypeptide backbone. It also explains why so many unrelated proteins form such fibrillar aggregates. The ensemble consists of rapidly interconverting compact conformations indicating the highly dynamic nature of protein conformational space. Tools are emerging which are capable of addressing the misfolding phenomenon at the level of a single molecule. The transient nature of misfolded conformations and self-propagating nature of amyloids highlights the importance of understanding what interactions between protein molecules drive the formation of a stable nucleus of aggregation. Misfolded aggregation-prone conformations of a protein molecule differ from other conformations by their enhanced propensity to associate with each other, promoting formation of nanoaggregates [135]. A monomeric protein should undergo structural reorganization to adopt an intermediate conformational state required for the initiation of aggregation.

Devices with names like tumour paint and Spectro Pen are in development, along with other advanced optical imaging systems that allow surgeons to "see" tumour cells during surgery. In preclinical studies, these agents spot fine-scale differences with a sensitivity that appears to surpass that of standard techniques, such as magnetic resonance imaging (MRI) and positron emission tomography-computed tomography (PET-CT).

None of these new imaging systems is in the clinic yet, but some have passed the proof-of-concept stage, and a few are in early clinical studies.

Optical imaging systems, which typically use fluorescent dyes or proteins, have obvious advantages over standard MRI or CT scans. Optical imaging systems can also scan a larger tissue area for tumour cells than pathologists can assess with the microscope. But current optical imaging systems have limitations. Subtle differences between tumour tissue and normal tissue combined with weak signalling can make it hard to see tumour margins (Diagram 11.7). The hope is that the nanotechnology-based contrast agents will overcome this problem and send strong, easily detectable signals from tumour cells. Gold nanoparticles, for instance, are particularly well suited to optical imaging since they strongly absorb or scatter light. The gold metal in the particle provides a signal that is more than 100 times brighter than the fluorescent beads used in other optical imaging devices. The Spectro Pen's signal from the tumour was nearly ten times higher than the signal from normal tissue. Fluorescent iron oxide nanoparticles combine the greater resolution and depth penetration of MRI with the greater sensitivity of optical imaging.

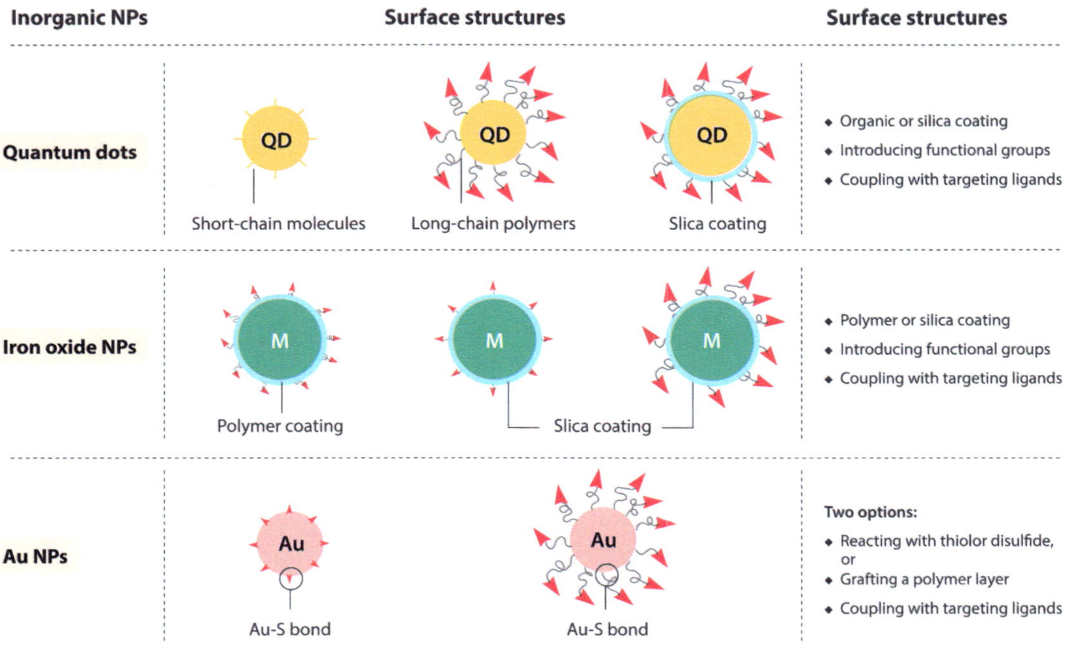

Diagram 11.7 Various inorganic particles and their surface structures

References

1. Kim BY, Rutka JT, Chan WC. Nanomedicine. N Engl J Med. 2010;363(25):2434–43.
2. Drexler KE. Engines of creation. New York, NY: Anchor; 1986.
3. Drexler KE. Nanosystems: molecular machinery, manufacturing, and computation. New York, NY: Wiley Interscience; 1992.
4. Ratner M, Ratner D. Size matters. In: Ratner M, Ratner D, editors. Nanotechnology. Upper Saddle River, NJ: Prentice Hall; 2003. p. 11–8.
5. Boverhof DR, Bramante CM, Butala JH, Clancy SF, Lafranconi M, West J, Gordon SC. Regul Toxicol Pharmacol. 2015;73:137–50. https://doi.org/10.1016/j.yrtph.2015.06.001.
6. Wickline SA, Lanza GM. Nanotechnology for molecular imaging and targeted therapy. Circulation. 2003;107:1092–5.
7. Bao C, Tian F, Estrada G. Improved visualisation of internalised carbon nanotubes by maximising cell spreading on nanostructured substrates. Nano Biomed Eng. 2010;2(4):201–7.
8. Shi Q, Huang Y, Chen X, Wu M, Sun J, Jing X. Haemoglobin conjugated micelles based on triblock biodegradable polymers as artificial oxygen carriers. Biomaterials. 2009;30(28):5077–85.
9. Marsh JN, Senpan A, Hu G, et al. Fibrin-targeted perfluorocarbon nanoparticles for targeted thrombolysis. Nanomedicine (Lond). 2007;2(4):533–43.
10. Culp WC, Porter TR, McCowan TC, et al. Microbubble-augmented ultrasound declotting of thrombosed arteriovenous dialysis grafts in dogs. J Vasc Interv Radiol. 2003;14(3):343–7.
11. Tiukinhoy-Laing SD, Buchanan K, Parikh D, et al. Fibrin targeting of tissue plasminogen activator loaded echogenic liposomes. J Drug Target. 2007;15(2):109–14.
12. Kong DF, Goldschmidt-Clermont PJ. Tiny solutions for giant cardiac problems. Trends Cardiovasc Med. 2005;15(6):207–11.
13. Nakano K, Egashira K, Masuda S, et al. Formulation of nanoparticle-eluting stents by a cationic electrodeposition coating technology: efficient nano-drug delivery via bioabsorbable polymeric nanoparticle eluting stents in porcine coronary arteries. JACC Cardiovasc Interv. 2009;2(4):277–83.
14. Bhargava B, Reddy NK, Karthikeyan G, et al. A novel paclitaxel-eluting porous carbon-carbon nanoparticle coated, nonpolymeric cobalt-chromium stent: evaluation in a porcine model. Catheter Cardiovasc Interv. 2006;67(5):698–702.
15. Guzman LA, Labhasetwar V, Song C, et al. Local intraluminal infusion of biodegradable polymeric nanoparticles: a novel approach for prolonged drug delivery after balloon angioplasty. Circulation. 1996;94(6):1441–8.
16. Winter PM, Caruthers SD, Kassner A, et al. Molecular imaging of angiogenesis in nascent Vx-2 rabbit tumors using a novel alpha(nu)beta3-targeted nanoparticle and 1.5 tesla magnetic resonance imaging. Cancer Res. 2003;63(18):5838–43.
17. Ellis-Behnke RG, Liang YX, Tay DK, et al. Nano hemostat solution: immediate haemostasis at the nanoscale. Nanomedicine. 2006;2(4):207–15.
18. Yang X. Interventional molecular imaging. Radiology. 2010;254(3):651–4.
19. Haley B, Frenkel E. Nanoparticles for drug delivery in cancer treatment. Urol Oncol 2008;26(1):57–64. 1462 September–October 2011 radiographics.rsna.org.
20. Ahmed M, Monsky WE, Girnun G, et al. Radiofrequency thermal ablation sharply increases intratumoral liposomal doxorubicin accumulation and tumor coagulation. Cancer Res. 2003;63(19):6327–33.
21. Ahmed M, Lukyanov AN, Torchilin V, Tournier H, Schneider AN, Goldberg SN. Combined radiofrequency ablation and adjuvant liposomal chemotherapy: effect of chemotherapeutic agent, nanoparticle size, and circulation time. J Vasc Interv Radiol. 2005;16(10):1365–71.
22. Hobbs SK, Monsky WL, Yuan F, et al. Regulation of transport pathways in tumor vessels: role of tumor type and microenvironment. Proc Natl Acad Sci U S A. 1998;95(8):4607–12.
23. Bechet D, Couleaud P, Frochot C, Viriot ML, Guillemin F, Barberi-Heyob M. Nanoparticles as vehicles for delivery of photodynamic therapy agents. Trends Biotechnol. 2008;26(11):612–21.
24. Hilger I, Hergt R, Kaiser WA. Use of magnetic nanoparticle heating in the treatment of breast cancer. IEE Proc Nanobiotechnol. 2005;152(1):33–9.
25. Johannsen M, Gneveckow U, Thiesen B, et al. Thermotherapy of prostate cancer using magnetic nanoparticles: feasibility, imaging, and three-dimensional temperature distribution. Eur Urol. 2007;52(6):1653–61.
26. Takamatsu S, Matsui O, Gabata T, et al. Selective induction hyperthermia following transcatheter arterial embolization with a mixture of nano-sized magnetic particles (ferucarbotran) and embolic materials: feasibility study in rabbits. Radiat Med. 2008;26(4):179–87.
27. Huang X, Qian W, El-Sayed IH, El-Sayed MA. The potential use of the enhanced nonlinear properties of gold nanospheres in photothermal cancer therapy. Lasers Surg Med. 2007;39(9):747–53.
28. Borm PJ, Robbins D, Haubold S, et al. The potential risks of nanomaterials: a review carried out for ECETOC. Part Fibre Toxicol. 2006;3:11.
29. Curtis J, Greenberg M, Kester J, Phillips S, Krieger G. Nanotechnology and nanotoxicology: a primer for clinicians. Toxicol Rev. 2006;25(4):245–60.
30. Monsky WL, Mouta Carreira C, Tsuzuki Y, Gohongi T, Fukumura D, Jain RK. Role of host microenvironment in angiogenesis and microvascular functions in human breast cancer xenografts: mammary fat pad versus cranial tumors. Clin Cancer Res. 2002;8(4):1008–13.

31. Al-Abd AM, Hong KY, Song SC, Kuh HJ. Pharmacokinetics of doxorubicin after intratumoral injection using a thermosensitive hydrogel in tumor-bearing mice. J Control Release. 2010;142(1):101–7.
32. Westphal M, Hilt DC, Bortey E, et al. A phase 3 trial of local chemotherapy with biodegradable carmustine (BCNU) wafers (Gliadel wafers) in patients with primary malignant glioma. Neuro Oncol. 2003;5(2):79–88.
33. Gadaleta CD, Ranieri G. Trans-arterial chemoembolization as a therapy for liver tumours: new clinical developments and suggestions for combination with angiogenesis inhibitors. Crit Rev Oncol Hematol. 2011;80(1):40–53. Epub 2010 Nov 8.
34. Husseini GA, Pitt WG. Micelles and nanoparticles for ultrasonic drug and gene delivery. Adv Drug Deliv Rev. 2008;60(10):1137–52.
35. Eisenhauer EA, Therasse P, Bogaerts J, et al. New response evaluation criteria in solid tumours: revised RECIST guideline (version 1.1). Eur J Cancer. 2009;45(2):228–47.
36. Nehoff H, Parayath NN, Domanovitch L, Taurin S, Greish K. Nanomedicine for drug targeting: strategies beyond the enhanced permeability and retention effect. Int J Nanomedicine. 2014;9:2539–55. https://doi.org/10.2147/IJN.S47129.
37. Kaittanis C, Shaffer TM, Thorek DL, Grimm J. Dawn of advanced molecular medicine: nanotechnological advancements in cancer imaging and therapy. Crit Rev Oncog. 2014;19:143–76.
38. Duncan R, Gaspar R. Nanomedicine(s) under the microscope. Mol Pharm. 2011;8(6):2101–41.
39. Lammers T, Aime S, Hennink WE, Storm G, Kiessling F. Theranostic nanomedicine. Acc Chem Res. 2011;44(10):1029–38.
40. Rizzo LY, Theek B, Storm G, Kiessling F, Lammers T. Recent progress in nanomedicine: therapeutic, diagnostic and theranostic applications. Curr Opin Biotechnol. 2013;24(6):1159–66.
41. Matsumura Y, Maeda H. A new concept for macromolecular therapeutics in cancer chemotherapy: mechanism of tumoritropic accumulation of proteins and the antitumor agent smancs. Cancer Res. 1986;46(12 Pt 1):6387–92.
42. Jain RK, Stylianopoulos T. Delivering nanomedicine to solid tumors. Nat Rev Clin Oncol. 2010;7(11):653–64.
43. Lammers T, Kiessling F, Hennink WE, Storm G. Drug targeting to tumors: principles, pitfalls and (pre-) clinical progress. J Control Release. 2012;161(2):175–87.
44. Kiessling F, Morgenstern B, Zhang C. Contrast agents and applications to assess tumor angiogenesis in vivo by magnetic resonance imaging. Curr Med Chem. 2007;14(1):77–91.
45. Heneweer C, Gendy SE, Peñate-Medina O. Liposomes and inorganic nanoparticles for drug delivery and cancer imaging. Ther Deliv. 2012;3(5):645–56.
46. Wagner M, Wagner S, Schnorr J, et al. Coronary MR angiography using citrate coated very small superparamagnetic iron oxide particles as blood-pool contrast agent: initial experience in humans. J Magn Reson Imaging. 2011;34(4):816–23.
47. Turetschek K, Preda A, Novikov V, et al. Tumor microvascular changes in antiangiogenic treatment: assessment by magnetic resonance contrast media of different molecular weights. J Magn Reson Imaging. 2004;20(1):138–44.
48. Wilson SR, Burns PN. Microbubble-enhanced US in body imaging: what role? Radiology. 2010;257(1):24–39.
49. Kim YK, Kwak HS, Kim CS, Chung GH, Han YM, Lee JM. Hepatocellular carcinoma in patients with chronic liver disease: comparison of SPIO-enhanced MR imaging and 16–detector row CT. Radiology. 2006;238(2):531–41.
50. Mack MG, Balzer JO, Straub R, Eichler K, Vogl TJ. Superparamagnetic iron oxide–enhanced MR imaging of head and neck lymph nodes. Radiology. 2002;222(1):239–44.
51. Schmitz SA, Taupitz M, Wagner S, Wolf KJ, Beyersdorff D, Hamm B. Magnetic resonance imaging of atherosclerotic plaques using superparamagnetic iron oxide particles. J Magn Reson Imaging. 2001;14(4):355–61.
52. Harisinghani MG, Barentsz J, Hahn PF, et al. Noninvasive detection of clinically occult lymph-node metastases in prostate cancer. N Engl J Med. 2003;348(25):2491–9.
53. Saleh A, Wiedermann D, Schroeter M, Jonkmanns C, Jander S, Hoehn M. Central nervous system inflammatory response after cerebral infarction as detected by magnetic resonance imaging. NMR Biomed. 2004;17(4):163–9.
54. Heesakkers RA, Jager GJ, Hövels AM, et al. Prostate cancer: detection of lymph node metastases outside the routine surgical area with ferumoxtran-10–enhanced MR imaging. Radiology. 2009;251(2):408–14.
55. Madru R, Kjellman P, Olsson F, et al. 99mTclabeled superparamagnetic iron oxide nanoparticles for multimodality SPECT/MRI of sentinel lymph nodes. J Nucl Med. 2012;53(3):459–63.
56. Desser TS, Rubin DL, Muller H, McIntire GL, Bacon ER, Toner JL. Blood pool and REVIEW: nanoparticles for imaging: top or flop? Kiessling et al radiology: volume 273: number 1—October 2014 n radiology.rsna.org 25 liver enhancement in CT with liposomal iodixanol: comparison with iohexol. Acad Radiol. 1999;6(3):176–83.
57. Krause W, Leike J, Sachse A, SchuhmannGiampieri G. Characterization of iopromide liposomes. Investig Radiol. 1993;28(11):1028–32.
58. Hallouard F, Anton N, Choquet P, Constantinesco A, Vandamme T. Iodinated blood pool contrast media for preclinical x-ray imaging applications: a review. Biomaterials. 2010;31(24):6249–68.

59. Aviv H, Bartling S, Kieslling F, Margel S. Radiopaque iodinated copolymeric nanoparticles for x-ray imaging applications. Biomaterials. 2009;30(29):5610–6.
60. Torchilin VP, Frank-Kamenetsky MD, Wolf GL. CT visualization of blood pool in rats by using long-circulating, iodine-containing micelles. Acad Radiol. 1999;6(1):61–5.
61. Rabin O, Manuel Perez J, Grimm J, Wojtkiewicz G, Weissleder R. An x-ray computed tomography imaging agent based on long-circulating bismuth sulphide nanoparticles. Nat Mater. 2006;5(2):118–22.
62. Aviv H, Bartling S, Grinberg I, Margel S. Synthesis and characterization of Bi2O3/HSA core-shell nanoparticles for x-ray imaging applications. J Biomed Mater Res B Appl Biomater. 2013;101(1):131–8.
63. Ocampo-García BE, FdeM R, Ferro-Flores G, et al. 99mTc-labelled gold nanoparticles capped with HYNIC-peptide/mannose for sentinel lymph node detection. Nucl Med Biol. 2011;38(1):1–11.
64. Kim S, Lim YT, Soltesz EG, et al. Near-infrared fluorescent type II quantum dots for sentinel lymph node mapping. Nat Biotechnol. 2004;22(1):93–7.
65. Cai X, Li W, Kim CH, Yuan Y, Wang LV, Xia Y. In vivo quantitative evaluation of the transport kinetics of gold nanocages in a lymphatic system by noninvasive photoacoustic tomography. ACS Nano. 2011;5(12):9658–67.
66. Sever AR, Mills P, Weeks J, et al. Preoperative needle biopsy of sentinel lymph nodes using intradermal microbubbles and contrast-enhanced ultrasound in patients with breast cancer. AJR Am J Roentgenol. 2012;199(2):465–70.
67. Sever AR, Mills P, Jones SE, et al. Preoperative sentinel node identification with ultrasound using microbubbles in patients with breast cancer. AJR Am J Roentgenol. 2011;196(2):251–6.
68. Morana G, Salviato E, Guarise A. Contrast agents for hepatic MRI. Cancer Imaging 2007;7(Spec No A):S24–S27.
69. Weissleder R, Elizondo G, Stark DD, et al. The diagnosis of splenic lymphoma by MR imaging: value of superparamagnetic iron oxide. AJR Am J Roentgenol. 1989;152(1):175–80.
70. Weissleder R. Liver MR imaging with iron oxides: toward consensus and clinical practice. Radiology. 1994;193(3):593–5.
71. Rappeport ED, Loft A, Berthelsen AK, et al. Contrast-enhanced FDG-PET/CT vs. SPIO-enhanced MRI vs. FDG-PET vs. CT in patients with liver metastases from colorectal cancer: a prospective study with intraoperative confirmation. Acta Radiol. 2007;48(4):369–78.
72. Ward J, Guthrie JA, Wilson D, et al. Colorectal hepatic metastases: detection with SPIO-enhanced breath-hold MR imaging— comparison of optimized sequences. Radiology. 2003;228(3):709–18.
73. Yamamoto H, Yamashita Y, Yoshimatsu S, Baba Y, Takahashi M. MR enhancement of hepatoma by superparamagnetic iron oxide (SPIO) particles. J Comput Assist Tomogr. 1995;19(4):665–7.
74. Ross RW, Zietman AL, Xie W, et al. Lymphotropic nanoparticle-enhanced magnetic resonance imaging (LNMRI) identifies occult lymph node metastases in prostate cancer patients prior to salvage radiation therapy. Clin Imaging. 2009;33(4):301–5.
75. Pandharipande PV, Harisinghani MG, Ozanne EM, et al. Staging MR lymphangiography of the axilla for early breast cancer: cost-effectiveness analysis. AJR Am J Roentgenol. 2008;191(5):1308–19.
76. Guimaraes AR, Tabatabei S, Dahl D, McDougal WS, Weissleder R, Harisinghani MG. Pilot study evaluating use of lymphotropic nanoparticle–enhanced magnetic resonance imaging for assessing lymph nodes in renal cell cancer. Urology. 2008;71(4):708–12.
77. Settles M, Etzrodt M, Kosanke K, et al. Different capacity of monocyte subsets to phagocytose iron-oxide nanoparticles. PLoS One. 2011;6(10):e25197.
78. Ye Q, Yang D, Williams M, et al. In vivo detection of acute rat renal allograft rejection by MRI with USPIO particles. Kidney Int. 2002;61(3):1124–35.
79. Yilmaz A, Dengler MA, van der Kuip H, et al. Imaging of myocardial infarction using ultrasmall superparamagnetic iron oxide nanoparticles: a human study using a multi-parametric cardiovascular magnetic resonance imaging approach. Eur Heart J. 2013;34(6):462–75.
80. Kircher MF, Gambhir SS, Grimm J. Noninvasive cell-tracking methods. Nat Rev Clin Oncol. 2011;8(11):677–88.
81. Alam SR, Shah AS, Richards J, et al. Ultrasmall superparamagnetic particles of iron oxide in patients with acute myocardial infarction: early clinical experience. Circ Cardiovasc Imaging. 2012;5(5):559–65.
82. Sosnovik DE, Nahrendorf M. Cells and iron oxide nanoparticles on the move: magnetic resonance imaging of monocyte homing and myocardial inflammation in patients with ST-elevation myocardial infarction. Circ Cardiovasc Imaging. 2012;5(5):551–4.
83. Kircher MF, Allport JR, Graves EE, et al. In vivo high resolution three-dimensional imaging of antigen-specific cytotoxic T-lymphocyte trafficking to tumors. Cancer Res. 2003;63(20):6838–46.
84. Pittet MJ, Grimm J, Berger CR, et al. In vivo imaging of T cell delivery to tumors after adoptive transfer therapy. Proc Natl Acad Sci U S A. 2007;104(30):12457–61.
85. Zhou R, Thomas DH, Qiao H, et al. In vivo detection of stem cells grafted in infarcted rat myocardium. J Nucl Med. 2005;46(5):816–22.
86. Grimm J, Swirski FK, Pittet M, Josephson L, Weissleder R. A nanoparticle-based cell labeling agent for cell tracking with SPECT/CT. Mol Imaging. 2006;5(Suppl 3):364.
87. de Vries IJ, Lesterhuis WJ, Barentsz JO, et al. Magnetic resonance tracking of dendritic cells in

melanoma patients for monitoring of cellular therapy. Nat Biotechnol. 2005;23(11):1407–13.
88. Saudek F, Jirák D, Girman P, et al. Magnetic resonance imaging of pancreatic islets transplanted into the liver in humans. Transplantation. 2010;90(12):1602–6.
89. Zhu J, Zhou L, XingWu F. Tracking neural stem cells in patients with brain trauma. N Engl J Med. 2006;355(22):2376–8.
90. Kuehnert N, Kraemer NA, Otto J, et al. In vivo MRI visualization of mesh shrinkage using surgical implants loaded with superparamagnetic iron oxides. Surg Endosc. 2012;26(5):1468–75.
91. Luderer F, Begerow I, Schmidt W, et al. Enhanced visualization of biodegradable polymeric vascular scaffolds by incorporation of gold, silver and magnetite nanoparticles. J Biomater Appl. 2013;28(2):219–31.
92. Nelson GN, Roh JD, Mirensky TL, et al. Initial evaluation of the use of USPIO cell labeling and non-invasive MR monitoring of human tissue-engineered vascular grafts in vivo. FASEB J. 2008;22(11):3888–95.
93. Perea H, Aigner J, Heverhagen JT, Hopfner U, Wintermantel E. Vascular tissue engineering with magnetic nanoparticles: seeing deeper. J Tissue Eng Regen Med. 2007;1(4):318–21.
94. Arifin DR, Long CM, Gilad AA, et al. Trimodal gadolinium-gold microcapsules containing pancreatic islet cells restore normoglycemia in diabetic mice and can be tracked by using US, CT, and positive-contrast MR imaging. Radiology. 2011;260(3):790–8.
95. Kiessling FM. Science to practice: are theranostic agents with encapsulated cells the key for diabetes therapy? Radiology. 2011;260(3):613–5.
96. Barnett BP, Ruiz-Cabello J, Hota P, et al. Fluorocapsules for improved function, immunoprotection, and visualization of cellular therapeutics with MR, US, and CT imaging. Radiology. 2011;258(1):182–91.
97. Jayapaul J, Arns S, Lederle W, et al. Riboflavin carrier protein-targeted fluorescent USPIO for the assessment of vascular metabolism in tumours. Biomaterials 2012;33(34):8822–8829. REVIEW: Nanoparticles for Imaging: Top or Flop? Kiessling et al Radiology: Volume 273: Number 1—October 2014 n radiology.rsna.org 27.
98. Tassa C, Shaw SY, Weissleder R. Dextran coated iron oxide nanoparticles: a versatile platform for targeted molecular imaging, molecular diagnostics, and therapy. Acc Chem Res. 2011;44(10):842–52.
99. Fréchou M, Beray-Berthat V, Raynaud JS, et al. Detection of vascular cell adhesion molecule-1 expression with USPIO-enhanced molecular MRI in a mouse model of cerebral ischemia. Contrast Media Mol Imaging. 2013;8(2):157–64.
100. Burtea C, Ballet S, Laurent S, et al. Development of a magnetic resonance imaging protocol for the characterization of atherosclerotic plaque by using vascular cell adhesion molecule-1 and apoptosis-targeted ultrasmall superparamagnetic iron oxide derivatives. Arterioscler Thromb Vasc Biol. 2012;32(6):e36–48.
101. Strijkers GJ, Kluza E, Van Tilborg GA, et al. Paramagnetic and fluorescent liposomes for target-specific imaging and therapy of tumor angiogenesis. Angiogenesis. 2010;13(2):161–73.
102. Kim YH, Jeon J, Hong SH, et al. Tumor targeting and imaging using cyclic RGDPEGylated gold nanoparticle probes with directly conjugated iodine-125. Small. 2011;7(14):2052–60.
103. Reuveni T, Motiei M, Romman Z, Popovtzer A, Popovtzer R. Targeted gold nanoparticles enable molecular CT imaging of cancer: an in vivo study. Int J Nanomedicine. 2011;6:2859–64.
104. Li J, Chaudhary A, Chmura SJ, et al. A novel functional CT contrast agent for molecular imaging of cancer. Phys Med Biol. 2010;55(15):4389–97.
105. Ghann WE, Aras O, Fleiter T, Daniel MC. Syntheses and characterization of lisinopril-coated gold nanoparticles as highly stable targeted CT contrast agents in cardiovascular diseases. Langmuir. 2012;28(28):10398–408.
106. Kiessling F, Bzyl J, Fokong S, Siepmann M, Schmitz G, Palmowski M. Targeted ultrasound imaging of cancer: an emerging technology on its way to clinics. Curr Pharm Des. 2012;18(15):2184–99.
107. Bzyl J, Lederle W, Rix A, et al. Molecular and functional ultrasound imaging in differently aggressive breast cancer xenografts using two novel ultrasound contrast agents (BR55 and BR38). Eur Radiol. 2011;21(9):1988–95.
108. Tardy I, Pochon S, Theraulaz M, et al. Ultrasound molecular imaging of VEGFR2 in a rat prostate tumor model using BR55. Investig Radiol. 2010;45(10):573–8.
109. Pysz MA, Foygel K, Rosenberg J, Gambhir SS, Schneider M, Willmann JK. Antiangiogenic cancer therapy: monitoring with molecular US and a clinically translatable contrast agent (BR55). Radiology. 2010;256(2):519–27.
110. Pochon S, Tardy I, Bussat P, et al. BR55: a lipopeptide-based VEGFR2-targeted ultrasound contrast agent for molecular imaging of angiogenesis. Investig Radiol. 2010;45(2):89–95.
111. Lewis AL, Dreher MR. Locoregional drug delivery using image-guided intra-arterial drug eluting bead therapy. J Control Release. 2012;161(2):338–50.
112. Van de Wiele C, Maes A, Brugman E, et al. SIRT of liver metastases: physiological and pathophysiological considerations. Eur J Nucl Med Mol Imaging. 2012;39(10):1646–55.
113. Wang X, Chen H, Zheng Y, et al. Au nanoparticle coated mesoporous silica nano capsule-based multifunctional platform for ultrasound mediated imaging, cytoclasis and tumor ablation. Biomaterials. 2013;34(8):2057–68.
114. Niu D, Wang X, Li Y, et al. Facile synthesis of magnetite/perfluorocarbon co-loaded organic/inorganic hybrid vesicles for dual modality ultrasound/magnetic resonance imaging and imaging-guided high-

intensity focused ultrasound ablation. Adv Mater. 2013;25(19):2686–92.
115. Maier-Hauff K, Ulrich F, Nestler D, et al. Efficacy and safety of intratumoral thermotherapy using magnetic iron-oxide nanoparticles combined with external beam radiotherapy on patients with recurrent glioblastoma multiforme. J Neuro-Oncol. 2011;103(2):317–24.
116. Xu QC, Zhang Y, Tan MJ, et al. AnticAngptl4 Ab-conjugated N-TiO(2)/NaYF(4):Yb, Tm nanocomposite for near infrared-triggered drug release and enhanced targeted cancer cell ablation. Adv Healthc Mater. 2012;1(4):470–4.
117. Shen H, You J, Zhang G, et al. Cooperative, nanoparticle-enabled thermal therapy of breast cancer. Adv Healthc Mater. 2012;1(1):84–9.
118. Su Y, Wei X, Peng F, et al. Gold nanoparticles–decorated silicon nanowires as highly efficient near-infrared hyperthermia agents for cancer cells destruction. Nano Lett. 2012;12(4):1845–50.
119. Yang K, Feng L, Shi X, Liu Z. Nano-graphene in biomedicine: theranostic applications. Chem Soc Rev. 2013;42(2):530–47.
120. Stone R, Willi T, Rosen Y, Mefford OT, Alexis F. Targeted magnetic hyperthermia. Ther Deliv. 2011;2(6):815–38.
121. Chertok B, David AE, Yang VC. Brain tumor targeting of magnetic nanoparticles for potential drug delivery: effect of administration route and magnetic field topography. J Control Release. 2011;155(3):393–9.
122. Janib SM, Moses AS, MacKay JA. Imaging and drug delivery using theranostic nanoparticles. Adv Drug Deliv Rev. 2010;62(11):1052–63.
123. Lammers T, Kiessling F, Hennink WE, Storm G. Nanotheranostics and image-guided drug delivery: current concepts and future directions. Mol Pharm. 2010;7(6):1899–912.
124. Xie J, Lee S, Chen X. Nanoparticle-based theranostic agents. Adv Drug Deliv Rev. 2010;62(11):1064–79.
125. Kiessling F, Heilmann M, Lammers T, et al. Synthesis and characterization of HE-24.8: a polymeric contrast agent for magnetic resonance angiography. Bioconjug Chem. 2006;17(1):42–51.
126. Lammers T, Subr V, Peschke P, et al. Image-guided and passively tumour-targeted polymeric nanomedicines for radio chemotherapy. Br J Cancer. 2008;99(6):900–10.
127. Koukourakis MI, Koukouraki S, Giatromanolaki A, et al. High intratumoral accumulation of stealth liposomal doxorubicin in sarcomas: rationale for combination with radiotherapy. Acta Oncol. 2000;39(2):207–11.
128. Lammers T, Rizzo LY, Storm G, Kiessling F. Personalized nanomedicine. Clin Cancer Res. 2012;18(18):4889–94.
129. Kaittanis C, Shaffer TM, Ogirala A, et al. Environment-responsive nanophores for therapy and treatment monitoring via molecular MRI quenching. Nat Commun. https://doi.org/10.1038/ncomms4384. Published online March 4, 2014.
130. de Smet M, Heijman E, Langereis S, Hijnen NM, Grüll H. Magnetic resonance imaging of high intensity focused ultrasound mediated drug delivery from temperature-sensitive liposomes: an in vivo proof-of-concept study. J Control Release. 2011;150(1):102–10.
131. Ranjan A, Jacobs GC, Woods DL, et al. Image-guided drug delivery with magnetic resonance guided high intensity focused ultrasound and temperature sensitive liposomes in a rabbit Vx2 tumor model. J Control Release. 2012;158(3):487–94.
132. Grüll H, Langereis S. Hyperthermia-triggered drug delivery from temperature sensitive liposomes using MRI-guided high intensity focused ultrasound. J Control Release. 2012;161(2):317–27.
133. Lammers T. Smart drug delivery systems: back to the future vs. clinical reality. Int J Pharm. 2013;454(1):527–9.
134. Knowles TP, Fitzpatrick AW, Meehan S, Mott HR, Vendruscolo M, Dobson CM, et al. Role of intermolecular forces in defining material properties of protein nanofibrils. Science. 2007;318:1900–3.
135. Kransnoslobodtsev AV, Shlyakhtenko LS, Ukraintsev E, Zaikova TO, Keana JF, Lyubchenko YL. Nanomedicine and protein misfolding diseases. Nanomedicine. 2005;1:300–5.

Nanoimaging II

12

Key Points (Abstract)

Nanotechnology is the newer field of the technology which is using the concept of the using the various atoms and molecules for the newer molecular components of very small size of the nanometre scale size. These newer avenues of the technologies have created the newer concepts of the diagnosis and treatment,. Various biomaterials will be used for the imaging as diagnostic imaging agents. They can be easily modifying due to their physical and chemical by various ligands which will be conjugated to the particle surface, site-specific ligand-molecule interaction, for the assessment molecular tissues. The therapeutic aspects will also have an impact for the various genes and drugs targeting as the nano- and microparticles for therapeutics also. Nanoimaging is the newer form of the molecular imaging modality which is based on the use of the various nanomaterials, like the nanoparticles, nanorods, nanosphere, nanoshells, and nanostars, which are seen mostly in oncological and biomedical imaging. These nano agents can be used as drug carriers, contrast agents for better resolution, photothermal agents, photoacoustic agents, and radiation dose enhancers. Due to the significant advancements and research, there are many nanotechnological advances which are being used in the functional imaging, cancer therapy, and various newer indications. The use of the nanomaterials can be done with all the imaging modalities including the magnetic resonance imaging, computed tomography, positron emission tomography, single-photon emission computerized tomography, optical imaging, ultrasound, and photoacoustic imaging. Along with these therapeutic options various photothermal therapy, photodynamic therapy, chemotherapy, and immunotherapy are there. Here the advances in various multimodality imaging with image-guided therapeutic options as well as various combination therapies can be used and considered.

Keywords

Nanomaterials · PET · MRI · Phototherapy

12.1 Introduction

Due to the significant advancements in the nanomaterials, various nanoparticles (NPs) probes are being developed which is being used for the molecular imaging. Magnetic resonance imaging (MRI), positron emission tomography (PET), and optical imaging are the imaging modalities which are commonly being used. In the MRI iron oxide, NPs are used in the T1-weighted and/or T2-weighted sequences, and various radioactive materials having capability to interact with the surface or core of the NP are being used in

S. Shaikh, *Advances in Imaging*, https://doi.org/10.1007/978-981-16-9535-3_12

PET. There will be development of the fluorescent NPs like carbon dots and NPs [1] (Diagram 12.1). The only limitations are the pharmacokinetic properties. The various aspects of the physiological principles of various diseases and their managements are based on specific NP. The use of the various therapeutic NPs will improve the better accumulation and release of pharmacologically active agents at the pathological site ultimately increasing the various therapeutic efficiencies along with the reduction of the various side effects. NPs also are important for the theranostic purposes which can be used for personalized nanomedicine-based therapies [2]. The magnetic or optical properties of these NP will make these agents an ideal for the various imaging modalities. They are also excellent contrast agents as they are very sensitive, along with their small size and composition. They can also be conjugated with targeting ligands on the surface of the particles.

12.2 Magnetic Resonance Imaging

Magnetic resonance imaging is an important well-established technique with the various multiparametric parameters which will have the precise information [3].

The ideal contrast agent is when injected will be excreted from the body without any side effects, but the available current contrast imaging agents are having various side effects from the minor to major also in some of the patients [4]. NPs are also having the great potential to be used as the contrast agent in MRI.

12.2.1 Gadolinium (Gd)

Gadolinium-based contrast agents are being used for the diagnostic use in MRI and also being used for the more functional applications. For example, the prostate has very high volume of Zn+2, which will increase the image contrast in MRI. The collagen is dysregulated in the diseased cell or cancer cells, with this excess production of this collagen is seen in the common liver conditions like alcohol and/or drug abuse. These can be easily used to detect the excess collagen with various Gd NP-based contrast agents.

12.2.2 Dendrimers

Dendrimers are having very important role in the nanoimaging and various MRI applications. The important properties are that they are rigid, have low polydispersity, and are capable of the surface

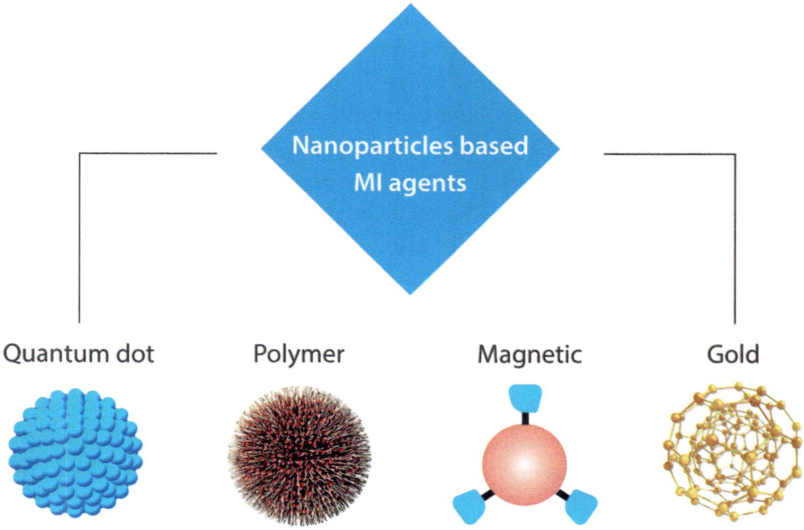

Diagram 12.1 Showing the various nanoparticle-based MI agents

modifications. The newer applications are cell tracking, lymph nodal imaging, blood pool imaging, and tumour-targeted theranostic imaging. Various paramagnetic agents like the gadolinium are having the highest relaxivity due to the correlation time of the large dendrimer molecules. In one of the studies, peptide complex is used as a targeting moiety for the combination with a multimodal Gd dendrimer contrast agent and gold nanoparticles (Au NPs) as carriers.

12.2.3 Super Paramagnetic Iron Oxide Nanoparticles (SPIONs)

The magnetic resonance imaging contrast agents are based on the T1 (positive) or T2 (negative) and preferable due to the T1 as it is easier for the identifying the haemorrhage and air in the tissue boundaries. T1 contrast agents are mainly the gadolinium-based agents which show very good enhancement. The superparamagnetic iron oxide nanoparticles are the combination of the various small crystals of iron oxide with the coating of organic compounds. Superparamagnetic iron oxide nanoparticles can be combined with the various antibodies and act as the drug carrier in various cancer therapies [5]. These particles can be used to label various cells and monitored using MRI [6]. Superparamagnetic iron oxide nanoparticles are T2 contrast agents based on their unique magnetic properties. Thus, the molecular imaging is the combination of the various modalities of medical physics, imaging technology, molecular biology, bioinformatics, and mathematics. As we all know, the basic concept of the molecular imaging is to study the molecular processes of the disease without disturbing them. With this property the magnetic resonance imaging is being established as the best imaging modality due to its non-invasive nature and very good spatial resolution. Various pathologies like inflammation, infection, ischaemia, atherosclerosis, and tumour metastasis, can also be used for the monitoring response to the various inflammatory process and therapies. Various target inflammatory cells are being tagged with the various SPIONs, and these nanoparticles tagged with the macrophages will invade the various inflammatory processes. Folate receptors are one of the particles which are overexpressed in cancerous tissues.

12.2.4 Carbon-13 (13C)

Carbon-13 (13C) is seen abundantly in various organic molecules in the body, and the use of the MRI will be the extremely useful metabolic imaging technique. When the hyperpolarization of 13C increases, the signal is increased significantly thus allowing the non-radioactive, real-time, safe, and specific investigation of the various metabolic and physiologic processes. Pyruvate is also an important imaging marker in the various diseases such as ischaemia inflammation and cancer. The proton-electron polarization transfer technique is the Overhauser effect technique which will enable the very high MRI of nanodiamond in water at room temperature and in an ultra-low magnetic field. This nanodiamond cannot be directly used due to the very low quantity and the small gyromagnetic ratio of spin of the 1 2 13C nuclei, which will be compromising the carbon lattice. The various electron paramagnetic resonance transitions are seen between the MRI signals and the transfers spin polarization of the various paramagnetic centres. The carbon nanotubes can also be synthesized with the single-walled or multiwalled of various diameters in the nm range and also in the μm range.

12.2.5 Graphene

Graphene is also the single layer of carbon atoms which will be in the 2D honeycomb lattice. Graphene-based nanoparticles are being used due to its very good physicochemical properties, excellent surface engineering, and various biological properties like the hydrodynamic size, very low toxicity, and the biocompatibility of the system all these can be used for the in vitro and in vivo imaging [7].

12.2.6 Manganese (Mn)

Manganese-based contrast agents are having the very good biocompatibility and are ideal for the MRI, with the short circulation time of Mn(II) ion chelate in the T1-weighted image. These manganese oxide NPs are having the very good toxicity and excellent T1-weighted contrast effects. The issue here is also the manganese oxide toxicity due to the retention in the reticuloendothelial system. This will have an important impact in the colloidal stability, with the excellent excretion capabilities, and relaxation performance. Silicon-based contrast agents are important for the various organic functional surface particles which will not reduce the nuclear magnetic resonance properties [8].

Atherosclerosis is one of the characteristic features of the chronic and inflammatory disease. Here the early identification and treatment will have more success rate in the management of the plaque. Magnetic resonance imaging is an important imaging modality used for the imaging and for the characterizing the blood vessel wall and plaque by the non-invasive nature without any ionizing radiation.

12.3 Computed Tomography

Computed tomography is based on the principle of the X-ray source and use of the detector array to form images. It is mostly used in the clinical imaging and produces an image with high spatial and temporal resolution. 3D anatomical information of the specific tissues and organs can be done non-invasively.

12.3.1 Gold Nanoparticles

Various gold nanoparticles are having the X-ray attenuation properties which can be easily modified. These nanoparticles along with the glucosamine are the more effective contrast agents [9]. As they are having very high X-ray absorption coefficient so they can be used to the imaging of the tumours by CT; this is due to the increased permeability (EPR]. A mesenchymal stem cell is a having very high potential for the regenerative and for treating the various pathologies like autoimmune, neurodegenerative, and cardiovascular diseases. Along with this they can also be used for the repair of the cartilage and bones. They can easily migrate to the various tissues, and this concept will play an important role in the evaluation of the metastases. The imaging with the computed tomography of porous Au NPs will have more enhancements as compared to the solid Au NPs [10].

12.3.2 Iodine (131I)

Iodine NP contrast agents are being used with the same concept of the very high affinity to the vascular contrast and tumour enhancement in these regions. They are having structure which will have better biodegradation and clearance as compared to the various other nanoparticle agents. And these agents will be accumulating in the various tumours to provide high vascular contrast in the tumour imaging [11]. In the thyroid diseases and radionuclide therapy, the iodine is routinely used as it is having more affinity towards the thyroid and also due to the longer half-life (8.01 days). Gamma emission will be used for the SPECT imaging with beta minus decay, for the various therapeutic purposes. Functional imaging of tumours has different characteristics where multiple contrast agents are used for the evaluation of the same cancers and also for the cancer progression and its development. These photon-counting detectors will be providing the lower background signal, for better characterization of the various signals for the tumour vasculature, and an intratumoral distribution pattern of NPs evaluation as compared to dual-energy micro-CT [12].

12.3.3 Bismuth I

This is used for the evaluation of the of the liver and spleen after 30 min and lasted for more than 4 h contrast enhancement in CT imaging. Significant good results are being seen and showing that it is having very good biocompatibility and the normal organ function is not hampered [13].

12.4 Positron Emission Tomography

Positron emission tomography (PET) is a functional imaging modality using the radiotracers, and based on this radionuclide distribution, the amount of the activity can be easily quantified. And these radiotracers are also seen in the biological pathways as it is a non-invasive method [14].

12.4.1 Gold Nanoparticles

Gold nanoparticles are also commonly used nanoparticles in PET. The visualization of the various dendritic cell migration also very highly sensitive, biocompatible, and also for the various stable imaging agents. The dendritic cell migration is very important in dendritic-based immunotherapy. Positron emission tomography in combination with the Cerenkov luminescent imaging confirmed that various tumour lesions at 1 h after an injection of NPs and signals remained visible in tumour lesions up to 24 h [15].

12.4.2 Copper (64Cu)

Copper sulphide (CuS) NPs are having the very complex, low toxicity and are of the small particle size, which makes them an ideal imaging agent. By the quantitative PET imaging, the macrophages in tumours showing the 64Cu-labelled polyglucose NPs (Marcin) were developed [16]. The single-chain antibodies are having the very high antigen which are very specific with more affinity to the modular structure and fast urinary clearance, which makes them ideal to be used as targeting ligands.

12.4.3 Nanoparticles

Various nanoparticles are also being used, having direct and indirect actions (Diagram 12.2) are being used in the inflammatory macrophages which are capable for the destruction which will be leading to the atherosclerosis, myocardial infarction, and heart failure. With this the monitoring of the macrophages in patients will be monitoring the early treatment of the various diseases. Macroflor NPs are having very high affinity towards the macrophages which will be enriching the various cardiac and plaque macrophages by significantly increasing the PET signal [17]. The pH-sensitive NPs are used for the white blood cells to be used in PET imaging. 68Ga3+ are also used for the labelling, showing very high spatial resolution for PET over SPECT [18].

Cerium oxide NPs are one of the particles having the unique chemistry. Cerium oxide NPs will

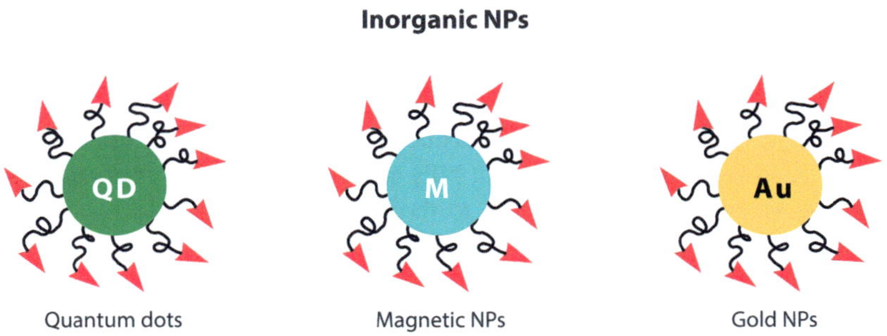

Diagram 12.2 Various inorganic nanoparticles

be coated with 89Zr, for the PET isotope, for PET imaging with great potential to be used [19].

12.5 Single-Photon Emission Computerized Tomography

Single-photon emission computerized tomography is a nuclear imaging modality which uses gamma rays for the evaluation of the molecular changes in the molecular target. Gold nanoparticles can be commonly used as the contrast agents in the SPECT imaging [20]. SPECT and MR fusion of the images will be used to identify the SLN on the MRI with more accurate results. Sentinel lymph node biopsy after injection of 99mTc-labelled nanocolloid within the tumour imaging of scintigraphy and SPECT/CT is also possible. But still the non-detection rates are very high [21].

12.6 Optical Imaging

The non-invasive optical imaging is useful for the evaluation of both macroscopic and microscopic levels. Optical imaging is seen in the fluorescence, chemiluminescence, and Raman imaging; these are all non-invasive 2D or multidimensional imaging.

Fluorescence imaging is being used to localize the molecule or various processes in various living organisms or cell culture. In this imaging the various excitation and absorption wavelengths should be there in the optical window for the very good signal detection. Various 700–750 nm excitation and 750–800 nm emission wavelengths are seen in the optimal range [22]. For the evaluation of the biomarker analysis, fluorescence imaging is being used, but there are some limitations due to the wavelength, photobleaching, and fluorescence self-quenching. Various fluorescent NPs are having the various shortcomings due to the various multiple fluorophore entities, causing more increased photoluminescent emission. The improved stability, with the reduced photobleaching and reduced toxicity, can be done by encapsulating them [23]. Indocyanine green (ICG) shows the NIRII fluorescence used for the evaluation of the different vascular structures in hindlimb and intracranial regions in vivo. Recent development of fluorescent probes is crucial for the diagnosis of the cancer and cancer surgery. Fluorescent probes which are fluorescent also can be used as contrast agents. Fluorine MRI will be detecting the various signatures by imaging a fluorinated tracer. This will be possible in the in vitro and in vivo, which can track and monitor the immune cells and cancer cells. Calcium-based fluorescent NPs can be correlated due to the different neuronal activity and with this the spatial, temporal and chemical resolution is improved, thus, resulting in the better application of the neurochemical circuit precisely [24].

12.7 Quantum Dots Fluorescence Imaging

This is the real-time evaluation of the details at a cellular level. The mesoporous silica NPs with graphene quantum dots will be able to monitor the monitor real-time localization of the doxorubicin (DOX) carrier for proper drug targeting as a fluorescent imaging agent.

12.7.1 Gold Nanoparticles

mRNA identification in the disease cells are of great significance for early diagnosis and treatment of various diseases. The agent like oligonucleotide-functionalized Au NPs will be more sensitive and stable and will increase intracellular delivery efficiency by endocytosis and high signal-to-background ratio for mRNA detection.

12.7.2 Persistent Luminescence Nanoparticles

The availability of the various nanoprobes is being used for the very early detection, for the accurate diagnosis, and monitoring the treatment based on the cellular and molecular level. PLNPs are the nanoparticles based on the various optical property which can be varied by chemical and physical variables like the composition, size, and surface nature [25].

12.8 Ultrasound

Ultrasound is a most commonly used modality which has the non-invasive nature that can provide to the assessment for the morphology, internal structure, orientation, and margins of the lesion from multiple planes with a high resolution both in predominantly fatty breast and dense glandular structures [26]. Various ultrasound-guided drug delivery agents like nanobubbles (NBs) are also showing promising results. Nanobubbles are usually composed of gas cores and stabilized shells. DOX is a cancer drug. Along with the diagnostic aspect therapeutic option, it can be done based on the theranostics.

The newer concept of the ultrasound-targeted NBs destruction technology will have no issue in systemic drug exposure and will maximize therapeutic efficacy. New non-invasive PAI is also used in the metastases by using the Au NPs (GC-Au NPs). Gold nanorods will be bestowing the wariest good biocompatibility and stability. Ultra-small 5 nm Au NPs can be used to develop molecular-activated plasmonic nanosensors for molecular-specific PAI [27].

12.9 Photoacoustic Tomography (PAT)

This can evaluate the cells with gadolinium image cells or tissue using contrast agents such as NPs and pigments. This contrast agent had strong optical absorption, which allowed for visualization of the agent using ultrasound-guided [28].

12.10 Carbon Nanotube (CNT)

Carbon-based NPs are unique in their specific physicochemical properties in nanotechnology [29]. Fluorescent imaging probe is made from the nanoprecipitation of biliverdin which is cross-linked with the amine linker. They will get accumulated due to the photoacoustic effect seen in the lymph node in mice for sentinel lymph node detection [30]. Photo-switchable hybrid probes along with the thermochromic dye and absorbing NPs seen in the temperature-sensitive spectral shifts in absorption can be switched through controllable photothermal heating of doped NPs providing the higher contrast in PEI [31].

The hypoxia is often associated with the tumour aggressiveness and poor treatment outcome. The early diagnosis of hypoxic tumour cells has a high potential in tumour control. Hypoxia-activated NPs can also increase the efficiency of the photoacoustic intensity, fluorescence, and chemotherapy. The hypoxia-activated NPs are usually not active in the blood circulation and the normal physiological conditions. The hypoxic condition will activate them with the extravasation into the hypoxic tumour microenvironment. Azobenzene hypoxia-activated fluorescence nanoparticles have high potential to be used in PAI [32].

12.11 Cancer Therapy

Cancer therapy is the treatment option for killing the cancer cells. Nanomaterials are now evolving in many ways for the therapeutic options of the various cancers.

12.11.1 Photothermal Therapy

Photothermal therapy is a hyperthermia-based cancer therapy. The goal of this therapy is to destroy tumour tissue while avoiding excessive heating of normal tissues. Biological tissue lacks NIR-absorbing chromophores. .Gold nanoparticles with thiol and amine groups can be added with the targeted antibodies and the drug products. Colloidal gold will be showing the surface resonance which is having the speciality to absorb the light at specific wavelengths, useful for the hyperthermic cancer management. Important mediators of the PTT are gold nanoparticles showing the higher level of the biocompatibility and capacity to absorb NIR light which can penetrate deeper in the tissues so that the tumour penetration will be more. The photothermal nanoparticle agents are the nanoshells, nanocages, nanorods, and nanostars. The PET-based nanoplatform will generate the heat of the plasmonic NPs leading to the anticancer agent. The various polymer-based NP systems are having limitations compared to the conventional agents. A suitable agent for the particular size and shape, with the better dispersion of the agent which will respond to the light in NIR range, prevents the damage to the adjacent tissues. It will have ability to have adequate diffusion and also the time to reach the tumour region before the photosensitivity and low cytotoxicity in the system. The various PTT agents are the metal NPs like the gold-, palladium-, silver-, germanium-, and carbon-based NPs. Red blood cell will have the photothermal conversion effect from inner cores and long blood retention due to the red blood cell coating.

12.11.2 Photodynamic Therapy (PDT)

Photodynamic therapy is the newer form of the light therapy using molecular oxygen, visible light, and photosensitizers (PS) for the destruction of the cancer cells and various pathogenic bacteria. Photodynamic therapy is non-invasive and very selectively cytotoxic agent to malignant cells by the direct cell damage which will be by apoptosis necrosis and autophagy. Photosensitizer is transferred into the tumour site by the systematic route by the vascular system. The molecular oxygen will cause the specific wavelength of the light to be applied in PDT which is followed by the production of reactive oxygen species (ROS), causing the damage to the cell. This had led to the cancer cell death. PS will act on the vascular system of the tumour, resulting in the haemostasis, vessel constriction, and breakdown. This has resulted in the decrease in oxygen and nutrient supply to the tumour, leading to cell death. Various conjugates of the antibodies like the proteins, peptide, and other ligands with specific cellular receptors are used in targeted PDT. This technique is being used for targeted delivery. The various photosensitizers like the mesoporous silica NPs are being excited in the chemical energy to generate singlet oxygen, where the glucose oxidase is being catalysed glucose into hydrogen peroxide in PDT. This technique will result in the starvation therapy and providing the hydrogen peroxide to synergistically enhance PDT [33]. These nanoparticle-based carriers are added to the targeted delivery. Serum glycoprotein is one of the targeting ligands used with NPs in chemotherapy drug delivery [34]. Gold nanoparticles will be having the very high stability, surface area-to-volume ratio, surface plasmon resonance, and multifunctionalities. This nontoxic, nonimmunogenic nature, having the very high permeability and associated retention effect of Au NPs, will enable higher penetration and accumulation of the drug at various tumour sites. Is the common agent used with radiation or other chemotherapeutic agents? Cisplatin is used along with the nanoparticles for reducing the delivery of the cisplatin to reduce toxicity. Various forms of the organic NPs which are being used for the transportation are liposomes, polymeric NPs, polymeric micelles, and dendrimers. Tumour-associated macrophages (TAMs) will be residing in the hypoxic region to promote and proliferate and also for the chemoresistance. Nanodandelions will be proliferating into the tumour tissue by the vascular barrier because of their small size. The sustained-released characteristics of NPs will be effective in the chemotherapy by drug concentrations for longer durations at the tumour site. Nanoparticles also will increase the penetration and accumulation of the inhaled drug in tumour tissue and cells. These features had made them the most suitable for chemotherapy for lung cancer [35].

12.11.3 Immunotherapy

Immunotherapy especially the cancer immune therapy has made significant change in the progress with the improvement in nanotechnology. Five types of the cancer immunotherapy are there based on their actions and use lymphocyte-promoting cytokines, agonistic antibodies against co-stimulatory receptors, checkpoint inhibitors, engineered T cells such as CAR T and T-cell receptor (TCR) T cells, and cancer vaccines. The use of the various nanoparticles is being used for the target T cells in the blood or transporting the mRNA to the cancer cell and other cell in the immunotherapy [36]. With recent advances the nanotechnology is being helpful in the antigen delivery which is the form of the peptide used to have stimulation effect on the immune response. These antigens when they are being presented with the cells with tumour antigen play an important role in the immune therapy initiation [37]. Thus, they are having various forms of the role in the recent immunotherapy regimes.

The immunotherapy is the important modalities for the cancer treatment. The tumour environment and the immune system are important for the various cancer treatments. The systematic delivery of immunotherapeutic agents by using NP delivery is of importance. The various nanoparticles which are being used in the immunotherapy are liposomes, Au NPs, polylactic-co-glycolic acid (PLGA) NPs, micelles, iron oxide NPs, and dendrimers.

One of the important immunotherapeutic agents like the cyclic dinucleotides (CDNs) is an important stimulator of the interferon receptor (STING) agonist. The efficacy is also of very small micromolar concentrations. Research on the various newer plant-based immunotherapies which will have lot of potential for the various types of the therapies is going on. Metallic NPs are there which will be showing the antitumour cytotoxic T-cell response and can be used in the form of the combination or the immunotherapy and PTT [38]. Immune-suppressive tumour microenvironment is an important challenge which needs to be addressed.

12.12 Theranostics

Theranostics is the combination of the various aspects of diagnosis. PET-MRI hybrid modality is the recent modality which is having the excellent spatial resolution and soft tissue contrast by MRI. Image-guided radiotherapy is the more focussed form of the treatment option which can have very good results [39–41]. The use of the theranostics where there is the combination of bismuth and gadolinium for the radiosensitization of the tumour and also for the image contrast enhancement. One of the studies showed that the various NPs are showing the contrast enhancement in the CT and MRI and also showed the significant tumour suppression with prolonged survival in non-small-cell lung carcinoma models with minimal off-target toxicity [42]. Theranostic tool in fluorescence and MRI can also be seen in the pancreatic cancer management [43]. Myocarditis is the common disease with higher mortality rate. These MnO-based NPs along with the MRI and NIR fluorescence imaging will be helpful for the combatting the minimal toxicity that is arising from it. These NPs can be used as the MRI contrast agent as well as the drug carrier and will have an important role to get accumulated in the infarcted myocardium, which has been seen in the fluorescence imaging [44].

Another example is the use of the paramagnetic chemical exchange saturation transfer (PARACEST) MRI contrast agent in the MRI-optical imaging which is again the dual modal MRI-optical glioma-imaging NPs.

12.13 Photoacoustic Imaging (PAI)

It is also based on the principle of the optical excitation. This imaging will be providing the deep tissue penetration along with the higher spatial resolution. Gold nanoparticles having the higher absorption coefficient will have enough fluoresce emission and can be used to label certain drugs and to carry the various drug components [45].

12.14 Image-Guided Therapy

The semiconducting plasmonic nanovesicle complex is the highly localized and will be having the very strong electromagnetic field which is between the adjacent Au NPs in the vesicular shell. When the radiotracer rGO-AuNRVe is labelled with 64Cu, it will be showing more accumulation of tumours via the passive accumulation in PET imaging [46]. The use of the pure bismuth NPs will have the ultrahigh X-ray attenuation coefficient with the light to heat conversion capabilities. These will make them more useful for the PAI and PTT. Various carbon nanotubes will be having the various optical, thermal, mechanical, electrical, and magnetic properties. CNT is being used as a combination of the heating agent, contrast agent, and drug delivery agent. The theranostic agent will be developing the perfluorohexane liquid and Au NPs which will make up the core and is stabilized by a polymer shell (poly(lactide-co-glycolic acid)(PLGA)).

Various gold nanoparticles will be having higher atomic number which will be strongly absorbing the various low and medium energy X-rays by the photoelectric effect [47–49]. In this photoelectric effect, the characteristic X-rays and Auger electrons will be released in the surroundings with the short, focussed range and can be capable to cause the local damage [50]. Gold nanoparticles are having the capability to get conjugated to targeting ligands and also can be selectively accumulated into the tumour, and due to this it will be having more potential effect in the better tumour radiotherapy and can also be used as a contrast agent in CT, thus leading to the better theranostic tool [51, 52]. The hyaluronic acid-functionalized bismuth oxide NP was being used as a targeted specific CT imaging and radiosensitizing of tumour. The carbon dots are also being used widely in optical imaging nanoprobes and labelled as the important and are used for the labelling of the cells in cancer treatment. The concept of the synergistic therapy and real-time imaging is being studied and is being used for the treatment of the cancer patients. Trastuzumab is being used as the targeting molecule which will be used in cancer therapy. These agents have the very good drug loading capabilities, excellent biocompatibility, strong X-ray attenuation of the bismuth element, and precise tumour targeting and accumulation. This will enhance the CT in deep tissue and is a therapeutic agent in synergistic photothermal chemotherapy [53]. Mesenchymal stem cells will be migrating more with more presentations within the tumours and also having the best antitumour efficacy in chemo photothermal therapy compared to other treatment groups in triple-negative breast cancer [54]. SPIONs will be having the very high r1and r2 relativities which can be excreted from the body. SPION-delivered chemotherapy is one of the possible excellent potentials being used along various small chemotherapeutic agents which have been incorporated into SPION-based nanocarriers. They will have a significant increase in blood circulation half-life, which will promote tumour retention, and enable real-time drug tracking.

12.15 Combination Therapy

Combination therapy is always the best option for the treatment of various cancers which is having the excellent clinical. They are capable of the synergistic drug action and important in relation to the drug resistance. There are several NPs used in combination therapy such as liposomes. Metallic NPs, dendrimers, nanodiamonds, carbon NPs, and CNT are the ones used in the combination therapy [55]. A mesoporous NP-based drug delivery system is there for the real-time imaging in photothermal/photodynamic therapy and nanozyme oxidative therapy. In vivo and vitro results showed the nanoprobe is evolving as the best tumour-targeting efficacy, due to longer tumour retention times and favourable therapeutic effect [56].

Chemotherapy is the most common cancer treatment option, but it has showed off-target toxicity issues. Theranostics NPs will be integrating both the diagnostic and therapeutic functions together, increasing the tumour selectivity for more effective therapy, and also for the assisting in diagnosis and monitoring of therapeutic response. Monotherapy of cancer is having the limitations of the therapeutic benefits. Gold nanoparticles in conjunction with PTT will destroy these cells and also the gold nanorods which will provide suitable contrast agents for PAI. The use of the NPs to pass beyond the blood-brain barrier and deliver the drug to the brain has various advantages [57]. Photoacoustic and fluorescence imaging in NIR-II is also having the very high potential as it is non-invasive with excellent spatial resolution properties. It is being used for the various image-guided synergistic chemo photodynamic therapies with gold nanorods. Photothermal therapy is also an important effective antitumour for the destruction of the tumour cells. Photothermal therapy along with the immunotherapy will significantly reduce the risk and also can be combined with the various blockage checkpoints for the antitumour effect. Metastatic breast cancer is usually the more dangerous form of the disease with the very less therapeutic options. These nanoparticle-based platforms are having the various aspects of the therapies. Nanoparticles also can offer the magnetothermal therapy where the multidimensional management will be offering the gene, immune, and PTT, and these agents will show the good gene transduction ability and combined treatment effect [58].

Thus, the recent advances in nanotechnology have revolutionized in various techniques with the benefit from the design of various materials like nanoparticles, nanocages, and nanodiamonds. These nanomaterials also will be delivering various drugs for specific target sites. Some limitations of nanomaterials are seen as the various drug carriers, contrast agents, and sensitizers, like the cytotoxicity and nonbiodegradability. With the advancements of imaging, in vitro and in vivo studies are having very much promising results. The newer challenges like the physicochemical properties, drug metabolism, cytotoxicity and biocompatibility, pharmacokinetic screening, surface engineering, in vivo efficacy, nanomaterial uptake, immunogenic issues, and preparation costs are all to be addressed. Future directions will be based on various mechanisms which will be focussed to the particular mechanisms for the various imaging and therapeutic effects, with the needed acceleration for the translation of various nanomaterials into clinical practice.

References

1. Rosado-De-Castro PH, Morales MDP, Pimentel-Coelho PM, Mendez-Otero R, Herranz F. Development and application of nanoparticles in biomedical imaging. Contrast Media Mol Imaging. 2018;2018:1403826.
2. Baetke SC, Lammers T, Kiessling F. Applications of nanoparticles for diagnosis and therapy of cancer. Br J Radiol. 2015;88(1054):20150207.
3. Yousaf T, Dervenoulas G, Politis M. Advances in MRI methodology. Int Rev Neurobiol. 2018;141:31–76.
4. Behzadi AH, Farooq Z, Newhouse JH, Prince MR. MRI and CT contrast media extravasation. Medicine. 2018;97(9):e0055.
5. Dulińska-Litewka J, Łazarczyk A, Hałubiec P, Szafrański O, Karnas K, Karewicz A. Superparamagnetic iron oxide nanoparticles-current and prospective medical applications. Materials. 2019;12(4):617.
6. Iyer SR, Xu S, Stains JP, Bennett CH, Lovering RM. Superparamagnetic iron oxide nanoparticles in musculoskeletal biology. Tissue Eng Part B Rev. 2017;23:373–85.
7. Garg B, Sung CH, Ling YC. Graphene-based nanomaterials as molecular imaging agents. Wiley Interdiscip Rev Nanomed Nanobiotechnol. 2015;7:737–58.
8. Kwiatkowski G, Jähnig F, Steinhauser J, Wespi P, Ernst M, Kozerke S. Nanometer size silicon particles for hyperpolarized MRI. Sci Rep. 2017;7:1–6.
9. Silvestri A, Zambelli V, Ferretti AM, Salerno D, Bellani G, Polito L. Design of functionalized gold nanoparticle probes for computed tomography imaging. Contrast Media Mol Imaging. 2016;11:405–14.
10. Farooq Aziz AI, Nazir A, Ahmad I, Bajwa SZ, Rehman A, Diallo A, Khan WS. Novel route synthesis of porous and solid gold nanoparticles for investigating their comparative performance as contrast agent in computed tomography scan and effect on liver and kidney function. Int J Nanomedicine. 2017;12:1555.
11. Hainfeld JF, Ridwan SM, Stanishevskiy Y, Smilowitz NR, Davis J, Smilowitz HM. Small, long blood half-life iodine nanoparticle for vascular and tumor imaging. Sci Rep. 2018;8:2–11.
12. Badea CT, Clark DP, Holbrook M, Srivastava M, Mowery Y, Ghaghada KB. Functional imaging of tumor vasculature using iodine and gadolinium-based nanoparticle contrast agents: a comparison of spectral micro-CT using energy integrating and photon counting detectors. Phys Med Biol. 2019;64:65007.
13. Chen J, Yang XQ, Qin MY, Zhang XS, Xuan Y, Zhao YD. Hybrid nanoprobes of bismuth sulfide nanoparticles and CdSe/ZnS quantum dots for mouse com-

puted tomography/fluorescence dual mode imaging. J Nanobiotechnol. 2015;13:1–10.
14. Santos BS, Ferreira MJ. Positron emission tomography in ischemic heart disease. Rev Port Cardiol. 2019;38:599–608.
15. Lee SB, Kumar D, Li Y, Lee IK, Cho SJ, Kim SK, Lee SW, Jeong SY, Lee J, Jeon YH. PEGylated crushed gold shell-radiolabeled core nanoballs for in vivo tumor imaging with dual positron emission tomography and Cerenkov luminescent imaging. J Nanobiotechnol. 2018;16:1–12.
16. Kim HY, Li R, Ng T, Courties G, Rodell CB, Prytyskach M, Kohler RH, Pittet MJ, Nahrendorf M, Weissleder R, et al. Quantitative imaging of tumor-associated macrophages and their response to therapy using (64)cu-labeled macrin. ACS Nano. 2018;12:12015–29.
17. Keliher EJ, Ye YX, Wojtkiewicz GR, Aguirre AD, Tricot B, Senders ML, Groenen H, Fay F, Perez-Medina C, Calcagno C, et al. Polyglucose nanoparticles with renal elimination and macrophage avidity facilitate PET imaging in ischaemic heart disease. Nat Commun. 2017;8:1–12.
18. Piras AM, Fabiano A, Sartini S, Zambito Y, Braccini S, Chiellini F, Cataldi AG, Bartoli F, de la Fuente A, Erba PA. pH-responsive carboxymethyl cellulose nanoparticles for 68Ga-WBC labelling in PET imaging. Polymers. 2019;11:1615.
19. McDonagh PR, Sundaresan G, Yang L, Sun M, Mikkelsen R, Zweit J. Biodistribution and PET imaging of 89-zirconium labeled cerium oxide nanoparticles synthesized with several surface coatings. Nanomedicine. 2018;14:1429–40.
20. Si-Mohamed S, Cormode DP, Bar-Ness D, Sigovan M, Naha PC, Langlois JB, Chalabreysse L, Coulon P, Blevis I, Roessl E, et al. Evaluation of spectral photon counting computed tomography K-edge imaging for determination of gold nanoparticle biodistribution in vivo. Nanoscale. 2017;9:18246–57.
21. De VeijMestdagh PD, Schreuder WH, Vogel WV, Donswijk ML, Van Werkhoven E, Van Der Wal JE, Dirven R, Karakullukcu B, Sonke JJ, Van Den Brekel MWM, et al. An analysis of SPECT/CT non-visualization of sentinel lymph nodes in renal tumors. EJNMMI Res. 2018; https://doi.org/10.1186/s13550-018-0460-y.
22. Boschi F, de Sanctis F. Overview of the optical properties of fluorescent nanoparticles for optical imaging. Eur J Histochem. 2017;61:245–8.
23. De-La-Cuesta J, González E, Pomposo JA. Advances in fluorescent single-chain nanoparticles. Molecules. 2017;22:1–14.
24. Kim EH, Chin G, Rong G, Poskanzer KE, Clark HA. Optical probes for neurobiological sensing and imaging. Acc Chem Res. 2018;51:1023–32.
25. Lecuyer T, Teston E, Ramirez-Garcia G, Maldiney T, Viana B, Seguin J, Mignet N, Scherman D, Richard C. Chemically engineered persistent luminescence nanoprobes for bioimaging. Theranostics. 2016;6:2488.
26. Guo R, Lu G, Qin B, Fei B. Ultrasound imaging technologies for breast cancer detection and management: a review. Ultrasound Med Biol. 2018;44:37–70.
27. Han S, Bouchard R, Sokolov KV. Molecular photoacoustic imaging with ultra-small gold nanoparticles. Biomed Opt Express. 2019;10:3472.
28. Hartman RK, Hallam KA, Donnelly EM, Emelianov SY. Photoacoustic imaging of gold nanorods in the brain delivered via microbubble-assisted focused ultrasound: a tool for in vivo molecular neuroimaging. Laser Phys Lett. 2019;16(2):025603.
29. Augustine S, Singh J, Srivastava M, Sharma M, Das A, Malhotra BD. Recent advances in carbon based nanosystems for cancer theranostics. Biomater Sci. 2017;5:901–52.
30. Fathi P, Knox HJ, Sar D, Tripathi I, Ostadhossein F, Misra SK, Esc MB, Chan J, Pan D. Biodegradable biliverdin nanoparticles for efficient photoacoustic imaging. ACS Nano. 2019;13:7690–704.
31. Harrington WN, Haji MR, Galanzha EI, Nedosekin DA, Nima ZA, Watanabe F, Ghosh A, Biris AS, Zharov VP. Photoswitchable non-fluorescent thermochromic dye-nanoparticle hybrid probes. Sci Rep. 2016;6:1–11.
32. Wang Y, Shang W, Niu M, Tian J, Xu K. Hypoxia-active nanoparticles used in tumor theranostic. Int J Nanomedicine. 2019;14:3705–22.
33. Yu Z, Zhou P, Pan W, Li N, Tang B. A biomimetic nanoreactor for synergistic chemiexcited photodynamic therapy and starvation therapy against tumor metastasis. Nat Commun. 2018;9:1–9.
34. Press D. Application of active targeting nanoparticle delivery system for chemotherapeutic drugs and traditional/herbal medicines in cancer therapy: a systematic review. Int J Nanomedicine. 2018;13:3921.
35. Mangal S, Gao W, Li T, Zhou QT. Pulmonary delivery of nanoparticle chemotherapy for the treatment of lung cancers: challenges and opportunities. Acta Pharmacol Sin. 2017;38:782–97.
36. Riley RS, June CH, Langer R, Mitchell MJ. Delivery technologies for cancer immunotherapy. Nat Rev Drug Discov. 2019;18:175–96.
37. Park W, Heo Y-J, Han DK. New opportunities for nanoparticles in cancer immunotherapy. Biomater Res. 2018;22:1–10.
38. Evans ER, Bugga P, Asthana V, Drezek R. Metallic nanoparticles for cancer immunotherapy. Mater Today. 2018;21:673–85.
39. Martelli S, Chow JCL. Dose enhancement for the flattening-filter-free and flattening-filter photon beams in nanoparticle-enhanced radiotherapy: a Monte Carlo phantom study. Nano. 2020;10:637.
40. Mututantri-Bastiyange D, Chow JCL. Imaging dose of cone-beam computed tomography in nanoparticle-enhanced image-guided radiotherapy: a Monte Carlo phantom study. AIMS Bioeng. 2020;7:1–11.
41. Chow JCL. Monte carlo nanodosimetry in gold nanoparticle-enhanced radiotherapy. In: Chan MF, editor. Recent advancements and applications applications in dosimetry. New York, NY: Nova Science

Publishers; 2018. Chapter 2. Nanomaterials 2020, 10, 1700 38 of 40.
42. Detappe A, Thomas E, Tibbitt MW, Kunjachan S, Zavidij O, Parnandi N, Reznichenko E, Lux F, Tillement O, Berbeco R. Ultrasmall silica-based bismuth gadolinium nanoparticles for dual magnetic resonance-computed tomography image guided radiotherapy. Nano Lett. 2017;17:1733–40.
43. Chen X, Zhou H, Li X, Duan N, Hu S, Liu Y, Yue Y, Song L, Zhang Y, Li D, et al. Plectin-1 targeted dual-modality nanoparticles for pancreatic cancer imaging. EBioMedicine. 2018;30:129–37.
44. Zheng Y, Zhang H, Hu Y, Bai L, Xue J. MnO nanoparticles with potential application in magnetic resonance imaging and drug delivery for myocardial infarction. Int J Nanomedicine. 2018;13:6177–88.
45. Zhang Y, Tang Z, Wu Y. The dual-mode imaging of nanogold-labeled cells by photoacoustic microscopy and fluorescence optical microscopy. Technol Cancer Res Treat. 2018;17:1–4.
46. Song J, Yang X, Jacobson O, Lin L, Huang P, Niu G, Ma Q, Chen X. Sequential drug release and enhanced photothermal and photoacoustic effect of hybrid reduced graphene oxide-loaded ultrasmall gold nanorod vesicles for cancer therapy. ACS Nano. 2015;9:9199–209.
47. Chow JCL. Photon and electron interactions with gold nanoparticles: a Monte Carlo study on gold nanoparticle-enhanced radiotherapy. In: Grumezescu AM, editor. Nanobiomaterials in medical imaging: applications of nanobiomaterials. Amsterdam: Elsevier; 2016.; Chapter 2. p. 45–70.
48. Chow JCL. Recent progress of gold nanomaterials in cancer therapy. In: Kharissova OV, Torres-Martínez LM, Kharisov BI, editors. Handbook of nanomaterials and nanocomposites for energy and environmental applications. Springer Nature: Cham; 2020. p. 1–30.
49. He C, Chow JC. Gold nanoparticle DNA damage in radiotherapy: a Monte Carlo study. AIMS Bioeng. 2016;3:352.
50. Wang Y, Strohm EM, Sun Y, Wang Z, Zheng Y, Wang Z, Kolios MC. Biodegradable polymeric nanoparticles containing gold nanoparticles and paclitaxel for cancer imaging and drug delivery using photoacoustic methods. Biomed Opt Express. 2016;7:4125. Nanomaterials 2020, 10, 1700 39 of 40
51. Ashton JR, Castle KD, Qi Y, Kirsch DG, West JL, Badea CT. Dual-energy CT imaging of tumor liposome delivery after gold nanoparticle-augmented radiotherapy. Theranostics. 2018;8:1782–97.
52. Siddique S, Chow JC. Gold nanoparticles for drug delivery and cancer therapy. Appl Sci. 2020;10:3824.
53. Li LH, Lu Y, Jiang CY, Zhu Y, Yang XF, Hu XM, Lin ZF, Zhang Y, Peng MY, Xia H, et al. Actively targeted deep tissue imaging and photothermal-chemo therapy of breast cancer by antibody-functionalized drug-loaded X-ray-responsive bismuth Sulfide@ Mesoporous silica core-shell nanoparticles. Adv Funct Mater. 2018;28(5):1704623.
54. Kim SJ, Lewis B, Steiner MS, Bissa UV, Dose C, Frank JA. Superparamagnetic iron oxide nanoparticles for direct labelling of stem cells and in vivo MRI tracking. Contrast Media Mol Imaging. 2016;11:55–64.
55. Gurunathan S, Kang MH, Qasim M, Kim JH. Nanoparticle-mediated combination therapy: two-in-one approach for cancer. Int J Mol Sci. 2018;19:1–37.
56. Zhang A, Pan S, Zhang Y, Chang J, Cheng J, Huang Z, Li T, Zhang C, De La Fuentea JM, Zhang Q, et al. Carbon-gold hybrid nanoprobes for real-time imaging, photothermal/photodynamic and nanozyme oxidative therapy. Theranostics. 2019;9:3443–58.
57. Ramanathan S, Archunan G, Sivakumar M, Selvan ST, Fred AL, Kumar S, Gulyás B, Padmanabhan P. Theranostic applications of nanoparticles in neurodegenerative disorders. Int J Nanomedicine. 2018;13:5561–76.
58. Zhang J, Zhao T, Han F, Hu Y, Li Y. Photothermal and gene therapy combined with immunotherapy to gastric cancer by the gold nanoshell-based system. J Nanobiotechnol. 2019;17:1–11.

13 Amyloid Imaging

Key Points (Abstract)

Amyloid imaging is the newer concept of molecular imaging which is related with the detection of b-amyloid plaques. Amyloid imaging is the important imaging component for the evaluation of the Alzheimer's disease by using the PET-CT. By this technique various patterns, forms, and stages of the Alzheimer plaques and the neurofibrillary tangles and their important neuropathologic features of Alzheimer's disease can be evaluated (AD). With the availability of the newer amyloid PET radiotracers, the diagnosis and evaluation of various suspected or diagnosed cases of the neurodegenerative disorders like Alzheimer's disease have become easier and precise. Amyloid PET imaging is now an important modality for providing the diagnostic and prognostic information in the patients of known or possible AD, having mild cognitive impairment (MCI), and various other clinical presentations.

Keywords

Amyloid plaques · PET-CT · Alzheimer's disease · Amyloid PET

13.1 Introduction

Amyloid imaging is the basis of the imaging for the diagnosis and evaluation of various stages of the AD or the response to the treatment after the management. Alzheimer's disease is an important neurodegenerative disorder which is progressive and manifested clinically by memory loss and cognitive decline. The neuropathologic presentation is the presence of extracellular amyloid plaques and neurofibrillary tangles (NFT) in the cells. Cerebral cortical atrophy also aids in the diagnosis of AD. The early detection of b-amyloid plaques is important and always correlates with the various degrees of the cognitive impairment (CI). The reverse is also true as the positive PET scan does not confirm the Alzheimer's disease or the cognitive impairment.

AD is the one of the most common forms of the neurocognitive disorder (NCD); first described by Alois Alzheimer in 1906, this was described based on the presence of the intracerebral neurotic plaques and neurofibrillary tangles (NFTs) in the post-mortem studies of the patients with chronic mental illness.

MRI was the important imaging modality for the evaluation and diagnosing the various aspects of the AD like the cortical atrophy, but not always consistent with the findings of the AD, as many other findings are also there which need to be differentiated from the cortical atrophy of AD. With the increasing age, there will be more overlaps of the various findings. Because of this functional imaging modalities will play an important role. PET-CT in dementia group evaluation is an important indication. The first and the foremost imaging modality is the

S. Shaikh, *Advances in Imaging*, https://doi.org/10.1007/978-981-16-9535-3_13

PET-CT now by using the FDG as the commonly used radiotracer. But again, it is based on the reduced uptake in the frontotemporal regions in AD, but again it is difficult for the later stages or the older age groups.

13.2 Clinical Indications of the Amyloid Imaging

- Assessing the cognitive impairment which can be mild, progressive, or regressive in manner
- Progressive dementia evaluation based on the early age of onset
- Clinical criteria of Alzheimer's disease for the identification of the specific aetiology which can again be typical, atypical or mixed presentations

13.3 Contraindications/Inappropriate Use

Pregnancy and breastfeeding are relative contraindications. According to Society of Nuclear Medicine and Molecular Imaging standards and European Association of Nuclear Medicine practice guidelines, the amyloid evaluation is not correct.

- Dementia severity evaluation
- Family history and asymptomatic individuals
- Asymptomatic individuals with APOE-e 4 genotype
- Asymptomatic individuals
- Cognitive impairment which is not confirmed
- Assessment of Alzheimer's disease
- Suspected autosomal dominant mutation carriers
- Symptoms, current medications, relevant personal history, and recent imaging procedures which are not known

The radiopharmaceuticals which are approved by the Food and Drug Administration for amyloid imaging are 18F-florbetapir, 18F-flutemetamol, and 18F-florbetaben.

Amyloid imaging is mostly done for the evaluation of the early AD diagnosis. This initial early evaluation is very important for the amyloid build-up which will be resulting into the neurodegeneration and dementia [1]. Frontotemporal dementia and other forms of dementias are usually amyloid-negative; despite of this they are considered as differentials for the dementia diagnosis.

B-amyloid accumulation in the brain is very early finding [2] and with pathobiochemical and pathophysiologic changes will lead to the neurodegeneration and further cognitive decline in AD [2, 3]. Still sometimes the dementia diagnosis can be missed and delayed [4, 5].

Various doses, metabolic uptake times, and the acquisition times are based on the specific radiopharmaceutical which will be used. After injection of the radiopharmaceutical, 5–15 mL of 0.9% sterile sodium chloride is also injected to make sure the proper dose delivery.

Recommended dose	Uptake time	Acquisition time
18F-florbetapir	10 mCi (370 MBq)	30–50 min 10 min
18F-flutemetamol	5 mCi (185 MBq)	60–120 min 10–20 min
18F-florbetaben	8.1 mCi (300 MBq)	45–130 min 15–20 min

The pathophysiology of the amyloid-β peptide and amyloid plaques is formed by the process of the cleavage of a transmembrane protein and amyloid precursor protein (APP), by the enzymes β- and γ-secretases, which will be resulting the Aβ species consisting of the [6–13] amino acid residues [14, 15]. During this procedure there will be release of the Aβ species, particularly Aβ40 and Aβ42, into the extracellular space [16]. These are the oligomers, which are specifically neurotoxic, and the mechanism is not completely understood [17–23]. It can possibly aggregate into larger insoluble β-sheet fibrils and dense fibrillary amyloid plaques which are classically seen in AD [19]. Not all amyloid plaques are pathologic or closely associated with AD [20, 24].

Thus, the amyloid plaques are seen in various other conditions like cerebral amyloid angiopathy (predominantly diffuse plaques), dementia with Lewy bodies (DLB), and Parkinson's disease [24, 25]. The Aβ and NFT molecular pathology of the neurodegeneration and AD is still not clear. The resulting amyloid cascade will show the abnormal accumulation of Aβ plaques and further leading into the pathological cascade causing the neurodegeneration and the clinical syndrome of AD [26]. Different molecular agents interact with the various genetic comorbid and also the various environmental factors. The higher levels of Aβ deposition in cognitively normal individuals associated with the subtle progressive deficits and greater risk of cognitive impairment will be able to modify the various cognitive factors along with the various genetic markers [27–29]. Other important biomarkers are hippocampal and adjacent cortical atrophy on MRI, hypometabolism on FDG-PET scans, and increased cerebrospinal fluid (CSF) concentration. The use of the 11C-PIB as the first amyloid radiotracer having very high specificity for fibrillar Aβ, dense amyloid plaques, and other extracellular Aβ forms, relative to intracellular Aβ (cf. 18F-FDDNP, the first amyloid radiotracer) [30–34].

Three 18F-labelled Aβ PET imaging agents have been approved by the US Food and Drug Administration (FDA) and the European Medicines Association (EMA): florbetapir, flutemetamol, and florbetaben. These show different kinetic behaviours with varying levels of specificity of Aβ and off-target WM binding [35, 36]. FDG-PET brain scan shows hypometabolism in the cortex of the temporal and posterior lobes and also frontal cortex in advanced cases of AD [37]. Hypometabolism in the posterior cingulate cortex also goes in the favour of the AD. Frontal hypometabolism or asymmetry in the metabolism will be suggestive of FTD [38]. Preserved cerebral FDG uptake and clinically diagnosed dementia make AD less likely, and other causes need to be investigated further [39, 40]. These FDA amyloid imaging tracers show nonspecific white matter retention in healthy controls (negative) and tracer retention seen in the cortical grey matter having more Aβ load (positive).

The use of the florbetaben can be useful in demonstrating the regions of importance. Comparison of the maximum WM and grey matter intensity form cerebellum; then lateral temporal and frontal lobes, followed by posterior cingulate cortex and praecuneus; and finally to the parietal lobe. The scoring is based in the region of interest showing (1) no binding, (2) minor binding, and (3) pronounced binding and then quantified into the overall three-grade score (negative, minor, or major Aβ load, for which the latter two are considered a positive amyloid PET scan).

These the three FDA-approved radiotracers are having the sensitivity of up to 92% and a specificity of 95% for detection of amyloid as compared to autopsy or procedure-related biopsy histopathology.

Mild cognitive impairment is defined as measurable cognitive deficits that are determined which will not interfere with the normal routine work and daily activities. MCI can come before AD dementia for a number of years [41, 42]. MCI phase and symptoms preceding the AD dementia is known as "MCI due to AD" or also the "prodromal AD", by two different workgroups which have categorized AD diagnostic criteria. Posterior cortical atrophy (PCA) is a rare, atypical variant of AD having the complex visual and cognitive changes, with selective progressive deterioration of visual association skills, FDG-PET hypometabolism predominantly in the occipital lobes [43, 44].

13.4 Limitations of Amyloid PET

Important limitation of amyloid imaging, a positive PET amyloid scan does confirm the diagnosis of AD without other clinical measures for AD. Amyloid imaging is an important diagnostic and prognostic component for the multimodal evaluation of MCI and AD, which improved diagnostic and prognostic accuracy as compared to the single biomarkers in research and some clinical settings [45–47].

13.5 Conclusion

Thus, the amyloid imaging is now the very important diagnostic and prognostic modality of imaging for the evaluation of the patients with AD and MCI. With further research in future newer PET radiotracers, techniques and other imaging and molecular biomarkers will be more helpful for a more precise evaluation and confirmation and also for the management of the possible therapeutic or preventative interventions for AD and MCI.

References

1. Jack CR Jr, Knopman DS, Jagust WJ, et al. Hypothetical model of dynamic biomarkers of the Alzheimer's pathological cascade. Lancet Neurol. 2010;9:119–28.
2. Braak H, Braak E. Neuropathological stageing of Alzheimer-related changes. Acta Neuropathol (Berl). 1991;82:239–59.
3. Public attitudes about diagnosis: value of knowing. Alzheimer Europe website. http://www.alzheimer-europe.org/Research/Value-of-Knowing/Publicattitudes-about-diagnosis. Updated July 13, 2011. Accessed August 21, 2017.
4. Bradford A, Kunik ME, Schulz P, Williams SP, Singh H. Missed and delayed diagnosis of dementia in primary care: prevalence and contributing factors. Alzheimer Dis Assoc Disord. 2009;23:306–14.
5. Bradford A, Upchurch C, Bass D, et al. Knowledge of documented dementia diagnosis and treatment in veterans and their caregivers. Am J Alzheimers Dis Other Dement. 2011;26:127–33.
6. Vandenberghe R, Van Laere K, Ivanoiu A, et al. 18F-flutemetamol amyloid imaging in Alzheimer disease and mild cognitive impairment: a phase 2 trial. Ann Neurol. 2010;68(3):319–29.
7. Landau SM, Breault C, Joshi AD, et al. Amyloid-β imaging with Pittsburgh compound B and florbetapir: comparing radiotracers and quantification methods. J Nucl Med. 2013;54(1):70–7.
8. Klunk WE, Koeppe RA, Price JC, et al. The Centiloid project: standardizing quantitative amyloid plaque estimation by PET. Alzheimers Dement 2015;11(1):1–15, e11–14.
9. Cselenyi Z, Jonhagen ME, Forsberg A, et al. Clinical validation of 18F-AZD4694, an amyloid-β-specific PET radioligand. J Nucl Med. 2012;53(3):415–24.
10. Kuhl DE. Imaging local brain function with emission computed tomography. Radiology. 1984;150(3):625–31.
11. Minoshima S, Frey KA, Koeppe RA, et al. A diagnostic approach in Alzheimer's disease using three-dimensional stereotactic surface projections of fluorine-18-FDG PET. J Nucl Med. 1995;36(7):1238–48.
12. Minoshima S, Giordani B, Berent S, et al. Metabolic reduction in the posterior cingulate cortex in very early Alzheimer's disease. Ann Neurol. 1997;42(1):85–94.
13. Bohnen NI, Minoshima S. FDG-PET and molecular brain imaging in the movement disorders clinic. Neurology. 2012;79(13):1306–7.
14. Thinakaran G, Koo EH. Amyloid precursor protein trafficking, processing, and function. J Biol Chem. 2008;283(44):29615–9.
15. O'Brien RJ, Wong PC. Amyloid precursor protein processing and Alzheimer's disease. Annu Rev Neurosci. 2011;34:185–204.
16. McLean CA, Cherny RA, Fraser FW, et al. Soluble pool of Aβ amyloid as a determinant of severity of neurodegeneration in Alzheimer's disease. Ann Neurol. 1999;46(6):860–6.
17. Jin M, Shepardson N, Yang T, et al. Soluble amyloid beta-protein dimers isolated from Alzheimer cortex directly induce tau hyperphosphorylation and neuritic degeneration. Proc Natl Acad Sci U S A. 2011;108(14):5819–24.
18. Aguzzi A. Neurodegeneration: Alzheimer's disease under strain. Nature. 2014;512(7512):32–4.
19. Finder VH, Glockshuber R. Amyloid-beta aggregation. Neurodegener Dis. 2007;4(1):13–27.
20. Braak H, Braak E. Demonstration of amyloid deposits and neurofibrillary changes in whole brain sections. Brain Pathol. 1991;1(3):213–6.
21. Nelson PT, Jicha GA, Schmitt FA, et al. Clinicopathologic correlations in a large Alzheimer disease center autopsy cohort: Neuritic plaques and neurofibrillary tangles "do count" when staging disease severity. J Neuropathol Exp Neurol. 2007;66(12):1136–46.
22. Thal DR, Sassin I, Schultz C, et al. Fleecy amyloid deposits in the internal layers of the human entorhinal cortex are comprised of N-terminal truncated fragments of Aβ. J Neuropathol Exp Neurol. 1999;58(2):210–6.
23. Rowe CC, Ellis KA, Rimajova M, et al. Amyloid imaging results from the Australian imaging, biomarkers and lifestyle (AIBL) study of aging. Neurobiol Aging. 2010;31(8):1275–83.
24. Ossenkoppele R, Jansen WJ, Rabinovici GD, et al. Prevalence of amyloid PET positivity in dementia syndromes: a meta-analysis. J Am Med Assoc. 2015;313(19):1939–49.

25. Johnson KA, Gregas M, Becker JA, et al. Imaging of amyloid burden and distribution in cerebral amyloid angiopathy. Ann Neurol. 2007;62(3):229–34.
26. Hardy JA, Higgins GA. Alzheimer's disease: the amyloid cascade hypothesis. Science. 1992;256(5054):184–5.
27. Mosconi L, Rinne JO, Tsui WH, et al. Amyloid and metabolic positron emission tomography imaging of cognitively normal adults with Alzheimer's parents. Neurobiol Aging. 2013;34(1):22–34. Clinical amyloid imaging 9
28. Vemuri P, Lesnick TG, Przybelski SA, et al. Effect of lifestyle activities on Alzheimer disease biomarkers and cognition. Ann Neurol. 2012;72(5):730–8.
29. Kemppainen NM, Aalto S, Karrasch M, et al. Cognitive reserve hypothesis: Pittsburgh compound B and fluorodeoxyglucose positron emission tomography in relation to education in mild Alzheimer's disease. Ann Neurol. 2008;63(1):112–8.
30. Agdeppa ED, Kepe V, Petri A, et al. In vitro detection of (S)-naproxen and ibuprofen binding to plaques in the Alzheimer's brain using the positron emission tomography molecular imaging probe 2-(1-[6- [(2-18F-fluoroethyl)(methyl)amino]-2-naphthyl]ethylidene)malononitrile. Neuroscience. 2003;117(3):723–30.
31. Fodero-Tavoletti MT, Brockschnieder D, Villemagne VL, et al. In vitro characterization of 18F-florbetaben, an Aβ imaging radiotracer. Nucl Med Biol. 2012;39(7):1042–8.
32. Ye L, Velasco A, Fraser G, et al. In vitro high affinity α-synuclein binding sites for the amyloid imaging agent PIB are not matched by binding to Lewy bodies in postmortem human brain. J Neurochem. 2008;105(4):1428–37.
33. Klunk WE, Engler H, Nordberg A, et al. Imaging brain amyloid in Alzheimer's disease with Pittsburgh compound-B. Ann Neurol. 2004;55(3):306–19.
34. Mathis CA, Mason NS, Lopresti BJ, et al. Development of positron emission tomography β-amyloid plaque imaging agents. Semin Nucl Med. 2012;42(6):423–32.
35. Landau SM, Thomas BA, Thurfjell L, et al. Amyloid PET imaging in Alzheimer's disease: a comparison of three radiotracers. Eur J Nucl Med Mol Imaging. 2014;41(7):1398–407.
36. Villemagne VL, Mulligan RS, Pejoska S, et al. Comparison of 11C-PIB and 18F-florbetaben for Aβ imaging in ageing and Alzheimer's disease. Eur J Nucl Med Mol Imaging. 2012;39(6):983–9.
37. Silverman DH, Small GW, Chang CY, et al. Positron emission tomography in evaluation of dementia: regional brain metabolism and long-term outcome. J Am Med Assoc. 2001;286(17):2120–7.
38. Rabinovici GD, Furst AJ, O'Neil JP, et al. 11C-PIB PET imaging in Alzheimer disease and frontotemporal lobar degeneration. Neurology. 2007;68(15):1205–12.
39. Dolan RJ, Grasby PM, Bench C, et al. Pharmacological challenge and PET imaging. Clin Neuropharmacol. 1992;15(Suppl 1 Pt A):216A–7A.
40. Rasgon NL, Kenna HA, Geist C, et al. Cerebral metabolic patterns in untreated postmenopausal women with major depressive disorder. Psychiatry Res. 2008;164(1):77–80.
41. Roe CM, Fagan AM, Grant EA, et al. Amyloid imaging and CSF biomarkers in predicting cognitive impairment up to 7.5 years later. Neurology. 2013;80(19):1784–91.
42. Morris JC, Storandt M, Miller JP, et al. Mild cognitive impairment represents early-stage Alzheimer disease. Arch Neurol. 2001;58(3):397–405.
43. Herholz K, Carter SF, Jones M. Positron emission tomography imaging in dementia. Br J Radiol. 2007;80:S160–7.
44. Ishii K. Clinical application of positron emission tomography for diagnosis of dementia. Ann Nucl Med. 2002;16(8):515–25.
45. Teipel S, Drzezga A, Grothe MJ, et al. Multimodal imaging in Alzheimer's disease: validity and usefulness for early detection. Lancet Neurol. 2015;14(10):1037–53.
46. Ossenkoppele R, Prins ND, Pijnenburg YA, et al. Impact of molecular imaging on the diagnostic process in a memory clinic. Alzheimers Dement. 2013;9(4):414–21.
47. Morris JC, Roe CM, Grant EA, et al. Pittsburgh compound B imaging and prediction of progression from cognitive normality to symptomatic Alzheimer disease. Arch Neurol. 2009;66(12):1469–75.

Hypoxia Imaging

14

Key Points (Abstract)

Oxygen is the most important component of living beings by the virtue of the nature's law. This oxygen plays an important role in the homeostasis in aerobic cells. Hypoxia is the clinical condition in which cells are devoid of the minimum required quantity of oxygen supply necessary for the normal functioning of cells. Changes in this vascular supply will show inadequate oxygen metabolism. Sometimes in many normal processes, there will be oxygen deprivation to the tissue resulting in the derangement of the metabolism. Pathogenesis of the hypoxic condition is the common factor which will result in the formation of the various pathologies. There are various pathways which will activate the hypoxic cells stimulating angiogenesis, altering the cellular metabolism leading to the slower growth rate, and preventing apoptosis. The altered metabolism in cancer cells by hypoxia will result in the more tumour phenotype development causing rapid tumour proliferations, treatment resistance, and poor prognosis.

O_2 supply to any tissue and cells is very important; if no supply then the cells will die in this process, and there will be more powerful regulating mechanism causing more production of numerous proteins playing an important role in the survival. With this there will be increased growth rate, causing the changed concept of mitochondria to glycolysis. Due to these mechanisms, hypoxia is an important causative factor. Few of the conditions are stroke, peripheral vascular disease, and ischaemic heart disease.

Keywords

Hypoxia · Tumour microenvironment · Angiogenesis · Tumour phenotypes · Glycolysis

14.1 Introduction

By definition hypoxia is lack of proper oxygenation of cells. This low level of oxygen concentration in the tissues leads to the mismatch between the oxygen supply and consumption. Again, there are two entities for these the physiological and pathological aspects for this hypoxia. In the physiological entity, there is the transient reduction of oxygen concentrations which is reverted back by various mechanisms in the body like vasodilation, reduction in oxygen consumption of the tissues, and cellular triggering of alternative metabolic pathways. Most of the times, there will be sufficient oxygen requirement so the oxygen to the tissues will be of enough quantity. When there are no mechanisms or not enough mechanisms to generate the required oxygen, then it will result in pathological changes. These pathological changes will result in derangement

S. Shaikh, *Advances in Imaging*, https://doi.org/10.1007/978-981-16-9535-3_14

of various functions of the body resulting various forms of diseases like cardiovascular disease, chronic renal disease, various diabetic pathologies (one of the common ones is retinopathy), and various inflammatory for example rheumatoid arthritis [1–5]. The reduced partial pressure of oxygen (PaO_2) of below 10 mmHg in the tumours is one of the important factors for the increased chances of the mortality and metastasis [6]. Some of the metabolites in the body like nitric oxide will cause sudden reduction of the O_2 concentration leading to cell death by necrosis or apoptosis resulting in hypoxia. This concept of poor perfusion in diabetic patients leads to retinopathy or arthritic changes in joints. There is no clear cutoff range to identify the exact level of O_2Hb concentration or % Hb saturation, tissue partial pressure, and PO_2 concentrations which will cause these changes from normoxia to hypoxia. Here as we know every cell is different and requires different amounts of nutrients including oxygen also so this hypoxia will be based on duration and also the specific requirements of these individual cells. After stroke or infarction, this hypoxic phenomenon plays an important role in the evaluation of the reperfusion. Hypoxia plays a very important and significant role in the evaluation of the oncology. The amount and duration of the oxygen deprivation in tumours are very important for diagnosis and for prognosis of these tumours. There is dysregulation of the microenvironment of the tumours with aggressive phenotypes which is an important factor for cancer development, thus leading to the increased risk of the invasion and poor prognosis of tumour and local and distant metastases [7, 8]. Tumour aggression is directly proportional to the amount of the delivery of the oxygenated blood which will be insufficient for the growing tumour cells leading to the hypoxia (Diagram 14.1).

14.2 Pathogenesis

Due to the increased requirement of the oxygen, there will be increased blood supply in the form of the angiogenesis. Various angiogenesis factors like interleukin-8, platelet-derived growth factor, cyclooxygenase-2, endothelin-1 and endothelin-2, fibroblast growth factor-3, and nitric oxide synthase will be released. There will be triggering of the various cellular responses leading to activation of various receptors like membrane tyrosine kinase receptors and various dimer and transphosphorylation processes [9]. This "angiogenic switch" mechanism has been important for the evaluation of the tumour metastasis due to microvasculature abnormalities resulting in reduced oxygen diffusion to the tumour cells and ultimately tumour oxygen deprivation [10–12]. Due to this deprivation, various adaptive mechanisms will be formed like changing gene expression impacting on the hypoxic environment. This will result in the upregulation of genes of the various metabolisms like glucose metabolism, pH regulation, cellular proliferation and apoptosis, and nitric oxide metabolism [13–17] (Diagram 14.2).

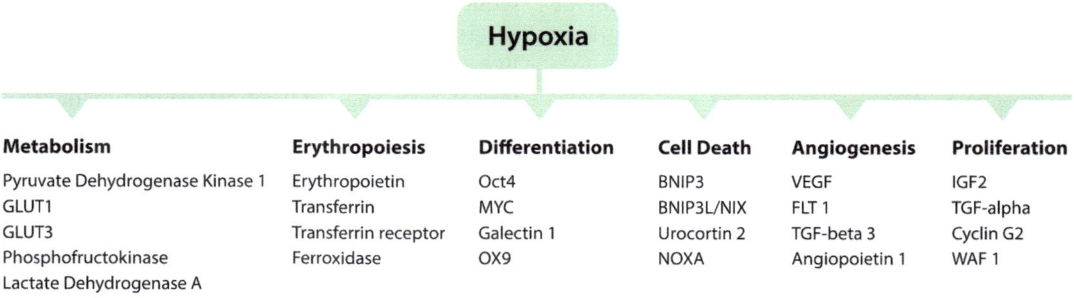

Diagram 14.1 Various causes of hypoxia and the pathogenesis involved in this

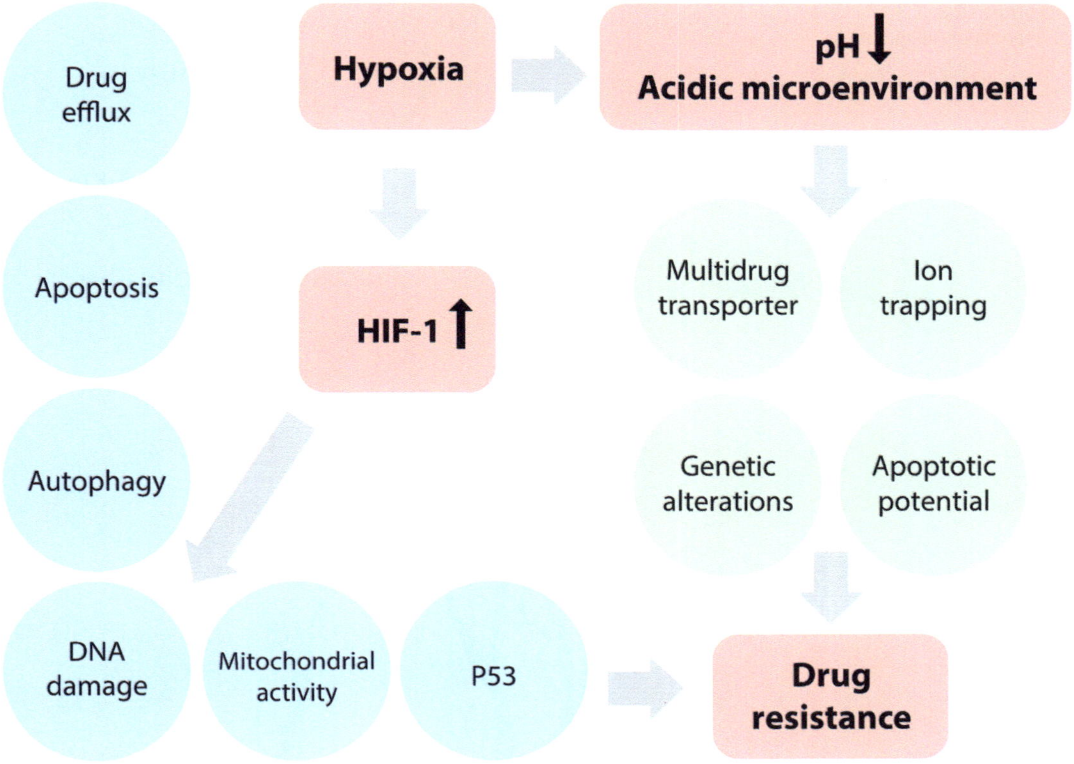

Diagram 14.2 Various components happening in the process of hypoxia

14.3 Biology of the Hypoxia

Gray's was the first who described the dangerous effects of the hypoxia in 1950 [5, 6, 18]. Here it was hypothesized that it will have an impact on gene expression which will be causing various conditions, impacting the cellular proliferation rates. Thus, this mechanism of hypoxia will precipitate the metastatic spread of tumour cells to distant sites (Diagram 14.3). DNA damage is one of the important aspects due to incoming high-energy photons resulting in direct damage to DNA due to these photons interacting with DNA, by the Compton effect due to ionization of the molecule. In this ionization high-energy electrons are released which will be causing significant damage to the tissues [19, 20].

Normal oxygen is consumed by cells, and then the oxygen concentration falls to zero, and in normal healthy tissues, there will be enough oxygen. But in cancer cells due to the abnormal growth of cells where the oxygen demand is more and supply less, this will result in hypoxia. The cells with higher OCR will have shorter diffusion lengths and with lower OCR will have longer diffusion lengths [21]. Majority of the tumours are heterogenous [22], and based on this heterogenicity, tumour vascularity will also have various changes in the vascularity, and few of them will have neovascularizing vessels with a greater number of vessels, and some of them will be torturous vessels; all these are not organized forms [23–29]. In this scenario the hypoxia will be starting even when there is significant amount of the compensatory mechanisms with variable perfusion resulting in the acute hypoxia. The long-term starvation of the tumours will cause chronic hypoxia due to limited diffusion and transient hypoxia mostly due to oxygen deprivation [30–41].

Diagram 14.3 Causes of hypoxia in the tumour cells

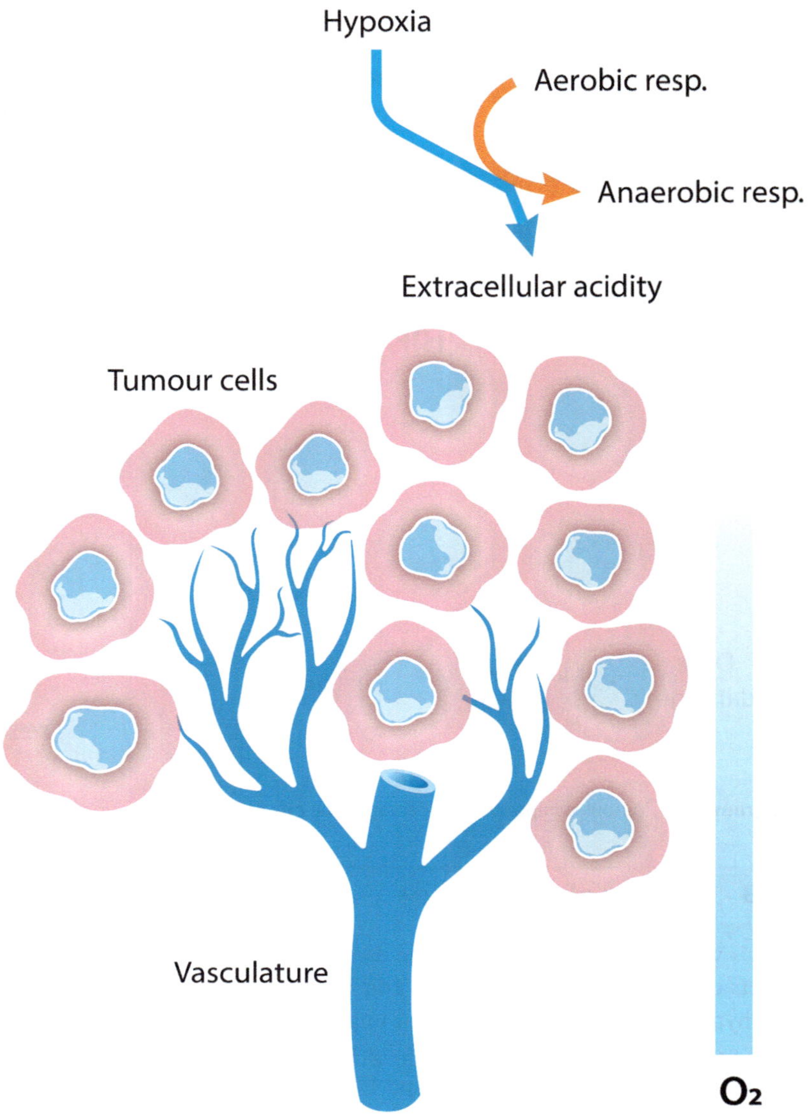

Molecular hypoxia imaging is the newer imaging concept for the evaluation of hypoxic process by various molecular imaging modalities. Positron emission tomography (PET) and single-photon emission CT are most commonly used imaging modalities by using the radiolabelled tracer which can be identified [42, 43]. In PET hypoxia imaging, Cu-ATSM is the first radiotracer used for hypoxia imaging with good binding and good amount of uptake [44–46]. The other newer hypoxia radiotracers are consisting of fluorine-18-labelled (18F) nitroimidazoles and include 18F-fluoroazomycin-arabinoside (18F-FAZA), 2-(2-Nitro-1H-imidazol-1-yl)-N-(2,2,3,3,3-[18F] pentafluoropropyl)-acetamide and 18F-fluoromisonidazole (18F-FMISO); these molecules bind with the intracellular macromolecules.

14.4 Hypoxia Non-invasive Imaging

The identification of the hypoxia is very important in the oncological settings for more accurate diagnosis and prognosis. Hypoxic tumours would improve patient outcomes by helping to adjust irradiation dose, thus selecting individuals for personalized management of the anti-hypoxia-directed therapies, and to increase the efficacy of drugs by increasing oxygen supply to the tumour (e.g. the administration of recombinant human erythropoietin) [47].

14.5 Radioisotope Techniques

PET and single-photon emission computed tomography (SPECT) are based on the basis of the single or dual gamma ray photons detection. Gamma-emitting radioisotopes are used in SPECT like technetium-99m, and radiopharmaceuticals which are labelled with fluorine-18 (18F) or carbon-11 are used in the PET. After injection these radiotracers are circulated by the systemic circulation and are delivered into the cells. These radiotracers will be emitting the energies which will be detected by the gamma camera in SPECT, and the pathological areas will be showing increased amount of the blood with corresponding increase in the metabolic activity. PET imaging is based on the principle of the annihilation after injecting the radionuclides after the injection of the radionuclides. Of these two modalities, SPECT is easier to acquire but has less sensitivity for the imaging of the hypoxia as compared with the PET. PET is having better special resolution and also shows in vivo physiological process better. Nitroimidazoles are the commonly used hypoxic agents for PET imaging of hypoxia. The delivery of these agents is by systemic circulation, and the entire process is reversible, but in the hypoxic conditions, the reduced molecules cannot be oxidized again. There will be binding to various other macromolecules which will be trapped inside viable hypoxic cells, and this forms the basis of the radioisotope imaging of hypoxia [48]. The commonly used radiotracer for PET is 18F-fluoromisonidazole (18F FMISO) for hypoxia evaluation [49–52]. The other radiotracers which are used in tumour hypoxia are 18F-fluoroazomycin arabinoside, 18F-flortanidazole, 18F-labeled fluoroerythronitroimidazole, 18F-fluoroazomycin arabinoside (18F FAZA), and 18F-flortanidazole [53]. These have faster clearances and can give more information of the tumour status and response to treatment. There are other thiosemicarbazones which can be labelled with a positron-emitting isotope of copper (Cu). During this process the c Cu^{2+} is reduced to Cu^{1+} within the cell cytoplasm in the presence of oxygen. In the process of hypoxia under low oxygen conditions, conversion of the Cu^{1+} to Cu^{2+} cannot be done [53] Diagram 14.4 and 14.5.

14.6 MRI Techniques

By using the contrast-enhanced MRI, the imaging of hypoxia can be done which will be having very high sensitivity and specificity. Dynamic contrast-enhanced (DCE) MRI is useful for the detection of the tumour hypoxia [54, 55]. This gives information related with the perfusion and permeability. But due to some limitations, functional MRI, 19F-oximetry, and magnetic resonance spectroscopy can also be used. The concept of the BOLD MRI is that tissue oxygen level-dependent MRI will be using the paramagnetic properties of deoxyhaemoglobin (deoxyHb), and using this concept there will be difference in the evaluation of the relaxivity of oxygenated and deoxygenated haemoglobin which is used to generate the signal. With BOLD direct evaluation of various signal estimations can be done of PaO_2. With the presence of deoxyHb in blood vessels, this will be resulting in the decrease in T2 resulting in dark signal in tissues having vessels in T2-weighted sequences. BOLD MRI is highly sensitive for the high spatial and temporal resolutions which can detect the oxygen levels in the tissues and the fluctuations in these tissues [56]. The biggest disadvantage of the BOLD is it measures the voxel which will include blood vessels and surrounding tissues, but there will be many small neovascularizations of the microcapillaries which will be difficult to interpret. Another limitation is that vascular oxygenation is being evaluated, and sometimes it will not be correlating to the tissue PaO_2 due to blood flow and oxygen

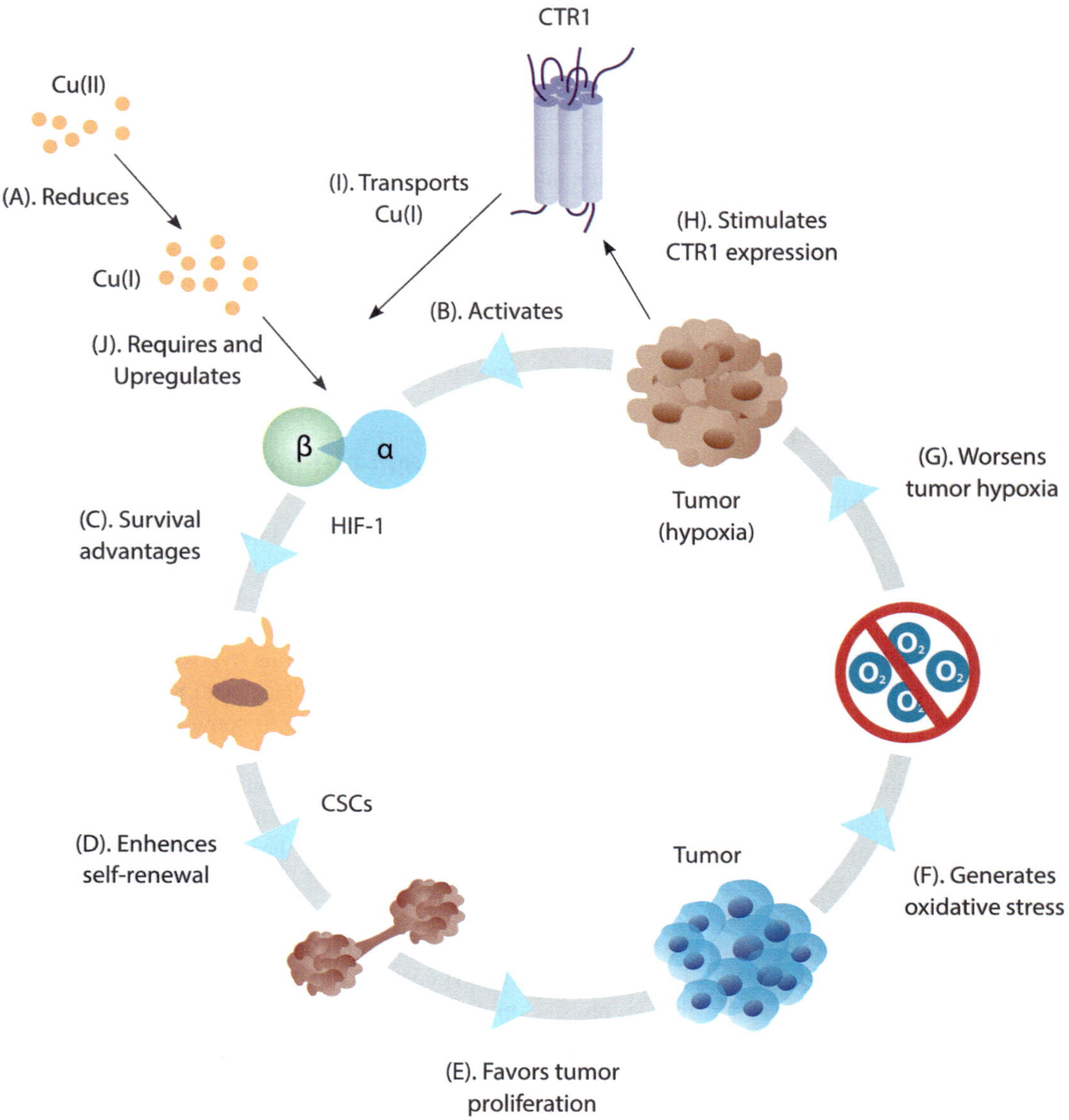

Diagram 14.4 Various mechanisms taking place in hypoxia imaging

[57]. Flow and oxygen dependent in contrast to tissue oxygen level-dependent (TOLD)/oxygen-enhanced MRI will give more precise information related to this [58]. With this newer concept the combination of the BOLD and TOLD MRI can give more precise information in tumour hypoxia [59, 60]. The basis of TOLD imaging is no contrast use and T1-weighted protocol will have short acquisition times which can monitor PaO_2 changes more precisely. Here oxygen is the contrast agent by virtue of the paramagnetic properties with T1 shortening having better correlation between PaO_2 and relaxation rates. T1 is being under the influence of various factors like temperature, tumour features, and basal blood oxygen saturation [61, 62]. Artefacts are one of the major limitations for these techniques which can result in the geometrical distortion in various tissues [63]. Multiparametric quantitative BOLD (qBOLD) is the newer technique for the

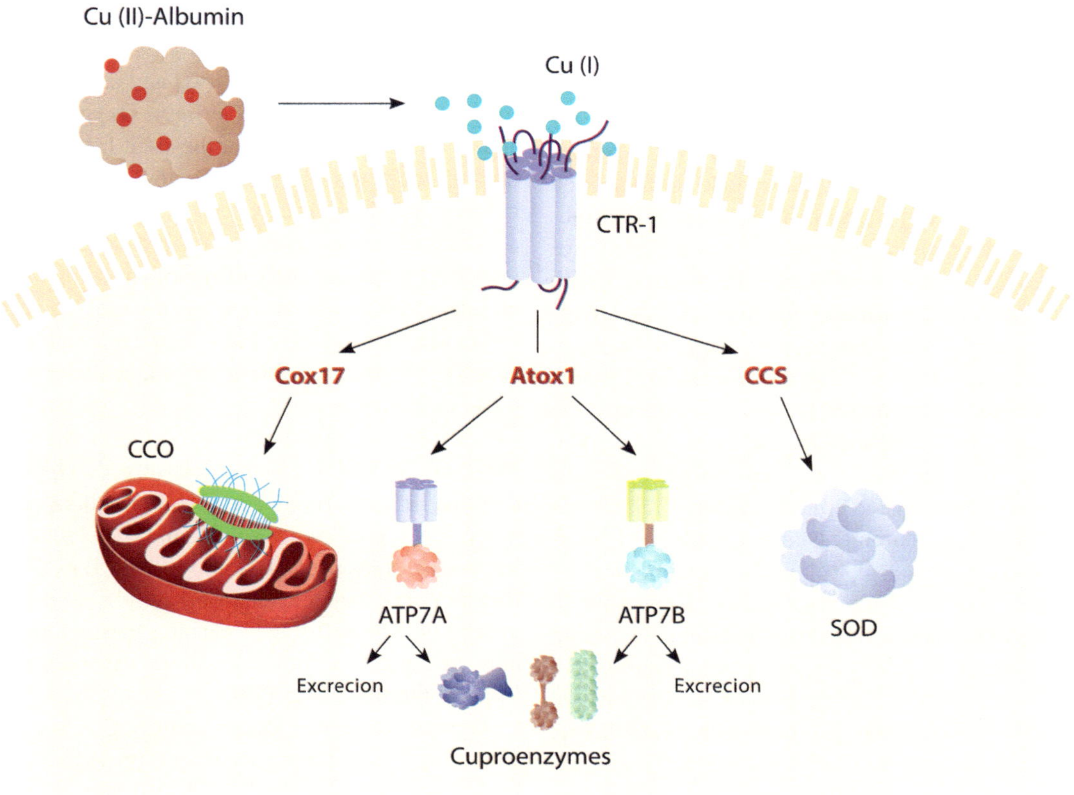

Diagram 14.5 Cu as an important molecular imaging parameter for the evaluation of the molecular aspects of hypoxia

quantitative mapping of tumour hypoxia by monitoring changes in tumour oxygenation [57].

MR oximetry is based on the use of F-labelled contrast which can be used alternatively to proton 1 H MRI, for the evaluation of hypoxia. The concept here is tumour hypoxia mapping by showing the heterogeneity in each tumour [64, 65]. T1 of fluorine agents is used which has biggest advantage to evaluate the in vivo oxygenation in tumour tissues. Perfluorocarbons (19F)-hexafluorobenzene is dependent on the amount of the dissolved oxygen which will be accumulating inside the macrophages [66, 67]. Another advantage of F-labelled agents is to quantify the oxygenation status based on the hormonal levels [68].

14.7 MR Spectroscopy

MRS is based on various nuclear spin properties of 1 H in a magnetic field, to absorb and emit radiofrequency. With these various metabolites when magnetic field is applied, the concentrations of that metabolite can be obtained. The suppression of the water signal is the basis for the MRS image acquisition as water proton signal is more powerful and is due to higher concentrations. Lactate is one of the important components used for MRS imaging [36]. 31P and 23Na MR spectroscopic imaging along with the choline will increase specificity and used to monitor the chemotherapy [69, 70].

14.8 Electron Paramagnetic Resonance or Electron Spin Resonance

In this MR technique, the quantitative evaluation of the PaO_2 in the tissue can be done. The electron paramagnetic resonance (EPR) oximetry is based on the principle of oxygen undergoing the spin exchange interaction with paramagnetic particles. Injection of a paramagnetic probe into the tumours has to be done where the unpaired oxygen electrons interact with the paramagnetic probe causing the changes in T2 depicted as line width of the spectrum and increased in peak-to-peak widths showing the oxygen concentrations [71].

These measurements are based on a non-invasive approach as well as the dynamic process which will show the response of the tumour to hyperoxic gas showing differences in PaO_2 within the tumour [72]. Various probe concentration and the paramagnetic properties of relaxation are used for evaluation. Combination of EPR/MR approach which uses low-field MR and paramagnetic contrast agent can be used. The tumour perfusion and oxygenation can be determined by using the probes like Oxo63. Here the image contrast is directly proportional to the concentration of the agent in the tumour perfusion, and this is inversely proportional to the oxygen concentration. The paramagnetic substances used as probes are of two types: soluble materials like nitroxides and triaryl methyl radicals and insoluble materials like coals, chars, and inks; the sensitivity of the insoluble agents is more for the oxygen [73].

14.9 Optical Imaging for Measuring Hypoxia

Optical imaging techniques for evaluation of the hypoxia are invasive which needs endogenous tumour markers to identify the hypoxia-inducible factors, [72], used to validate other biomarkers of hypoxia. By introducing transgenes with hypoxic response elements, hypoxia transgenes can be used as promoters to reporter genes and by bioluminescent imaging technique can use the luciferase or green fluorescent proteins [74–76]. Visible light photons can also be used to obtain imaging of cells and tissues. The bigger advantage is that the ionizing radiation is not used and can be used based on the light colours of light. Oxygen concentration in the tissues can be used by absorption of the contrast from haemoglobin-oxygen binding and luminescence properties. Different absorption contrast imaging can be done on the principle of the property of the oxyhaemoglobin and deoxyHb to absorb light with variable spectral range; and this correlates with the amount of the oxygen saturation. With variable wavelengths pulse oximetry is commonly used by measuring the differential absorption in the blood vessels; PaO_2 in the blood can be determined. Optical contrast between oxyhaemoglobin and deoxyHb when combined with ultrasound detectors is known as photoacoustic tomography. Based on this principle, molecule absorbs light, and the energy will be distributed causing thermal pressure emitting detectable ultrasonic waves known as photothermal effect [77].

Optical coherence tomography (OCT) is also a non-invasive imaging technique providing the high-resolution images. Broadband light is used as source, to create cross-sectional images measuring echo time delay and intensity of the reflected and backscattered light, depending on the depth of the tissue [78]. Spectral-domain OCT is the newer form of the spectral detectors which will allow the inference of oxygen saturation depicted in the spectra [79]. Newer luminescent probes are under research for the assessment of hypoxia-induced factors and for hypoxia detection [80].

Radioactive decay light emission of positron-emitting radionuclides is a new method known as Cherenkov luminescence imaging based on the phenomenon of the annihilation. This is based on the property of the positron velocity which exceeds the speed of light leading to the production of Cherenkov radiation. These are produced when a charged particle travels with speed more than the light which will produce polarization. Cherenkov luminescence imaging uses selective probes which is now the important technique to measure hypoxia in vivo and also to monitor tumour response to hypoxia-targeted drugs [81, 82].

14.10 Conclusion

The information of the tumour oxygenation evaluation is very important for both treatment efficacy and patient prognosis. Hypoxia is a complex and interrelated problem and needs lot of research. But with available resources, hypoxia imaging has definitely highlighted the various aspects of diagnosis, therapeutic options, and prognosis also.

References

1. Hultén LM, Levin M. The role of hypoxia in atherosclerosis. Curr Opin Lipidol. 2009;20:409–14.
2. Taylor PC, Sivakumar B. Hypoxia and angiogenesis in rheumatoid arthritis. Curr Opin Rheumatol. 2005;17:293–8.
3. Ishida S, Shinoda K, Kawashima S, Oguchi Y, Okada Y, Ikeda E. Coexpression of VEGF receptors VEGF-R2 and neuropilin-1 in proliferative diabetic retinopathy. Invest Ophthalmol Vis Sci. 2000;41:1649–56.
4. Mateo J, Izquierdo-Garcia D, Badimon JJ, Fayad ZA, Fuster V. Noninvasive assessment of hypoxia in rabbit advanced atherosclerosis using 18f-fluoromisonidazole PET imaging. Circ Cardiovasc Imaging. 2014;7:312–20.
5. Vaupel P, Thews O, Hoeckel M. Treatment resistance of solid tumours. Med Onco. 2001;18:243–59. https://doi.org/10.1385/mo:18:4:243.
6. Vaupel P, Mayer A, Hockel M. Tumor ¨ hypoxia and malignant progression. Methods Enzymol. 2004;381:335–54.
7. Mujcic H, Hill RP, Koritzinsky M, Wouters BG. Hypoxia signaling and the metastatic phenotype. Curr Mol Med. 2014;14:565–79.
8. Sullivan R, Graham CH. Hypoxia-driven selection of the metastatic phenotype. Cancer Metastasis Rev. 2007;26:319–31.
9. Gomes A, Guillaume L, Grimes DR, Fehrenbach J, Lobjois V, Ducommun B. Oxygen partial pressure is a rate-limiting parameter for cell proliferation in 3d spheroids grown in physioxic culture condition. PLoS One. 2016;11:e0161239.
10. Harris AL. Hypoxia--a key regulatory factor in tumour growth. Nat Rev Cancer. 2002;2:38–47.
11. Vaupel P, Harrison L. Tumor hypoxia: causative factors, compensatory mechanisms, and cellular response. Oncologist. 2004;9(Suppl 5):4–9.
12. Bristow RG, Hill RP. Hypoxia and metabolism. Hypoxia, DNA repair and genetic instability. Nat Rev Cancer. 2008;8:180–92.
13. Shaw RJ. Glucose metabolism and cancer. Curr Opin Cell Biol. 2006;18:598–608.
14. Dang CV, Semenza GL. Oncogenic alterations of metabolism. Trends Biochem Sci. 1999;24:68–72.
15. Semenza GL. Hydroxylation of HIF-1: oxygen sensing at the molecular level. Physiology (Bethesda). 2004;19:176–82.
16. Adamaki M, Georgountzou A, Moschovi M. Cancer and the cellular response to hypoxia. Pediatr Therapeut. 2012;S1:002.
17. Gatenby RA, Smallbone K, Maini PK, Rose F, Averill J, Nagle RB, et al. Cellular adaptations to hypoxia and acidosis during somatic evolution of breast cancer. Br J Cancer. 2007;97:646–53.
18. Vaupel P, Briest S, Höckel M. Hypoxia in breast cancer: pathogenesis, characterization, and biological/therapeutic implications. Wien Med Wochenschr. 2002;152:334–42. https://doi.org/10.1046/j.1563-258x.2002.02032.x.
19. Wilson WR, Hay MP. Targeting hypoxia in cancer therapy. Nat Rev Cancer. 2011;11:393–410. https://doi.org/10.1038/nrc3064.
20. Gray LH, Conger AD, Ebert M, Partridge M. A mechanistic investigation of the oxygen fixation hypothesis and oxygen enhancement ratio. Biomed Phys Eng Express. 2015;1:045209.
21. Kreuzer F. Oxygen supply to tissues: the Krogh model and its assumptions. Experientia. 1982;38:1415–26.
22. Grimes DR, Fletcher AG, Partridge M. Oxygen consumption dynamics in steadystate tumour models. R Soc Open Sci. 2014;1:140080.
23. Carmeliet P, Jain RK. Angiogenesis in cancer and other diseases. Nature. 2000;407:249–57. https://doi.org/10.1038/35025220.
24. Shibuya K, Hoshino H, Chiyo M, Iyoda A, Yoshida S, Sekine Y, et al. High magnification bronchovideoscopy combined with narrow band imaging could detect capillary loops of angiogenic squamous dysplasia in heavy smokers at high risk for lung cancer. Thorax. 2003;58:989–95. https://doi.org/10.1136/thorax.58.11.989.
25. Baluk P, Hashizume H, McDonald DM. Cellular abnormalities of blood vessels as targets in cancer. Curr Opin Genet Dev. 2005;15:102–11. https://doi.org/10.1016/j.gde.2004.12.005.
26. Secomb TW, Hsu R, Dewhirst M, Klitzman B, Gross J. Analysis of oxygen transport to tumor tissue by microvascular networks. Int J Radiat Oncol Biol Phys. 1993;25:481–9. https://doi.org/10.1016/0360-3016(93)90070-c.
27. Secomb TW, Hsu R, Ong ET, Gross JF, Dewhirst MW. Analysis of the effects of oxygen supply and demand on hypoxic fraction in tumors. Acta Oncol. 1995;34:313–6. https://doi.org/10.3109/02841869509093981.
28. Secomb TW, Hsu R, Braun R, Ross J, Gross J, Dewhirst M, et al. Theoretical simulation of oxygen transport to tumors by three dimensional networks of microvessels. Oxygen transport to tissue XX. New York: US, Springer; 1998. p. 629–34.
29. Grimes DR, Kannan P, Warren DR, Markelc B, Bates R, Muschel R, et al. Estimating oxygen distribution from vasculature in three-dimensional tumour tissue. J R Soc Interface. 2016;13:20160070.

30. Mueller-Klieser W. Method for the determination of oxygen consumption rates and diffusion coefficients in multicellular spheroids. Biophys J. 1984;46:343–8.
31. Groebe K, Vaupel P. Evaluation of oxygen diffusion distances in human breast cancer xenografts using tumor-specific in vivo data: role of various mechanisms in the development of tumor hypoxia. Int J Radiat Oncol Biol Phys. 1988;15:691–7. https://doi.org/10.1016/0360-3016(88)90313-622.
32. Grimes DR, Kelly C, Bloch K, Partridge M. A method for estimating the oxygen consumption rate in multicellular tumour spheroids. J R Soc Interface. 2014;11:20131124. https://doi.org/10.1098/rsif.2013.1124.
33. Grimes DR, Kannan P, McIntyre A, Kavanagh A, Siddiky A, Wigfield S, et al. The role of oxygen in avascular tumor growth. PLoS One. 2016;11:1–19.
34. Chaplin DJ, Durand RE, Olive PL. Acute hypoxia in tumors: implications for modifiers of radiation effects. Int J Radiat Oncol Biol Phys. 1986;12:1279–82. https://doi.org/10.1016/0360-3016(86)90153-7.
35. Denekamp J, Daşu A. Inducible repair and the two forms of tumour hypoxia—time for a paradigm shift. Acta Oncol. 1999;38:903–18. https://doi.org/10.1080/028418699432590.
36. Toma-Dasu I, Dasu A. Modelling tumour oxygenation, reoxygenation and implications on treatment outcome. Comput Math Methods Med. 2013;2013:141087.
37. Kallinowski F, Zander R, Hoeckel M, Vaupel P. Tumor tissue oxygenation as evaluated by computerized-PO2-histography. Int J Radiat Oncol Biol Phys. 1990;19:953–61.
38. Griffiths JR, Robinson SP. The OxyLite: a fibre-optic oxygen sensor. Br J Radiol. 1999;72:627–30. https://doi.org/10.1259/bjr.72.859.10624317.
39. Toma-Daşu L, Waites A, Dasu A, Denekamp J. Theoretical simulation of oxygen tension measurement in tissues using a microelectrode: I. The response function of the electrode. Physiol Meas. 2001;22:713–25.
40. Toma-Dasu I, Dasu A, Waites A, Denekamp J, Fowler JF. Theoretical simulation of oxygen tension measurement in the tissue using a microelectrode: II. Simulated measurements in tissues. Radiother Oncol. 2002;64:109–18.
41. Kazanzides P, Chang J, Iordachita I, Li J, Ling CC, Fichting. J Nucl Med. 2012;53(10):1608–15.
42. Mees G, Dierckx R, Vangestel C, Van De Wiele C. Molecular imaging of hypoxia with radiolabelled agents. Eur J Nucl Med Mol Imaging. 2009;36:1674–86. https://doi.org/10.1007/s00259-009-1195-9.
43. Sun X, Niu G, Chan N, Shen B, Chen X. Tumor hypoxia imaging. Mol Imaging Biol. 2011;13:399–410. https://doi.org/10.1007/s11307-010-0420-z.
44. Rahmim A, Zaidi H. PET versus SPECT: strengths, limitations and challenges. Nucl Med Commun. 2008;29:193–207. https://doi.org/10.1097/mnm.0b013e3282f3a515.
45. Vavere AL, Lewis JS. Cu-ATSM: a radiopharmaceutical for the PET imaging of hypoxia. Dalton Trans. 2007;43:4893.
46. Padhani AR, Krohn KA, Lewis JS, Alber M. Imaging oxygenation of human tumours. Eur Radiol. 2007;17:861–72. https://doi.org/10.1007/s00330-006-0431-y.
47. Overgaard J. Hypoxic radiosensitization: adored and ignored. J Clin Oncol. 2007;25:4066–74.
48. Wardman P. Chemical radiosensitizers for use in radiotherapy. Clin Oncol (R Coll Radiol). 2007;19:397–417.
49. Fleming IN, Manavaki R, Blower PJ, West C, Williams KJ, Harris AL, et al. Imaging tumour hypoxia with positron emission tomography. Br J Cancer. 2015;112:238–50.
50. Ueda S, Saeki T, Osaki A, Yamane T, Kuji I. Bevacizumab induces acute hypoxia and cancer progression in patients with refractory breast cancer: multimodal functional imaging and multiplex cytokine analysis. Clin Cancer Res. 2017;23:5769–78.
51. Quintela-Fandino M, Lluch A, Manso L, Calvo I, Cortes J, García-Saenz JA, et al. 18F-fluoromisonidazole PET and activity of neoadjuvant nintedanib in early HER2-negative breast cancer: a window-of opportunity randomized trial. Clin Cancer Res 2017;23:1432–41. https://ejbc.kr. https://doi.org/10.4048/jbc.2019.22.e26 168 Hypoxia Assessment and Its Importance in Breast Cancer.
52. Cheng J, Lei L, Xu J, Sun Y, Zhang Y, Wang X, et al. 18F-fluoromisonidazole PET/CT: a potential tool for predicting primary endocrine therapy resistance in breast cancer. J Nucl Med. 2013;54:333–40.
53. Reischl G, Dorow DS, Cullinane C, Katsifis A, Roselt P, Binns D, et al. Imaging of tumor hypoxia with [124I]IAZA in comparison with [18F]FMISO and [18F]FAZA--first small animal PET results. J Pharm Pharm Sci. 2007;10:203–11.
54. Jensen RL, Mumert ML, Gillespie DL, Kinney AY, Schabel MC, Salzman KL. Preoperative dynamic contrast-enhanced MRI correlates with molecular markers of hypoxia and vascularity in specific areas of intratumoral microenvironment and is predictive of patient outcome. Neuro Oncol. 2014;16:280–91.
55. Halle C, Andersen E, Lando M, Aarnes EK, Hasvold G, Holden M, et al. Hypoxia-induced gene expression in chemoradioresistant cervical cancer revealed by dynamic contrast-enhanced MRI. Cancer Res. 2012;72:5285–95.
56. Baudelet C, Gallez B. How does blood oxygen level-dependent (BOLD) contrast correlate with oxygen partial pressure (pO2) inside tumors? Magn Reson Med. 2002;48:980–6.
57. Christen T, Lemasson B, Pannetier N, Farion R, Remy C, Zaharchuk G, et al. Is T2* enough to assess oxygenation? Quantitative blood oxygen level-dependent analysis in brain tumor. Radiology. 2012;262:495–502.
58. Howe FA, Robinson SP, Rodrigues LM, Griffiths JR. Flow and oxygenation dependent (FLOOD)

contrast MR imaging to monitor the response of rat tumors to carbogen breathing. Magn Reson Imaging. 1999;17:1307–18.
59. Mason RP, Zhao D, Pacheco-Torres J, Cui W, Kodibagkar VD, Gulaka PK, et al. Multimodality imaging of hypoxia in preclinical settings. Q J Nucl Med Mol Imaging. 2010;54:259–80.
60. White DA, Zhang Z, Li L, Gerberich J, Stojadinovic S, Peschke P, et al. Developing oxygen-enhanced magnetic resonance imaging as a prognostic biomarker of radiation response. Cancer Lett. 2016;380:69–77.
61. Ding Y, Mason RP, McColl RW, Yuan Q, Hallac RR, Sims RD, et al. Simultaneous measurement of tissue oxygen level-dependent (TOLD) and blood oxygenation level-dependent (BOLD) effects in abdominal tissue oxygenation level studies. J Magn Reson Imaging. 2013;38:1230–6.
62. O'Connor JP, Robinson SP, Waterton JC. Imaging tumour hypoxia with oxygen-enhanced MRI and BOLD MRI. Br J Radiol 2019;92:20180642. https://ejbc.kr. https://doi.org/10.4048/jbc.2019.22.e26 169 Hypoxia Assessment and Its Importance in Breast Cancer.
63. Maril N, Collins CM, Greenman RL, Lenkinski RE. Strategies for shimming the breast. Magn Reson Med. 2005;54:1139–45.
64. Hunjan S, Zhao D, Constantinescu A, Hahn EW, Antich PP, Mason RP. Tumor oximetry: demonstration of an enhanced dynamic mapping procedure using fluorine-19 echo planar magnetic resonance imaging in the dunning prostate R3327-AT1 rat tumor. Int J Radiat Oncol Biol Phys. 2001;49:1097–108.
65. Zhao D, Jiang L, Hahn EW, Mason RP. Comparison of 1 H blood oxygen level-dependent (BOLD) and 19F MRI to investigate tumor oxygenation. Magn Reson Med. 2009;62:357–64.
66. Le D, Mason RP, Hunjan S, Constantinescu A, Barker BR, Antich PP. Regional tumor oxygen dynamics: 19F PBSR EPI of hexafluorobenzene. Magn Reson Imaging. 1997;15:971–81.
67. Procissi D, Claus F, Burgman P, Koziorowski J, Chapman JD, Thakur SB, et al. In vivo 19F magnetic resonance spectroscopy and chemical shift imaging of tri-fluoro-nitroimidazole as a potential hypoxia reporter in solid tumors. Clin Cancer Res. 2007;13:3738–47.
68. Bartusik D, Tomanek B, Siluk D, Kaliszan R, Fallone G. The application of 19F magnetic resonance ex vivo imaging of three-dimensional cultured breast cancer cells to study the effect of δ-tocopherol. Anal Biochem. 2009;387:315–7.
69. Pinker K, Helbich TH, Morris EA. The potential of multiparametric MRI of the breast. Br J Radiol. 2017;90:20160715.
70. O'Flynn EA, DeSouza NM. Functional magnetic resonance: biomarkers of response in breast cancer. Breast Cancer Res. 2011;13:204.
71. Velan SS, Spencer RG, Zweier JL, Kuppusamy P. Electron paramagnetic resonance oxygen mapping (EPROM): direct visualization of oxygen concentration in tissue. Magn Reson Med. 2000;43:804–9.
72. Krohn KA, Link JM, Mason RP. Molecular imaging of hypoxia. J Nucl Med. 2008;49(Suppl 2):129S–48S.
73. Roussakis E, Li Z, Nichols AJ, Evans CL. Oxygen-sensing methods in biomedicine from the macroscale to the microscale. Angew Chem Int Ed Engl. 2015;54:8340–62.
74. Shibata T, Giaccia AJ, Brown JM. Development of a hypoxia-responsive vector for tumor-specific gene therapy. Gene Ther. 2000;7:493–8.
75. Vordermark D, Shibata T, Brown JM. Green fluorescent protein is a suitable reporter of tumor hypoxia despite an oxygen requirement for chromophore formation. Neoplasia 2001;3:527–34. https://ejbc.kr https://doi.org/10.4048/jbc.2019.22.e26 170 Hypoxia Assessment and Its Importance in Breast Cancer.
76. Harada H, Kizaka-Kondoh S, Hiraoka M. Optical imaging of tumor hypoxia and evaluation of efficacy of a hypoxia-targeting drug in living animals. Mol Imaging. 2005;4:182–93.
77. Wang LV, Hu S. Photoacoustic tomography: in vivo imaging from organelles to organs. Science. 2012;335:1458–62.
78. Nam HS, Yoo H. Spectroscopic optical coherence tomography: a review of concepts and biomedical applications. Appl Spectrosc Rev. 2018;53:91–111.
79. Schuman JS. Spectral domain optical coherence tomography for glaucoma (an AOS thesis). Trans Am Ophthalmol Soc. 2008;106:426–58.
80. Sandhu S, Kydd L, Jaworski J. Luminescent probe based techniques for hypoxia imaging. J Nanomed Res. 2017;6:00160.
81. Ciarrocchi E, Belcari N. Cerenkov luminescence imaging: physics principles and potential applications in biomedical sciences. EJNMMI Phys. 2017;4:14.
82. Desvaux E, Courteau A, Bellaye PS, Guillemin M, Drouet C, Walker P, et al. Cherenkov luminescence imaging is a fast and relevant preclinical tool to assess tumour hypoxia in vivo. EJNMMI Res. 2018;8:111.

15 Translational Imaging

Key Points (Abstract)

Biomedical imaging has significantly increased due to various translational approaches formed due to in vitro to clinical imaging. Various aspects of disciplines, scales, and scopes through translational imaging will combine to reach the in vivo context (e.g. through animal models), which ideally then leads to direct evaluation, validation, and application in humans. The importance of the various translational aspects for the new biomarkers for their clinical applications, for diagnosis to therapy planning and follow-up. There are different aspects of the imaging in the broad sense for the biomarkers and novel diagnostics agents for bridging the gaps between research, instrumentation, imaging devices, and in vitro imaging for the various clinical applications.

With advancements in the technologies, imaging has "infiltrated" in all aspects of science, along with the cell and developmental biologists, pathobiologists, physicists, material scientists, chemists, pharmaceutical specialists, and clinicians; thus the bases of "translational" methods are invented.

Keywords

Biomedical imaging · Biomarkers · PET · MRI · Optical imaging · Anticancer agents · Translational imaging

15.1 Introduction

Translational medicine is seen as the interdisciplinary branch of biomedicine, aiming for the translation of the results in preclinical to the clinical setting, with the concept of the "from bench to bedside" aspect [1]. The main goal of this is to improve prevention, better diagnosis, and more specific treatment options for the various human diseases which can be managed efficiently along with the concept from the preclinical to the clinical setting. This translational research aims for the better discovery process, with excellent experimental design with its more specific application in our clinical practice [2].

The perfect combination of the experimental model along with the study design is seen more relevantly. Animal model imaging is still the basis of any studies which will be done in vitro. They are still an essential source of the information [3] (Diagram 15.1).

The biomedical imaging concept involves the use of the energy for the body and measuring, with the excellent spatial localization, so that the energy, which is transmitted through and emitted from, is reflected back from various organs and tissues. Electromagnetic energy is the most common form of the energy like X-rays or lights; along with this the other form of the energy like the mechanical sound energy will be used for ultrasound scans. As we all know imaging started

S. Shaikh, *Advances in Imaging*, https://doi.org/10.1007/978-981-16-9535-3_15

Diagram 15.1 Systematic diagram showing the translational science and regulatory science in various aspects

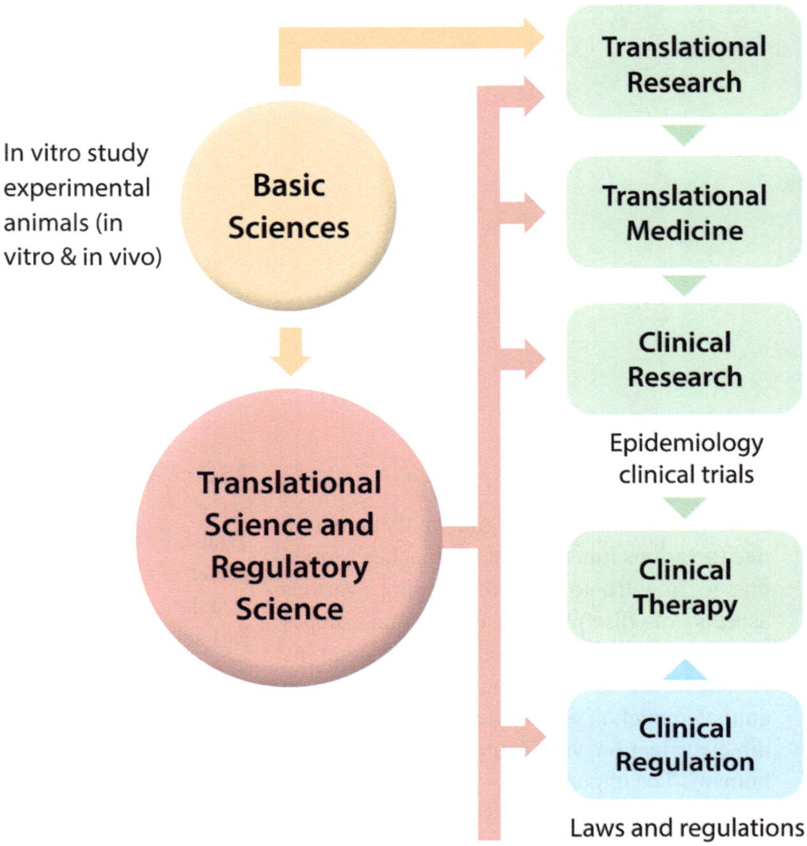

with the use of the X-ray imaging by the Roentgen [4].The use of computerized tomography is being more widely used for various pathologies for the diagnosis and its measure and also to monitor the sequence of events in the various pathologies. The same concept is being used in the nuclear medicine for the use of positron emission tomography (PET) and single-photon emission computed tomography (SPECT). Magnetic resonance imaging (MRI) is the soft tissue modality with excellent soft tissue contrast with excellent resolution. Along with this the ultrasound (US) imaging and the newer optical imaging (OI) are also having the better sensitivity. Of these existing modalities, the majority of them will be for the clinical imaging, while the optical imaging is the modality which will be used for the preclinical animal applications. One of the important aspects of the imaging in animal imaging of the mice is important due to the use of genetically engineered mice for the biomedical research and also to measure the various anatomic, functional, and molecular phenotypes. Animal in vivo imaging will be more successfully used for the more precise non-destructive as each animal serves as its own control; it can image the whole animal and lastly provide a bigger gap between the translational bridge from animal to human studies [3, 4]. Increased research and the advanced technologies which are there for the imaging of small animals can be used in the similar manner for human imaging thus can be translated for the various clinical applications. Oncologic imaging will provide the researchers and clinicians for the assessment of cancer progression, especially with the availability of the novel anticancer agents. Various aspects of the quantitative data related with the various aspects of the tumour size, metastases, physiology and metabolism, molecular markers, and specific targets for various malignancies. The concept of personalized medicine has been developed for the oncological practice which was once having the cytotoxic agents which were not selective and now the newer targeted agents in the form of the various signal transduction inhibitors, STIs, which can further block specific pathways which are for neoplastic transformation, growth, and metastasis. The newer concept is the use of the already established imaging modalities for the development of various novel imaging protocols and also for the pharmacodynamic imaging to access the end-point results [5–10]. The various newer protocols in the evaluation of the various tumour metabolic activities, like cellularity and vascularization can be done more precisely (Diagram 15.2).

The available imaging technologies are used for anatomical, physiological, and metabolic evaluation based on various principles. The imaging modalities which are based on the physical components will be having interaction of external energy in form of radiofrequency waves (MRI), X-rays (CT), radiation decay (PET, SPECT), or sound waves (US) having significant more spatial and time-based reconstruction of the various anatomical, physiological, or molecular images.

15.2 Magnetic Resonance Imaging and Spectroscopy (MRI and MRS)

MRI images are generated by the use of the external magnetic field to the body. This is the most complex technique based on many physical interactions. The use of magnetic field will align the hydrogen atoms with parallel and antiparallel directions to the magnetic field. By the applications of the radio wave pulse to the body by the use of the surface coils, the distribution of the magnetism will decide the property of these techniques [11–13]. Various hydrogen atoms will have different relaxation properties which can be detected by the radiofrequency MR receivers. This MRI of tissue relaxation will be helpful for the radiofrequency pulse energy which is being translated into the mobility and chemical bonding of hydrogen. Two basic types of the images are T1- and T2-weighted MRI. As we all know, T1-weighted images will be showing the fat as a white bright signal, on contrary the water and cerebrospinal fluid (CSF) are dark. Fat is grey on

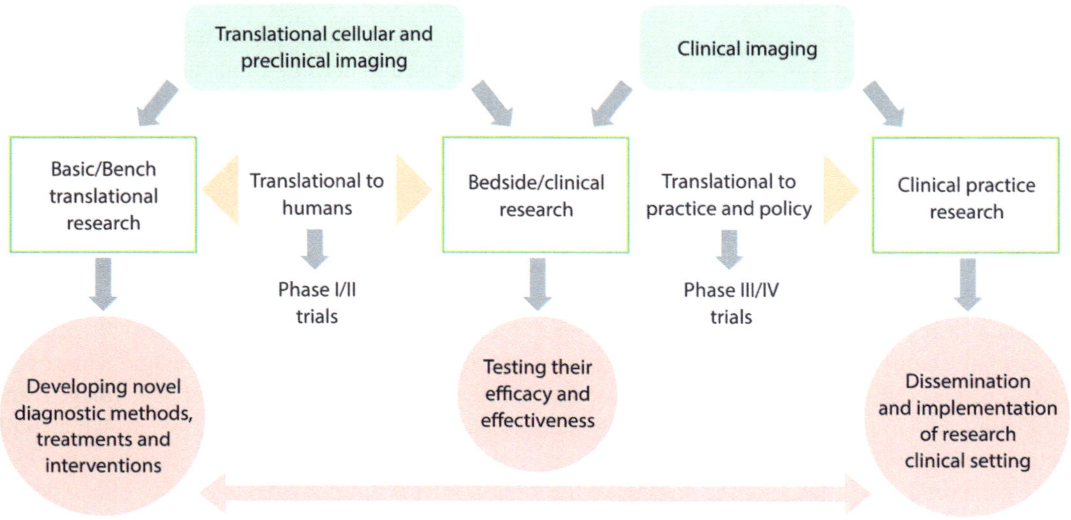

Diagram 15.2 The relation between the translational preclinical imaging and the clinical imaging

T2-weighted image, and blood, oedema, and CSF appear white. MR is also important for the perfusion and permeability of various organs after injecting gadolinium-based contrast agents [14]. Iron oxide-based nanoparticles like superparamagnetic iron oxide, SPIOs, and ultra-superparamagnetic iron oxide, USPIOs, will also have the molecular imaging properties on the T2-weighted scans [15]. In various hydrogen-containing molecules or other atoms like 31P and 13C, the metabolic information is also being given by magnetic resonance spectroscopy (MRS) scan [16, 17]. MRS is also based on the amount of protons. MRI is preferred for the imaging of the central nervous system, musculoskeletal system, and stationary soft tissues. Recent applications of the MR are use in the lung, in the form of the hyperpolarized 129Xe or 3He gas to evaluate the pulmonary gas transfer and to access the gaseous exchange in lung [18]. The use of the hyperpolarized pyruvate will be used for the faster and in vivo assessment of cancer metabolism [19]. Thus, with the capabilities of the better spatial resolution, higher soft tissue contrast, no ionizing radiation, and the applications for the anatomic, metabolic, physiological, and molecular imaging. Some of the drawbacks are that it is a very expensive and challenging imaging modality and has long scan times for large volume/high resolution.

15.3 X-Ray and Computed Tomography (CT)

X-ray and CT are based on the various intrinsic properties of physical and electron density. X-rays are absorbed in different amounts by various tissues or materials in the body. The process of the absorption and the scattering will be there, and small amount will be striking the detector [20]. The basis of Ct is similar to X-ray production from the X-ray tube passing through the detectors. The CT image quantification can be done on various densities, and the basics are the air is black, fat is dark grey, soft tissue is light grey, and bone or calcium and contrast agents are white. So, CT is superior to bone and lung scans. With various advantages the CT is a faster scanning modality with widespread availability and excellent high spatial resolution, whole-body scan, moderate costs, and shorter duration of the scans. Various disadvantages of CT are the very high radiation dose, anatomic information only no functional information, and poor soft tissue contrast.

15.4 Positron Emission Tomography (PET)

PET and SPECT are the nuclear medicine modalities which will be having the higher spatial and temporal distribution by the use of specific target-specific radiotracers and pharmaceuticals. In PET, positron-emitting radioisotopes are injected in small doses usually less than 0.3 mCi for a mouse and less than 20 mCi for a patient intravenously [4, 21]. There are various aspects of the glucose metabolism, blood volume and flow, tissue uptake, receptor binding, and oxygen utilization. Various radiopharmaceuticals or the molecular probes like carbon-11-, nitrogen-13-, oxygen-15-, and fluorine-18-based tracers to evaluate the different protocols of pathophysiology and biology are being used . The basic information of the increased uptake of glucose in malignant cells which was described by Otto Warburg in 1930, based on the uptake of FDG, will be used to detect various tumour lesions and metastases [21]. Every organ will be having FDG uptake including the brain, heart, kidney, and bladder and, in mice, by brown fat on FDG-PET [22]. Molecular function assessment is the important aspect of this modality but having very poor spatial resolution due to which the anatomical location of the lesion cannot be specifically located. With the use of the CT, it will become the hybrid scanner PET/CT scanner. These two modality images of PET and CT images are obtained by the fusion of these images which will give the physiological and molecular data [23]. PET/MRI is nowadays the modality of choice for the evaluation of the physiologic and biochemical information. The disadvantage is the use of radiation.

PET is very sensitive (nM-pM), for various labelling of small molecules will be having the whole-body 3D volumetric imaging, quantitative, and also the clinical use of these parameters. Ionizing radiation, and the use of the radiolabelled molecules, with the shorter half-life radionuclides (need for cyclotrons), lower spatial resolution can be used.

15.5 Ultrasound (US)

Ultrasound uses high-frequency sound waves for imaging. This imaging is based on the principle of the ultrasound energy reflected from interfaces in the body ("echoes") with different tissue interfaces and different acoustic impedances based on various physical density and velocity of the sound in the tissue [24]. Cyst is sonolucent as it contains water, solid organs like the liver and spleen which have homogenous echo texture. The concept of hyperechoic structures will be calcification, fat, and air. It has no ionizing radiation, is real-time imaging, easily available and is not expensive [25]. The various advantages of US are it is real-time, has no ionizing radiation, is low-cost, has good spatial resolution, is easily available, and has good physiological information. Limited field of view is one of the limitations.

15.6 Optical Imaging (OI)

OI modalities are very sensitive for the detectors for the bioluminescent or fluorescent light which is transmitted from internal sources. The use of the optical filters will select both excitation and emission of wavelengths [26]. Excitation of light in bioluminescence imaging in the range of (400–600 nm) will emit various fluorescence levels. Bioluminescence imaging based on the expression of luciferases, which are isolated from organisms modifying the substrates to produce the light, can be used for the detection of the various cameras. Fluorescence imaging is another entity for the bioluminescence which is very sensitive. The lower the depth of penetration (1–2 mm) is due to scattering and absorption of the emitted photons. The advantages of OI are they are easily accessible having the low cost with high-throughput, significantly sensitive for the targets and contrast agents without the ionizing radiation. These imaging are difficult to translate to clinical use, 3D is very difficult, it is not quantitative, and size of fluorophores can be the limiting factor.

Every modality has its advantages and disadvantages

- Spatial resolution: is the resolution so that the smallest object I can visualize?,
- Signal-to-noise: Is it the precision of the measurement?
- Quantitation: is the measurement correct?
- Contrast-to-noise: Different image intensity for the clear depiction of the object of interest?
- Sensitivity: is the detection precise for the object ?

Contrast Agents (CAs): These are the tracers which are administered in the modality which is seen based on the tissue and/or lesion contrast. Dynamic functional information of tissue/lesion and its characteristics for the perfusion and permeability like the dynamic contrast-enhanced DCE-MRI, CE-CT, or CEUS. The use of the bioluminescence, radioactive and luciferase-tracers are used for the detection of the signal [27, 28].

CT CAs: The intravenous, oral, or rectal contrast agents use the X-ray and CT images for the proper depiction of the neoplastic lesions and angiography for various disease pathologies and for the dynamic perfusion studies. In the study of the molecular imaging, there is the use of gold nanoparticles.

MRI CAs: Gadolinium (Gd)-based chelates which are having the paramagnetic properties will be used for the reduction of the T1 relaxation times thus having the brightness of T1-weighted images. Another one is the iron oxide nanoparticle-based like SPIO, USPIO superparamagnetic agents, having the characteristics of the specified T2 relaxation times causing decreased signal intensity on T2-weighted images.

PET CAs: Radiolabelled short-life molecules, peptides, and antibodies are produced by the cyclotrons having the smaller half-life periods like 18F 110 min, 11C 20 min, 13N 9.9 min, and 15O 120 s.

US CAs: There is the more specific application of the various gas or air-filled microbubbles or lipid microspheres having more scatters on the ultrasound, and some of the agents like Optison, Definity, Levovist, Echogen, and Biosphere are administered intravascular, while SonoRx is used orally.

OI CAs: These are based on various fluorescent proteins or enzymes, which will be facilitating the bioluminescent molecules/dyes for labelling various biomolecules and cells. Various newer targeted agents like the PET radiotracers, MRI nanoparticles, and luciferase constructs will be used for the visualization of the genes [3], proteins [15], tumour pH, and microenvironment [29].

15.7 Oncologic Imaging for Assessment of Therapy Response

With the advent of the various newer therapeutic options in the oncology which are being increasingly used to specifically target the various metabolic pathways for the tumour growth and tumour proliferation and to evaluate the metastasis. Biomarkers are increasingly utilized in the early clinical development for identification, for validation and better optimization of therapeutic targets and agents, for the determination of various mechanisms of pharmacodynamic properties for the prediction, and to monitor and also for the response to the treatment or resistance [30].

The response evaluation criteria in solid tumours (RECIST) and World Health Organization (WHO) criteria are being used for the evaluation of therapeutic response to cytotoxic chemotherapy regimens [31, 32]. The anatomical criteria are being used for the evaluation of the response to the treatment. The use of cytotoxic drugs demonstrates various imaging protocols for the novel signal transduction inhibitors (STIs) which will be exhibiting cytotoxic properties. For better evaluation it is not only the anatomical tumour evaluation but also the important and novel and physiological imaging points will be informative to estimate early therapy response and/or resistance development.

15.8 Cytotoxic and Cytostatic Anticancer Agents

The use of the various cytotoxic anticancer agents for the treatment of solid tumours along with the various neo-adjuvant and adjuvant therapies in the palliative care can be evaluated. The basic mechanism of action for the chemotherapeutic agents is the destruction of cell proliferation.

15.9 DNA Synthesis and Cell Division

These will have an important effect on cell death by either apoptosis or necrosis [33, 34]. Various factors of tumour growth, angiogenesis, invasion, and metastasis will be regulated by various growth factors by their receptor tyrosine kinases. The suppression of the inhibition of these signalling pathways which are being used for the therapeutic approach is recently used [35, 36]. Various novel targeted agents will be a signal transduction inhibitor (STIs) along with various anti-growth factor antibodies, anti-receptor monoclonal antibodies, antisense, and small molecule tyrosine kinase inhibitors [35, 37]. Some of them will be there for the introduction of imatinib and many modulators and kinases [38, 39]. The major problem here is the development of resistance to various targets [40]. Metastatic breast disease with containing trastuzumab will experience disease progression and the effectiveness of salvage therapy by 10% [39, 41]. Even in this modern era, once the resistance to the anticancer drugs emerges, it will be difficult to salvage the various aspects of the functional imaging to identify the effectiveness of the therapy response. The use of targeted imaging will help for the development of the translational and clinical drug development [30].

Functional and molecular imaging—especially MRI and PET role is to evaluate the response to the therapy. As already mentioned, the role of the morphological assessment of cytotoxic treatment by the RECIST and WHO criteria is being commonly used for the evaluation of antitumour cytotoxic therapies; these can be done on some of the parameters of measurement so the particular lesions like size and number of primary as well as the secondary lesions [31, 32, 42, 43]. Other criteria's of the diffusion-weighted (DW) MRI is to access the various parameters due to the impact by the chemotherapeutic agents and along with the anti-angiogenic regimens. The principle of the DW-MRI is based on the motion of water molecules in the tissue which are detected due to the additional changes in various physical properties when there is the mobility of the agents [44]. DW-MRI is very sensitive for the detection and changes in various dynamics in cell membranes. The tumours will be having significant increased cellularity as well as water diffusion due to the increased proliferation and cell density in tumours. Tumour cellularity is also evaluated by the apparent diffusion coefficients (ADCs) from malignant areas to the ADCs of normal tissues [45, 46]. There will be significant increase in the ADC values based on the increase in proton diffusion and decreased cellularity or necrosis development [47–49]. Thus, tumour T1 relaxation times will be correlating with hypocellularity and necrosis and also the quantitative imaging parameter for the identification of various cytotoxic agents [50].

The imaging of the anti-angiogenic treatment will show the microvasculature of tumours, as compared to the normal tissue, which are structurally and functionally abnormal, tortuous, and poorly organized, making the vessels "leaky" [51, 52]. Dynamic contrast-enhanced (DCE) MRI is being now widely used for the evaluation of vascular properties [14, 53]. Fast T1-weighted dynamic MRI is taken before, during, and after gadolinium contrast injection. The concept here is that the hypoxic tumours are resistant to radiation and chemotherapy. The heterogeneous tumour blood flow may affect the efficacy of systemic chemotherapeutics; methods for assessing tumour blood flow and tumour perfusion will be the identification factors of the hypoxia, and this can be used for the more precise prediction of the response to treatment or require another alternative therapeutic approach [54, 55]. By increasing the use of anti-angiogenic agents, which will reduce the significant tumour volume, DCE-MRI is an alternative quantitative method for the monitoring and for the evaluation for therapeutic response [5, 56–59]. DCE-MRI uses tumour microvasculature enhancement in T1-weighted images; due to this it is being widely used for in vivo staging of tumours and therapy response. And this can be correlated with the microvasculature with pathology, therapeutic response, and prognosis [60]. Many preclinical and clinical trials are showing the significant use of the DCE-MRI for earlier evaluation as early as 2 weeks of treatment, before tumour regression [5, 58, 61, 62]. Quantitative contrast-enhanced (CE) CT like DCE is also based on various contrast enhancement patterns after injection of iodine-based contrast which can be performed [63]. For the potential toxicity of various contrast agents, the CECT is not routinely used [64].

The earlier early evaluation of the ultrasound by the use of microbubbles is showing remarkable results in gastrointestinal stromal tumours (GISTs) and renal tumours. It used in the significant reduction in the contrast for the evaluation [65]. The response criteria are seen as significant change in the progression-free survival [66–68]. Qualitative analysis by the ultrasound has been there in clinical practice for very long. And it is used in the evaluation of the neovascularity in primary tumours like the prostate cancers [69, 70]. Now the second-generation contrast agents along with the perfusion software are being used [71, 72]. The microbubbles' contrast agents will be using the contrast by ultrasound probe [73, 74]. This availability of data is seen for the actual perfusion of the tumours, various parameters for the characterizing the perfusion agents which will be used for the quantitative analysis.

15.10 Metabolic Response to Anticancer Agents

This is the important aspect for the tumour biochemistry and physiology for the in vivo evaluation in PET where the malignancies will show the significantly increased glucose uptake and glycolytic metabolism. The common and mostly use radiotracer is the 18FDG, which is a marker for hexokinase activity. Here the glucose dependence in various malignancies describes the overexpression of glucose transporters along with various key enzymes of glycolytic pathways, like hexokinase, pyruvate kinase, and phosphofructokinase. FDG when trapped inside the cell cannot be metabolized by glucose-6-phosphate isomerase [75], and thus it will be accumulated in cancer cells having very high expression and activity of GLUT-1. FDG-PET is also used for the monitoring response to the therapy [76]. The quantitative changes in tumour ideally are seen in 2–3 weeks post-therapy which will correlate with tumour response and ultimately the patient survival [77–79]. FDG uptake quantification for therapy assessment is seen in the head and neck carcinoma, lymphoma, breast, lung, and colorectal cancers [21, 80–83]. Normal PET is with no abnormal FDG uptake, and partial response shows the significant reduction in the FDG uptake. Decrease of SUV (standard uptake values) of the primary tumour of at least 20% suggests the response to the therapy. This also includes radiation and chemotherapy and also includes various factors for tumour response to the FDG uptake. For the majority of tumours, metabolic PET was superior to CT in radiotherapy planning and assessment of therapy response [84]. Several studies have indicated that in response to tumours. The FDG uptake is significantly reduced in the first chemotherapy cycle or after 14 days of treatment [82, 83, 85, 86]. Gastric cancers show the histopathological response in majority along with the various favourable prognosis, whereas metabolic non-responders have a poor prognosis and showed histopathologic response in only 17% [87]. Some of the favourable responses is seen in the use of imatinib in gastrointestinal stromal tumour (GIST) even in the first hours after treatment begins and can be used to adjust a patient's daily dose [88].

References

1. Cohrs RJ, Martin T, Ghahramani P, Bidaut L, Higgins PJ, Shahzad A. Translational medicine definition by the European Society for Translational Medicine. New Horiz Transl Med. 2015;2:86–8. https://doi.org/10.1016/j.nhtm.2014.12.002.
2. Rubio DM, Schoenbaum EE, Lee LS, Schteingart DE, Marantz PR, Anderson KE, Platt LD, Baez A, Esposito K. Defining translational research: implications for training. Acad Med. 2010;85:470–5. https://doi.org/10.1097/ACM.0b013e3181ccd618.
3. De Jong M, Maina T. Of mice and humans: are they the same?—implications in cancer translational research. J Nucl Med. 2010;51:501–4. https://doi.org/10.2967/jnumed.109.065706.
4. Gambhir SS. Molecular imaging of cancer with positron emission tomography. Nat Rev Cancer. 2002;2:683–93. [PubMed: 12209157]
5. Spratlin JL, Cohen RB, Eadens M, et al. Phase I pharmacologic and biologic study of Ramucirumab (IMC-1121B), a fully human immunoglobulin G1 monoclonal antibody targeting the vascular endothelial growth factor receptor-2. J Clin Oncol. 2010;28:780–7. [PubMed: 20048182]
6. Nayak TK, Garmestani K, Milenic DR, et al. HER1-targeted Y-panitumumab possesses superior targeting characteristics than Y-cetuximab for PET imaging of human malignant mesothelioma tumors xenografts. PLoS One. 2011;6:e18198. [PubMed: 21464917]
7. Mileshkin L, Hicks RJ, Hughes BG, et al. Changes in FDG- and FLT-PET imaging in patients with non-small cell lung cancer treated with erlotinib. Clin Cancer Res. 2011. [Epub ahead of print]; https://doi.org/10.1158/1078-0432.CCR-10-2763.
8. Zander T, Scheffler M, Nogova L, et al. Early prediction of non-progression in advanced non-small-cell lung cancer treated with erlotinib by using 18F-fluorodeoxyglucose and 18F-fluorothymidine positron emission tomography. J Clin Oncol. 2011. [Epub ahead of print]; https://doi.org/10.1200/JCO.2010.32.4939.
9. Pope WB, Young JR, Ellingson BM. Advances in MRI assessment of gliomas and response to antiVEGF therapy. Curr Neurol Neurosci Rep. 2011;11:336–44. [PubMed: 21234719]
10. Krause BJ, Souvatzoglou M, Treiber U. Imaging of prostate cancer with PET/CT and radioactively labelled choline derivates. Urol Oncol. 2011. [Epub ahead of print]; https://doi.org/10.1016/j.urolonc.2010.08.008.
11. Tidwell AS, Jones JC. Advanced imaging concepts: a pictorial glossary of CT and MRI technology. Clin

Tech Small Anim Pract. 1999;14:65–111. [PubMed: 10361360]
12. Lauterbur PC. Nobel lecture: all science is interdisciplinary—from magnetic moments to molecules to men. Biosci Rep. 2004;24:165–78. [PubMed: 16209126]
13. Mansfield P. Snapshot magnetic resonance imaging (Nobel lecture). Angew Chem Int Ed Engl. 2004;43:5456–64. [PubMed: 15384128]
14. Hylton N. Dynamic contrast-enhanced magnetic resonance imaging as an imaging biomarker. J Clin Oncol. 2006;24:3293–8. [PubMed: 16829653]
15. Serkova NJ, Renner B, Larsen BA, Stoldt CR, Hasebroock KM, Bradshaw-Pierce EL, Holers VM, Thurman JM. Renal inflammation: targeted iron oxide nanoparticles for molecular MR imaging in mice. Radiology. 2010;255:517–26. [PubMed: 20332377]
16. Gillies RJ, Morse DL. In vivo magnetic resonance spectroscopy in cancer. Annu Rev Biomed Eng. 2005;7:287–326. [PubMed: 16004573]
17. Leach MO. Magnetic resonance spectroscopy (MRS) in the investigation of cancer at The Royal Marsden Hospital and The Institute of Cancer Research. Phys Med Biol. 2006;51:R61–82. [PubMed: 16790921]
18. Deppe MH, Parra-Robles J, Ajraou S, Wild JM. Combined measurement of pulmonary inert gas washout and regional ventilation heterogeneity by MR of a single dose of hyperpolarized 3He. Magn Reson Med. 2011;65:1075–83. [PubMed: 21413071]
19. Kurhanewicz J, Vigneron DB, Brindle K, Chekmenev EY, Comment A, Cunningham CH. Analysis of cancer metabolism by imaging hyperpolarized nuclei: prospects for transition to clinical research. Neoplasia. 2011;13:81–97. [PubMed: 21403835]
20. Vaughan CL, Mayosi BM. Origins of computed tomography. Lancet. 2007;369:1168. [PubMed: 17416259]
21. Kapoor V, Fukui MB, McCook BM. Role of 18FFDG PET/CT in the treatment of head and neck cancers: principles, technique, normal distribution, and initial staging. AJR Am J Roentgenol. 2005a;184:579–87. [PubMed: 15671384]
22. Fueger BJ, Czernin J, Hilderbrandt I, Tran C, Halpern BS, Stout D, Phelps ME, Weber WA. Impact of animal handling on the results of 18F-FDG-PET studies in mice. J Nucl Med. 2006;47:999–1006. [PubMed: 16741310]
23. Blodgett TM, Meltzer CC, Townsend DW. PET/CT: form and function. Radiology. 2007;242:360–85. [PubMed: 17255408]
24. Bolondi L, Correas JM, Lencioni R, Weskott HP, Piscaglia F. New perspectives for the use of contrast-enhanced liver ultrasound in clinical practice. Dig Liver Dis. 2007;39:187–95. [PubMed: 17208526]
25. Blomley MJ, Eckersley RJ. Functional ultrasound methods in oncologic imaging. Eur J Cancer. 2002;38:2108–15. [PubMed: 12387836]
26. Weissleder R, Ntziachristos V. Shedding light into live molecular targets. Nat Med. 2003;9:123–8. [PubMed: 12514725]
27. Hasebroock KM, Serkova NJ. Toxicity of MRI and CT contrast agents. Expert Opin Drug Metab Toxicol. 2009;5:403–16. [PubMed: 19368492]
28. Dobrucki L, de Muinck ED, Lindner JR, Sinusas AJ. Approaches to multimodality imaging of angiogenesis. J Nucl Med. 2010;51(Suppl):66S–79S.
29. Zhang X, Lin Y, Gillies RJ. Tumor pH and its measurement. J Nucl Med. 2010;51:1167–70. [PubMed: 20660380]
30. Evelhoch J, Garwood M, Vigneron D, Knopp M, Sullivan D, Menkens A, Clarke L, Liu G. Expanding the use of magnetic resonance in the assessment of tumor response to therapy: workshop report. Cancer Res. 2005;65:7041–4. [PubMed: 16103049]
31. Jaffe CC. Measures of response: RECIST, WHO, and new alternatives. J Clin Oncol. 2006;24:3245–51. [PubMed: 16829648]
32. Jaffe CC. Response assessment in clinical trials: implications for sarcoma clinical trial design. Oncologist. 2008;13:14–8. [PubMed: 18434633]
33. Kerbel RS, Kamen BA. The anti-angiogenic basis of metronomic chemotherapy. Nat Rev Cancer. 2004;4:423–36. [PubMed: 15170445]
34. Brunelle JK, Zhang B. Apoptosis assays for quantifying the bioactivity of anticancer drug products. Drug Resist Updat. 2010;13:172–9.
35. Levitzki A, Gazit A. Tyrosine kinase inhibition: an approach to drug development. Science. 1995;267:782–28. [PubMed: 17813884]
36. Hollande F, Pannequin J, Joubert D. The long road to colorectal cancer therapy: searching for the right signals. Drug Resist Updat. 2010;13:44–56.
37. Dancey J, Sausville EA. Issues and progress with protein kinase inhibitors for cancer treatment. Nat Rev Drug Discov. 2003;2:296–331. [PubMed: 12669029]
38. Dent P, Curiel DT, Fisher PB, Grant S. Synergistic combinations of signaling pathway inhibitors: mechanisms for improved cancer therapy. Drug Resist Updat. 2009;12:65–73.
39. Zhang S, Huang WC, Li P, Guo H, Poh SB, Brady SW, et al. Combating trastuzumab resistance by targeting SRC, a common node downstream of multiple resistance pathways. Nat Med Publ. 2011; https://doi.org/10.1038/nm.2309.
40. Broxterman HJ, Gotink KJ, Verheul HM. Understanding the causes of multidrug resistance in cancer: a comparison of doxorubicin and sunitinib. Drug Resist Updat. 2009;12:114–26.
41. Nahta R, Esteva RJ. Trastuzumab: triumphs and tribulations. Oncogene. 2007;26:3637–43. [PubMed: 17530017]
42. Eisenhauer EA, Therasse P, Bogaerts J, Schwartz LH, Sargent D, Ford R, et al. New response evaluation criteria in solid tumours: revised RECIST guideline (version 1.1). Eur J Cancer. 2009;45:228–47. [PubMed: 19097774]
43. Ramasamy K, Nield L, Serkova NJ, Hasebroock KM, Tyagi A, Raina K, et al. Silibinin prevents lung tumorigenesis in wild-type but not in iNOS-/- mice: potential of real-time microCT in lung cancer chemo-

prevention studies. Clin Cancer Res. 2011;17:753–61. [PubMed: 21148748]
44. Koh DM, Collins DJ. Diffusion-weighted MRI in the body: application and challenges in oncology. Am J Roentgenol. 2007;188:622–35. [PubMed: 17312045]
45. Desouza NM, Reinsberg SA, Scurr ED, Brewster JM, Payne GS. Magnetic resonance imaging in prostate cancer: the value of apparent diffusion coefficient for identifying malignant nodules. Br J Radiol. 2007;80:90–5. [PubMed: 17303616]
46. Reinsberg SA, Payne GS, Riches SF, et al. Combined use of diffusion-weighted MRI and 1H-MR spectroscopy to increase accuracy in prostate cancer detection. Am J Roentgenol. 2007;188:91–8. [PubMed: 17179350]
47. Padhani AR, Liu G, Koh DM, et al. Diffusion-weighted magnetic resonance imaging as a cancer biomarker: consensus and recommendations. Neoplasia. 2009;11:102–25. [PubMed: 19186405]
48. Rozel S, Galban CJ, Nicolay K, et al. Synergy between anti-CCL2 and docetaxel as determine by DWMRI in a metastatic bone cancer model. J Cell Biochem. 2009;107:58–64. [PubMed: 19259948]
49. Thoeny HC, Ross BD. Predicting and monitoring treatment response with diffusion-weighted MRI. J Magn Reson Imaging. 2010;32:2–16. [PubMed: 20575076]
50. McSheehy PMJ, Weidensteiner C, Cannet C, et al. Quantified tumor T1 is a generic early-response imaging biomarker for chemotherapy reflecting cell viability. Clin Cancer Res. 2009;16:212–25. [PubMed: 20008843]
51. Jain RK. Molecular regulation of vessel maturation. Nat Med. 2003;9:685–93. [PubMed: 12778167]
52. Folkman J. What is the evidence that tumors are angiogenesis dependent? J Natl Cancer Inst. 1990;82:4–6. [PubMed: 1688381]
53. Thomassin-Naggara I, Bazot M, Darai E, et al. Epithelial ovarian tumors: values of dynamic contrast-enhanced MR imaging and correlation with tumor angiogenesis. Radiology. 2008;248:148–59. [PubMed: 18458244]
54. Semple SIK, Staff RT, Heys SD, et al. Baseline MRI delivery characteristics predict change in invasive ductal breast carcinoma PET metabolism as a result of primary chemotherapy administration. Ann Oncol. 2006;17:1393–8. [PubMed: 16788001]
55. Zahara MA, Hollingsworth KG, Sala E, Lomas DJ, Tan LT. Dynamic contrast-enhanced MRI as a predictor of tumor response to radiotherapy. Lancet Oncol. 2007;8:63–74. [PubMed: 17196512]
56. Robinson SP, McIntyre DJO, Checkley D, et al. Tumor dose response to the antivascular agent ZD6126 assessed by magnetic resonance imaging. Br J Cancer. 2003;88:1592–7. [PubMed: 12771928]
57. Marzola P, Degrassi A, Calderan L, et al. In vivo assessment of antiangiogenic activity of SU6668 in an experimental colon carcinoma model. Clin Cancer Res. 2004;10:739–50. [PubMed: 14760097]
58. Troiani T, Serkova NJ, Gustafson DL, et al. Investigation of two dosing schedules of Vandetanib (ZD6474), an inhibitor of VEGFR and EGFR signaling, in combination with Irinotecan in a human colon cancer xenograft model. Clin Cancer Res. 2007;13:6450–8. [PubMed: 17975157]
59. Moasser MM, Wilmes LJ, Wong CH, et al. Improved vascular function following high-dose epidermal growth factor receptor tyrosine kinase inhibitor therapy. J Magn Reson Imaging. 2007;26:1618–25.
60. Leach MO, Brindle KM, Evelhoch JL, et al. The assessment of antiangiogenic and antivascular therapies in early-stage clinical trials using magnetic resonance imaging: issues and recommendations. Br J Cancer. 2005;92:1599–610. [PubMed: 15870830]
61. Morgan B, Thomas AL, Drevs J, et al. Dynamic contrast-enhanced magnetic resonance imaging as a biomarker for the pharmacological response of PTK787/ZK 222584, an inhibitor of the vascular endothelial growth factor receptor tyrosine kinases, in patients with advanced colorectal cancer and liver metastases: results from two phase I studies. J Clin Oncol. 2003;21(21):3955–64.
62. Liu G, Rugo HS, Wilding G, et al. Dynamic contrast-enhanced magnetic resonance imaging as a pharmacodynamic measure of response after acute dosing of AG-013736, an oral angiogenesis inhibitor, in patients with advanced solid tumors: results from a phase I study. J Clin Oncol. 2005;23:5464–73. [PubMed: 16027440]
63. Miles KA, Young H, Chica SL, Esser PD. Quantitative contrast-enhanced computed tomography: is there a need for system calibration? Eur Radiol. 2007;17:919–26. [PubMed: 17008987]
64. Bisdas S, Medov L, Baghi M, et al. A comparison of tumor perfusion assessed by deconvolution-based analysis of dynamic contrast-enhanced CT and MR imaging in patients with squamous cell carcinoma of the upper aerodigestive tract. Eur Radiol. 2008;18:843–50. [PubMed: 18175123]
65. Lassau N, Lamuraglia M, Chami L, Leclere J, Bonvalot S, Terrier P, Roche A, Le Cesne A. Gastrointestinal stromal tumors treated with imatinib: monitoring response with contrast-enhanced sonography. Am J Roentgenol. 2006;187:1267–73. [PubMed: 17056915]
66. Lamuraglia M, Escudier B, Vhami L, Schwartz B, Leclere J, Roche A, Lassau N. To predict progression-free survival and overall survival in metastatic renal cancer treated with sorafenib: pilot study using contrast-enhanced Doppler ultrasound. Eur J Cancer. 2006;42:2472–9. [PubMed: 16965911]
67. Escudier B, Lassau N, Angevin E, Soria JC, Chami L, Lamuraglia M, et al. Phase I trial of sorafenib in combination with IFN aplha-2a in patients with unresectable and/or metastatic renal cell carcinoma or malignant melanoma. Clin Cancer Res. 2007;13:1801–9. [PubMed: 17363536]

68. Lassau N, Chami L, Benatsou B, Peronneau P, Roche A. Dynamic contrast-enhanced ultrasonography (DCE-US) with quantification of tumor perfusion: a new diagnostic tool to evaluate the early effects of antiangiogenic treatment. Eur Radiol Suppl. 2007;17:F89–98.
69. Halpern E. Contrast-enhanced ultrasound imaging of prostate cancer. Rev Urol. 2006;8:S29–37. [PubMed: 17021624]
70. Padhani AR, Harvey CJ, Cosgrove DO. Angiogenesis imaging in the management of prostate cancer. Nat Clin Pract Urol. 2005;2:596–607. [PubMed: 16474547]
71. Greenbaum L, Burns P, Copel J, et al. American Institute of Ultrasound in Medicine recommendations for contrast-enhanced liver ultrasound imaging clinical trials. J Ultrasound Med. 2007;26:705–16. [PubMed: 17526602]
72. Turnbull LW. Dynamic contrast-enhanced MRI in the diagnosis and management of breast cancer. NMR Biomed. 2009;22:28–39. [PubMed: 18654999]
73. Wilson SR, Greenbaum LD, Goldberg BB. Contrast-enhanced ultrasound: what is the evidence and what are the obstacles? Am J Roentgenol. 2009;193:55–60.
74. Wilson SR, Burns PN. Microbubble-enhanced US in body imaging: what role? Radiology. 2010;257:24–39. [PubMed: 20851938]
75. Gambhir SS, Czernin J, Schwimmer J, et al. A tabulated summary of the FDG-PET literature. J Nucl Med. 2001;42:1S–93S. [PubMed: 11483694]
76. Shanka LK, Hoffman JM, Bacharach S, et al. Consensus recommendations for use of 18F-FDG PET as an indicator of therapeutic response in patients in National Cancer Institute trials. J Nucl Med. 2006;47:1059–66. [PubMed: 16741317]
77. Weber WA. Use of PET for monitoring cancer therapy and for predicting outcome. J Nucl Med. 2005;46:983–95. [PubMed: 15937310]
78. Weber W, Figlin R. Monitoring cancer treatment with PET/CT: does it make a difference? J Nucl Med. 2007;48:36S–44S. [PubMed: 17204719]
79. Castell F, Cook GJ. Quantitative techniques in 18FDG-PET scanning in oncology. Br J Cancer. 2008;98:597–60.
80. Kostakoglu L, Goldsmith SJ. PET in the assessment of therapy response in patients with sarcoma of the head and neck and of the esophagus. J Nucl Med. 2004;45:56–68. [PubMed: 14734674]
81. Kapoor V, Fukui MB, McCook BM. Role of 18FDG PET/CT in the treatment of head and neck cancers: posttherapy evaluation and pitfalls. AJR Am J Roentgenol. 2005b;184:589–97. [PubMed: 15671385]
82. Evilevitch V, Weber WA, Tap WD, et al. Reduction in glucose metabolic activity is more accurate than change in size at predicting histopathologic response to neoadjuvant therapy in high-grade soft-tissue sarcomas. Clin Cancer Res. 2008;14:715–20. [PubMed: 18245531]
83. Leibold T, Akhurst TJ, Chessin DB, et al. Evaluation of 18F-FDG-PET for early detection of suboptimal response of rectal cancer to perioperative chemoradiotherapy: a prospective analysis. Ann Surg Oncol. 2011. [Epub ahead of print]; https://doi.org/10.1245/s10434-011-1634-2.
84. Gregoire V, Haustermans K, Geets X, Roels S, Lonneux M. PET-based treatment planning in radiotherapy: a new standard? J Nucl Med. 2007;48:68S–77S. [PubMed: 17204722]
85. Kostakoglu L, Goldsmith SJ, Leonard JP, et al. FDG-PET after cycle 1 of therapy predicts outcome in diffuse large cell lymphoma and classic Hodgkin disease. Cancer. 2006;107:2678–87. [PubMed: 17063502]
86. Lippert TH, Ruoff HJ, Volm M. Current status of methods to assess cancer drug resistance. Int J Med Sci. 2011;23:245–53. [PubMed: 21487568]
87. Ott K, Herrmann K, Lordick F, et al. Early metabolic response evaluation by fluorine-18 fluorodeoxyglucose positron emission tomography allows in vivo testing of chemosensitivity in gastric cancer: long-term results of a prospective study. Clin Cancer Res. 2008;14:2012–8. [PubMed: 18381939]
88. Hughes B, Yip D, Goldstein D, et al. Cerebral relapse of metastatic gastrointestinal stromal tumor during treatment with imatinib mesylate: case report. BMC Cancer. 2004;4:1–7. [PubMed: 14725718]

16 Multiparametric Imaging

Key Points (Abstract)

Multiparametric magnetic resonance imaging (mp-MRI) is the newer concept of MR which is evolving and being used widely for various applications. This will be more helpful for more precise diagnosis and localization of the lesions, risk stratification, and staging of clinically significant cancers like prostate cancer. With this the newer options of the local management of the prostate cancer are being explored and used. Various combinations of T2-weighted imaging, diffusion imaging, perfusion, and spectroscopic and functional imaging are being used widely in mp-MRI assessment of prostate cancer. The basic sequence T2 for the anatomic assessment and newer functional evaluation by the diffusion-weighted sequences is important for the prostate cancer diagnosis on mp-MRI. One of the drawbacks here that (this is still to be validated) there are subjective possibilities which are not uniform. For this the Prostate Imaging and Reporting Archiving Data System PI-RADS scoring system is being established and used for the accurate diagnosis.

Keywords

mp-MRI · DWI · DCE · MRS · T2

16.1 Introduction

Multiparametric magnetic resonance imaging (mp-MRI), where there will be the combination of the T2-weighted imaging (T2WI) for the morphological assessment along with the diffusion-weighted imaging (DWI) and use of the dynamic contrast-enhanced (DCE) perfusion imaging and spectroscopic imaging (MRSI) are already in use [1–6]. In this the potential of the T2WI and DWI is very important and is showing excellent results for the detection, localization, risk stratification, and staging of prostate cancer [7–10].

The most commonly recommended technique in prostate cancer mp-MRI is the high-resolution T2WI along with this at least two functional MRI techniques [11]. We all know the limitation of the T1-wegithed sequence for the assessment of the prostatic morphology or identifying tumour within the gland. The important use of the T1-weighted sequence is for the evaluation of the haemorrhage in post-biopsy scenarios. Another fallacies are bowel peristalsis where bowel motion artefacts have to be minimized by the administering of the anti-peristaltic agents. At 3T benefits as there will be higher signal-to-noise ratio this will be more beneficial for prostate imaging. The endorectal coil (ERC) will be more advantageous and will give better results, but still

S. Shaikh, *Advances in Imaging*, https://doi.org/10.1007/978-981-16-9535-3_16

it is not an absolute requirement for cancer detection protocol. 1.5T [12] ERC is more recommended for staging purposes. ERC balloon has to be inflated with air, but again this air will be the cause of distortion in DWI. For this the use of liquids like the perfluorocarbon or barium suspension can limit these artefacts. Around 60 cc of air or fluid is needed for the distension of the balloon.

16.2 T2 Sequence

T2WI is one of the most important sequence of prostate MRI which is having very high spatial resolution. Due to this T2W sequence the evaluation of the zonal anatomy as well as differentiation of the different zones of the prostate, ejaculatory ducts, anterior fibromuscular stroma, seminal vesicles and the urethra can be done more precisely [13]. The differentiation of the neurovascular bundle can also be done very clearly. Due to higher amount of water content in the peripheral zone, it will be showing higher signal intensity on T2WI. The same principle is also used for the evaluation of cancer which appears as a lower-signal area. But this low T2 signal in the peripheral zone is common in prostatitis, fibrosis, scar tissue, post-biopsy haemorrhage, or postirradiation.

The associated multiple nodules with BPH (benign prostate hyperplasia or benign enlargement of the prostate) will be more difficult for the evaluation of various zones especially the transition zone, and this will be a little difficult to evaluate the difference with prostatic cancers due to their heterogenicity [14]. The role of functional imaging for the transition zone tumour versus benign stromal or proliferating hyperplasia will be difficult as both will show heterogenous enhancement on DCE with restricted diffusion on DWI [15, 16]. One of the features is the "erased charcoal" appearance which will be seen due to ill-defined margins of the nodule, presentation of low signal into peripheral zone, lenticular shape, and local infiltration into the fibromuscular stroma, few of the criteria to differentiate tumour from benign tissue. But the BPH nodules are sometimes not clearly demarcated or encapsulated, so the clear demarcation is not possible with mp-MRI. T2WI is an important sequence of all the mp-MRI sequences for detection of cancer especially in the transition zone. But again, the degree of intensity which will be decreasing on T2WI in the peripheral zone is also being correlated with Gleason grade of tumour. The Gleason score will be based on lower-signal intensities on T2WI which will be playing an important role for risk evaluation of the tumour [17]. The bigger advantage of this sequence is the high spatial resolution of T2WI making it an important sequence for the local staging of disease [18]. The local infiltration in the form of the low signal intensity involving the adjacent seminal vesicles, recto-prostatic angle involvement, and also the neurovascular bundle involvement are all signs of extracapsular extension (ECE) of tumour on T2WI.

16.3 DWI Sequence

Diffusion-weighted MRI is a functional imaging sequence which is based on random Brownian motion of water molecules in tissue. The apparent diffusion coefficient (ADC) on MRI in which the molecules will be displaced shows the restricted diffusion.

And this is quantified by the two sets of the images in different fields of the magnet.

Two b factors are needed for the calculation of ADC. The multipoint b-value analyses will be showing increased accuracy of the calculated ADC, but there will be increased scan time and decreased in signal-to-noise ratio (SNR). The previous studies show the use of maximal b-value of 1000 s/mm^2, but in 3T MR this can be increased to 2000 s/mm^2, which can be obtained on 3T scanners. By suppressing the signal of the normal prostate tissue, the cancerous areas can be better seen hyperintense [19].

High b-values >1000 s/mm^2 DWI can be used along with the ADC, and the low ADC is one of the characteristic features of the cancer and having high b-value DWI images ($\geq$1400 s/mm^2). If higher b-values are there, DWI includes increased noise and anatomic distortion of the image.

More and more research is going on the inverse correlation between quantitative ADC values and Gleason score, and based on this the risk stratification for selection and also for the therapeutic options is more accurate [7, 20, 21]. But, there is significant overlap in confidence intervals that most of the clinical cases will be having ADC value of <1000 [14, 22].

DWI is a now more commonly used technique of the functional imaging sequence in mp-MRI.

Functional imaging components like DWI, DCE, and magnetic resonance spectroscopic imaging [MRSI] can easily be able to diagnose and differentiate the specific pathologies. DWI is helpful for the differentiation of cancer from benign conditions like prostatitis, fibrosis, scar tissue, post-biopsy haemorrhage, or postirradiation in the peripheral zone; due to this the identification of the DWI is more sensitive to the tumours in the peripheral zone [23]. Along with this it also has more sensitivity for tumour detection in the transition zone. Various multiple studies as being labelled with the mp-MRI are being done for the evaluation of the detected prostate cancer, thereby improving the diagnostic performance of mp-MRI [24–28].

DCE-MRI is the one of the commonest fast T1-weighted sequences before, during, and after rapid intravenous (IV) administration (2–4 mL/s) of gadolinium-based contrast agent to assess and also for monitoring tumour angiogenesis. This tumour is diagnosed early and also has high-amplitude enhancement with the rapid washout as compared to the normal tissue.

DCE-MRI images can be evaluated by simple visual analysis. These data will be via scrolling for the obtained images or on subtraction images and also for the early nodular and focal enhancement. Various parameters like upslope gradient, peak enhancement, and washout gradient can be calculated for the generation of the slope curve (Types A, B, and C) for assessment. Quantitative metric assessment may also be performed using pharmacokinetic (Tofts) models to estimate contrast concentration within the tissue. The microvascular permeability and blood flow, V_e, and the extracellular-extravascular compartment volume fraction or leakage can be analysed [29]. Visual analysis of images or semi-quantitative assessment of enhancement curve are being used for the various types and also seen as the image inter and also for the image interpretation. The assessment for the response to therapy can be done easily even when there are no morphological appearances.

There are many times and conditions where there is the overlap of the findings like the enhancement pattern in benign conditions like prostatitis which is seen in the peripheral zone and also in the benign nodules in the transition zone; DCE-MRI is not the important sequence for the assessment of cancer, in all the zones, and is seen as the complimentary sequence to T2WI and DWI in mp-MRI. DCE is helpful in cases when the T2WI/DWI imaging is equivocal and also when other sequences are suboptimal due to image distortion on DWI.

There is also the poor correlation of the DCE-MRI parameters with Gleason grade.

DCE-MRI is more sensitive for the detection of the residual/recurrent tumour post-therapy.

DCE-MRI in the post-treatment scenario generally doesn't give any information, but in the case of the prostatectomy, this sequence can be useful to evaluate the local recurrence [30].

MRSI of the prostate, the peak in the spectrum, is having the resonance from the protons in citrate (resonates at 2.6 ppm), creatine (resonates at 3.0 ppm), and the choline compounds (resonates at 3.2 ppm). Choline elevated and citrate reduction is seen in the malignant tissues. The choline and the creatine-to-citrate ratio is more precise for the malignancies. MRSI and MRI together will be giving more information of prostate cancer [31, 32]. Various MRSI studies are showing more sensitivity for cancer detection in cases of elevated PSA levels [33]. Even the malignant potential and the aggressiveness of the cancer can be seen better by the MRSI [34–36] also for the evaluation of the recurrence and monitoring therapy response [37, 38]. The only issue is the time which is around 10 min for the spectroscopic acquisition. Magnetic field distortions due to biopsy can be seen immediately after the procedure so comfortable time span lapse has to be there. MRSI is time-consuming in comparison with all other sequences. So, it is not done more often.

16.4 Accuracy of mp-MRI

As MRI has many sequences and all the sequences are relevant for particular applications. T2WI along with the two functional sequences is having better sensitivity for the evaluation of the tumours of the prostate [39–41]. In one of the studies, de Rooij et al. showed higher sensitivity and specificity of mp-MRI by using T2WI, DWI, and DCE-MRI. The combined pooled sensitivity and specificity were 0.74 and 0.88, respectively, negative predictive value (NPV) from 0.65 to 0.94 range [42]. mp-MRI has very good sensitivity and specificity in detecting as well as ruling out the cancer, having the NPV of 95% by using the transperineal biopsy [43]. These authors thus concluded that mp-MRI will act like the triage test when the biopsy is negative. One of the studies showed the NPV of mp-MRI at 89.6% for cancer in the follow-up of 5 years [44]. Shakir et al. showed the higher sensitivity of the MRI, and targeted biopsy increases when PSA levels are significantly increased with the increased chances of biopsy when the PSA level is 5.2 ng/mL [45].

The functional imaging is more precise for the evaluation in prostate cancer especially when it is in the peripheral zone [23, 28, 46], but in another way the functional imaging will have limited sensitivity in the transition zone lesions on mp-MRI due to the heterogenous appearance and also the pattern of the enhancement which will be secondary to benign prostatic hyperplasia. Hoeks et al. [47] showed that DCE-MRI does not have any advantage over the T2WI cancer detection in the transition zone. The accuracy of mp-MRI for detecting Gleason grades in the 4 and 5 in the transitional zones was 79% for T2WI and 72% when DWI and DCE-MRI are combined. In the low-risk disease, the accuracy levels were 66% for T2WI and 62% when combined with functional imaging. One study showed that DWI to T2WI showed more accuracy for the detection of the prostate cancer in the transition zone [48].

The tumour volume estimation is one of the prognostic factors, and the correct estimation will show the success in cases of the focal therapy [49]. With newer techniques, the focal therapy ablation is selectively done for the involved local tissue and sparing the adjacent tissues which are normal.

As we all know, the tumour will be affecting the quantitative MRI findings and is the major predictor of tumour visibility on mp-MRI [50, 51]. The tumour in combination with the normal tissue will appear like MRI-visible "dense" tumour. The greatest tumour volume on mp-MRI is determined by various individual sequences as accurate as that of the histology [52] and also in the larger tumours over 10 mm [53] and >0.5 cc [54] in volume than for small tumours [49].

Due to the larger variabilities in the MRI interpretation the MRI (Prostate Imaging and Reporting Archiving Data System [PI-RADS]) is there on the 1- to 5-point scale for the MRI interpretation and reporting [11]. The Likert scoring system is a more subjective form of evaluation. Despite of this there are many inter-observer variations seen in both PI-RADS and the Likert scoring systems [14]. The recent meta-analysis of 14 studies evaluating use of the PI-RADS scoring system for prostate cancer detection on mp-MRI showed good diagnostic accuracy [55]. PI-RADS scoring system is being used widely, and PI-RADS version 2 has recently been published [56].

mp-MRI in men with no previous biopsy with cost-effectiveness and the true value are studied in some group of populations. National Health Services in the United Kingdom showed that prostate MRI even in biopsy-naïve patients may be cost-effective [57]. De Rooij et al. [58] showed the quality of life and healthcare costs for the TRUS-guided biopsy, and the imaging-based MR-guided biopsies were performed.

16.5 mp-MRI in Biopsy-Naïve Patients

In one of the randomized trials showing the prospective study by Panebianco et al. [1], prostate cancer was detected in 215/570 (38%) patients in the TRUS biopsy. Of the 355/570 patients wherein the TRUS biopsy is negative, mp-MRI after the biopsy, which was showing doubtful focal lesion in 208 patients, 186 were positive on biopsy (i.e. 52% of patients after an initial negative biopsy). In another study, Haffner et al. showed the cancer detection rate of 54% in the systematic biopsy versus 63% in the MRI [59]. Various studies have shown the tumour detection more in the MRI as compared to the systematic biopsy, thus improving the biopsy results after the MR imaging for the diagnosis of cancer [59–62].

16.6 mp-MRI Following Biopsy

In a meta-analysis including 14 studies and 698 patients, the significant higher cancer detection rate was 37.5% (range 19.2–68.3%) in biopsy-negative patients [63]. The combined pooled sensitivity and specificity by site-by-site analysis were 57% and 90%, respectively. The positive predictive value of mp-MRI is in the range from 17 to 92. Hoeks et al. showed the cancer detection rate of 25% (108/438) in patients having at least negative biopsy at least once for increased PSA and mp-MRI- and MRI-guided in bore biopsy, with 87% of these cancers found to be clinically significant [64]. The positive predictive value was 41% (108/265) by patient analysis and 33% (123/368) by site analysis by mp-MRI. Similarly, Vourganti et al. showed the cancer detection rate of 37% (73/195) with suspicious mp-MRI but negative biopsy. Recently, Sonn et al. [65] detected cancer in 34% (36/105) of patients using MRI-TRUS fusion with the negative biopsy; of these 72% were clinically significant. The positive predictive value of mp-MRI for PI-RAD scores of 4 and 5 was 50% (24/48 patients).

16.7 Role of MRI in Active Surveillance

Various studies are there for the upgrading (range 17–72%) after the targeted biopsy in men having the low-risk disease on biopsy and increasing various treatment options [66]. Margel et al. reported that 32% of patients have higher risk for the disease after the mp-MRI targeted biopsy in a cohort of 60 active surveillance patients [67]. Turkbey et al. retrospectively studied 133 patients who underwent mp-MRI prior to radical prostatectomy. Mp-MRI sensitivity of 93%, positive predictive value of 57%, and overall accuracy of 92% improved the appropriate selection of therapeutic option (AS versus radical treatment) [68]. The absence of a visible lesion on mp-MRI with low-risk disease is showing the good prognostic indicator for men on as thus reducing the disease [69] (Fig. 16.1a–f).

16.8 mp-MRI in BREAST

Multiparametric breast MR imaging which will be showing the very high quantitative pharmacokinetic DCE-MR imaging models and also functional MR imaging techniques like diffusion-weighted imaging (DWI) and magnetic resonance spectroscopy (MRS), for the specific biological properties, with abnormal vessel permeability, cellularity, and chemical composition, can be used for the advanced MRI imaging techniques.

The high-quality breast MR imaging, with the multiparametric MR imaging acquisition, can be done. However, the MR imaging using the high-field (B0) magnet (1.5T) should be used covering the bilateral breasts and bilateral axillae. The use of the breast surface coils with the breast MR imaging application built-in body coil will give the signal-to-noise ratio (SNR) for high-quality breast imaging.

DCE-MR imaging acquisition along with the breast MR imaging protocols with the ACR Breast MRI Accreditation Program (BMRAP) shows the use of the multiphase T1-weighted acquisition for the clinical breast MR imaging. DCE-MR imaging protocols are using the higher spatial resolution with high temporal resolution in imaging with contrast uptake kinetics in the breast.

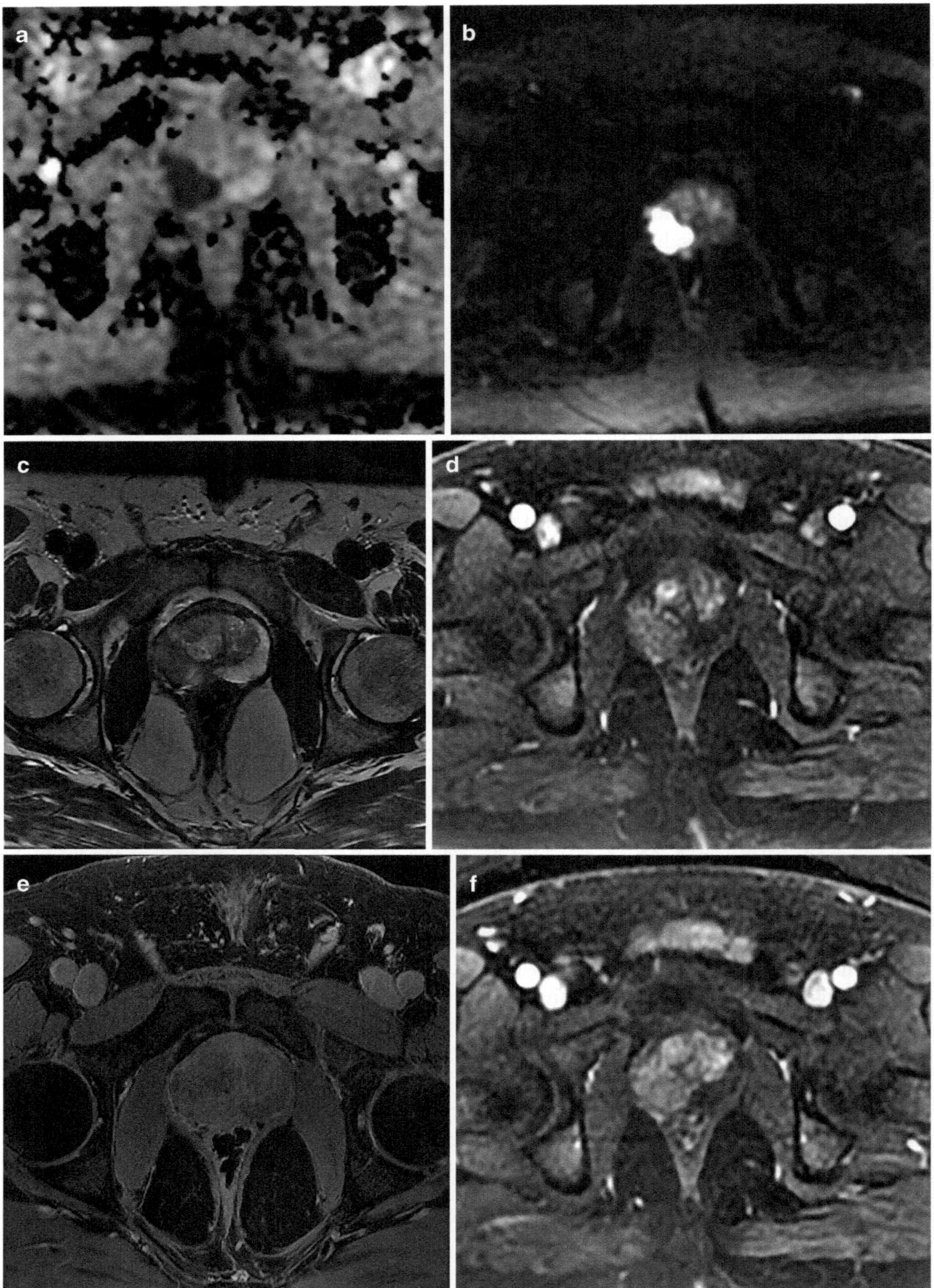

Fig. 16.1 (**a**–**f**) mp-MRI role by using the different parameters of the prostatic lesion imaging DWI, post-contrast different phase contrast images. This technique is more specific for the earlier and precise diagnosis of the prostatic lesions. Here the lesion is seen in the right lateral lobe of the prostate. Image courtesy: Dr. Amit Chaudhari, Assistant Professor, Department of Radiology, Tata Medical Hospital, Mumbai

16.9 Dynamic Contrast-Enhanced Kinetic Enhancement Features

The pattern of the enhancement of malignancies in the breast tissue is based on the concept of the neovascularization of the tumour cells for the growth. These abnormal vessels can be analysed and assessed by using various kinetic enhancement curves of DCE-MR imaging.

DWI will reduce the false-positive results and also the unnecessary biopsies widely used for breast imaging. Various studies had shown the restricted water diffusion in breast malignancies with significant differences in ADC values between the benign and malignant lesions [70–73].

The possibility of the spatial distortion and low resolution and one-to-one mapping of DCE-MR imaging and DWI features limit clinical implementation of breast DWI [74–77]. More information can be used by doing the breast DWI scans which includes the intravoxel incoherent motion (IVIM) modelling, giving the information about the perfusion status in addition to the diffusion [78–81]. The diffusion kurtosis modelling can be characterized due to the deviation at high b-values >1500 s/mm^2 accounting for tissue complexity and various physical barriers to diffusion in the tissue parenchyma.

MRS is a non-invasive technique based on the chemical composition of the tissue. MRS shows the signal spectrum, based on various structure and concentration of different chemical compounds in region of interest. MRS is very sensitive for the differentiation of tissue characteristics for normal, malignant, necrotic, or hypoxic, and the analysis can be based on the amount of the metabolites. Proton MRSs of the breast show the elevated levels of choline in malignant lesions when compared with the benign lesions and normal breast parenchyma [82–85]. The choline peak at approximately 3.2 ppm will be representing the different choline-containing compounds like the free choline, phosphocholine, and glycerophosphocholine, by in vivo methods [86] labelled as the total choline (tCho). Choline indicates the cell membrane turnover and is a marker of cell proliferation. Elevated choline in malignancies is due to the combination of both increased intracellular phosphocholine concentration and increased cell density in the lesion [86, 87].

Breast magnetic resonance spectroscopy increases the chances of various suspicious breast lesions on MR imaging. The hydrogen (1 H)-MRS of choline levels in suspicious breast lesions will provide very high specificity in benign versus malignant lesion differentiation [88–90]. The major limitation of breast MRS is low sensitivity for detecting choline levels in smaller lesions (Fig. 16.2).

In prostate cancer, ADC mapping and T2-weighted images show the increased cellularity with the loss of extracellular space/fluid. Different tissue components show different MR properties [91], and this is based on the Gleason score which will be correlating with the MR signal [92]. DCE-MR imaging in cancer patients shows early enhancement [23, 24]. The uptake is based on the contrast important for the tissue components [93]. Different MR biophysical properties of tissue will play an important role in the development of new imaging techniques to evaluate the tumour microenvironment [94].

The total combination of clinical findings, imaging features, pathological aspects, and the genomics data will further increase cancer diagnosis. Prostate-specific membrane antigen PSMA radiotracer is also more sensitive. PET combined with MR imaging has excellent soft-tissue contrast, with high spatial resolution for morphological imaging and functional and molecular information by PET [95], which will be more helpful in the diagnosis [96]. PSMA increases prostate cancer diagnosis as compared with FDG along with various other treatment options [97, 98]. Different new molecular markers like the Ki-67, hypoxia inducible factor-1a, and vascular endothelial growth factor are being used widely for multiparametric MR imaging helping for the better sensitivity for tumour proliferation, tumour hypoxia, and tumour angiogenesis [99]. Genetic profiling with the transcriptase polymerase chain reaction assay also is more precise for the evaluation of the multiparametric MR [100]. Other

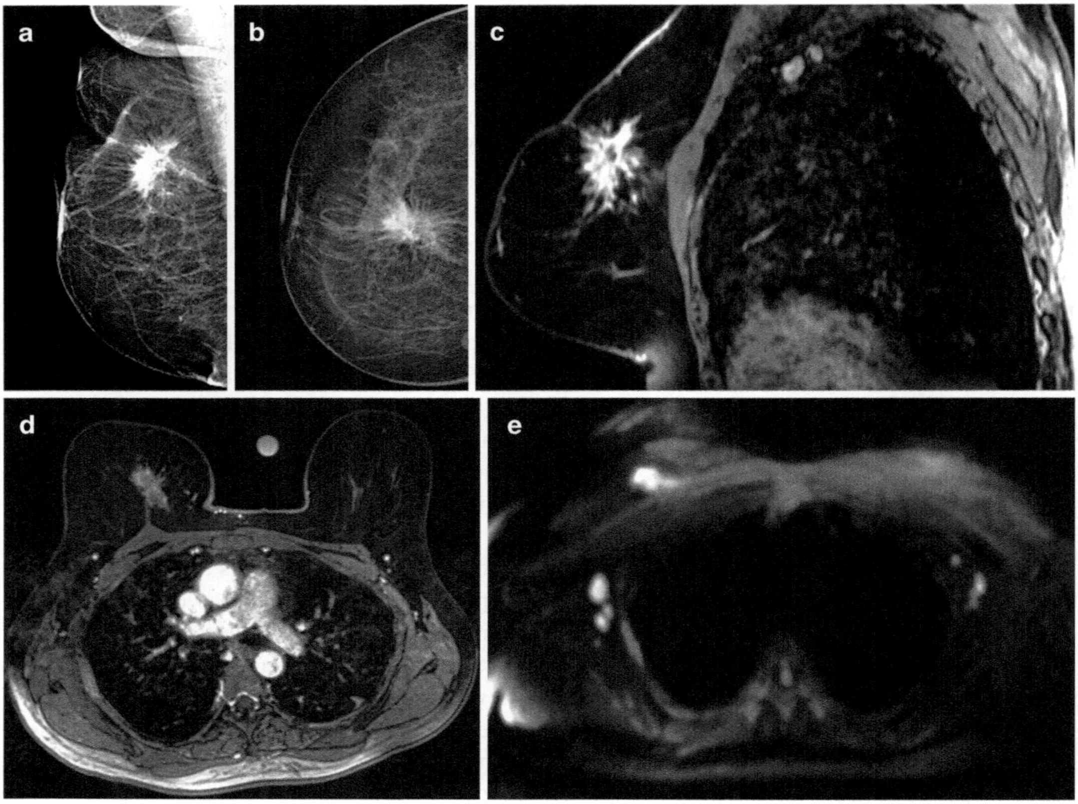

Fig. 16.2 More specific evaluation of the right breast lesion as seen in the mammographic image and compared with the pre- and post-contrast MRI image, delineating the tumour better. Image (**a**) and (**b**) are the Mammographic images showing spiculated lesion in right breast parenchyma. (**c, d**) and (**e**) MR images showing corresponding spiculated lesion which is clearly defined. Image courtesy: Dr. Amit Chaudhari, Assistant Professor, Department of Radiology, Tata Medical Hospital, Mumbai

genetic markers like phosphatase and tensin homolog gene are also more useful for the prostate cancer with excellent results.

Thus, by various data studies, multiparametric MRI (mp-MRI) is the established imaging technique for easy and precise diagnosis of prostate cancer [101] and cystic renal masses differentiation [102]. Newer concept of the urinary bladder cancer evaluation is by Vesical Imaging-Reporting and Data System (VI-RADS) score [103]. The urinary bladder cancer management is based on clinical T stage followed by transurethral resection of bladder tumour (TURBT) [104]. Based on the TURBT findings, the radical cystectomy or any other procedure shows very high morbidity [105–107]. Thus, mp-MRI to evaluate the sensitivity for TURBT is more precise. T2-weighted (T2W) MRI, diffusion-weighted imaging (DWI), and dynamic contrast enhancement (DCE) are important to confirm the infiltration of the surrounding muscle. Post-procedural bladder wall oedema has to be differentiated from the tumour infiltration. Ideally the MRI should be performed before or ≥2 weeks after TURBT or after intravesical instillation [108]. Post-procedural gas collection along with the antispasmodic agent for preventing artefacts from the bowel peristalsis is used [109]. Important is that the urinary bladder should be well distended before the MRI scan [110]. In the 1.5 T MR T2W, DWI, and DCE-MRI images are the routinely used sequences for mp-MRI. There is a field of view to include the entire urinary bladder, proximal urethra, pelvic region, and prostate if the patient is a male and in females genital organs uterus, ovaries, fallopian tubes, and vagina. The 5-point VI-RADS score is based on the structural category (SC), diffusion-weighted (DW) category, and contrast-enhanced (CE) category from T2W, DWI, and DCE-MRI to involvement of the various structures. In VI-RADS 1 score, muscle invasion is not there: SC, CE, and DW category 1.

In VI-RADS 2 score, muscle invasion is less likely present: SC, CE, and DW category 2, both CE and DW category 2 with SC category 3.

In VI-RADS 3 score, muscle invasion is equivocal: SC, CE, and DW category 3, or SC category 3 CE or DW category 3, the remaining sequence category 2.

In VI-RADS 4 score, muscle invasion is likely: at least SC and/or DW and CE category 4, the remaining category 3 or 4; SC category 3 plus DW and/or CE category 4; SC category 5 plus DW and or CE category 4.

In VI-RADS 5 score, invasion of muscle and beyond the bladder is very likely: at least SC plus DW and/or CE category 5, the remaining category 4 or 5.

Thus, the mp-MRI helps in differentiating the NMIBC from MIBC, and the ability of VI-RADS to discriminate NMIBC from MIBC is presented [103, 111–115]. NMIBC and MIBC are important for counselling patients with bladder cancer. mp-MRI will help reduce costs and complications.

The current guidelines TURBT in patients diagnosed with high-risk NMIBC or in cases of T1 bladder cancer without muscle in the specimen [104]. Del Giudice et al. [111] studied the VI-RADS system in diagnosing residual MIBC and showing the sensitivity, specificity, PPV, and NPV of 85%, 93.6%, 74.5%, and 96.6%, respectively.

16.10 mp-MRI in Cerebral Lesions

mp-MRI in the evaluation of brain tumours is there for the evaluation of the various parameters which are based on the cerebral blood flow (CBF), cellularity of the cells, mobility of the water, and different compositions of the biochemical elements which are known as markers. These biomarkers are capable for evaluation of various normal and abnormal biological processes along with various responses to the treatment as well as the interventions. The histopathology is the final diagnosis, but still the role of the various imaging biomarkers is being widely used in neuro-oncology. The various biomarkers are the cerebral blood volume (CBV), volume transfer of the plasma and extracellular extravascular space (Ktrans), cerebral blood flow, apparent diffusion coefficient (ADC), fractional anisotropy (FA), and metabolite analysis by MRS.

The role of rCBV is for the evaluation of the neoangiogenesis that is flow-related and the sequence which is being used in DSC-MR imaging; these sequences are T1-weighted steady-state dynamic contrast-enhanced (DCE) and perfusion DSC-MR imaging, using the T2-weighted sequence for the contrast difference. The Ktrans is there for the measurement of the neoangiogenesis depicting the permeability and is being done by the DCE-MR imaging. ADC is for the evaluation of the cellularity and is done by sequence DWI. The fractional anisotropy is for the white matter integrity and the sequence is the DTI. Choline will be depicting the cellular turnover by MR spectroscopy [116, 117].

The evaluation of the various lesions especially the primary brain tumour versus the metastatic lesions is to be differentiated. The metastases will be having higher permeability as compared to the GBM. The basis of the no blood-brain barrier (BBB) infiltration is seen in the metastases, while the GBM will be having the deranged or damaged BBB (Fig. 16.3a, b). The CBV which will be on the higher side will be seen as the hyperintense area around the enhancing component of a GBM; these are infiltrative neoplastic cells. The signal intensity recovery curve is greater in patients with GBM compared with metastasis.

The concept of the angiogenesis is based on vascular proliferation due to the tumoral growth. The various factors which are responsible are the vascular endothelial growth factor (VEGF) and vascular permeability factor (VPF) which will depict the various measurements of the angiogenesis, and these can be identified by DSC-MR imaging and DCE-MR imaging. The CBV and Ktrans are being derived by the perfusion and permeability imaging, which will be correlating with the factors like VEGF/VPF. The relative

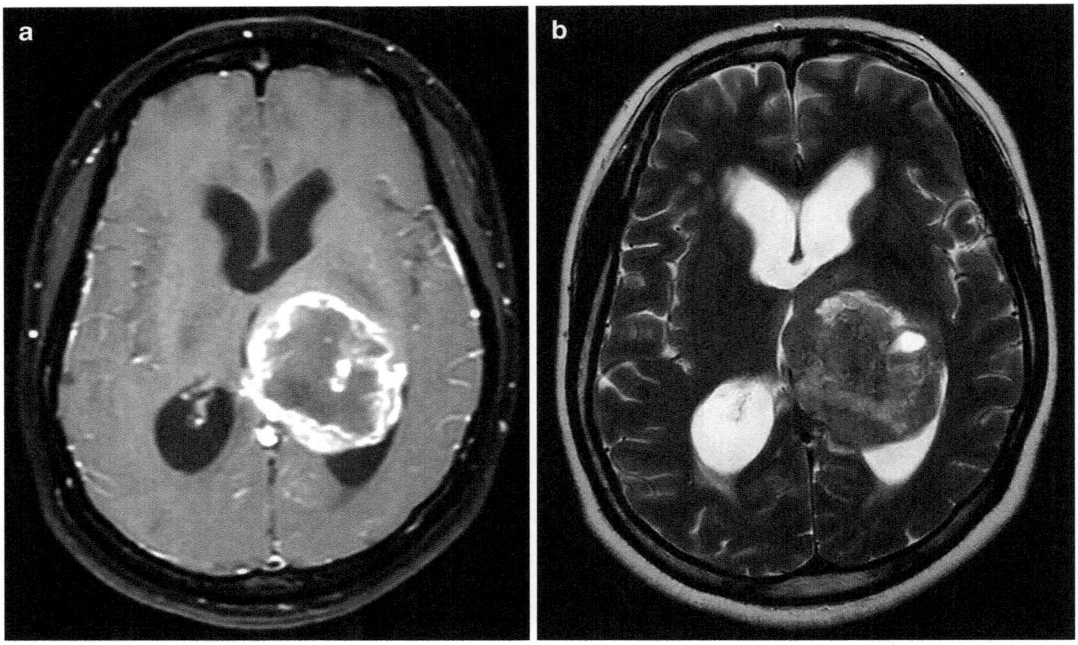

Fig. 16.3 (**a**, **b**) Post-contrast and T2w sequences of glioblastoma multiforme. Image courtesy: Dr. Amit Chaudhari, Assistant Professor, Department of Radiology, Tata Medical Hospital, Mumbai

CBV (rCBV) measurements are helpful for the evaluation of the grading of the tumour and the vascularity of the tumour [118, 119].

16.11 Perfusion MR

The use of perfusion MR imaging is important for the differentiation and overall assessment of solitary brain lesions. This is possible with various biomarkers which will be useful for the differentiation of various lesions, and based on these the therapeutic options can be planned. One of the differentiating factors is the lymphoma vs glioblastoma multiforme (GBM) tumours which will have same features but can be easily differentiated by these perfusion scans. The rCBV ratio of primary intracranial lymphomas was 1.72:0.59, whereas the rCBV ratio of high-grade gliomas (HGGs) was 4.86:2.18 [120, 121] (Fig. 16.4).

16.11.1 Tumour Necrosis

The post-treatment analysis of various aspects needs to be explained in relation to tumour necrosis versus tumour recurrence/growth; they can be there, or both can be there. This scenario is not possible with routine examinations of the MRI but possible with the multiparametric MR imaging, and this is very important for the evaluation as the standard adjuvant management line has to be there which needs to be differentiated from the recurrence. The delayed radiation necrosis in relation to the occlusive vasculopathy causing the various endothelial cell proliferation can represent the pseudo-progression and can be analysed by the radio necrosis; this can also cause various aspects of fibrinoid necrosis of small vessels, associated with the endothelial thickening, causing the hyalinization, and also vascular thrombosis. The recurrence of tumours needs to be

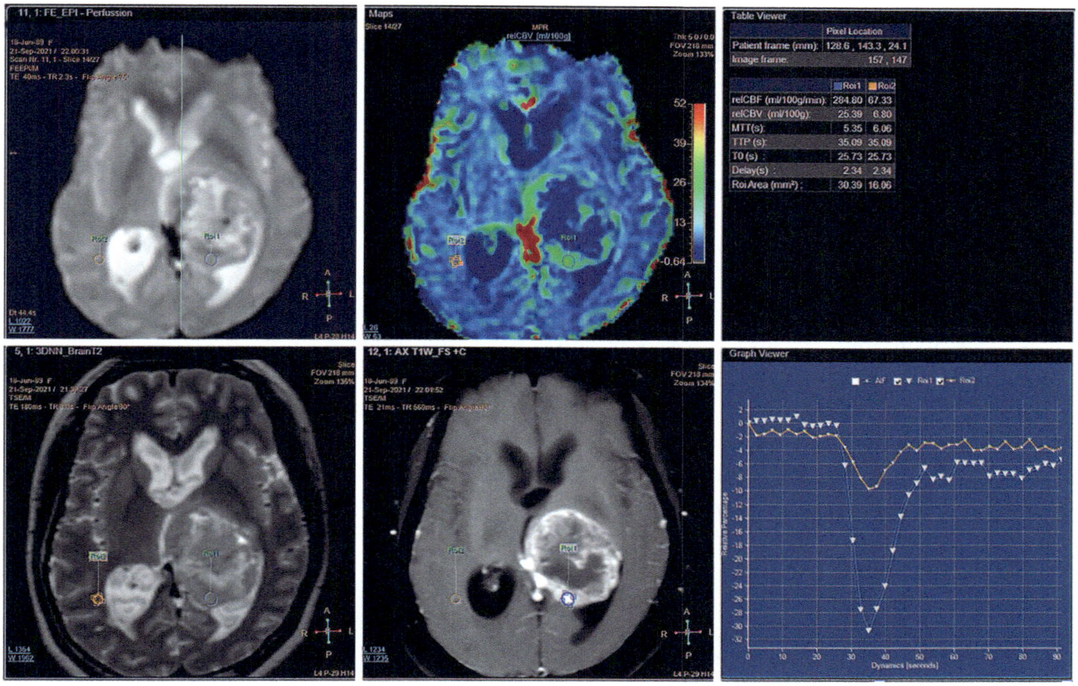

Fig. 16.4 mp-MRI sequences showing the advantage of various MR protocols for better sensitivity and earlier diagnosis. Image courtesy: Dr. Amit Chaudhari, Assistant Professor, Department of Radiology, Tata Medical Hospital, Mumbai

associated with vascular proliferation causing the angiogenesis. CBV and Ktrans can be used to differentiate radiation necrosis from recurrent tumour [122–124].

16.12 Diffusion-Weighted Imaging

DWI is the important modality which is based on the function of water movement at the molecular level like random or Brownian motion of water molecules thus can quantify the diffusion of water molecules. Echo-planar imaging (EPI) spin echo T2-weighted sequence is mostly used as it will reduce motion artefacts and the acquisition is faster. The diffusion can be seen by using less diffusion in one image and another with the more amount of diffusion, and the ADC is calculated on voxel-by-voxel basis. The quantification of various values will help in characteristics of various tumours. Low ADC values will represent the increasing cellularity which is directly proportional to the increasing grade of tumour and which is being identified by the increasing Ki-67 cellular proliferation index. Due to this aspect, it is being used for assessing the response to the tumour after various therapies like chemotherapy, radiotherapy, and antiangiogenic therapy [125–128].

16.13 Diffusion Tensor Imaging

DTI is a one of the fascinating modalities with many limitations of this technique. In one of the tensor models, the mobility of the water is 3 by 3 matrix. The fractional anisotropy will be measuring the total magnitude of diffusion anisotropy. Thus, the DTI is used for the delineation of the white matter fibre tracts. This is possible due to each voxel connection in relation to another direction. DTI is able to distinguish the tumour and the local infiltration of the tumour in peritumoral oedema along with the adjacent normal brain parenchyma by identifying the adjacent various fibre tracts which will give more precise information to the surgeon, so there will be surgical options to prevent the loss of various functions [126, 129]. Various patterns of the DTI involvement are seen in white matter involvement. The main four categories based on FA maps are the displaced, infiltrated, disrupted, and oedematous patterns. When the lesion has displaced fibres of the main tract, the FA will be normal or only slightly reduced. In the infiltration category, the FA values are clearly reduced by the lesion, but the affected tracts can be identified. In the disrupted category, the fibre tracts cannot have anatomically and significantly reduced FA values. Significantly reduced FA values in peritumoral region are seen with oedematous white matter involvement where there can be tumoral infiltration or not [130, 131].

In the post-treatment evaluation, the role of the MRS is very important to differentiate the radiation injury and the tumour recurrence in the clinical settings of radiation therapy, with various types of the surgery like gamma knife radiosurgery or brachytherapy. As we all know, the Cho/Cr or Cho/NAA ratio will be favouring the recurrent tumour. On the other hand, the reduction in Cho and Cr ratio will be consistent with the radiation necrosis. Still the MRS cannot differentiate between the mixed tumour/radiation necrosis tissues either from the tumour or radiation necrosis; still it can definitely differentiate between the complete necrosis versus complete tumour [132–134] (Fig. 16.5a, b).

16.14 fMRI

In BOLD imaging, after the stimulation of the particular area of the brain, there will be significantly increased blood flow corresponding to the increased oxyhaemoglobin supply which will have the diamagnetic effect leading to the increased signal intensity in that region. This technique is used to analyse the functional assessment of the various motor, visual, and auditory areas and also for the analysis of the other motor functions like language areas [135] (Fig. 16.6).

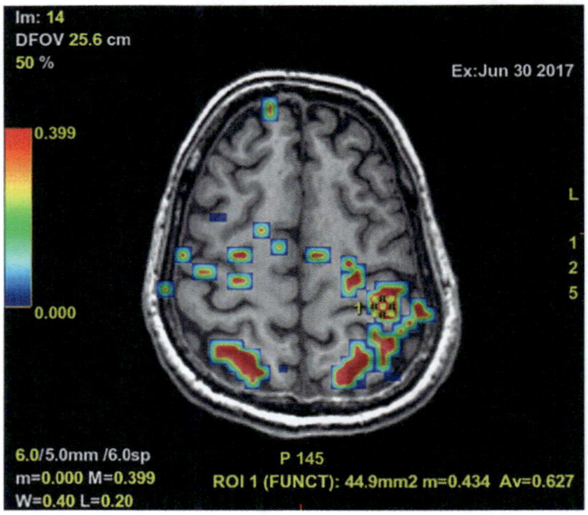

Fig. 16.6 Showing the functional aspects of the MRI that will be depicting the brain activity. Image courtesy: Dr. Amit Chaudhari, Assistant Professor, Department of Radiology, Tata Medical Hospital, Mumbai

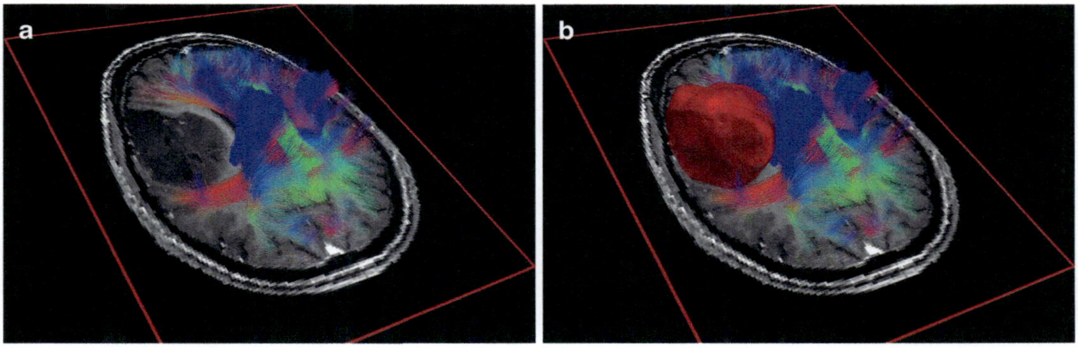

Fig. 16.5 (**a**, **b**) Showing the tumour displacing the fibre tracts on left side. Image courtesy: Dr. Amit Chaudhari, Assistant Professor, Department of Radiology, Tata Medical Hospital, Mumbai

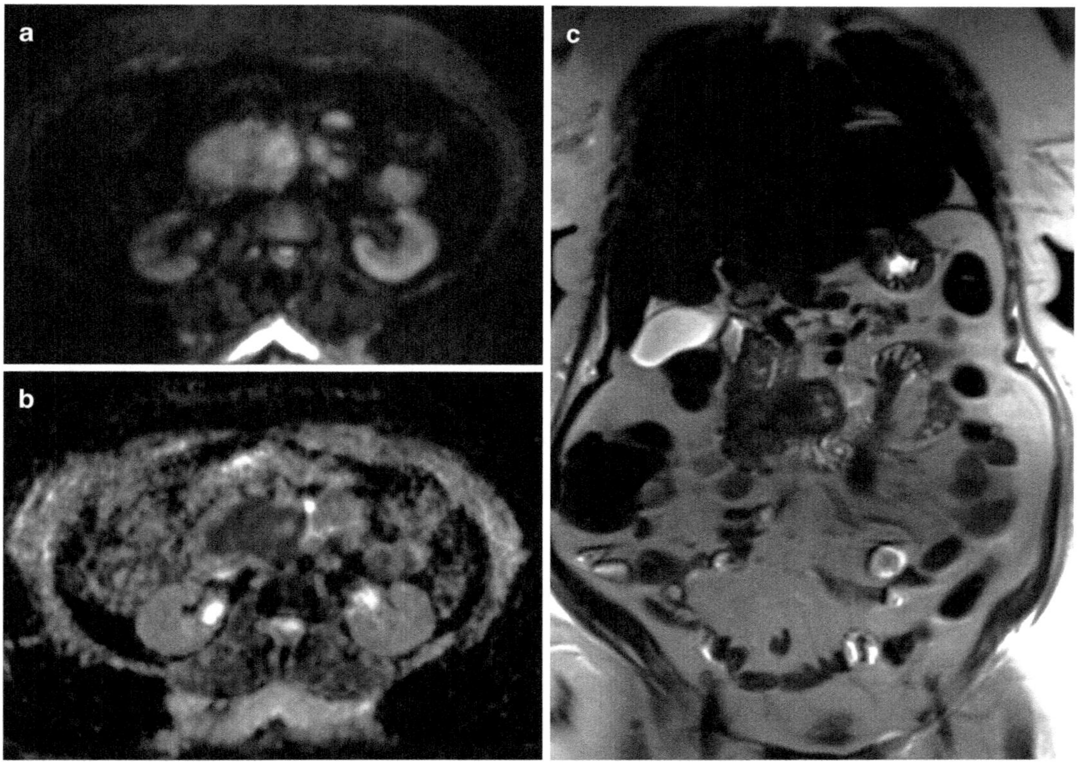

Fig. 16.7 Precaval node in the DWI and the T2W sequence depicting the better clarity of the lesion. Image courtesy: Dr. Amit Chaudhari, Assistant Professor, Department of Radiology, Tata Medical Hospital, Mumbai

Some of the other aspects of the mp-MRI have also been used in the some of the retroperitoneal tumours or various abdominal pathologies commonly seen in the hepatic lesions. The advantage of the various sequences is that it can be an allied factor for the more precise and early diagnosis as compared to the single MR protocols (Fig. 16.7).

16.15 Conclusion

Thus, mp-MRI has evolved as an important imaging technique for the evaluation of various cancers. But it is well established in neurological tumours and breast and prostatic cancers.

This had led to the newer techniques evolved based on newer reported criteria like PI-RADS and VI-RADS.

And fast-growing biomarkers in various modalities as well as in MR the concept of the functional and molecular imaging will also be ascertained leading to the precision medicine concept.

References

1. Panebianco V, Barchetti F, Sciarra A, Ciardi A, Indino EL, Papalia R, et al. Multiparametric magnetic resonance imaging vs. standard care in men being evaluated for prostate cancer: a randomized study. Urol Oncol. 2015;33(17):e1–7.
2. Schimmöller L, Quentin M, Arsov C, Hiester A, Buchbender C, Rabenalt R, et al. MR-sequences for prostate cancer diagnostics: validation based on the PI-RADS scoring system and targeted MR-guided in-bore biopsy. Eur Radiol. 2014;24:2582–9.
3. Petrillo A, Fusco R, Setola SV, Ronza FM, Granata V, Petrillo M, et al. Multiparametric MRI for prostate cancer detection: performance in patients with prostate-specific antigen values between 2.5 and 10 ng/mL. J Magn Reson Imaging. 2014;39:1206–12.

4. Penzkofer T, Tempany-Afdhal CM. Prostate cancer detection and diagnosis: the role of MR and its comparison with other diagnostic modalities—a radiologist's perspective. NMR Biomed. 2014;27:3–15.
5. Park SY, Kim CK, Park BK, Kwon GY. Comparison of apparent diffusion coefficient calculation between two-point and multipoint B value analyses in prostate cancer and benign prostate tissue at 3 T: preliminary experience. AJR Am J Roentgenol. 2014;203:W287–94.
6. Manenti G, Nezzo M, Chegai F, Vasili E, Bonanno E, Simonetti G. DWI of prostate cancer: optimal b-value in clinical practice. Prostate Cancer. 2014;2014:868269.
7. Nowak J, Malzahn U, Baur AD, Reichelt U, Franiel T, Hamm B, et al. The value of ADC, T2 signal intensity, and a combination of both parameters to assess Gleason score and primary Gleason grades in patients with known prostate cancer. Acta Radiol. 2014. Epub ahead of print. https://doi.org/10.1177/0284185114561915.
8. Marcus DM, Rossi PJ, Nour SG, Jani AB. The impact of multiparametric pelvic magnetic resonance imaging on risk stratification in patients with localized prostate cancer. Urology. 2014;84:132–7.
9. Lawrence EM, Gallagher FA, Barrett T, Warren AY, Priest AN, Goldman DA, et al. Preoperative 3-T diffusion-weighted MRI for the qualitative and quantitative assessment of extracapsular extension in patients with intermediate- or high-risk prostate cancer. AJR Am J Roentgenol. 2014;203:W280–6.
10. Jie C, Rongbo L, Ping T. The value of diffusion-weighted imaging in the detection of prostate cancer: a meta-analysis. Eur Radiol. 2014;24:1929–41.
11. Barentsz JO, Richenberg J, Clements R, Choyke P, Verma S, Villeirs G, et al. European Society of Urogenital Radiology. ESUR prostate MR guidelines 2012. Eur Radiol. 2012;22:746–57.
12. Shah ZK, Elias SN, Abaza R, Zynger DL, DeRenne LA, Knopp MV, et al. Performance comparison of 1.5-T endorectal coil MRI with 3-T nonendorectal coil MRI in patients with prostate cancer. Acad Radiol. 2015;22:467–74.
13. Choi YJ, Kim JK, Kim N, Kim KW, Choi EK, Cho KS. Functional MR imaging of prostate cancer. Radiographics. 2007;27:63–77.
14. Rosenkrantz AB, Lim RP, Haghighi M, Somberg MB, Babb JS, Taneja SS. Comparison of interreader reproducibility of the prostate imaging reporting and data system and Likert scales for evaluation of multiparametric prostate MRI. AJR Am J Roentgenol. 2013;201:W612–8.
15. Hoeks CM, Vos EK, Bomers JG, Barentsz JO, Hulsbergen-van de Kaa CA, Scheenen TW. Diffusion-weighted magnetic resonance imaging in the prostate transition zone: histopathological validation using magnetic resonance-guided biopsy specimens. Invest Radiol. 2013;48:693–701.
16. Oto A, Kayhan A, Jiang Y, Tretiakova M, Yang C, Antic T, et al. Prostate cancer: differentiation of central gland cancer from benign prostatic hyperplasia by using diffusion-weighted and dynamic contrast-enhanced MR imaging. Radiology. 2010;257:715–23.
17. Wang L, Mazaheri Y, Zhang J, Ishill NM, Kuroiwa K, Hricak H. Assessment of biologic aggressiveness of prostate cancer: correlation of MR signal intensity with Gleason grade after radical prostatectomy. Radiology. 2008;246:168–76.
18. Hoeks CM, Barentsz JO, Hambrock T, Yakar D, Somford DM, Heijmink SW, et al. Prostate cancer: multiparametric MR imaging for detection, localization, and staging. Radiology. 2011;261:46–66.
19. Kitajima K, Takahashi S, Ueno Y, Yoshikawa T, Ohno Y, Obara M, et al. Clinical utility of apparent diffusion coefficient values obtained using high b-value when diagnosing prostate cancer using 3 tesla MRI: comparison between ultra-high b-value (2000 s/mm^2) and standard high b-value (1000 s/mm^2). J Magn Reson Imaging. 2012;36:198–205.
20. Hambrock T, Somford DM, Huisman HJ, van Oort IM, Witjes JA, Hulsbergen-van de Kaa CA, et al. Relationship between apparent diffusion coefficients at 3.0-T MR imaging and Gleason grade in peripheral zone prostate cancer. Radiology. 2011;259:453–61.
21. Turkbey B, Shah VP, Pang Y, Bernardo M, Xu S, Kruecker J, et al. Is apparent diffusion coefficient associated with clinical risk scores for prostate cancers that are visible on 3-T MR images? Radiology. 2011;258:488–95.
22. Kumar V, Jagannathan NR, Kumar R, Thulkar S, Gupta SD, Dwivedi SN, et al. Apparent diffusion coefficient of the prostate in men prior to biopsy: determination of a cut-off value to predict malignancy of the peripheral zone. NMR Biomed. 2007;20:505–11.
23. Haider MA, van der Kwast TH, Tanguay J, Evans AJ, Hashmi AT, Lockwood G, et al. Combined T2-weighted and diffusion-weighted MRI for localization of prostate cancer. AJR Am J Roentgenol. 2007;189:323–8.
24. Tan CH, Wei W, Johnson V, Kundra V. Diffusion-weighted MRI in the detection of prostate cancer: meta-analysis. AJR Am J Roentgenol. 2012;199:822–9.
25. Wu LM, Xu JR, Gu HY, Hua J, Chen J, Zhang W, et al. Usefulness of diffusion-weighted magnetic resonance imaging in the diagnosis of prostate cancer. Acad Radiol. 2012;19:1215–24.
26. Wu LM, Xu JR, Ye YQ, Lu Q, Hu JN. The clinical value of diffusion-weighted imaging in combination with T2-weighted imaging in diagnosing prostate carcinoma: a systematic review and meta-analysis. AJR Am J Roentgenol. 2012;199:103–10.
27. Katahira K, Takahara T, Kwee TC, Oda S, Suzuki Y, Morishita S, et al. Ultra-high-b-value diffusion-weighted MR imaging for the detection of prostate cancer: evaluation in 201 cases with histopathological correlation. Eur Radiol. 2011;21:188–96.

28. Osugi K, Tanimoto A, Nakashima J, Shinoda K, Hashiguchi A, Oya M, et al. What is the most effective tool for detecting prostate cancer using a standard MR scanner? Magn Reson Med Sci. 2013;12:271–80.
29. Bonekamp D, Jacobs MA, El-Khouli R, Stoianovici D, Macura KJ. Advancements in MR imaging of the prostate: from diagnosis to interventions. Radiographics. 2011;31:677–703.
30. Kitajima K, Murphy RC, Nathan MA, Froemming AT, Hagen CE, Takahashi N, et al. Detection of recurrent prostate cancer after radical prostatectomy: comparison of 11C-choline PET/CT with pelvic multiparametric MR imaging with endorectal coil. J Nucl Med. 2014;55:223–32.
31. Umbehr M, Bachmann LM, Held U, Kessler TM, Sulser T, Weishaupt D, et al. Combined magnetic resonance imaging and magnetic resonance spectroscopy imaging in the diagnosis of prostate cancer: a systematic review and meta-analysis. Eur Urol. 2009;55:575–90.
32. Villeirs GM, De Meerleer GO, De Visschere PJ, Fonteyne VH, Verbaeys AC, Oosterlinck W. Combined magnetic resonance imaging and spectroscopy in the assessment of high grade prostate carcinoma in patients with elevated PSA: a single-institution experience of 356 patients. Eur J Radiol. 2011;77:340–5.
33. Javali TD, Dwivedi DK, Kumar R, Jagannathan NR, Thulkar S, Dinda AK. Magnetic resonance spectroscopy imaging-directed transrectal ultrasound biopsy increases prostate cancer detection in men with prostate-specific antigen between 4-10 ng/mL and normal digital rectal examination. Int J Urol. 2014;21:257–62.
34. Kobus T, Hambrock T, Hulsbergen-van de Kaa CA, Wright AJ, Barentsz JO, Heerschap A, et al. *In vivo* assessment of prostate cancer aggressiveness using magnetic resonance spectroscopic imaging at 3 T with an endorectal coil. Eur Urol. 2011;60:1074–80.
35. Kobus T, Wright AJ, Van Asten JJ, Heerschap A, Scheenen TW. *In vivo* (1) H MR spectroscopic imaging of aggressive prostate cancer: can we detect lactate? Magn Reson Med. 2014;71:26–34.
36. Selnaes KM, Gribbestad IS, Bertilsson H, Wright A, Angelsen A, Heerschap A, et al. Spatially matched *in vivo* and *ex vivo* MR metabolic profiles of prostate cancer—investigation of a correlation with Gleason score. NMR Biomed. 2013;26:600–6.
37. Sciarra A, Panebianco V, Salciccia S, Osimani M, Lisi D, Ciccariello M, et al. Role of dynamic contrast-enhanced magnetic resonance (MR) imaging and proton MR spectroscopic imaging in the detection of local recurrence after radical prostatectomy for prostate cancer. Eur Urol. 2008;54:589–600.
38. Pucar D, Shukla-Dave A, Hricak H, Moskowitz CS, Kuroiwa K, Olgac S, et al. Prostate cancer: correlation of MR imaging and MR spectroscopy with pathologic findings after radiation therapy-initial experience. Radiology. 2005;236:545–53.
39. Fütterer JJ, Heijmink SW, Scheenen TW, Veltman J, Huisman HJ, Vos P, et al. Prostate cancer localization with dynamic contrast-enhanced MR imaging and proton MR spectroscopic imaging. Radiology. 2006;241:449–58.
40. Tanimoto A, Nakashima J, Kohno H, Shinmoto H, Kuribayashi S. Prostate cancer screening: the clinical value of diffusion-weighted imaging and dynamic MR imaging in combination with T2-weighted imaging. J Magn Reson Imaging. 2007;25:146–52.
41. Turkbey B, Pinto PA, Mani H, Bernardo M, Pang Y, McKinney YL, et al. Prostate cancer: value of multiparametric MR imaging at 3 T for detection-histopathologic correlation. Radiology. 2010;255:89–99.
42. de Rooij M, Hamoen EH, Fütterer JJ, Barentsz JO, Rovers MM. Accuracy of multiparametric MRI for prostate cancer detection: a meta-analysis. AJR Am J Roentgenol. 2014;202:343–51.
43. Abd-Alazeez M, Ahmed HU, Arya M, Charman SC, Anastasiadis E, Freeman A, et al. The accuracy of multiparametric MRI in men with negative biopsy and elevated PSA level-can it rule out clinically significant prostate cancer? Urol Oncol. 2014;32:45.e17–22.
44. Itatani R, Namimoto T, Atsuji S, Katahira K, Morishita S, Kitani K, et al. Negative predictive value of multiparametric MRI for prostate cancer detection: outcome of 5-year follow-up in men with negative findings on initial MRI studies. Eur J Radiol. 2014;83:1740–5.
45. Shakir NA, George AK, Siddiqui MM, Rothwax JT, Rais-Bahrami S, Stamatakis L, et al. Identification of threshold prostate specific antigen levels to optimize the detection of clinically significant prostate cancer by magnetic resonance imaging/ultrasound fusion guided biopsy. J Urol. 2014;192:1642–9.
46. Delongchamps NB, Rouanne M, Flam T, Beuvon F, Liberatore M, Zerbib M, et al. Multiparametric magnetic resonance imaging for the detection and localization of prostate cancer: combination of T2-weighted, dynamic contrast-enhanced and diffusion-weighted imaging. BJU Int. 2011;107:1411–8.
47. Hoeks CM, Hambrock T, Yakar D, Hulsbergen-van de Kaa CA, Feuth T, Witjes JA, et al. Transition zone prostate cancer: detection and localization with 3-T multiparametric MR imaging. Radiology. 2013;266:207–17.
48. Jung SI, Donati OF, Vargas HA, Goldman D, Hricak H, Akin O. Transition zone prostate cancer: incremental value of diffusion-weighted endorectal MR imaging in tumor detection and assessment of aggressiveness. Radiology. 2013;269:493–503.
49. Cornud F, Khoury G, Bouazza N, Beuvon F, Peyromaure M, Flam T, et al. Tumor target volume for focal therapy of prostate cancer-does multiparametric magnetic resonance imaging allow for a reliable estimation? J Urol. 2014;191:1272–9.

50. Rosenkrantz AB, Mendrinos S, Babb JS, Taneja SS. Prostate cancer foci detected on multiparametric magnetic resonance imaging are histologically distinct from those not detected. J Urol. 2012;187:2032–8.
51. Langer DL, van der Kwast TH, Evans AJ, Sun L, Yaffe MJ, Trachtenberg J, et al. Intermixed normal tissue within prostate cancer: effect on MR imaging measurements of apparent diffusion coefficient and T2—sparse versus dense cancers. Radiology. 2008;249:900–8.
52. Bratan F, Melodelima C, Souchon R, Hoang Dinh A, Mège-Lechevallier F, Crouzet S, et al. How accurate is multiparametric MR imaging in evaluation of prostate cancer volume? Radiology. 2015;275:144–54.
53. Nakashima J, Tanimoto A, Imai Y, Mukai M, Horiguchi Y, Nakagawa K, et al. Endorectal MRI for prediction of tumor site, tumor size, and local extension of prostate cancer. Urology. 2004;64:101–5.
54. Coakley FV, Kurhanewicz J, Lu Y, Jones KD, Swanson MG, Chang SD, et al. Prostate cancer tumor volume: measurement with endorectal MR and MR spectroscopic imaging. Radiology. 2002;223:91–7.
55. Hamoen EH, de Rooij M, Witjes JA, Barentsz JO, Rovers MM. Use of the prostate imaging reporting and data system (PI-RADS) for prostate cancer detection with multiparametric magnetic resonance imaging: a diagnostic meta-analysis. Eur Urol. 2015;67:1112–21.
56. American College of Radiology. MR prostate imaging reporting and data system version 2.0. Accessed Jan 2015 from http://www.acr.org/Quality-Safety/Resources/PIRADS/.
57. Mowatt G, Scotland G, Boachie C, Cruickshank M, Ford JA, Fraser C, et al. The diagnostic accuracy and cost-effectiveness of magnetic resonance spectroscopy and enhanced magnetic resonance imaging techniques in aiding the localisation of prostate abnormalities for biopsy: a systematic review and economic evaluation (1-281). Health Technol Assess. 2013;17:vii–xix.
58. de Rooij M, Crienen S, Witjes JA, Barentsz JO, Rovers MM, Grutters JP. Cost-effectiveness of magnetic resonance (MR) imaging and MR-guided targeted biopsy versus systematic transrectal ultrasound-guided biopsy in diagnosing prostate cancer: a modelling study from a health care perspective. Eur Urol. 2014;66:430–6.
59. Haffner J, Lemaitre L, Puech P, Haber GP, Leroy X, Jones JS, et al. Role of magnetic resonance imaging before initial biopsy: comparison of magnetic resonance imaging-targeted and systematic biopsy for significant prostate cancer detection. BJU Int. 2011;108:E171–8.
60. Mozer P, Rouprêt M, Le Cossec C, Granger B, Comperat E, de Gorski A, et al. First round of targeted biopsies using magnetic resonance imaging/ultrasonography fusion compared with conventional transrectal ultrasonography-guided biopsies for the diagnosis of localised prostate cancer. BJU Int. 2015;115:50–7.
61. Puech P, Rouvière O, Renard-Penna R, Villers A, Devos P, Colombel M, et al. Prostate cancer diagnosis: multiparametric MR-targeted biopsy with cognitive and transrectal US-MR fusion guidance versus systematic biopsy—prospective multicenter study. Radiology. 2013;268:461–9.
62. Schoots IG, Roobol MJ, Nieboer D, Bangma CH, Steyerberg EW, Hunink MG. Magnetic resonance imaging-targeted biopsy may enhance the diagnostic accuracy of significant prostate cancer detection compared to standard transrectal ultrasound-guided biopsy: a systematic review and meta-analysis. Eur Urol. 2014. Epub ahead of print. https://doi.org/10.1016/j.eururo.2014.11.037.
63. Zhang ZX, Yang J, Zhang CZ, Li KA, Quan QM, Wang XF, et al. The value of magnetic resonance imaging in the detection of prostate cancer in patients with previous negative biopsies and elevated prostate-specific antigen levels: a meta-analysis. Acad Radiol. 2014;21:578–89.
64. Hoeks CM, Schouten MG, Bomers JG, Hoogendoorn SP, Hulsbergen-van de Kaa CA, Hambrock T, et al. Three-Tesla magnetic resonance-guided prostate biopsy in men with increased prostate-specific antigen and repeated, negative, random, systematic, transrectal ultrasound biopsies: detection of clinically significant prostate cancers. Eur Urol. 2012;62:902–9.
65. Sonn GA, Chang E, Natarajan S, Margolis DJ, Macairan M, Lieu P, et al. Value of targeted prostate biopsy using magnetic resonance-ultrasound fusion in men with prior negative biopsy and elevated prostate-specific antigen. Eur Urol. 2014;65:809–15.
66. Bjurlin MA, Meng X, Le Nobin J, Wysock JS, Lepor H, Rosenkrantz AB, et al. Optimization of prostate biopsy: the role of magnetic resonance imaging targeted biopsy in detection, localization and risk assessment. J Urol. 2014;192:648–58.
67. Margel D, Yap SA, Lawrentschuk N, Klotz L, Haider M, Hersey K, et al. Impact of multiparametric endorectal coil prostate magnetic resonance imaging on disease reclassification among active surveillance candidates: a prospective cohort study. J Urol. 2012;187:1247–52.
68. Turkbey B, Mani H, Aras O, Ho J, Hoang A, Rastinehad AR, et al. Prostate cancer: can multiparametric MR imaging help identify patients who are candidates for active surveillance? Radiology. 2013;268:144–52.
69. Dianat SS, Carter HB, Pienta KJ, Schaeffer EM, Landis PK, Epstein JI, et al. Magnetic resonance-invisible versus magnetic resonance-visible prostate cancer in active surveillance: a preliminary report on disease outcomes. Urology. 2015;85:147–53.
70. Guo Y, Cai YQ, Cai ZL, et al. Differentiation of clinically benign and malignant breast lesions using diffusion-weighted imaging. J Magn Reson Imaging. 2002;16(2):172–8.
71. Rubesova E, Grell AS, De Maertelaer V, et al. Quantitative diffusion imaging in breast cancer: a

clinical prospective study. J Magn Reson Imaging. 2006;24(2):319–24.
72. Sinha S, Lucas-Quesada FA, Sinha U, et al. In vivo diffusion-weighted MRI of the breast: potential for lesion characterization. J Magn Reson Imaging. 2002;15(6):693–704.
73. Woodhams R, Matsunaga K, Kan S, et al. ADC mapping of benign and malignant breast tumors. Magn Reson Med Sci. 2005;4(1):35–42.
74. Bogner W, Pinker K, Zaric O, et al. Bilateral diffusion-weighted MR imaging of breast tumors with submillimeter resolution using readout-segmented echo-planar imaging at 7 T. Radiology. 2015;274(1):74–84.
75. Lee SK, Tan ET, Govenkar A, et al. Dynamic slice-dependent shim and center frequency update in 3 T breast diffusion weighted imaging. Magn Reson Med. 2014;71(5):1813–8.
76. Singer L, Wilmes LJ, Saritas EU, et al. High-resolution diffusion-weighted magnetic resonance imaging in patients with locally advanced breast cancer. Acad Radiol. 2012;19(5):526–34.
77. Teruel JR, Fjosne HE, Ostlie A, et al. Inhomogeneous static magnetic field-induced distortion correction applied to diffusion weighted MRI of the breast at 3T. Magn Reson Med. 2014; https://doi.org/10.1002/mrm.25489.
78. Bokacheva L, Kaplan JB, Giri DD, et al. Intravoxel incoherent motion diffusion-weighted MRI at 3.0 T differentiates malignant breast lesions from benign 236 Rahbar & Partridge lesions and breast parenchyma. J Magn Reson Imaging. 2014;40(4):813–23.
79. Iima M, Yano K, Kataoka M, et al. Quantitative non-Gaussian diffusion and intravoxel incoherent motion magnetic resonance imaging: differentiation of malignant and benign breast lesions. Invest Radiol. 2015;50(4):205–11.
80. Liu C, Liang C, Liu Z, et al. Intravoxel incoherent motion (IVIM) in evaluation of breast lesions: comparison with conventional DWI. Eur J Radiol. 2013;82(12):e782–9.
81. Sigmund EE, Cho GY, Kim S, et al. Intravoxel incoherent motion imaging of tumor microenvironment in locally advanced breast cancer. Magn Reson Med. 2011;65(5):1437–47.
82. Roebuck JR, Cecil KM, Schnall MD, et al. Human breast lesions: characterization with proton MR spectroscopy. Radiology. 1998;209(1):269–75.
83. Gribbestad IS, Singstad TE, Nilsen G, et al. In vivo 1H MRS of normal breast and breast tumours using a dedicated double breast coil. J Magn Reson Imaging. 1998;8(6):1191–7.
84. Cecil KM, Schnall MD, Siegelman ES, et al. The evaluation of human breast lesions with magnetic resonance imaging and proton magnetic resonance spectroscopy. Breast Cancer Res Treat. 2001;68(1):45–54.
85. Yeung DK, Cheung HS, Tse GM. Human breast lesions: characterization with contrast-enhanced in vivo proton MR spectroscopy—initial results. Radiology. 2001;220(1):40–6.
86. Sitter B, Sonnewald U, Spraul M, et al. High-resolution magic angle spinning MRS of breast cancer tissue. NMR Biomed. 2002;15(5):327–37.
87. Haddadin IS, McIntosh A, Meisamy S, et al. Metabolite quantification and high-field MRS in breast cancer. NMR Biomed. 2009;22(1):65–76.
88. Bartella L, Morris EA, Dershaw DD, et al. Proton MR spectroscopy with choline peak as malignancy marker improves positive predictive value for breast cancer diagnosis: preliminary study. Radiology. 2006;239(3):686–92.
89. Meisamy S, Bolan PJ, Baker EH, et al. Adding in vivo quantitative 1H MR spectroscopy to improve diagnostic accuracy of breast MR imaging: preliminary results of observer performance study at 4.0 T. Radiology. 2005;236(2):465–75.
90. Bartella L, Thakur SB, Morris EA, et al. Enhancing nonmass lesions in the breast: evaluation with proton (1H) MR spectroscopy. Radiology. 2007;245(1):80–7.
91. Bourne RM, Kurniawan N, Cowin G, et al. Microscopic diffusivity compartmentation in formalin-fixed prostate tissue. Magn Reson Med. 2012;68(2):614–20.
92. Chatterjee A, Watson G, Myint E, et al. Changes in epithelium, stroma, and lumen space correlate more strongly with Gleason pattern and are stronger predictors of prostate ADC changes than cellularity metrics. Radiology. 2015;277(3):751–62.
93. Mustafi D, Gleber S-C, Ward J, et al. IV administered gadodiamide enters the lumen of the prostatic glands: x-ray fluorescence microscopy examination of a mouse model. AJR Am J Roentgenol. 2015;205(3):W313–9.
94. Bourne R, Power C, Chatterjee A, et al. Distinctive water diffusion properties of epithelia may be the key to better cancer imaging techniques. Paper presented at Sydney Cancer Conference, Sydney, 27–28 Nov 2014.
95. Wetter A, Lipponer C, Nensa F, et al. Simultaneous 18F choline positron emission tomography/magnetic resonance imaging of the prostate: initial results. Invest Radiol. 2013;48(5):256–62.
96. de Perrot T, Rager O, Scheffler M, et al. Potential of hybrid (1)(8)F-fluorocholine PET/MRI for prostate cancer imaging. Eur J Nucl Med Mol Imaging. 2014;41(9):1744–55.
97. Mehralivand S, Shih JH, Rais-Bahrami S, et al. A magnetic resonance imaging-based prediction model for prostate biopsy risk stratification. JAMA Oncol. 2018;4(5):678–85.
98. Li J, Weng Z, Xu H, et al. Support Vector Machines (SVM) classification of prostate cancer Gleason

score in central gland using multiparametric magnetic resonance images: a cross-validated study. Eur J Radiol. 2018;98:61–7.
99. Ma T, Yang S, Jing H, et al. Apparent diffusion coefficients in prostate cancer: correlation with molecular markers Ki-67, HIF-1alpha and VEGF. NMR Biomed. 2018;31(3):9.
100. Leapman MS, Westphalen AC, Ameli N, et al. Association between a 17-gene genomic prostate score and multi-parametric prostate MRI in men with low and intermediate risk prostate cancer (PCa). PLoS One. 2017;12(10):e0185535.
101. Padhani AR, Weinreb J, Rosenkrantz AB, et al. Prostate imaging-reporting and data system steering committee: PI-RADS v2 status update and future directions. Eur Urol. 2019;75:385–96.
102. Ferreira AM, Reis RB, Kajiwara PP, et al. MRI evaluation of complex renal cysts using the Bosniak classification: a comparison to CT. Abdom Radiol. 2016;41:2011–9.
103. Panebianco V, Narumi Y, Altun E, et al. Multiparametric magnetic resonance imaging for bladder cancer: development of VI-RADS (Vesical Imaging-Reporting And Data System). Eur Urol. 2018;74(3):294–306.
104. Babjuk M, Böhle A, Burger M, et al. EAU guidelines on non-muscle-invasive urothelial carcinoma of the bladder: update 2016. Eur Urol. 2017;71:447–61.
105. Moschini M, Simone G, Stenzl A, et al. Critical review of outcomes from radical cystectomy: can complications from radical cystectomy be reduced by surgical volume and robotic surgery? Eur Urol Focus. 2016;2:19–29.
106. Tourinho-Barbosa RR, Tobias-Machado M, CastroAlfaro A, et al. Complications in robotic urological surgeries and how to avoid them: a systematic review. Arab J Urol. 2018;16:285–92.
107. Rangarajan K, Somani BK. Trends in quality of life reporting for radical cystectomy and urinary diversion over the last four decades: a systematic review of the literature. Arab J Urol. 2019;17:181–94.
108. Kim B, Semelka RC, Ascher SM, et al. Bladder tumor staging: comparison of contrast-enhanced CT, T1- and T2-weighted MR imaging, dynamic gadolinium-enhanced imaging, and late gadolinium-enhanced imaging. Radiology. 1994;193:239–45.
109. Johnson W, Taylor MB, Carrington BM, et al. The value of hyoscine butylbromide in pelvic MRI. Clin Radiol. 2007;62:1087–93.
110. Panebianco V, Barchetti F, de Haas RJ, et al. Improving staging in bladder cancer: the increasing role of multiparametric magnetic resonance imaging. Eur Urol Focus. 2016;2:113–21.
111. Del Giudice F, Barchetti G, De Berardinis E, et al. Prospective assessment of Vesical Imaging Reporting and Data System (VI-RADS) and its clinical impact on the management of high-risk non-muscle-invasive bladder cancer patients candidate for repeated transurethral resection. Eur Urol. 2020;77:101–9.
112. Hafeez S, Koh M, Sohaib A, Huddart R. PD-0464: assessing response to chemotherapy with diffusion weighted MRI (DW-MRI) in muscle invasive bladder cancer (MIBC). Radiother Oncol. 2013;106(Suppl 2):S180–1.
113. Panebianco V, Barentsz J, Narumi Y, Catto J. Multiparametric magnetic resonance imaging for bladder cancer: development of VI-RADS (Vesical ImagingReporting and Data System). Eur Urol 2018;74:294-306. Eur Urol. 2018;74(5):e109.
114. Teoh JYC, Herrmann TRW, Babjuk M. Re: Valeria Panebianco, Yoshifumi Narumi, Ersan Altun, et al. Multiparametric magnetic resonance imaging for bladder cancer: development of VI-RADS (Vesical Imaging-Reporting and Data System). Eur Urol 74, 2018, 294-306. Eur Urol. 2019;75(2):e27–8.
115. Thoeny HC, Bellin MF, Comperat EM, Thalmann GN. Vesical imaging-reporting and data system (VI-RADS): added value for management of bladder cancer patients? Eur Urol. 2018;74(3):307–8.
116. Lacerda S, Law M. Magnetic resonance perfusion and permeability imaging in brain tumors. Neuroimaging Clin N Am. 2009;19:527–57.
117. Hu LS, Baxter LC, Pinnaduwage DS, et al. Optimized preload leakage correction methods to improve the diagnostic accuracy of dynamic susceptibility-weighted contrast-enhanced perfusion MR imaging in posttreatment gliomas. AJNR Am J Neuroradiol. 2010;31(1):40–8.
118. Barajas RF, Hodgson JG, Chang JS, et al. Glioblastoma multiform regional genetic and cellular expression patterns: influence on anatomic and physiologic MR imaging. Radiology. 2010;254(2):564–76.
119. Provenzale JM, Schmainda K. Perfusion imaging for brain tumor characterization and assessment of treatment response. In: Newton HB, Jolesz FA, editors. Handbook of neuro-oncology neuroimaging. New York: Elsevier; 2008. p. 264–77.
120. Hygino da Cruz LC Jr, Rodriguez I, Domingues RC, et al. Pseudoprogression and pseudoresponse: imaging challenges in the assessment of post treatment glioma. AJNR Am J Neuroradiol. 2011;32(11):1978–85.
121. Cha S. Update on brain tumor imaging: from anatomy to physiology. AJNR Am J Neuroradiol. 2006;27:475–87.
122. Hu LS, Baxter LC, Smith KA, et al. Relative cerebral blood volume values to differentiate high-grade glioma recurrence from posttreatment radiation effect: direct correlation between image-guided tissue histopathology and localized dynamic susceptibility-weighted contrast-enhanced perfusion MR imaging measurements. AJNR Am J Neuroradiol. 2009;30(3):552–8.
123. Mangla R, Singh G, Ziegelitz D, et al. Changes in relative cerebral blood volume 1 month after radiation-temozolomide therapy can help predict overall survival in patients with glioblastoma. Radiology. 2010;256:575–84.

124. Cruz LC, Vieira IG, Domingues R. Diffusion MR imaging: an important tool in the assessment of brain tumors. Neuroimaging Clin N Am. 2011;21(1):27–49.
125. Pope WB, Qiao XJ, Kim HJ, et al. Apparent diffusion coefficient histogram analysis stratifies progression-free and overall survival in patients with recurrent GBM treated with bevacizumab: a multicenter study. J Neurooncol. 2012;108:491–8.
126. Hwang EJ, Cha Y, Leum Lee A, et al. Early response evaluation for recurrent high grade gliomas treated with bevacizumab: a volumetric analysis using diffusion-weighted imaging. J Neurooncol. 2013;112:427–35.
127. Chapman CH, Nazem-Zadeh M, Lee OE, et al. Regional variation in brain white matter diffusion index changes following chemoradiotherapy: a prospective study using tract-based spatial statistics. PLoS One. 2013;8(3):e57768.
128. Brunberg JA, Chenevert TL, McKeever PE, et al. In vivo MR determination of water diffusion coefficients and diffusion anisotropy: correlation with structural alteration in gliomas of the cerebral hemispheres. AJNR Am J Neuroradiol. 1995;16:361–71.
129. Jellinson BJ, Field AS, Medow J, et al. Diffusion tensor imaging of cerebral white matter: a pictorial review of physics, fiber tract anatomy, and tumor imaging patterns. AJNR Am J Neuroradiol. 2004;23:356–69.
130. Goebell E, Paustenbach S, Vaeterlein O, et al. Low-grade and anaplastic gliomas: differences in architecture evaluated with diffusion-tensor MR imaging. Radiology. 2006;239:217–22.
131. Hall WA, Galicich W, Bergman T, et al. 3-Tesla intraoperative MR imaging for neurosurgery. J Neurooncol. 2006;77(3):297–303.
132. Saraswathy S, Crawford FW, Lamborn KR, et al. Evaluation of MR markers that predict survival in patients with newly diagnosed GBM prior to adjuvant therapy. J Neurooncol. 2009;91(1):69–81.
133. Smith EA, Carlos RC, Junck LR, et al. Developing a clinical decision model: MR spectroscopy to differentiate between recurrent tumor and radiation change in patients with new contrast-enhancing lesions. AJR Am J Roentgenol. 2009;192:W45–52, 119.
134. Chernov MF, Hayashi M, Izawa M, et al. Multivoxel proton MRS for differentiation of radiation-induced necrosis and tumor recurrence after gamma knife radiosurgery for brain metastases. Brain Tumor Pathol. 2006;23:19–2.
135. Bizzi A, Blasi V, Falini A, et al. Presurgical functional MR imaging of language and motor functions: validation with intraoperative electrocortical mapping. Radiology. 2008;248(2):579–89.

Immunoimaging

17

Key Points (Abstract)

Immunoimaging is one of the most rapidly growing imaging modalities of molecular imaging, and this is because of the major success of immunotherapy in various conditions. Based on the advantage of this immunotherapy, various components like the response to the treatment by immunotherapy, differentiating them into the responders and non-responders, can differentiate various inflammations along with the various roles of the immune system like for diagnosis and therapy. Various immunoimaging techniques are being developed due to the impact based on the sensitivity, specificity, and various ligands and also for the concept of the newer multifunctionality/multimodality imaging. Thus, immunoimaging is a newer concept of imaging for the evaluation of the immunological status of the patients which will help in the diagnosis of various pathologies and further evaluation and post-treatment assessment. Positron emission tomography can be used with the radiolabelled immunoglobulin-derived targeting probes for the evaluation of the immunological status. Nanobodies which are the smallest antigen-binding antibody fragments and have fast and specific targeting to tissues in vivo can be used for evaluation. These probes are like magic bullets for immunoimaging. Various radiolabelled nanobodies are also used as targeting probes for immunoimaging.

Keywords

Immune response · PET-CT · PET-MR
Interleukins · Interferon · Targeting probe

17.1 Introduction

The immune system function is based on the various complex mechanisms which are important for the evaluation of various processes which will be impacting the immune system in various diseases. This imaging is based on the non-invasive structure for monitoring of various processes in vivo. This imaging technique is of more help for various pathologies and most commonly will be the cancer imaging for immunotherapies, and these can be done with the help of specifically targeted tumour-associated antigens, which will be modulating the immune activation, by suppressing the various signalling pathways to enhance immune activity. The immune responses show the proliferation of leukocytes at the site of injury, can recognize the insult, and respond accordingly. Various sets of methods and analytical tools will be used to see various immune responses at the cellular and molecular level like the real-time orientation. With application of various newer techniques and advances in optical imaging, the molecular and cellular responses can be studied more precisely and earlier compared to other modalities especially on the neutrophils, macrophages, and lymphocytes.

S. Shaikh, *Advances in Imaging*, https://doi.org/10.1007/978-981-16-9535-3_17

Molecular imaging is the imaging at the molecular and cellular level. The most important aspect here is the study of normal physiological environment and changes in the body which happen in various pathological diseases [1]. The targeting probe is labelled with radioisotope which will be circulated in the body and will interact with the specific molecular target , bind with it, and will be at the site; the remaining radiotracer which is free will be excreted from the body. Various classes of immunoglobulins and derived proteins are the routinely used probes for molecular imaging based on various targets and can be engineered in different forms. Hybrid scanners are more sensitive for the detection of these molecular signals with the high-resolution anatomical maps in the single imaging procedure. These signals will be detected by positron emission tomography (PET), and the hybrid imaging modality can evaluate the anatomical information. The sensitivity of these hybrid systems, PET/CT or PET/MRI, is being more revolutionized and is capable of measuring the picomolar concentrations of a tracer molecule, and whole-body scan can be done within 30 min [2]. The various targets here are membrane antigens which are more specific for a particular disease. With this the exact phenotype of the particular disease can be defined clearly and is also for the diagnosis of the selective therapy [3]. During this process various antibodies will be produced against these biomarkers, and due to this the antigen-binding fragments will be of more relevance in immunoimaging.

PET uptake is based on various aspects, and the most common is the difference or contrast seen between the target site and the surrounding tissues. Again, the target site will be dependent on the interaction between radiolabelled probe and the molecular agent which is used for the evaluation of the uptake. The "specific contrast" development for the new molecular imaging probe is based on the tracer retention in the area of interest which is again based on various factors like amount of the radiotracer injected. Thus, the molecular imaging is different from the targeted therapy where high dose of a therapeutic moiety is delivered to the target tissue to obtain therapeutic effect. The non-specific accumulation of the tracer at the target site or with the high background signals will give false-positive results. The ideal therapeutic agent should interact with larger number of targets for effective therapy; however, molecular imaging detects the molecular target which requires a small number of the target molecules without disturbing the cells and tissues.

17.2 Immunotherapy and Immunoimaging

There are various aspects of mechanism, various applicable indications, and available therapeutic drugs used by the immune system for the evaluation of cancer. First immunomodulator Coley's toxin was used in the late nineteenth century, to induce the response in various tumours [4]. In the late twentieth century, this was followed by various vaccines, cytokines, and immune-stimulating agents. Interferon and interleukin-2 were approved by the FDA for treating kidney cancer and melanoma [5, 6]. Enhancing the immune system has revolutionized cancer immunotherapy treatments. This immune checkpoint activation will prevent the host immune system to react from various tumours cells; these are recognized as foreign bodies based on the neoantigen expression [7, 8]. The use of cytotoxic T lymphocyte-associated protein 4 (CTLA-4) for lymph node level prevents the responses from the tumour site [9, 10]. To prevent the interaction of CTLA-4 and PD-1, various antibodies are used to prevent the adaptive immune mechanism against cancer.

Various other components are required for effective antitumor response, tumour antigenicity (neoantigens), T-cell infiltration, and various immune-responsive microenvironments. Ipilimumab which was used for the melanoma in 2013 [11] and then another anti-PD-1 agent, pembrolizumab, also were approved by the FDA. For early phases of the disease, these drugs were used for neoadjuvant or adjuvant therapies [12]. Despite of this a lot of fallacies are there which are not completely effective for all patients [13].

Various immune-related side effects were also documented despite the antitumour properties. Few of them are like blocking intrinsic downregulators of immunity causing the immune system to hyperactivate through T lymphocytes causing various side effects like autoimmune diseases. The immunologic homeostasis has to be maintained despite of the autoimmune process, which can have an impact due to inflammation. Autoimmune reactions are usually mild, but few are life-threatening for which the ICI therapy and active treatment need to be stopped further preventing various complications [14–16]. Clinically they may not be relevant. Ipilimumab is one of the drugs which will show significant symptoms in the first 3 months of treatment. The most common is dermatologic effects first (within 2–3 weeks), followed by gastrointestinal or hepatic effects (within 6–7 weeks), pulmonary effects (within 9 weeks), and endocrine-related effects (within 9–11 weeks). By using anti-CTLA-4 drugs, these various manifestations will occur earlier than ICIs [15–17]. By this any organ or system can be affected.

Molecular imaging of the cells and molecules will help significantly in evaluating various mechanisms of action, and failure, of immunotherapies. The detailed structured immunoimaging comprises of the hardware, software, and biologic components for the dynamic and non-invasive visualization of immune responses and also the imaging probes [1, 2, 18]. Various probes can be targeted to endogenous immune cell biomarkers which can be binded or selectively taken up by endogenous immune molecules or immune cells, respectively. CD markers are the immune target markers which will identify various immune cell classes of CD cells (e.g. CD3-positive T cells) to specific cell subsets (e.g. CD3-positive, CD4-positive, FoxP3-positive regulatory T cells) and immune cell states (e.g. CD3-positive, CD4-positive, CD25-positive, CD279-high, FOXP3-positive activated regulatory T cells) (Diagram 17.1). The deoxyguanosine kinase and deoxycytidine kinase can be impacted for nucleoside salvage pathways.

Different antibodies can be there for various immunotherapeutic applications which can be changed tagging it to contrast agent or radionuclide and imaged. New biological components are being developed for improved pharmacokinetics of various newer agents like minibodies, diabodies, and scFv fragments [3, 19]. Various ligands will be having more affinity towards the matured and modified versions to be used as probes [4], and aptamers, adnectins, and cystine knots are the newer brands of immunoimaging agents. T cells, B cells, natural killer cells, dendritic cells, macrophage, monocytes, and hematopoietic stem cells will be monitoring the response to immune cells. The direct impact will be on the cell function.

By using direct labelling, this has become the important imaging technique for immune cell reconstitution and cell homing to sites of disease or damage. Indirect labelling can be done by viral transduction or transfection of a reporter gene into the immune cell area of interest.

17.3 Immunoimaging Applications Towards Immunotherapy

Various immunoimaging protocols will be useful to clearly predict and monitor response to immunotherapy. In normal physiologic conditions, various mechanisms will be there to prevent the negative impact on the tissues. However, the mechanism of various cancers is to upregulate various immune checkpoint molecules ultimately leading to their non-detection and destruction. By the use of various immunosuppressive signalling pathways with therapeutic drugs, various blockade strategies of the immune mechanism can enable the formation of an optimal therapeutic antitumor immune response. This blockade of checkpoints is seen in late-stage melanoma, non-small-cell lung cancer, and bladder cancer. Different types of probes which will be targeting various endogenous biomarkers of immune mechanism will help in the dynamic and heterogeneous expression of immune checkpoint molecules. Various imaging agents include PD-1, PD-L1, and CTLA-4 expression. Chimeric antigen receptor T cells (CAR-Ts)

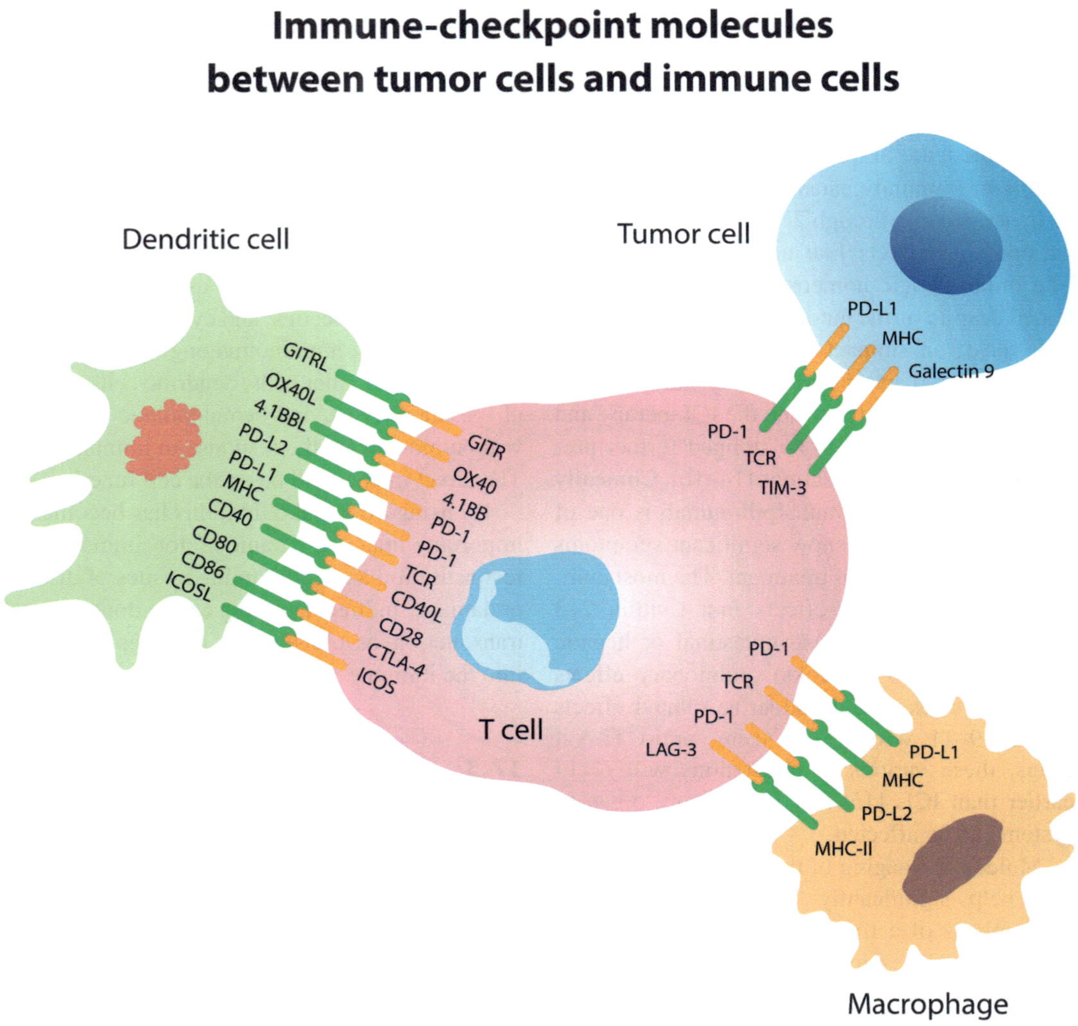

Diagram 17.1 Immune checkpoint molecules between the tumour cells and immune cells

CAR-Ts are being developed to have the therapeutic approach by which the T cells are removed from a patient (Diagram 17.2).

17.4 Dendritic Cell Vaccines

Dendritic cell vaccines are also the form of immunotherapy where the antigen-presenting cells, dendritic cells, are attached to the antigen and again transferred back to the patient. Adaptive immune response is created against the region of the interest.

Direct cell labelling and imaging are done to evaluate various impacts on the cells for example dendritic cells after injection. Direct cell labelling by MRI is being used for monitoring dendritic cell vaccines for immunotherapy. MRI evaluation of the dendritic cells by using superparamagnetic iron oxide nanoparticles can be seen in the melanoma for evaluation [20]. Newer applications of the immunoimaging for graft versus host disease [21] and rheumatoid arthritis and neurodegenerative diseases like multiple sclerosis [22] and Alzheimer's disease can be evaluated

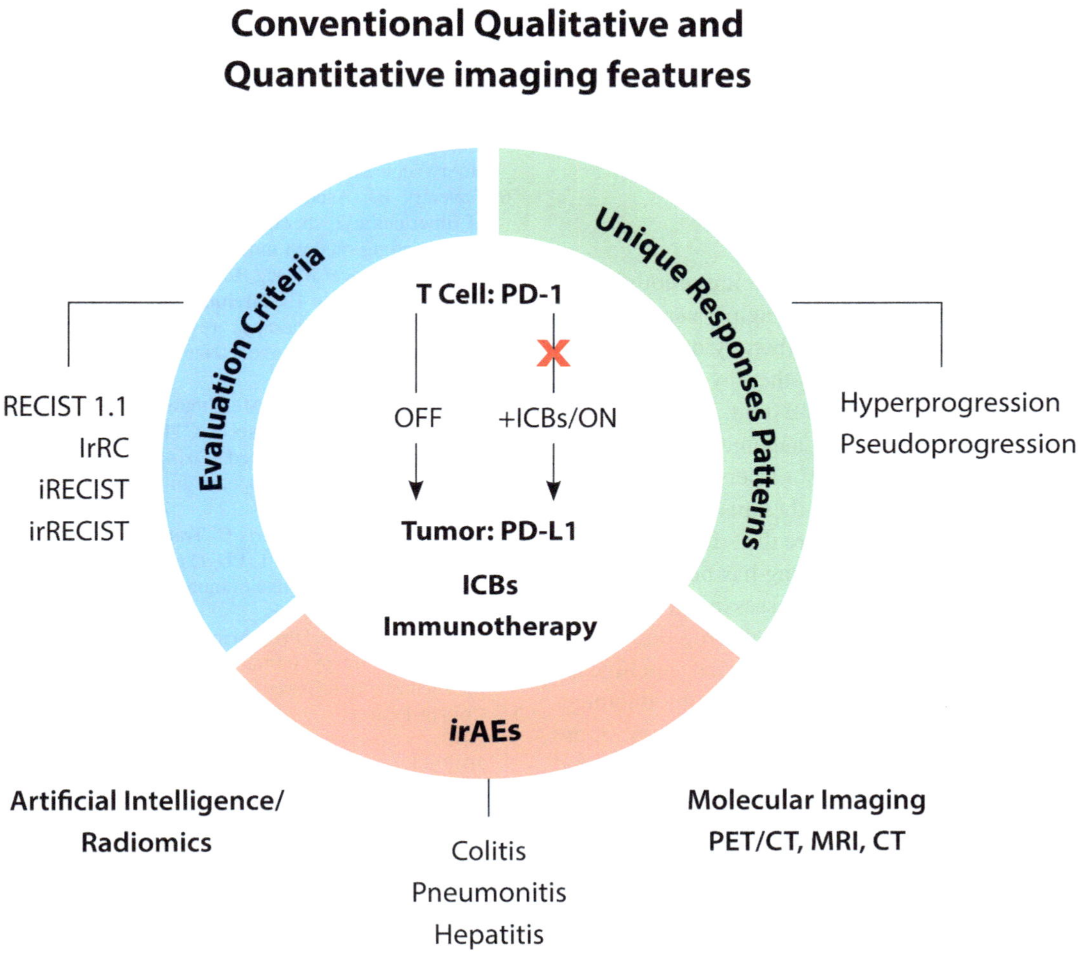

Diagram 17.2 Conventional quantitative and qualitative features of immunoimaging

17.5 ImmunoPET

Immuno-positron emission tomography (immunoPET) is the newer concept of the molecular imaging modality which is combining the excellent specificity of monoclonal antibody (mAb) along with the sensitivity of the PET. ImmunoPET probes are being seen as the development of various radiochemistry and conjugation strategies. Various nanobodies along with more specific binding affinity are used for the design of various novel immunoPET probes. Due to the dynamic and the non-invasive expression of heterogeneous tumour antigens, this modality has changed the theranostic aspect of these malignancies. With this the immunoPET has become the modality of choice for the evaluation of specific tumour markers, immune cells, immune checkpoints, and various inflammatory processes. Combination of the immunoPET imaging for antibody drug development is done by antibody-targeting abilities and distribution profiles [23–29].

17.6 Immunotheranostics

The immunotheranostics is the newer concept where immunotherapy is being used for the combination of the therapeutic, diagnostic, and various screening technologies. This is again based on various entities like small molecules, peptides, antibodies, and nanoparticles and also various cells of the targets [30–34].

17.7 Expanding Roles for Immunoimaging

The basic aim here is to have immunotherapies to succeed. By immunoimaging various other applications like immunotherapy drug development and for the immunotherapy strategies can be evaluated to the larger extent. By early evaluation of the disease, management will become more specific. In this era of personalized medicine, the highly targeted therapeutics can evolve better to target drug before the administration of the drug. Here PET imaging has better sensitivity for the quantitative assessment of target expression, drug selection, and drug dosing.

Machine learning and artificial intelligence will also have an important role in immunoimaging in the future which will again be more focussed towards the concept of the personalized medicine.

17.8 Conclusion

Technological innovations have defined the use of various concepts of immunoimaging for various pathologies. By the emergence of the different biomarkers, also it helps in the more focussed analysis of various disease processes acting as the theranostic approach for various disease entities.

References

1. Pysz MA, Gambhir SS, Willmann JK. Molecular imaging: current status and emerging strategies. Clin Radiol. 2010;65:500–16.
2. Sauter AW, Wehrl HF, Kolb A, Judenhofer MS, Pichler BJ. Combined PET/MRI: one step further in multimodality imaging. Trends Mol Med. 2010;16:501–8.
3. Liu H, Saxena A, Sidhu SS, Wu D. Fc engineering for developing therapeutic bispecific antibodies and novel scaffolds. Front Immunol. 2017;8:38. https://doi.org/10.3389/fimmu.2017.00038.
4. Tsung K, Norton JA. Lessons from Coley's toxin. Surg Oncol. 2006;15(1):25–8.
5. Gardner TA, Elzey BD, Hahn NM. Sipuleucel-T (Provenge) autologous vaccine approved for treatment of men with asymptomatic or minimally symptomatic castrate-resistant metastatic prostate cancer. Hum Vaccine Immunother. 2012;8(4):534–9.
6. Coventry BJ, Ashdown ML. The 20th anniversary of interleukin-2 therapy bimodal role explaining long-standing random induction of complete clinical responses. Cancer Manag Res. 2012;4:215–21.
7. Drake CG, Lipson EJ, Brahmer JR. Breathing new life into immunotherapy: review of melanoma, lung and kidney cancer. Nat Rev Clin Oncol. 2014;11(1):24–37.
8. Snyder A, Makarov V, Merghoub T, et al. Genetic basis for clinical response to CTLA-4 blockade in melanoma. N Engl J Med. 2014;371(23):2189–99 [Published correction appears in N Engl J Med. 2018;379(22):2185].
9. Constantinidou A, Alifieris C, Trafalis DT. Targeting programmed cell death-1 (PD-1) and ligand (PD-L1): a new era in cancer active immunotherapy. Pharmacol Ther. 2019;194:84–106.
10. Zang X. 2018 Nobel Prize in medicine awarded to cancer immunotherapy: immune checkpoint blockade—a personal account. Genes Dis. 2018;5(4):302–3.
11. Couzin-Frankel J. Breakthrough of the year 2013: cancer immunotherapy. Science. 2013;342(6165):1432–3.
12. Oliveira LJC, Gongora ABL, Jardim DLF. Spectrum and clinical activity of PD-1/PD-L1 inhibitors: regulatory approval and under development. Curr Oncol Rep. 2020;22(7):70.
13. Topalian SL, Taube JM, Anders RA, Pardoll DM. Mechanism-driven biomarkers to guide immune checkpoint blockade in cancer therapy. Nat Rev Cancer. 2016;16(5):275–87.
14. Postow MA, Sidlow R, Hellmann MD. Immune-related adverse events associated with immune checkpoint blockade. N Engl J Med. 2018;378(2):158–68.
15. Sosa A, Lopez Cadena E, Simon Olive C, Karachaliou N, Rosell R. Clinical assessment of immune-related adverse events. Ther Adv Med Oncol. 2018; https://doi.org/10.1177/1758835918764628.
16. June CH, Warshauer JT, Bluestone JA. Is autoimmunity the Achilles' heel of cancer immunotherapy? Nat Med. 2017;23(5):540–7. [Published correction appears in Nat Med 2017;23(8):1004].
17. Chan KK, Bass AR. Autoimmune complications of immunotherapy: pathophysiology and management. BMJ. 2020;369:m736.
18. Ngen EJ, Artemov D. Advances in monitoring cell-based therapies with magnetic resonance imaging: future perspectives. Int J Mol Sci. 2017;18:14–22.
19. Liao F, Xu H, Torrey N, Road P, Jolla L. In vivo imaging with antibodies and engineered fragments. Mol Immunol. 2015;2:142–52.
20. de Vries IJM, Lesterhuis WJ, Barentsz JO, et al. Magnetic resonance tracking of dendritic cells in mel-

anoma patients for monitoring of cellular therapy. Nat Biotechnol. 2005;23:1407–13.
21. Ronald JA, Kim BS, Gowrishankar G, et al. A PET imaging strategy to visualize activated T cells in acute graft-versus-host disease elicited by allogenic hematopoietic cell transplant. Cancer Res. 2017;77:2893–902.
22. James ML, Hoehne A, Mayer AT, et al. Imaging B cells in a mouse model of multiple sclerosis using 64 Cu-rituximab-PET. J Nucl Med. 2017;58:1845–51.
23. James ML, Gambhir SS. A molecular imaging primer: modalities, imaging agents, and applications. Physiol. Rev. 2012;92:897–965.
24. Rahmim A, Lodge MA, Karakatsanis NA, Panin VY, Zhou Y, McMillan A, Cho S, Zaidi H, Casey ME, Wahl RL. Dynamic whole-body PET imaging: principles, potentials and applications. Eur J Nucl Med Mol Imaging. 2019;46:501–18.
25. Scott AM, Wolchok JD, Old LJ. Antibody therapy of cancer. Nat Rev Cancer. 2012;12:278–87.
26. Khalil DN, Smith EL, Brentjens RJ, Wolchok JD. The future of cancer treatment: immunomodulation, CARs and combination immunotherapy. Nat Rev Clin Oncol. 2016;13:273–90.
27. Sanmamed MF, Chen L. A paradigm shift in cancer immunotherapy: from enhancement to normalization. Cell. 2018;175:313–26.
28. Pimlott SL, Sutherland A. Molecular tracers for the PET and SPECT imaging of disease. Chem Soc Rev. 2011;40:149–62.
29. Cho SY, Lipson EJ, Im HJ, Rowe SP, Gonzalez EM, Blackford A, Chirindel A, Pardoll DM, Topalian SL, Wahl RL. Prediction of response to immune checkpoint inhibitor therapy using early-Time-Point (18) F-FDG PET/CT imaging in patients with advanced melanoma. J Nucl Med. 2017;58:1421–8.
30. Raimondi MT, Donnaloja F, Barzaghini B, Bocconi A, Conci C, Parodi V, et al. Bioengineering tools to speed up the discovery and preclinical testing of vaccines for SARS-CoV-2 and therapeutic agents for COVID-19. Theranostics. 2020;10:7034–52.
31. Chen X. Introducing Theranostics journal—from the editor-in-chief. Theranostics. 2011;1:1–2.
32. Li J, Van Valkenburgh J, Hong X, Conti PS, Zhang X, Chen K. Small molecules as theranostic agents in cancer immunology. Theranostics. 2019;9:7849–71.
33. Su T, Zhang Y, Valerie K, Wang XY, Lin S, Zhu G. STING activation in cancer immunotherapy. Theranostics. 2019;9:7759–71.
34. Zhang L, Huang Y, Lindstrom AR, Lin TY, Lam KS, Li Y. Peptide-based materials for cancer immunotherapy. Theranostics. 2019;9:7807–25.

18 Optical Imaging

Key Points (Abstract)

Optical imaging is the newer novel imaging technique which is important for the evaluation of various pathologies which routine conventional imaging modalities cannot diagnose. This optical imaging is based on the concept of bioluminescence and fluorescence and is the newer imaging modality for the evaluation of the disease and therapy. This innovative concept of the molecular biology and chemistry is using various optical methods for the evaluation of various cellular and molecular. Various mechanisms in the form of protein interactions, protein degradation, and protease activity are noted by different algorithms. Optical imaging is already being used for research in small animal models, as a concept of molecular imaging.

Keywords

Bioluminescence · Planar fluorescence imaging · Fluorescence molecular tomography · Optoacoustics · Multispectral optoacoustic tomography · Multispectral imaging Hybrid systems · Data processing

Diffuse optical imaging (DOI) is a newer imaging modality which is label-free, very safe, and cheap and has features of quantitative imaging having the property of metabolic and molecular contrasts by using visible or near-infrared light. These modalities have excellent resolution which can image up to several centimetres deep in tissues so that the imaging of human tissues and organ can be easily done. This imaging modality is already existing for academic research, having very good depth, very good resolution, field of view, blend of the spectral content, and various specific imaging criteria. Acquisition and processing speeds are less, and this is the disadvantage for clinical exploration and implementation.

Optical imaging is advantageous as it is very safe, simple to use, and very cost-effective. Another aspect is also the very high scattering and high absorption in various living tissues. These will be having different modalities which can be easily differentiated: planar imaging comprising of the fluorescence and bioluminescence in vivo imaging, optical tomography, and optoacoustic approaches. Here the latest advantages of various optical in vivo imaging along with the various pharmacological applications, and also for the development of the new optical imaging probes. This will have a very strong absorption for the different tissue like the haemoglobin thus overcoming the limitations due to scattering.

18.1 Introduction

Optical imaging is the newer concept of non-invasive imaging which doesn't have ionizing radiation by using the visible light which has

S. Shaikh, *Advances in Imaging*, https://doi.org/10.1007/978-981-16-9535-3_18

specific properties for getting more detailed images of specific organs as well as the tissues and also of the cells and molecules. Here it uses the special properties of light as well as photons which are particles of light as well as that of electromagnetic radiation. It is minimally invasive or non-invasive in nature and is using the visible, ultraviolet, and infrared light, and due to this the optical imaging is safe and can be used for repeated use. Thus, optical imaging is used for the soft tissue evaluation as the soft tissues are capable of absorbing and scattering the light. Based on this principle, optical imaging is capable of measuring the metabolic changes of the functions of the tissues. The principle of this imaging modality is based on light generation, like bioluminescence or fluorescence imaging, which is on the principle of light absorption like optoacoustics (Diagram 18.1). These all-imaging modalities are in vivo imaging having higher sensitivities; they are safe, more sensitive, and have the non-ionizing wavelengths. These are also very cost-effective in comparison with other conventional imaging modalities [1, 2]. Scattering and absorption of tissue are the drawbacks [3–7]. Scattering will deviate the direction of light causing the blurring of the image. The presence of melanin and blood reduces the intensity causing decreased signal-to-noise ratio in the visible range [5–7]. Absorption will lead to signal loss due to the excitation and emission of the wavelengths and comprising of the haemoglobin, melanin, water, and lipids which are least absorbed [8, 9]. High scattering can obtain a very good 3D image or quantitative information of the living organism.

Various imaging approaches which are seen in the optical in vivo imaging are categorized in three categories: (1) planar optical imaging, (2) optical tomography, and (3) optoacoustic tomography.

18.2 Planar Optical Imaging

Planar optical imaging is the very commonly used technique because it is very simple to use and is of very low cost. This source of the light generation in the two planar imaging modalities will be on the basis of the bioluminescence and fluorescence. These modalities will have a camera with very high sensitivity (CCD mainly) with aperture camera taking the single long exposure image.

18.2.1 Bioluminescence

Oxidation of a substrate (luciferin) which is mediated by an enzyme (luciferase) is the principle of bioluminescence imaging. Here the luciferase will use the ATP and magnesium leading to

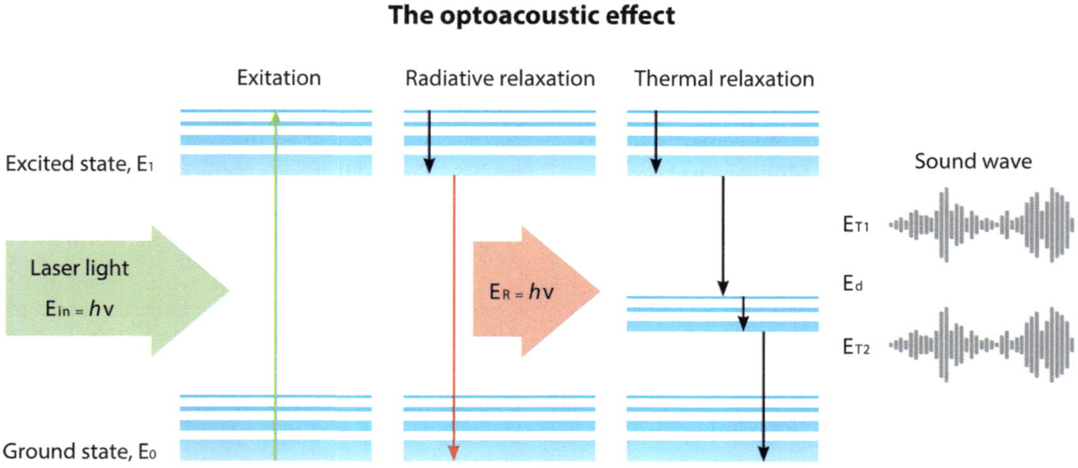

Diagram 18.1 Basic concept of the optoacoustic effect for the use of optical imaging

the emission of light, based on the pH, the polarity of the solvent, and the microenvironment of the enzyme [10]. As this luciferase is cloned [11], this luc gene is being used for gene regulation studies. Thus, the newer bioluminescent probes are used to detect specific activities of the enzyme. Thus, bioluminescence is the important component of the in vivo imaging with the biggest advantage of absent background signal (Diagram 18.2).

18.2.2 Fluorescence In Vivo Imaging

The important concept of the fluorescent agent is that in the presence of the light source, there will be fluorescence as a result of radiative transition from the excited singlet state higher energy to lower energy as followed by the Stoke's law [12, 13]. The biggest advantage is the higher sensitivity, and with the latest advances in fluorescence, this is used for non-invasive imaging. Image generation due to the excitation the size should be that of the fluorophore. Pharmacological studies [14] showed the use of planar fluorescence for the monitoring response to the therapy in murine models of Alzheimer's disease.

Autofluorescence and planar fluorescence imaging are similar (Diagram 18.3). In this prior anatomical information and various optical properties will significantly improve the image quality and quantitation.

18.3 Optoacoustic In Vivo Imaging

Based on the principle of the emission of sound due to the transient increase in volume due to light absorption, photoacoustic effect will be used to image in 3D location with fluorescence probe concentration by using the advanced acoustic transducers and various light sources. This will cause image blurring due to less scattering and increased penetration depth with no significant loss of signal to noise. Pulsed lasers can be used by ultrasound wave for the localized absorption of pulse of light by the tissue. Multiple

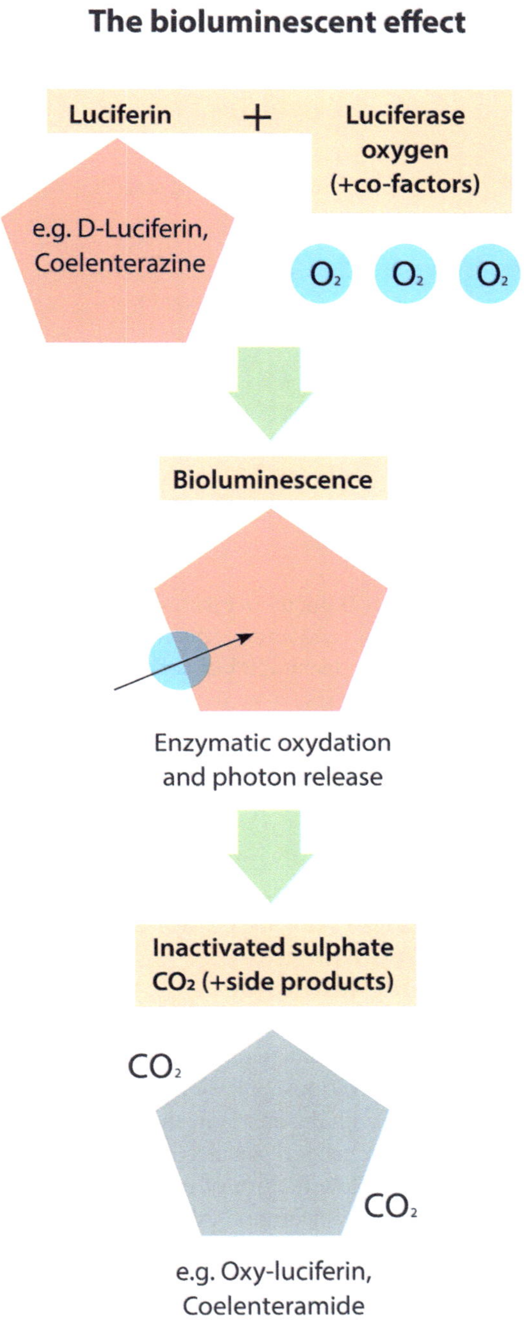

Diagram 18.2 Bioluminescence effect for optical imaging

locations and the various tomographic methods will be used for the multispectral optoacoustic tomography (MSOT), and with these different fluorophores can be separated with the quantification

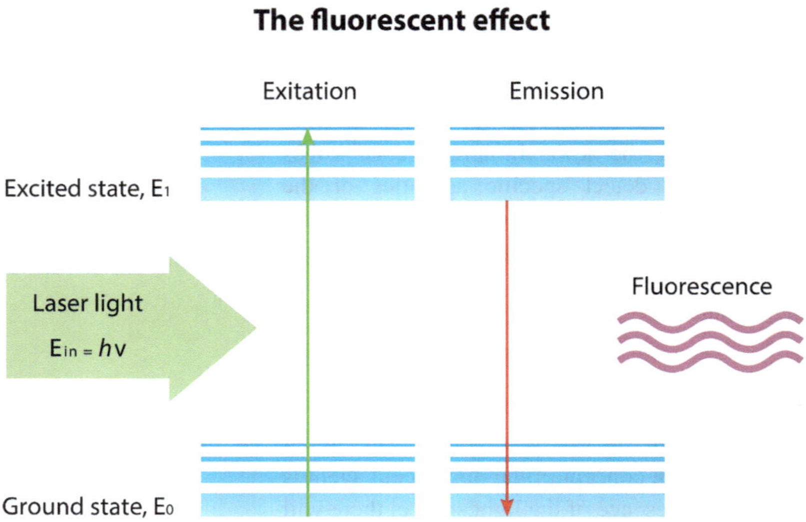

Diagram 18.3 Fluorescent imaging concepts

methods [15–17], focussing the use of the MSOT for quantitative and more specific for in vivo imaging. As the haemoglobin is having stronger absorber properties, the use of optoacoustic tomography will be there for differentiating vascular structures and also for measuring oxygen saturation and blood volume in a particular tissue [18, 19].

18.4 Latest Advances to Improve Quantification and Resolution

The quantification and resolution can be changed by using the various emission spectra of the probes along with the anatomical information.

Bioluminescence resonance energy transfer (BRET) will allow the use of excitation sources and the emission spectrum in the optical window of the spectrum; in this the blood absorption is minimum [8, 9]. In optoacoustics, fluorescent probe advances are related to the probes of high absorption properties and quantum yield. These optoacoustic imaging principles are based on the new acoustic probes consisting of various metallic nanoparticles like gold having very higher absorption [20, 21]. Cherenkov-excited luminescence imaging (CELSI) is also there to improve resolution and avoid the effect of absorption in fluorophores [22–24]. This technique of the Cherenkov-emitted NIR light forms the ionizing radiation which is generated in a linear accelerator where the imaging fluorescent markers can have penetration deep in tissue and have higher resolution.

Hybrid Systems: Optical imaging modalities can be combined with structural imaging modalities like X-ray, CT, and MRI for using the anatomical information for improving the resolution as well as sensitivity [25]. The technical aspects of these hybrid systems will be compatible with different imaging modalities and also in sequential imaging [26].

18.5 Future Outlook

The optical imaging modalities with the essential tools in pharmacological studies can be used for in vivo imaging of the animals. Each modality is having advantages as well as disadvantages due to the effect of absorption as well as the scattering of light which will be propagating in various living tissues. In quantitative imaging, the location of the probe and tomography are combined with routine anatomical imaging modalities like MRI or X-ray/CT. Thus, optoacoustic tomography in particular MSOT is better and has the best resolution, except for the imaging of the lung where it has limitations. More specific near-infrared fluorescent probes and proteins with distinct spectral features and specific nanoparticles for high and specific optoacoustic signal generation are generated with further improvement of the performance of the technologies opening newer opportunities for various newer applications. Optical imaging will be having very high sensitivity and specificity for offering the fullest potential for the 3D quantitative imaging.

Various photon-tissue interactions form the basis for most of medical imaging modalities (Diagram 18.4). The various aspects of optical microscopy, optical coherence tomography, mammography, and X-ray computed tomography will be relying on the various aspects. Various high-resolution imaging modalities will be using the lower-energy photons and penetration of few millimetres due to optical scattering. Diffuse optical imaging (DOI) will multiply scattered photons and then will interact with the tissue for the several centimetres below the surface [27]. The increase in penetration depth will cause increased uncertainty about the probing volume, thus limiting the spatial resolution for approximately 0.5–10 mm depending on the measurement geometry and tissue type [28, 29]. The DOI is considered as safe and inexpensive modality of imaging which is more sensitive to haemoglobin and other tissue chromophores, still with limited spatial resolution. The recent developments will be causing major improvements with the potential to bring metabolic and molecular information directly and immediately to the treating physician.

The change in the arterial volume is based on various phases of the cardiac cycle and venous volume changes during the respiratory cycle [30, 31]. The use of the photoplethysmographic (PPG) waveform for the evaluation of the hemodynamic information, helping the substantially faster rates to capture these dynamics [32, 33]. Fast optical scattering changes or event-related optical signals (EROS) will be used to study neuronal activation [34–36]. The oxygenation cycles which are seen in the timescales of about 15 min [37] will show the cycles as fast as one cycle per minute [38]. The use of various DOI methods will show that the breast tumour haemodynamic will behave differently than normal breast tissue in breath hold [39]. For this the DOI data should be

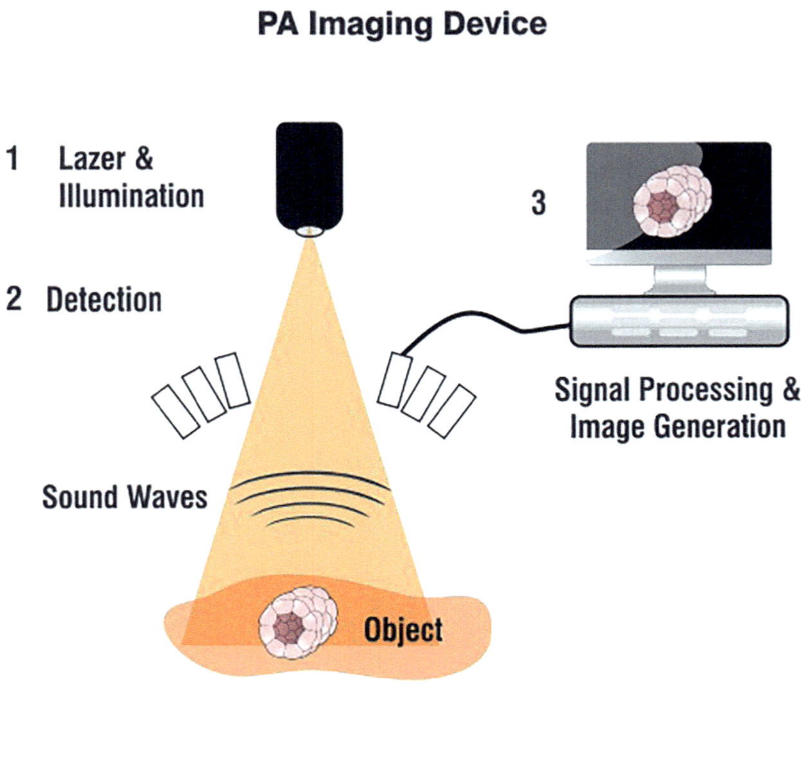

Diagram 18.4 Photo-acoustic imaging technique

processed easily to image larger volumes of tissue at very high speed. This will clear the regulation in the diseased tissues like tumours and also for the more specific tissue brain.

18.6 Overview of Diffuse Optical Imaging Methodologies

DOI instruments are of three main categories: continuous wave (CW), time-domain (TD), and frequency domain (FD). CW techniques are simple in design, are least expensive, and can take the rapid measurements. CW measurements can only measure the relative changes in various tissue chromophore concentrations [40]. The other FD and TD techniques can separate the scattering from absorption, thus enabling the direct measurement of the tissue absorption coefficient (μa). To quantify the absolute molar concentration, various oxy- and deoxyhaemoglobins in tissue are also marked with the spectra and near-infrared (NIR), time-domain diffuse optical imaging (TD-DOI), frequency domain diffuse optical spectroscopy (FD-DOS), diffuse optical topography/tomography (DOT), and spatial frequency domain imaging (SFDI). TD-DOI uses short pulses of light to measure the temporal point spread function (TPSF) of tissue, whereas FD-DOS uses temporally modulated light to measure how a sample changes the amplitude and phase of a propagating photon density wave. Both of these techniques can be used to extract tissue absorption and scattering. DOT uses measurements made at many different locations of the tissue to reconstruct the spatial variation of absorbers in the sampled region.

18.7 Time-Domain Diffuse Optical Imaging

Traditional TD-DOI principle is based on the short pulse of near-infrared light into the tissue. With the scattered photons which can be detected by the time-correlated single photon counting (TCSPC), these can evaluate the temporal point spread function (TPSF) [41, 42]. This is also important for the depth-sensitive imaging which will be helpful in functional activation of the brain. The acquisition time needs to be developed in such a way that it will develop new sources and detectors, thus leading to faster measurements and multiplexing [42].

18.8 Frequency Domain Diffuse Optical Spectroscopy

The frequency domain diffuse optical spectroscopy (FD-DOS) uses various light sources which will be modulated at various radiofrequencies (typically 50 MHz to 1 GHz). These options of the optical absorption and scattering will be quantified by the measurement of the amplitude and phase of the propagating photon density wave that will be travelling [43–46]. There is no need for the pulsed laser or photon counting detector.

18.9 Diffuse Optical Topography and Tomography

The newer techniques can be more precise for generating 3D images of the brain, breast, and other tissues in order to improve the spatial localization of DOI contrast [47–49]. CW is commonly used as it is very simple and speed afforded by CW measurements [50–52]. There will be constant intensity of the light source into tissue, by an array of optical sources and/or optical fibres impinging on the tissue over a wide area.

18.10 Spatial Frequency Domain Imaging

Spatial frequency domain imaging (SFDI) is a wide-field DOI technique which will be providing the absorption and scattering on a pixel-by-pixel basis, having the shallow tissue depth (i.e. 2–5 mm). These will be using various spatial patterns of light which will be projected to detect diffusely the scattered light over a wide area 2.97. The tissue should be measured by using these two spatial frequencies to accurately estimate both μa and μs. SFDI method is a common method which will collect images in different phases for each spatial frequency. This can be used more computationally to isolate the tissue response at each spatial frequency 2 T [53–55].

18.11 Conclusion

Thus, the use of optical imaging is the future of molecular imaging for the precise diagnosis of the various pathologies as described. Still, most of them are in infancy, but a lot more can happen for the evaluation.

References

1. Ntziachristos V, Leroy-Willig A, Tavitian B, editors. Textbook of in-vivo imaging in vertebrates. West Sussex: Wiley; 2007.
2. Stuker F, Ripoll J, Rudin M. Fluorescence molecular tomography: principles and potential for pharmaceutical research. Pharmaceutics. 2011;3:229–74. https://doi.org/10.3390/pharmaceutics3020229.
3. Boas DA, Pitris C, Ramanujam N, editors. Handbook of biomedical optics. Boca Raton: CRC; 2011.
4. Branchini BR, Ablamsky DM, Davis AL, Southworth TL, Butler B, Fan F, et al. Red-emitting luciferases for bioluminescence reporter and imaging applications. Anal Biochem. 2010;396:290–7. https://doi.org/10.1016/j.ab.2009.09.009.
5. Ripoll J, Arranz A. Advances in optical imaging for pharmacological studies. Front Pharmacol. 2015;6:189.
6. Ripoll J. Principles of diffuse light propagation. Singapore: World Scientific; 2012.
7. Sadikot RT, Blackwell TS. Bioluminescence imaging. Proc Am Thorac Soc. 2005;2:537–40, 511–2. https://doi.org/10.1513/pats.200507-067DS.
8. Ntziachristos V, Ripoll J, Wang LV, Weissleder R. Looking and listening to light: the evolution of whole-body photonic imaging. Nat. Biotechnol. 2005;23:313–20. https://doi.org/10.1038/nbt1074.
9. Jacques SL. Optical properties of biological tissues: a review. Phys. Med. Biol. 2013;58:5007–8. https://doi.org/10.1088/0031-9155/58/14/5007.
10. Li J, Chen L, Du L, Li M. Cage the firefly luciferin!—a strategy for developing bioluminescent probes. Chem. Soc. Rev. 2013;42:662–76. https://doi.org/10.1039/C2CS35249D.
11. de Wet JR, Wood KV, Helinski DR, DeLuca M. Cloning of firefly luciferase cDNA and the expression of active luciferase in Escherichia coli. Proc Natl Acad Sci USA. 1985;82:7870–3. https://doi.org/10.1073/pnas.82.23.7870.
12. Sauer M, Hofkens J, Enderlein J, editors. Handbook of fluorescence spectroscopy and imaging: from ensemble to single molecules. Weinheim: Wiley VCH; 2011.
13. Shcherbo D, Merzlyak EM, Chepurnykh TV, Fradkov AF, Ermakova GV, Solovieva EA, et al. Bright far-red fluorescent protein for whole-body imaging. Nat Methods. 2007;4:741–6. https://doi.org/10.1038/nmeth1083.
14. Zhang X, Tian Y, Zhang C, Tian X, Ross AW, Moir RD, et al. Near-infrared fluorescence molecular imaging of amyloid beta species and monitoring therapy in animal models of Alzheimer's disease. Proc Natl Acad Sci USA. 2015;112:9734–9. https://doi.org/10.1073/pnas.1505420112.
15. Laufer J, Delpy D, Elwell C, Beard P. Quantitative spatially resolved measurement of tissue chromophore concentrations using photoacoustic spectroscopy: application to the measurement of blood oxygenation and haemoglobin concentration. Phys Med Biol. 2007;52:141–68. https://doi.org/10.1088/0031-9155/52/1/010.
16. Ma R, Taruttis A, Ntziachristos V, Razansky D. Multispectral optoacoustic tomography (MSOT) scanner for whole-body small animal imaging. Opt Express. 2009;17:21414–26. https://doi.org/10.1364/OE.17.021414.
17. Tzoumas S, Deliolanis N, Morscher S, Ntziachristos V. Unmixing molecular agents from absorbing tissue in multispectral optoacoustic tomography. IEEE Trans Med Imaging. 2014;33:48–60. https://doi.org/10.1109/TMI.2013.2279994.
18. Lao Y, Xing D, Yang S, Xiang L. Noninvasive photoacoustic imaging of the developing vasculature during early tumor growth. Phys Med Biol. 2008;53:4203–12. https://doi.org/10.1088/0031-9155/53/15/013.
19. Hu S, Wang LV. Photoacoustic imaging and characterization of the microvasculature. J Biomed Opt. 2010;15:1–15. https://doi.org/10.1117/1.3281673.
20. Bao C, Beziere N, Del Pino P, Pelaz B, Estrada G, Tian F, et al. Gold nanoprisms as optoacoustic signal nanoamplifiers for in vivo bioimaging of gastrointestinal cancers. Small. 2013;9:68–74. https://doi.org/10.1002/smll.201201779.
21. Vonnemann J, Beziere N, Böttcher C, Riese SB, Kuehne C, Dernedde J, et al. Polyglycerol sulfate functionalized gold nanorods as optoacoustic signal nanoamplifiers for in vivo bioimaging of rheumatoid arthritis. Theranostics. 2014;4:629–41. https://doi.org/10.7150/thno.8518.
22. Zhang R, Glaser A, Esipova TV, Kanick SC, Davis SC, Vinogradov S, et al. Čerenkov radiation emission and excited luminescence (CREL) sensitivity during external beam radiation therapy: Monte Carlo and tissue oxygenation phantom studies. Biomed Opt Express. 2012;3:2381–94. https://doi.org/10.1364/BOE.3.002381.

23. Zhang R, Davis SC, Demers J-LH, Glaser AK, Gladstone DJ, Esipova TV, et al. Oxygen tomography by Čerenkov-excited phosphorescence during external beam irradiation. J Biomed Opt. 2013;18:50503. https://doi.org/10.1117/1.JBO.18.5.050503.
24. Zhang R, D'Souza AV, Gunn JR, Esipova TV, Vinogradov SA, Glaser AK, et al. Cherenkov-excited luminescence scanned imaging. Opt Lett. 2015;40:827–30. https://doi.org/10.1364/OL.40.000827.
25. Ale A, Ermolayev V, Herzog E, Cohrs C, de Angelis MH, Ntziachristos V. FMT-XCT: in vivo animal studies with hybrid fluorescence molecular tomography-X-ray computed tomography. Nat Methods. 2012;9:615–20. https://doi.org/10.1038/nmeth.2014.
26. McCann CM, Waterman P, Figueiredo JL, Aikawa E, Weissleder R, Chen JW. Combined magnetic resonance and fluorescence imaging of the living mouse brain reveals glioma response to chemotherapy. Neuroimage. 2009;45:360–9. https://doi.org/10.1016/j.neuroimage.2008.12.022.
27. O'Sullivan TD. Diffuse optical imaging using spatially and temporally modulated light. J Biomed Opt. 2012;17:071311.
28. Cuccia DJ, Bevilacqua F, Durkin AJ, Ayers FR, Tromberg BJ. Quantitation and mapping of tissue optical properties using modulated imaging. J Biomed Opt. 2009;14(2):024012.
29. Boas DA, Dale AM, Franceschini MA. Diffuse optical imaging of brain activation: Approaches to optimizing image sensitivity, resolution, and accuracy. NeuroImage. 2004;23(Suppl. 1):S275–88.
30. Tromberg BJ, et al. Predicting responses to neoadjuvant chemotherapy in breast cancer: ACRIN 6691 trial of diffuse optical spectroscopic imaging. Cancer Res. 2016;76(20):5933–44.
31. Franceschini MA, et al. Near-infrared spiroximetry: Noninvasive measurements of venous saturation in piglets and human subjects. J. Appl. Physiol. 2002;92(1):372–84.
32. Murray W, Foster PA. The peripheral pulse wave: Information overlooked. J Clin Monit. 1996;12(5):365–77.
33. Allen J, Murray A. Age-related changes in the characteristics of the photoplethysmographic pulse shape at various body sites. Physiol Meas. 2003;24(2):297–307.
34. Gratton G, Fabiani M. The event-related optical signal: A new tool for studying brain function. Int J Psychophysiol. 2001;42(2):109–21.
35. Gratton G, Fabiani M. Fast optical imaging of human brain function. Front Hum Neurosci. 2010;4:1–9.
36. Franceschini MA, Boas DA. Non-invasive measurement of neuronal activity with near-infrared optical imaging. NeuroImage. 2004;21(1):372–86.
37. Michiels C, Tellier C, Feron O. Cycling hypoxia: A key feature of the tumor microenvironment. Biochim Biophys Acta Rev Cancer. 2016;1866(1):76–86.
38. Yu B, et al. Measuring tumor cycling hypoxia and angiogenesis using a side firing fibre optic probe. J Biophotonics. 2014;7(7):552–64.
39. Flexman ML, et al. Optical biomarkers for breast cancer derived from dynamic diffuse optical tomography. J Biomed Opt. 2013;18(9):096012.
40. Sassaroli A, Fantini S. Comment on the modified Beer–Lambert law for scattering media. Phys Med Biol. 2004;49(14):N255–7.
41. Mora AD, et al. Towards next-generation time-domain diffuse optics for extreme depth penetration and sensitivity. Biomed Opt Express. 2015;6(5):1749.
42. Pifferi A, Contini D, Mora AD, Farina A, Spinelli L, Torricelli A. New frontiers in time-domain diffuse optics, a review. J Biomed Opt. 2016;21(9):091310.
43. Tromberg BJ, Svaasand LO, Tsay T-T, Haskell RC. Properties of photon density waves in multiple-scattering media. Appl Opt. 1993;32(4):607.
44. Roblyer D, et al. Optical imaging of breast cancer oxyhemoglobin flare correlates with neoadjuvant chemotherapy response one day after starting treatment. Proc Natl Acad Sci USA. 2011;108(35):14626–31.
45. Tromberg BJ, Svaasand LO, Tsay T-T, Haskell RC, Berns MW. Optical property measurements in turbid media using frequency-domain photon migration. Proc SPIE. 1991;1525:52–8.
46. No K-S, Kwong R, Chou PH, Cerussi A. Design and testing of a miniature broadband frequency domain photon migration instrument. J Biomed Opt. 2008;13(5):050509.
47. Culver JP, et al. Three-dimensional diffuse optical tomography in the parallel plane transmission geometry: Evaluation of a hybrid frequency domain/continuous wave clinical system for breast imaging. Med Phys. 2003;30(2):235–47.
48. Corlu A, et al. Three-dimensional in vivo fluorescence diffuse optical tomography of breast cancer in humans. Opt Express. 2007;15(11):6696–716.
49. Durduran T, Choe R, Baker WB, Yodh AG. Diffuse optics for tissue monitoring and tomography. Rep Prog Phys. 2010;73(7):076701.
50. Corlu A, et al. Uniqueness and wavelength optimization in continuous-wave multispectral diffuse optical tomography. Opt Lett. 2003;28(23):2339–41.
51. Li A, Zhang Q, Culver JP, Miller EL, Boas DA. Reconstructing chromosphere concentration images directly by continuous-wave diffuse optical tomography. Opt Lett. 2004;29(3):256–8.
52. Xu Y, Iftimia N, Jiang H, Key LL, Bolster MB. Imaging of in vitro and in vivo bones and joints with continuous-wave diffuse optical tomography. Opt Express. 2001;8(7):447–51.
53. Zhao Y, et al. Deep learning model for ultrafast multifrequency optical property extractions for spatial frequency domain imaging. Opt Lett. 2018;43(22):5669–72.
54. Bodenschatz N, et al. Detecting structural information of scatters using spatial frequency domain imaging. J Biomed Opt. 2015;20(11):116006.
55. Rohrbach DJ, et al. Preoperative mapping of the nonmelanoma skin cancer using spatial frequency domain and ultrasound imaging. Acad Radiol. 2014;21(2):263–70.

19 Gene-Mediated Imaging

Key Points (Abstract)

Molecular imaging is now a very broad entity including the various aspects like various processes like proteomic, metabolic, cellular biologic, and also genetic imaging. Molecular imaging also is now defined as genetic imaging leading to molecular genetic imaging. The basic concept here is the role of imaging reporter genes which is crucial in molecular genetic imaging. The major three modalities of the molecular genetic imaging are optical imaging, MRI, and nuclear medicine imaging. Every modality has its own reporter genes and probes which will be helpful for bench to bedside applications. These reporter genes can quantify the levels of expression of specific exogenous and endogenous genes along the various intracellular biological phenomena. This includes various signal transduction pathways, various associated nuclear receptor activities, and different protein-protein interactions. By virtue of this technique, it will be easier to monitor the tumour mass by in vivo target cells, like immune cells and stem cells. Evolution of drug discovery and development also has impacted on the imaging reporter gene which is being used now for the drug and stem cell therapy development. By the advancements of imaging instrumentation, the use of novel targets and genes, along with the imaging probe developments, will have an important role in the future for diagnosis and therapy of cancer.

Keywords

Molecular imaging · Genomics · Fluorescence resonance energy transfer · MRI probes Fluorescence and bioluminescent imaging Biomarker probes · MRI · PET · SPECT

19.1 Introduction

Imaging the genetics along with molecular genetics for biological mechanisms by the use of technology is crucial for the diagnosis of various disorders. By this technique it will be easier to understand various complex pathways and mechanisms for studying genes, the brain, and associated aspects in various pathologies. As we all know, the important aspect of genetic studies is to inform the risk and apply it for studying the development or disorders

Various genome projects are involved in studying human genome projects [1]. The study of genomics will allow to show manipulation of genes which will have an impact on various developmental processes, cell physiology, and ultimately the cell fate. But with the advancements the basic function is to see the functionality of genes in various cellular processes and diseases. Due to the advancements in the translational and clinical research various changes in the gene expression the subsequent events in the genetic and molecular is seen.

S. Shaikh, *Advances in Imaging*, https://doi.org/10.1007/978-981-16-9535-3_19

Genetic and molecular imaging is now important as it will depict the earliest during the disease progression and development in the form of the changes in the gene expression and also the activation of enzymatic activities as all these changes will be seen before anatomical changes. The availability of the various molecular imaging techniques can be useful to diagnose the changes in cellular activity especially in the pre-pathologic state for earlier disease detection and intervention. This also can be useful to intervene in the form of specific molecular markers for earlier therapy assessment response. By the development of various molecular newer imaging probes in optical and magnetic resonance imaging, it has become an important for in vivo detection of reporter genes for the identification of individual various different cell types, organelles, or proteins. The identification of various endogenous gene expressions and enzymatic activity also can be done in vivo. By this it will be easier to understand cancer progression, various infectious pattern of the diseases and their management options, various protein-protein interactions, different signalling events, and also various disease progression patterns.

Molecular imaging which is also defined as "the spatially localized and/or temporally resolved sensing of molecular and cellular processes in vivo" [2] and here with the combination of the various multiple disciplines which will be involving the engineering, biomedical physics, chemistry, molecular biology, genetics, and medical imaging these all will based on the basic, translational, and clinical research. This reporter gene imaging is based on the concept of various encoding proteins which will be acting like surrogate markers when combined with regions of interest of the genes. Thus, it is the indirect method for the evaluation of the process of gene expression. With this various reporter gene components like various membrane transporters, along with the intra- and extracellular receptors and enzymes, play an important role in the evaluation of various biomarkers. DNA plasmid is the reporter gene which will be attached to the target gene and thus the regulation of the activity of the target gene which is seen as the triggering effect leading to the endogenous promoters and transcription factors. The process will be involved in the gamma emission, ionic oscillation, or positron emission, which can be detected by SPECT, MRI, or PET. Again, based on the properties, these can again be expressed by various luminescent proteins which are being imaged by various optical imaging modalities. There is significant technological development in the imaging instrumentation in magnetic resonance (MR) imaging, ultrasound (US), microscopic single-photon emission tomography (SPECT), and positron emission tomography (PET), and all these are being used as in vivo imaging techniques with various advantages and disadvantages. All these imaging modalities like MRI and optical imaging are not standardized to the extent of very high sensitivity but are having variable spatial resolution, temporal resolution, and also sensitivities [3–5]. By the use of reporter probe developments for cell tracking, gene expression and protease activity all these will be enhancing the possibility of better diagnosis (Diagram 19.1). The use of fluorescent dyes and proteins in the optical fluorescence techniques, by using tissue-penetrating near-infrared light, bioluminescence, and tomographic techniques, is also equally useful and sensitive [6, 7].

The use of various molecular genetic imaging components like use of the reporter gene expression which will be providing the more precise information on the location, duration, and levels of gene expression [8]. Small animal imaging technologies has shown the significant use of the reporter gene imaging by using real-time high-resolution imaging [9]. Reporter gene imaging for the detection of gene expression is based on the indirect method [9]. These genes are genetically encoded as tag or promoter genes for the expression of the specific molecular event [9, 10] (Diagram 19.2). By using various light fluorescent proteins or a specific chemical, the reporter genes can be identified. The biggest advantage of the use of reporter genes is that they can be used at any time including the development, subcellular localization, split-protein complementation assays, and visualizing protein-protein interactions [9, 11].

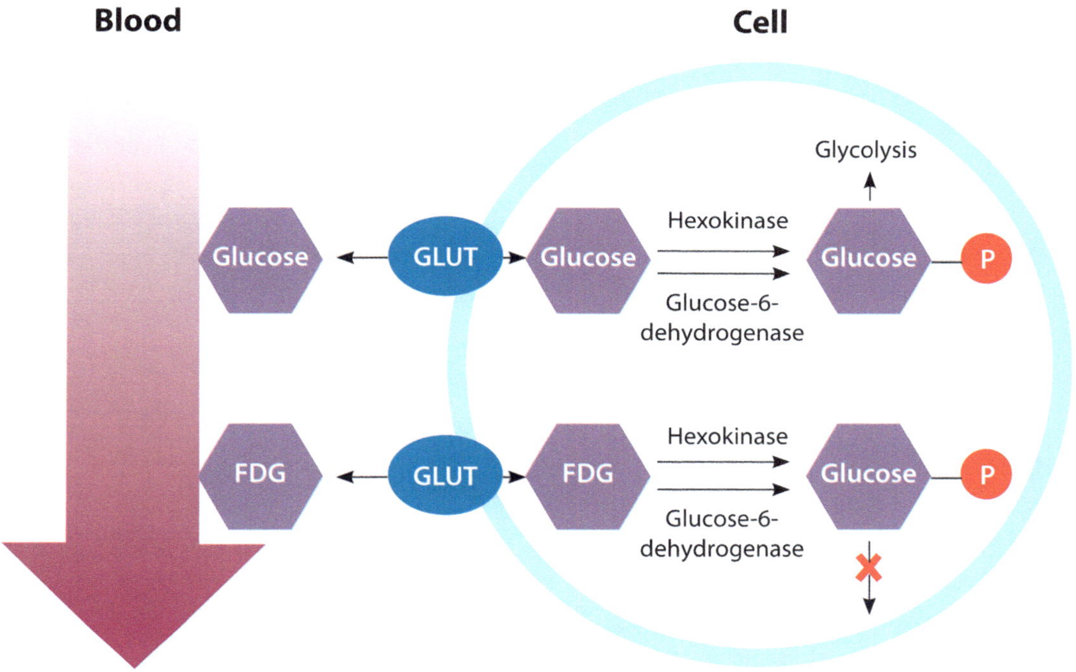

Diagram 19.1 Basic metabolism of the cell

19.2 Optical Imaging

The two optical imaging are fluorescence imaging (FI) and bioluminescence imaging (BLI), and these utilize luciferases as enzymes [3]. The bigger advantage of these imaging modalities is that they have very short acquisition times which will be ranging from few milliseconds to several minutes and having the very high spatial resolution, and on the other hand, they are being limited by various penetration issues, the amount of autofluorescence, light scattering, and absorption of light by haemoglobin [3]. Thus, the optical imaging can be used for the oncolytic virus evaluation in the preclinical setting.

Various fluorescent reporter proteins are used by cloning of GFP in the 1990s and are used to examine subcellular localization of various proteins, gene expression, and track cells [12]. This GFP along with the associated various mutagenic variants is used due to their stability in range of the pH and temperature, and they are less toxic [9, 13]. Usually, the GFP is emitting green light (507 nm) or blue light (488 nm) when it is excited by UV light. The mutation of GFP to yield blue FP (BFP), cyan FP (CFP), and yellow FP (YFP) has resulted in greater stability and spectral properties [14–16]. Thus, fluorescent proteins can be used for the characterization of different spectral properties which will be causing multi-protein labelling by using different colours for depicting various changes for localization and interactions [17]. The spectral shift of fluorescent proteins also will change the depth penetration in various tissue for in vivo studies [18]. The use of genetically encoded FRET fluorescence resonance energy transfer biosensors made up of the fluorescent proteins will be used for better functional understanding of proteins and interactions of various molecules [19, 20]. The basic principle of the FRET is that it is a quantum mechanical process where the non-radiative transfer of energy can be done between a donor and an acceptor molecule by using the Förster mechanism [21, 22]. This energy transfer will require a significant overlap between the

Diagram 19.2 Molecular imaging showing the role of the promoter gene and reporter gene

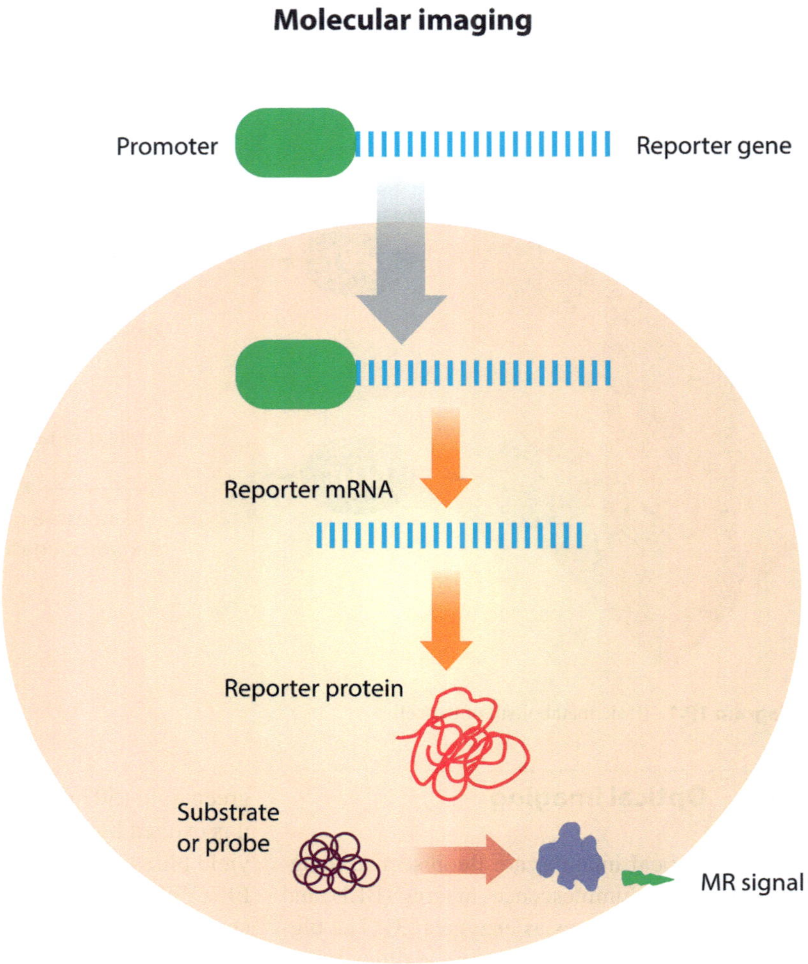

emission spectrum of the donor and the excitation spectrum of the acceptor molecule [22]. When donor and acceptor molecular win close proximity, the excitation of the donor will excite the acceptor molecule, by emitting the light of a particular wavelength [23]. For analysing the most efficient FRET quantification, the donor to acceptor ratio should be one to one. If this ratio is not 1:1, then the observed fluorescent signal is not accurate. FRET also is being used to visualize various changes in protein conformation and quantify protein-protein interactions in vivo [11, 24]. FRET biosensors which are based on fluorescent proteins are being utilized as GFP pairs [25, 26]. Various sensors like Ca(II) probe can utilize the modified GFPs [27, 28].

19.3 Bioluminescence

Bioluminescence is another technique which is used for the transmission of light into the tissues and emitting the luciferase enzymes which will be capable of tracking cells and possible various genetic changes [29]. The luciferase genes by genetic manipulations can be encoded in cells [29]. The principle is that luciferase enzymes will catalyse the oxidation of a substrate producing photons of light. The use of luciferase chemiluminescence is having more significant advantages over fluorescent proteins for the detection of the reporter genes in vivo: (1) as we all know that mammalian tissues do not naturally emit light; due to this the in vivo bioluminescence will have very low background [30]. (2) Luciferases have increased tissue permeability and have the broad spectrum of emission [31]. (3) No interaction of the molecules is there as the principle here is chemiluminescent reaction and not fluorescence. (4) Luciferase is non-toxic and can be used repeatedly. (5) The luciferin is seen in all tissues [32]. Renal excretion is very quick [33]. The process of the bioluminescence was first developed by bacterial infection model [34, 35]. For better stability the lux operon is introduced into pathogenic bacteria as a plasmid integrating into the chromosome [34]. Various processes of the labelling different infectious bacteria with a light-producing signal can be used to detect the location and the extent of infection and can define the efficacy of various antibiotic therapies [36, 37]. Bioluminescence is also used to visualize various viral infections [38, 39]. The efficacy of antiviral treatments also can be studied efficiently [40]. Bioluminescence can also quantify the efficacy of the vector delivery for gene therapy [32, 41, 42]. Gene delivery tracking and quantifying tumour growth in real-time can be done by the use of bioluminescent reporter genes [43]. Tumour size and ultimately tumour burden can be quantified by bioluminescence [44]. Small tumours and metastases can also be seen with higher sensitivity as compared to X-ray in detecting micrometastases in the bone with foci as small as 0.5 mm^3 [45].

19.4 Bioluminescence Resonance Energy Transfer (BRET)

Bioluminescence resonance energy transfer (BRET) is based on the similar principle to FRET that is non-radiative energy transfer between the electromagnetic dipoles of a luminescent donor molecular and a fluorescent protein acceptor [46]. Based on luciferase the three main classes of BRET reporters are there. BRET1, RLuc, is attached to yellow fluorescent protein (EYFP) as the acceptor. BRET3 is the most recently developed [47]. BRET3 is highly sensitive for the single cell and small micrometastases due to better light output and significant tissue penetration [47]. BRET is more sensitive than FRET as it is having very less cell toxicity [46]. External light is used for donor excitation, and there is no cellular scattering of excitation light or cellular autofluorescence [10]. This helps in the monitoring of the short, phasic transient events in signalling pathways. Various transcriptional activities are being visualized in tumour-bearing mice using a mCherry-Luc BRET fusion reporter with HIF1-α-inducible promoter [48]. mCherry fluorescence is another technique used to detect only when tumour cells co-expressed HIF1-α by using the genetically engineered probe to see the deep tissue events having the heterogeneous environment of the tumour [48]. MRI reporter genes are based on metalloproteins, and due to this high spatial and temporal resolution of MRI, it can visualize in better way the internal organs of whole animals [49]. These metalloproteins are transgenes and have the reporter which is made up of the superparamagnetic properties due to the iron component [50, 51]. Ferritin is a metalloprotein made up of ferric oxyhydroxide core [52]. Ferritin is the main iron storage of the body. By the co-expression of the iron transporter, there will be significant increase in the transferrin cellular uptake of iron while maintaining the iron cellular levels to cellular equilibrium [53]. Superparamagnetic iron oxide MRI contrast agent in the form of cellular accumulation by bacterial MagA iron transport protein [54] can be used. The use of a bacterial gene is the one of the biggest advantages. NIR fluorescent β-galactosidase optical contrast agent is very much sensitive for better gene expression by 2D reflectance imaging [55–57].

Various bioluminogenic probes are also used as they are having significant advantage due to bioluminescence spectral property. β-lactamase is the bacterial enzyme used in various infectious diseases as a reporter gene [58]. Thus the fluorescence and bioluminescent imaging of β-lactamase activity as a reporter gene is very important for the detection of the bacterial infection and also to assess the treatment options for antibiotics, [58, 59].

Thus, with these different types of reporter genes, molecular imaging is more specific for tumour progression, identification and the levels of expression of proteases [60, 61], various cell surface markers [62], steroid and different specified growth factor receptors [63], and other modulating signal transduction proteins. Usually, the two general classes of molecular imaging probes are used for endogenous gene expression [64]. Bioactivated probes are based on the detected signal and also after interaction with the target protein. Most of the tumours are having elevated levels of proteolytic enzymes and are directly related to the aggressiveness of the various carcinomas [65]. These proteases promote invasion, metastasis, and angiogenesis, and due to this the protease inhibitors can be used as anticancer therapeutic option [66–68]. Protease activity can be easily identified by optical NIRF and MRI probes for identifying the protease synthase activity in vivo, for tumour progression, and also for the evaluation of the therapeutics. Cleavage of the peptide in relation to the contrast agent shows MMP-2 positive and MMP-2 clearance in knockdown tumours [69]. Thus, it signifies that the cleavage is specific based on the solubility and enhancement protease activity which can be assessed and identified.

MRI is the well-established modality for various preclinical and translational evaluations of cell delivery and gene expression. These MR probes are being used for the evaluation of various exogenous and endogenous gene expressions which will be more specific in identifying various signal transduction pathways and also receptor status or protein-protein interactions. The use of the MR-based receptor genetic imaging will be used for cell migration, for the retention and survival, and also for the monitoring response to the gene expression (Diagram 19.3). Various MRI-

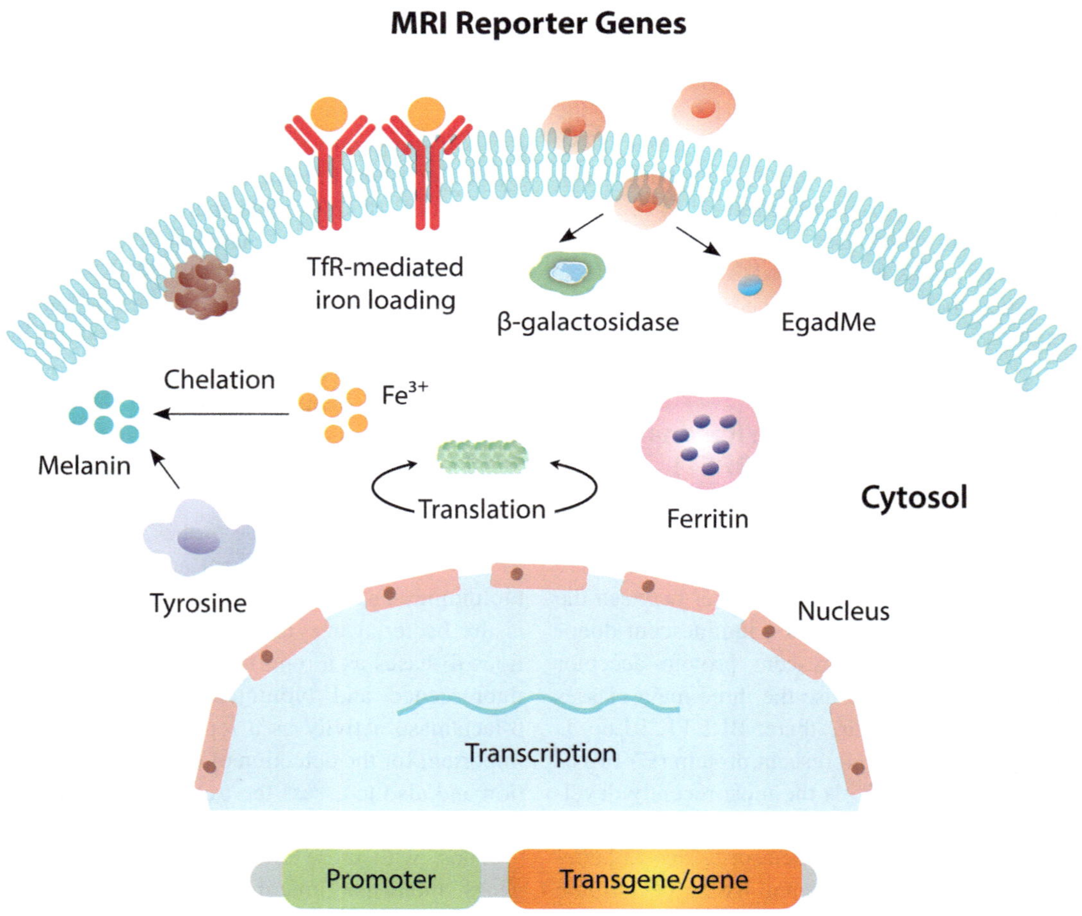

Diagram 19.3 MRI-based reporter genes and their various interactions

based RGI will be using the reporter genes which further can encode various enzymes like the tyrosinase and β-galactosidase, along with various cell receptors like transferrin receptor and also for the endogenous ferritin which has affinity towards the iron and will be binding the iron which will be the MR contrast agent for imaging like T2-W sequences [70].

Various MRI reporter genes are combined with various bioluminescent, fluorescent, and/or PET reporters, which can have high depth penetration leading to higher sensitivities for the profiling of various imaging techniques leading to the newer concept of the multimodality protocol for monitoring gene expression in gene therapy for the assessment of various aspects of the stem cells also (Diagram 19.4).

Thus, the futuristic approach will be to visualize protein-protein interaction, spontaneous signalling events, and various proteolytic events. The use of the exogenous contrast agents like β-galactosidase and β-lactamase activity by optical imaging and MRI will allow tailored management of the disease. With these techniques the valuable information on tumour grade can be evaluated more precisely by using these contrast agents.

19.5 Conclusion

Thus, the development of various molecular imaging probes and their applications will be the landmark in vivo molecular imaging. The analy-

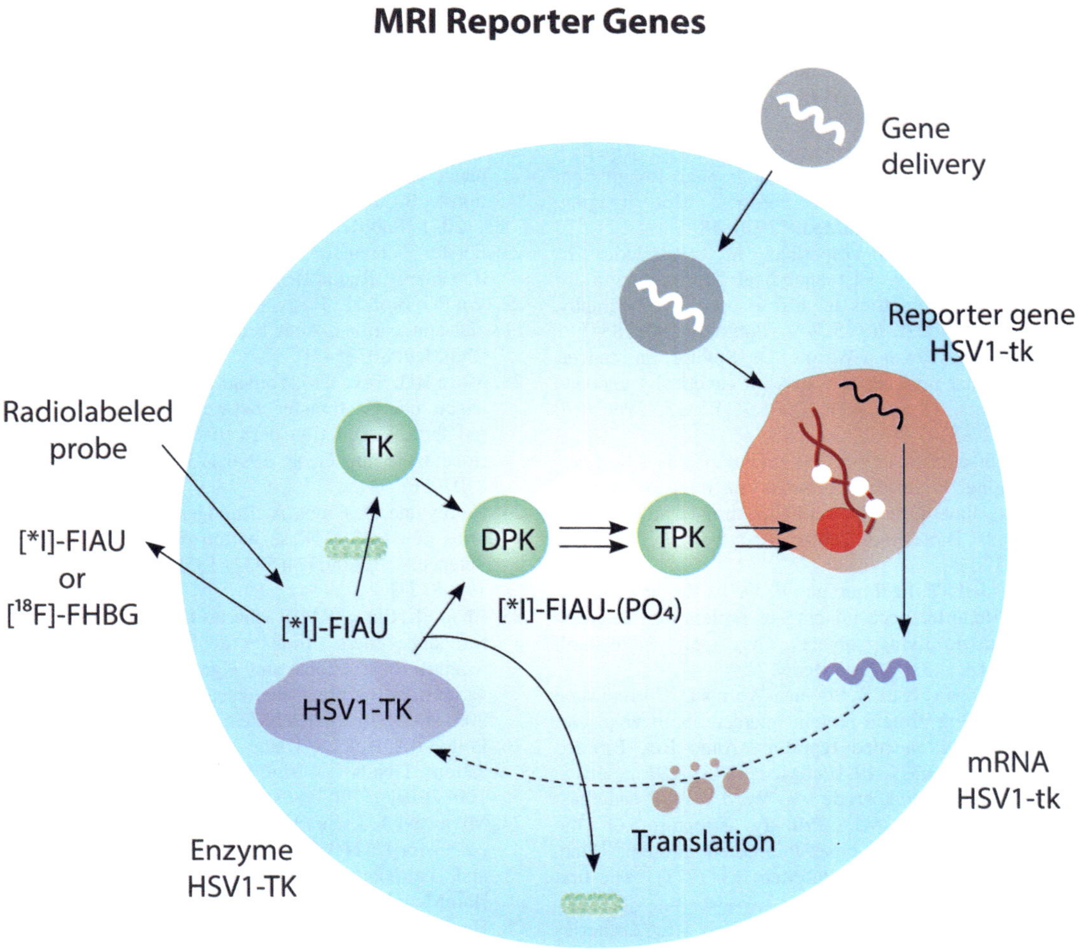

Diagram 19.4 MRI-based herpes simplex virus thymidine kinase reporter gene

sis of the DNA, RNA, or other genetic components can be done more precisely. Again, this is based on the position and intensity of the signal of reporter genes, technologies, and probes which will have a significant impact in the concept of precision medicine.

References

1. Collins FS, Mckusick VA. Implications of the human genome project for medical science. JAMA. 2001;285(5):540–4. [PubMed: 11176855]
2. Piwnica-Worms DR. Introduction to molecular imaging. J Am Coll Radiol. 2004;1(1, Suppl 1):2–3. [PubMed: 17411748]
3. Weissleder R, Mahmood U. Molecular imaging. Radiology. 2001;219(2):316–33. [PubMed: 11323453]
4. Weissleder R. Scaling down imaging: molecular mapping of cancer in mice. Nat Rev Cancer. 2002;2(1):11–8. [PubMed: 11902581]
5. Tsien RY. Imagining imaging's future. Nat Rev Mol Cell Biol. 2003;(Suppl):SS16–21 [PubMed: 14587522].
6. Ntziachristos V, Bremer C, Graves EE, Ripoll J, Weissleder R. In vivo tomographic imaging of near-infrared fluorescent probes. Mol Imaging. 2002;1(2):82–8. [PubMed: 12920848]
7. Ripoll J, Nieto-Vesperinas M, Weissleder R, Ntziachristos V. Fast analytical approximation for arbitrary geometries in diffuse optical tomography. Opt Lett. 2002;27(7):527–9. [PubMed: 18007854]
8. Gross S, Piwnica-Worms D. Spying on cancer: molecular imaging in vivo with genetically encoded reporters. Cancer Cell. 2005;7(1):5–15. [PubMed: 15652745]
9. Nowotschin S, Eakin GS, Hadjantonakis AK. Live-imaging fluorescent proteins in mouse embryos: multi-dimensional, multi-spectral perspectives. Trends Biotechnol. 2009;27(5):266–76. [PubMed: 19339068]
10. Massoud TF, Paulmurugan R, De A, Ray P, Gambhir SS. Reporter gene imaging of protein-protein interactions in living subjects. Curr Opin Biotechnol. 2007;18(1):31–7. [PubMed: 17254764]
11. Villalobos V, Naik S, Piwnica-Worms D. Current state of imaging protein-protein interactions in vivo with genetically encoded reporters. Annu Rev Biomed Eng. 2007;9:321–49. [PubMed: 17461729]
12. Prasher DC, Eckenrode VK, Ward WW, Prendergast FG, Cormier MJ. Primary structure of the Aequorea victoria green-fluorescent protein. Gene. 1992;111(2):229–33 [PubMed: 1347277] *The first cloning of GFP.
13. Griesbeck O, Baird GS, Campbell RE, Zacharias DA, Tsien RY. Reducing the environmental sensitivity of yellow fluorescent protein. Mechanism and applications. J Biol Chem. 2001;276(31):29188–94. [PubMed: 11387331]
14. Heim R, Prasher DC, Tsien RY. Wavelength mutations and posttranslational autoxidation of green fluorescent protein. Proc Natl Acad Sci U S A. 1994;91(26):12501–4. [PubMed: 7809066]
15. Heim R, Tsien RY. Engineering green fluorescent protein for improved brightness, longer wavelengths and fluorescence resonance energy transfer. Curr Biol. 1996;6(2):178–82. [PubMed: 8673464]
16. Rizzo MA, Springer GH, Granada B, Piston DW. An improved cyan fluorescent protein variant useful for fret. Nat Biotechnol. 2004;22(4):445–9. [PubMed: 14990965]
17. Nowotschin S, Eakin GS, Hadjantonakis AK. Dual transgene strategy for live visualization of chromatin and plasma membrane dynamics in murine embryonic stem cells and embryonic tissues. Genesis. 2009;47(5):330–6. [PubMed: 19358158]
18. Chudakov DM, Lukyanov S, Lukyanov KA. Fluorescent proteins as a toolkit for in vivo imaging. Trends Biotechnol. 2005;23(12):605–13. [PubMed: 16269193]
19. Truong K, Ikura M. The use of FRET imaging microscopy to detect protein-protein interactions and protein conformational changes in vivo. Curr Opin Struct Biol. 2001;11(5):573–8. [PubMed: 11785758]
20. Didenko VV. DNA probes using fluorescence resonance energy transfer (FRET): designs and applications. Biotechniques. 2001;31(5):1106–16, 1118, 1120–1 [PubMed: 11730017]
21. Forster T. Transfer mechanisms of electronic excitation energy. Radiat Res Suppl. 1960;2:326–39.
22. Wu PG, Brand L. Resonance energy transfer: methods and applications. Anal Biochem. 1994;218(1):1–13. [PubMed: 8053542]
23. Mitra RD, Silva CM, Youvan DC. Fluorescence resonance energy transfer between blue-emitting and red-shifted excitation derivatives of the green fluorescent protein. Gene. 1996;173(1):13–7. [PubMed: 8707050]
24. Kamiyama D, Chiba A. Endogenous activation patterns of cdc42 GTPase within drosophila embryos. Science. 2009;324(5932):1338–40. [PubMed: 19498173]
25. Chan FK, Siegel RM, Zacharias D, et al. Fluorescence resonance energy transfer analysis of cell surface receptor interactions and signalling using spectral variants of the green fluorescent protein. Cytometry. 2001;44(4):361–8. [PubMed: 11500853]
26. Pollok BA, Heim R. Using GFP in FRET-based applications. Trends Cell Biol. 1999;9(2):57–60. [PubMed: 10087619]
27. Miyawaki A, Llopis J, Heim R, et al. fluorescent indicators for Ca2+ based on green fluorescent proteins and calmodulin. Nature. 1997;388(6645):882–7. [PubMed: 9278050]
28. Hara M, Bindokas V, Lopez JP, et al. Imaging endoplasmic reticulum calcium with a fluorescent biosen-

sor in transgenic mice. Am J Physiol Cell Physiol. 2004;287(4):C932–8. [PubMed: 15163621]
29. Sato A, Klaunberg B, Tolwani R. In vivo bioluminescence imaging. Comp Med. 2004;54(6):631–4. [PubMed: 15679260]
30. De Wet JR, Wood KV, Deluca M, Helinski DR, Subramani S. Firefly luciferase gene: structure and expression in mammalian cells. Mol Cell Biol. 1987;7(2):725–37. [PubMed: 3821727]
31. Bhaumik S, Gambhir SS. Optical imaging of Renilla luciferase reporter gene expression in living mice. Proc Natl Acad Sci U S A. 2002;99(1):377–82. [PubMed: 11752410]
32. Leo BM, Li X, Balian G, Anderson DG. In vivo bioluminescent imaging of virus-mediated gene transfer and transduced cell transplantation in the intervertebral disc. Spine (Phila Pa 1976). 2004;29(8):838–44. [PubMed: 15082981]
33. Berger F, Paulmurugan R, Bhaumik S, Gambhir SS. Uptake kinetics and biodistribution of 14C-D-luciferin—a radiolabelled substrate for the firefly luciferase catalysed bioluminescence reaction: impact on bioluminescence based reporter gene imaging. Eur J Nucl Med Mol Imaging. 2008;35(12):2275–85. [PubMed: 18661130]
34. Contag CH, Contag PR, Mullins JI, Spilman SD, Stevenson DK, Benaron DA. Photonic detection of bacterial pathogens in living hosts. Mol Microbiol. 1995;18(4):593–603. [PubMed: 8817482]
35. Hutchens M, Luker GD. Applications of bioluminescence imaging to the study of infectious diseases. Cell Microbiol. 2007;9(10):2315–22. [PubMed: 17587328]
36. Mook-Kanamori B, Rouse M, Kang C-I, Van De Beek D, Steckelberg J, Patel R. Daptomycin in experimental murine pneumococcal meningitis. BMC Infect Dis. 2009;9(1):50. [PubMed: 19405978]
37. Thorn RMS, Nelson SM, Greenman J. Use of a bioluminescent pseudomonas aeruginosa strain within an in vitro microbiological system, as a model of wound infection, to assess the antimicrobial efficacy of wound dressings by monitoring light production. Antimicrob Agents Chemother. 2007;51(9):3217–24. [PubMed: 17638701]
38. Dothager RS, Flentie K, Moss B, Pan M-H, Kesarwala A, Piwnica-Worms D. Advances in bioluminescence imaging of live animal models. Curr Opin Biotechnol. 2009;20(1):45–53. [PubMed: 19233638]
39. Luker KE, Luker GD. Applications of bioluminescence imaging to antiviral research and therapy: multiple luciferase enzymes and quantitation. Antiviral Res. 2008;78(3):179–87. [PubMed: 18358543]
40. Luker GD, Bardill JP, Prior JL, Pica CM, Piwnica-Worms D, Leib DA. Non-invasive bioluminescence imaging of herpes simplex virus type 1 infection and therapy in living mice. J Virol. 2002;76(23):12149–61. [PubMed: 12414955]
41. Mizuno T, Mohri K, Nasu S, Danjo K, Okamoto H. Dual imaging of pulmonary delivery and gene expression of dry powder inhalant by fluorescence and bioluminescence. J Control Release. 2009;134(2):149–54. [PubMed: 19100298]
42. Zincarelli C, Soltys S, Rengo G, Rabinowitz JE. Analysis of AAV serotypes 1–9 mediated gene expression and tropism in mice after systemic injection. Mol Ther. 2008;16(6):1073–80. [PubMed: 18414476]
43. Klerk CP, Overmeer RM, Niers TM, et al. Validity of bioluminescence measurements for non-invasive in vivo imaging of tumor load in small animals. Biotechniques. 2007;43(1 Suppl):7–13, 30. [PubMed: 17936938]
44. Paroo Z, Bollinger RA, Braasch DA, et al. Validating bioluminescence imaging as a high throughput, quantitative modality for assessing tumor burden. Mol Imaging. 2004;3(2):117–24. [PubMed: 15296676]
45. Wetterwald A, Van Der Pluijm G, Que I, et al. Optical imaging of cancer metastasis to bone marrow: a mouse model of minimal residual disease. Am J Pathol. 2002;160(3):1143–53. [PubMed: 11891210]
46. Xu Y, Piston DW, Johnson CH. A bioluminescence resonance energy transfer (BRET) system: application to interacting circadian clock proteins. Proc Natl Acad Sci U S A. 1999;96(1):151–6. [PubMed: 9874787]
47. De A, Ray P, Loening AM, Gambhir SS. BRET3: a red-shifted bioluminescence resonance energy transfer (BRET)-based integrated platform for imaging protein-protein interactions from single live cells and living animals. FASEB J. 2009;23(8):2702–9. * The most recently published class of BRET reporters with red-shifted emission for enhanced tissue penetration.
48. Iglesias P, Costoya JA. A novel BRET-based genetically encoded biosensor for functional imaging of hypoxia. Biosens Bioelectron. 2009;24(10):3126–30. [PubMed: 19423327]
49. Seemann MD. Whole-body PET/MRI: the future in oncological imaging. Technol Cancer Res Treat. 2005;4(5):577–82. [PubMed: 16173829]
50. Gilad AA, Winnard PT Jr, Van Zijl PCM, Bulte JWM. Developing MR reporter genes: promises and pitfalls. NMR Biomed. 2007;20(3):275–90. [PubMed: 17451181]
51. Cohen B, Ziv K, Plaks V, Harmelin A, Neeman M. Ferritin nanoparticles as magnetic resonance reporter gene. Wiley Interdiscip Rev Nanomed Nanobiotechnol. 2009;1(2):181–8. [PubMed: 20049789]
52. St. Pierre TG, Chan P, Bauchspiess KR, et al. Synthesis, structure and magnetic properties of ferritin cores with varying composition and degrees of structural order: models for iron oxide deposits in iron-overload diseases. Coord Chem Rev. 1996;151:125–43.
53. Deans AE, Wadghiri YZ, Bernas LM, Yu X, Rutt BK, Turnbull DH. Cellular MRI contrast via coexpression of transferrin receptor and ferritin. Magn Reson Med. 2006;56(1):51–9. [PubMed: 16724301]
54. Zurkiya O, Chan AW, Hu X. MagA is sufficient for producing magnetic nanoparticles in mammalian

cells, making it an MRI reporter. Magn Reson Med. 2008;59(6):1225–31. [PubMed: 18506784]
55. Tung C-H, Zeng Q, Shah K, Kim D-E, Schellingerhout D, Weissleder R. In vivo imaging of {beta}-galactosidase activity using far red fluorescent switch. Cancer Res. 2004;64(5):1579–83. [PubMed: 14996712]
56. Josserand V, Texier-Nogues I, Huber P, Favrot MC, Coll JL. Non-invasive in vivo optical imaging of the LacZ and Luc gene expression in mice. Gene Ther. 2007;14(22):1587–93. [PubMed: 17882264]
57. Zhang G-J, Chen T-B, Connolly B, et al. In vivo optical imaging of lacz expression using LacZ transgenic mice. Assay Drug Dev Technol. 2009;7(4):391–9. [PubMed: 19689207]
58. Zlokarnik G, Negulescu PA, Knapp TE, et al. Quantitation of transcription and clonal selection of single living cells with beta-lactamase as reporter. Science. 1998;279(5347):84. [PubMed: 9417030]
59. Xing B, Khanamiryan A, Rao J. Cell-permeable near-infrared fluorogenic substrates for imaging beta-lactamase activity. J Am Chem Soc. 2005;127(12):4158–9. [PubMed: 15783183]
60. Lee S, Park K, Kim K, Choi K, Kwon IC. Activatable imaging probes with amplified fluorescent signals. Chem Commun (Camb). 2008;36:4250–60. [PubMed: 18802536]
61. Maxwell D, Chang Q, Zhang X, Barnett EM, Piwnica-Worms D. An improved cell-penetrating, caspase-activatable, near-infrared fluorescent peptide for apoptosis imaging. Bioconjug Chem. 2009;20(4):702–9. [PubMed: 19331388]
62. Sega EI, Low PS. Tumor detection using folate receptor-targeted imaging agents. Cancer Metastasis Rev. 2008;27(4):655–64. [PubMed: 18523731]
63. Ke S, Wen X, Gurfinkel M, et al. Near-infrared optical imaging of epidermal growth factor receptor in breast cancer xenografts. Cancer Res. 2003;63(22):7870–5. [PubMed: 14633715]
64. Mahmood U, Weissleder R. Near-infrared optical imaging of proteases in cancer. Mol Cancer Ther. 2003;2(5):489–96. [PubMed: 12748311]
65. Stearns ME, Wang M. Type IV collagenase (Mr 72,000) expression in human prostate: benign and malignant tissue. Cancer Res. 1993;53(4):878–83. [PubMed: 7679051]
66. Hu L, Roth JM, Brooks P, Luty J, Karpatkin S. Thrombin up-regulates cathepsin D which enhances angiogenesis, growth, and metastasis. Cancer Res. 2008;68(12):4666–73. [PubMed: 18559512]
67. Hotary K, Allen E, Punturieri A, Yana I, Weiss SJ. Regulation of cell invasion and morphogenesis in a three-dimensional type I collagen matrix by membrane-type matrix metalloproteinases 1, 2, and 3. J Cell Biol. 2000;149(6):1309–23. [PubMed: 10851027]
68. Whittaker M, Floyd CD, Brown P, Gearing AJH. Design and therapeutic application of matrix metalloproteinase inhibitors. Chem Rev. 1999;99(9):2735–76. [PubMed: 11749499]
69. Lebel R, Jastrzebska B, Therriault H, et al. Novel solubility-switchable MRI agent allows the non-invasive detection of matrix metalloproteinase-2 activity in vivo in a mouse model. Magn Reson Med. 2008;60(5):1056–65.
70. Jurgielewicz P, et al. New imaging probes to track cell fate: reporter genes in stem cell research. Cell Mol Life Sci. 2017;74:4455–69.

Molecular Imaging and Stem Cell Imaging

20

Key Points (Abstract)

Stem cell (SC) is the newer concept of the regenerative medicine. This is being established as an important component of the cells having capability of the excellent proliferation, having very high differentiation potential and with the important property of the self-renewal. The stem cell imaging is based on the various concepts of the harvesting of the cells at various sites of interest, then purification, and lastly implantation of the cells. Now in this era, the stem cell therapies have become one of the most advanced forms of the treatment options having the excellent results. Here the basic aim of these stem cells is the evaluation of the functioning of the cell and then differentiating the various stages of the pathologies and their exact location detection and for also for the characterization of the various pathologies in the tissues at the early molecular level. These stem cells are playing a significant role in the development of the tissues, their pathological basis, having option for the various medical therapies, and for the cell regeneration therapeutics. Due to various safety issues, still this type of therapy is few in number and still being used widely. These types of therapies are important for cell survival and cell distribution and for cell which needs to be analysed. These stem cells can be imaged in relation to various existing modalities like MRI, scintigraphy, PET, ultrasound, and optical imaging.

Keywords

In vivo imaging · Stem cell tracking · PET · SPECT · MRI · Magnetic particle imaging · Radionuclides · Ultrasound · Microbubbles · Optical imaging · Photoacoustic imaging approach

20.1 Introduction

Stem cell transplantation SCT has been possible due to the biology development and newer drug discoveries and in the regenerative medicine and various imaging techniques which will help in the establishing the purity, differentiation of the cells, their numbers, and the exact location. SCT are the specific forms of the treatment options for the use of various pathologies like various cancers, neurological diseases, and many newer pathologies as well which are still in trial. By the use of the cell labelling and cell tracking technologies, it has become easier for stem cells to track the distribution of these cells to specific targets. Stem cell (SC) therapy use has changed the entire scenario of the management of the various diseases which are not having marked results with the existing line of the management [1]. These stem cells are again quantified into the

S. Shaikh, *Advances in Imaging*, https://doi.org/10.1007/978-981-16-9535-3_20

cell-specific types of the based on the immunophenotypic, morphological, and functional aspects.

Due to the significant technological changes and the research in the microscopy, various advancements in the fluorescent probes and various morphological changes along with the functional aspects of the stem cells are under research for the various applications. As we all know, various specific cell therapies are being used replacing or restoring various damaged tissues which are having significant impact on the disease progression. These stem cells are of various types, embryonic stem cells (ESCs) [2], mesenchymal stem cells (MSCs) [3], neuroprogenitor stem cells (NSCs) origin [4], and induced pluripotent stem cells (iPSCs) [2, 5, 6]. This stem cell imaging plays a vital role in the evaluation of the behaviour, various functions, their precise location, various protein expression levels, and viability of the cells including the amount of the viable cells, in differentiating between the cells, and finally the cell environment associations in the adjacent tissues and the interactions as well. These MSCs comprise 0.01% of the total mononuclear cells which are basically found in the bone marrow. The bone marrow, cord blood, and dental pulp are the most common sources of the mesenchymal stem cells. These stem cells are having significant therapeutic potential and are also used for the regeneration of many tissues. These SCs have been used for the management of the conditions like Parkinson's disease [7] and liver disease [8] and to regenerate the infarcted and ischemic tissues [9, 10]. The basis of the mechanism of the SC therapy is based on the genetic changes by the use of the cytokines [11]; these will cause significant changes in the SC function and their behaviour in different environments, but along with this, we can also have unwanted side effects [12]. The most important aspect is that the entire therapeutic efficiency is based on various factors like the stem cell origin, route of administration, their biodistribution in the body, and the amount of the cell viability after the therapy [12, 13]. The safety of these SC is based on the biodistribution of these particles in various target tissues, where their accumulation will depend on the viability of the SC and the specific functions of the SC which will have access to the target tissues non-invasively [14, 15]. The first process starts with the preparation of the cells, then the labelling of cells, and then the sorting of the cells based on the specific requirements. For MSCs once they are ready, these cells need to be purified from the components like the bone marrow aspirate, which needs to be further expanded, and lastly labelled for the identification. For this the labelling of the SCs can be done with the reporter genes for their easy identification so that with this their functional assessment will be easier so that more and more promising results will be there in the future [16].

20.2 SC Labelling Techniques

SC labelling is one of the important components for the imaging based on this the imaging and tracking of the SC [12], and also for studying their functionalities in the preclinical studies [17]. The labelling of SC can be done by two methods like direct labelling or indirect labelling with various molecular probes which are having significant advantages and disadvantages for each of these approaches [14, 17].

20.2.1 Direct Labelling

Direct labelling of SCs by the reporter for easy detection by using the modality of choice for easy localization. The direct labelling can be done by the quantum dots, various fluorophores, radionuclides, and super paramagnetic iron oxide as well as paramagnetic nanoparticles. Direct labelling advantages are the simplicity, the use of the exact amount concentration of label, and very short processing times. There should be optimal amount of the SC for a very good spatial and temporal resolution. Again, it is based on the cell division, cell migration, and SC tracking as this will be very important for the identification of the viability and function of the stem cell. As we know this direct labelling does not provide the information of the cells' viability and proliferation, so the dead cells cannot be identified from the viable cells, and this is the biggest disadvantage which will be limiting the direct use of these for longer duration tracking of the cells which are labelled .

20.2.2 Indirect Labelling

The indirect labelling is by the reporter gene when introduced in the genome of the cell which is the area of the interest for the various functions like the expression of the receptors, various enzymes, or the fluorescent/bioluminescent proteins. These are all being more useful for the imaging of the exact cell location, number of the cells, and the exact functions. These can be done by the incorporation of a reporter gene in the SC which will be used for the viral or non-viral carriers to detect these expressed reporters when engrafted in various tissues and based on these this gene which is introduced by live cells for the detection will be used for cell viability. Reporter genes are in the form of the expressed proteins like fluorescent proteins which will generate the contrast by the concept of the emitting of the fluorescence when excited and can be imaged directly having very high sensitivity [18]; they can also trap iron for identification [19], also used as a receptor to target reporter [20] enzyme which will induce the reporter trapping [21, 22]. The indirect labelling is useful for the long-term monitoring of cell viability which can be done by various reporter gene transfections.The reporter genes are also capable of integrating various tissues randomly which can cause the changes in the MSCs which are being used from their parent cells. But due to the technological advancements in gene-editing technologies, this had resulted in the site-specific DNA integration which will have better results.

After labelling the process of the sorting and purification will be done. These process do not have any specificity of 100%. The sorting is based on the properties on the surface, amount of the dose used, the exact cell type, the various coatings of the cell membrane, the incubation time of the cells after labelling, and the cell transfection factor. Fluorescence-activated cell sorting and magnetic-activated cell sorting are the two important methods used for the sorting. After sorting the cell purification is done.

The contrast agents which are used should be in the optimum quantity, and any higher will lead to toxicity. Even though there is direct relation between the increased contrast agent, it will have increased signal, but the balanced quantification needs to be done which should have best resolution with optimum contrast agent without any side effects.

20.3 SC Imaging Technologies

All imaging modalities are having their sensitivities which are based on various reporters used, the labelling characteristics, the optimal amount of the cell required for the detection, the resolution of the modality, the average time needed for the imaging, and various applications for which it will be used. The spatial resolution is also based on various reporter concentrations of the signal: voxel ratios, noise reduction, and detection of the signals. The sensitivity of the imaging is directly proportional to the reporters: voxel required for the optimal visualization of the signal. The optical fluorescence imaging (FLI) is having the highest sensitivity of detecting the various nanomolar concentrations.

Delivery of the stem cell agents: The most important aspect in the stem cell therapies is the delivery of the agents to the specific target tissues. The main aim is to deliver these agents more accurately, efficiently, and effectively. These agents should be delivered more accurately to the site of the injury, preventing the damage to the surrounding tissues and most importantly the viability and the proliferation of stem cell after implantation. Again, these delivery options are variable depending on the region of the interest in therapeutics.

20.4 Ultrasound

Ultrasound (US) is having the advantage of having the higher spatial resolution and increased sensitivity for the reporters and microbubbles. And the biggest advantage is the less cost, no radiation, easy availability, and real time, and also it can be used for the bedside applications. Here the depth is inversely proportional to the depth of the penetration. Perfluorocarbon (PFC) microbubbles are very small 3 μm in diameter, which are highly elastic in nature oscillating at μm causing the US transmitters. These oscillations will have specific characteristic frequencies so that it will be possible for the detection of single microbubble [23] and also the single cell both in vitro and in vivo [24]. This microbubble US imaging has similarities to the photoacoustic imaging (PAI), with the only difference that the MB uses sound generation, whereas the photoacoustic imaging uses the light which is transmitted in the tissues so that it reaches the desired target. After reaching the target, there will be a blend of mechanisms which will have various effects like heating which will expand and then cool very rapidly; the generation of the sound waves is detectable by various transducers. This detected sound is used for the generation of the image in the particular field of view. Photoacoustic imaging PAI is a hybrid technique which is similar to optical imaging rather than the use of US. PAI advantage over the optical imaging is that light absorption is based on the generated sound which will have depth; images will be of higher spatial resolution than standard ultrasound. PAI is depth limited; but the external light source will use the amount of the energy into tissues to generate the sound. When MSCs are loaded with gold nanoparticles, an ideal PAI reporter, SCs can be detected in vivo [25]. The routine conventional imaging modalities like PET, CT and MRI, the sensitivity and sensitivity of these modalities is based on the type of the scan machine, its resolution, the various technicalities related with machine, various factors that will have impact because of the patient like size of the patient, etc. The ultrasound will not provide the exact MB concentration required between various tissues, but the recently available MB are having very good resolutions which are depending on the entire field of view [26, 27]. The combination and amalgamation of the imaging modalities PET and CT will be having the highest sensitivities due to increased resolutions of even these modalities CT or MRI in fusion with the PET. The newer fusion that is the ultrasound fusion which is being done over the existing modalities like PET, CT, or MRI

20.5 Advantages and Challenges of Stem Cell Imaging

Radionuclide imaging (PET and SPECT) is nowadays having very high sensitivity due to technological developments and increased in vivo sensitivity; various labelling procedures can be done for these protocols. The increased sensitivity of the PET has more advantage for the stem cell imaging for the evaluation of the various cells' viability [9, 12–14, 17]. PET and SPECT are the different technological modalities which will be using various radiotracers [9, 12–14, 17]. Many newer PET imaging radiotracers are being used which will have variable half-life from 1–2 h to approximately 13 h (64Cu). The advantage of the various SC labelling and evaluation by these modalities is that it will be easier to label and track the cells by which there is a proper time for them to get evaluated. Various SPECT radiotracers are used for evaluation due to this property [28, 29]. SPECT is known to have a lower spatial resolution, and based on this, there is more attenuation of the gamma rays, and the half-life of these radiotracers used is more from hours to days which is more favourable for the SC labelling and tracking [17, 29]. 111In is being used for the labelling especially for the trafficking and studying the large animal models [30, 31]. Diverse tracers have been used for SC imaging with PET and SPECT, such as 18FDG, 64Cu-PTSM, 111In-oxine, and 99mTc-HMPAO [12, 14, 17, 32]. 18FDG the amount of the uptake is directly proportional to the amount of the metabolic rate [33]. Due to the lesser half-life, this is not much of use for the monitoring of the SC [12,

34]. SPECT has the property of the gamma—emitting the variable different energies for the radiotracers; this SPECT is an excellent example for the dual-energy evaluation of the 99mTc (149.5 KeV) and 111In (144 and 218 KeV) which have been used to track different SC populations [35, 36]. 99mTc can be done on the higher doses due to its shorter half-life but with the higher spatial resolution [14, 29]. The most commonly used are the NSCs and MSCs along with the FDG [37, 38] and 99mTc-HMPAO [39]. The direct labelling of the stem cells with radiotracers can be done [13, 14, 17, 30, 35]. With this technique it is very difficult to differentiate them from the living cells to the dead cells; due to the cell division and migration, it is very small, and due to the ionizing radiation, this will have an impact on the SCs [13, 14, 17, 30, 35]. Due to this the agents with the longer half-lives have excellent stability and high potential labelling [29, 40, 41].

Reporter genes are used to detect gene expression for the SCs imaging multiple and also to confirm the cell viability [12, 14, 17]. Reporter genes for PET and SPECT imaging are herpes simplex virus type 1 thymidine kinase (HSV1-tk) where cell accumulation is very high. Stem cell reporters are used for the iodine transport in thyroid cells. SCs expression of the receptor like the dopamine D2 receptor is commonly seen in the substantia nigra [42–44]. Gene reporters can be used to scan the various radiotracers numerously [14, 16, 45]. NIS imaging can also be done with 124I for PET and 123I for SPECT [45].

20.6 MRI

MRI-based SC imaging is an important component for the evaluation of various SCs non-invasively [46, 47]. This is also used for the monitoring of the structural and various stem cell engraftment [14, 17]. MRI-based SC labelling is based on T1 and more common T2 agents, [31]. Superparamagnetic iron oxide nanoparticles are very small in size and are commonly used T2 agents due to very high relaxation and biocompatibility [19]. MR is very less sensitive than the PET/SPECT in the molecular level but still can have excellent resolution based on the magnetic properties of various ferromagnetic, paramagnetic, or superparamagnetic markers as well as the strength which can easily identify the SC migration and differentiation. SCs in cell cultures can be added to these particles with no significant effect on the SC viability and therapeutic efficacy [48]. Contrast agent here is highly sensitive ^{19}F, whose signal intensity is proportional to the amount of ^{19}F. Imaging reporter gene will enhance the overall signal of MRI by the principle of the gene which will be targeted to for the substance to be formed. Report genes are the lacZ, transferrin gene, and ferritin gene which are used in MRI. The superparamagnetic iron oxides (SPIOs) are the type of the iron oxide nanoparticles which will be exhibiting the super paramagnetic properties which will be having significantly high sensitivity and due to this component can be used in very small concentrations, and this is the reason for the very less side effects. Another important aspect of the SPIOs is that they will be coated with various polymers, and due to this the stability and biocompatibility are increased to the greater extent. SPION labelling is used for MSCs in patients with multiple sclerosis and amyotrophic lateral sclerosis [49] and can be used for the evaluation of various conditions [4, 50–52]. The impact of the T2 shortening will have an important role where the larger micron particles are having better effect as compared to the smaller counterparts. With this various MPIOs will have better labelling efficiency and particle retention [53]. These labelled SCs are more commonly used in various cell-based therapies, for the regenerative medicine, and as well as major cancers of the body [54]. However, despite of this these iron oxide-based will have lower particle dilution, less cell proliferation, and lower cell migration, due to the decreased retention [55]. Chelated gadoliniums are commonly used T1 agents by increasing the various MR signals [14]. Conjugating Gd gold nanoparticles will be used as MRI contrast agents which will be having more sensitivity [56–58]. Gd hybrid iron oxide (GdIO) nanocomposites can be used for the dual T1- and T2-weighted imaging of stem cells [59]. They demonstrated that SC viability, proliferation, or differentiation can't be done [59].

19F is widely available and its resonating frequency is similar to the commonly used RF coils in the MR systems. 19F signal is very low as compared to various hydrogen-based contrast agents for detection [60, 61]. PFCs are the highest level of the concentrations where carbon and fluorine are being given as the emulsions [62, 63]. They are inert in living systems and exhaled from the body from a couple of minutes to years of PFC emulsion particles when added to the cells, and then they can be easily tracked in vivo (d) [14, 17, 64, 65]. As they are very small and inert, then they do not have any characteristics [66]. 19F agent has a very good sensitivity and depth [67]. Low signal with lesser loading capacity of cells for detection [68] can be done for the shortening relaxation time [69, 70]. Emulsion particles are based on the dilution which is secondary to the proliferation and migration of the cells. The use of aquaporin 1 (AQP1) will facilitate the water diffusion rate, with increased contrast on diffusion-weighted MRI [71, 72]. Chemical exchange saturation transfer (CEST) is now a very important biomarker [73, 74] and can monitor the exact distribution of an extracellular hydrogel matrix [75].

20.7 MPI

MPI is a MR technique which is capable of detecting the superparamagnetic nanoparticles, with MPI which is being commonly used for the detection, localization and recognizing the better specificity than MRI. High-contrast images are being detected and being used as various signals. MPI direct imaging is to image the reporter and will be suffering from various signal losses when the cells divide and migrate. MPI is having the property to image the superparamagnetic particles [76]. Faster imaging is needed for this [77]. MPI is used for the SC tracking and also the [78–80]. Another important aspect is the labelling with CFC labelling.

20.8 Ultrasound

Whereas several US contrast agents are being used to be seen on the B-mode imaging [81], various SCs are to be added to the PFC vapour as the single cell to be diagnosed [24]. MB are intracellular and not viable if in the circulation and are destroyed [24]. US can also track MB-labelled SCs for days [82, 83]. US tracking can be done by the liposomes and theranostic mesoporous silica nanoparticles which are active in the sound [84, 85]. Various gene expressions can also be used to detect the SCs [86]. Engrafted endothelial progenitor cells (EPCs) are used as surface receptors for the specific ligand to detect the implanted SCs [86]. Interaction with MB can happen with the SC in the blood due to the smaller size of the 1–3 μm; due to this it will be confined in the intravascular space [87, 88]. MB can be attached to surface receptors [87, 88]. High-intensity-focused HIFU has greater efficacy of SC therapy [89]. Shapiro et al. used the gas-based vesicles and showed the activeness in US and MRI contrast agents [90–92]. The genetic protein vesicles are used as a US and MRI gene reporter system [92]. High sensitivity is a very important technique for the labelling and tracking the SCs. Localized heating will be increasing the US signal [25]. Optical absorption is seen better in the infrared region [93]. Based on these properties, the adequate sensitivity is determined. Further, the administration of the MSCs in the labelled mouse hearts are having the semiconducting polymers [94].

20.9 Optical Imaging

Fluorescence and bioluminescence are two methods of the optical imaging used for identifying the location and functional status of SCs [17, 72]. Fluorescence uses the light and transmits it into various tissues by exciting the various fluorophores by the principle of fluorescence. Here the use of the various reporter genes which are fluorescent like green fluorescent protein (EGFP) is being used widely for the labelling. The advantage is that no substrate will be needed, and the excitation of the light is mandatory for the higher levels of the energy and also to emit longer-wavelength emission light. And these fluorescent reporter genes can be used alone and do not require any other substrates. These reporter genes can be used for both living and fixed cells and tissues. Fluorescent dye labelled cells will emit the various infrared ranges for imaging at the better depth [95]. Reporter labelling by various fluorescent polymeric NPs and quantum dot (QD) accumulation in wound healing will be done by the chemoattractants [96]. Reporter can be introduced in the cytoplasm US and MB, by sonoporation technique [97]. By the use of the photoporation, Xiong et al. increased efficiency and longer duration of accumulation [97].

20.10 Bioluminescence Imaging

Bioluminescence imaging (BLI) principle uses detection of the amount of the light generated in tissues. The source of light is luciferase catalyses luciferin. Majority of the cells are configured for the luciferase and luciferin expressions. The emitted photons are having different wavelengths, and on this principle the different SC can be evaluated [98]. This technique of the BLI will be more useful in tracking the various SCs in vivo in small animals [16, 99–101]. By administration of this substrate, this can be evaluated (e) [98, 99]. Photon generation is based on the energy required that is ATP-dependent [99], and the adequate amount of the oxygen is required [102]. The substrate should be efficiently administered so that along the blood flow, binding capacity of the protein and the inhibitory effect anaesthetics can be done [103, 104]. Gene expression is more efficient and can emit so as to reach the detector from the deeper regions of the various tissues [105].

20.11 Multimodality Imaging Hybrid Imaging

Multimodality imaging hybrid imaging modalities are advantageous for various imaging techniques [83, 106]. The most developed and clinically used is PET-CT which combines the high spatial resolution of CT with the high reporter sensitivity of PET [13]. PET is more advantageous due to softer tissue sensitivities of the MRI. Here the advantage of hybrid imaging has advantages along with the PET imaging which is based on X-ray attenuation in the case of CT [107]. This has added the new dimensions for the multimodality multiparametric imaging [66, 108]. Thus PET-MR is having significant increased sensitivities due to various applications [109]. Various modality combinations are there like BLI with MRI and SPECT with FLI [110, 111]. MRI and BLI combination has led to better sensitivities leading to better evaluation of these conditions [112]. The available concept of the non-invasive SC imaging and monitoring will provide the comprehensive aspect of the imaging. Again, these are based on the changes in the physiology, pharmacokinetics, their basal metabolic rates, and also the basal metabolic rates [113]. These are along with the SC doses, their administration schedule and pattern, route of administration, and target organs [114]. The various labelling aspects for the short-term monitoring time, destination, and various aspects for the migration, proliferation, function, and survival. Usually, SCs are administered intravenously for the mimic of the physiological SC delivery. But significant amount will be adherent to the lung parenchyma [115, 116]. Optimal delivery of the SCs to tissues and organs will increase the efficiency and the dose [117–120]. These techniques are used in the SC delivery, in the heart [121], brain [122], spinal cord [123], liver [124], and kidney [125]. Various local injections are capable of the disruption of the native tissues structure and will result in various adverse effects [126]. SCs are completely based on the structure of the environment where it is injected even causing the SC death and decreased potency [127]. Various SC genetic modifications can be done [128–130].

As we all know mesenchymal stem cells (MSCs), also known as mesenchymal stromal cells [131], are commonly used in the regenerative medicine and accounts for ~38% of all SC trials [132] (Diagram 20.1). MSCs are having the significant property of the genetic manipula-

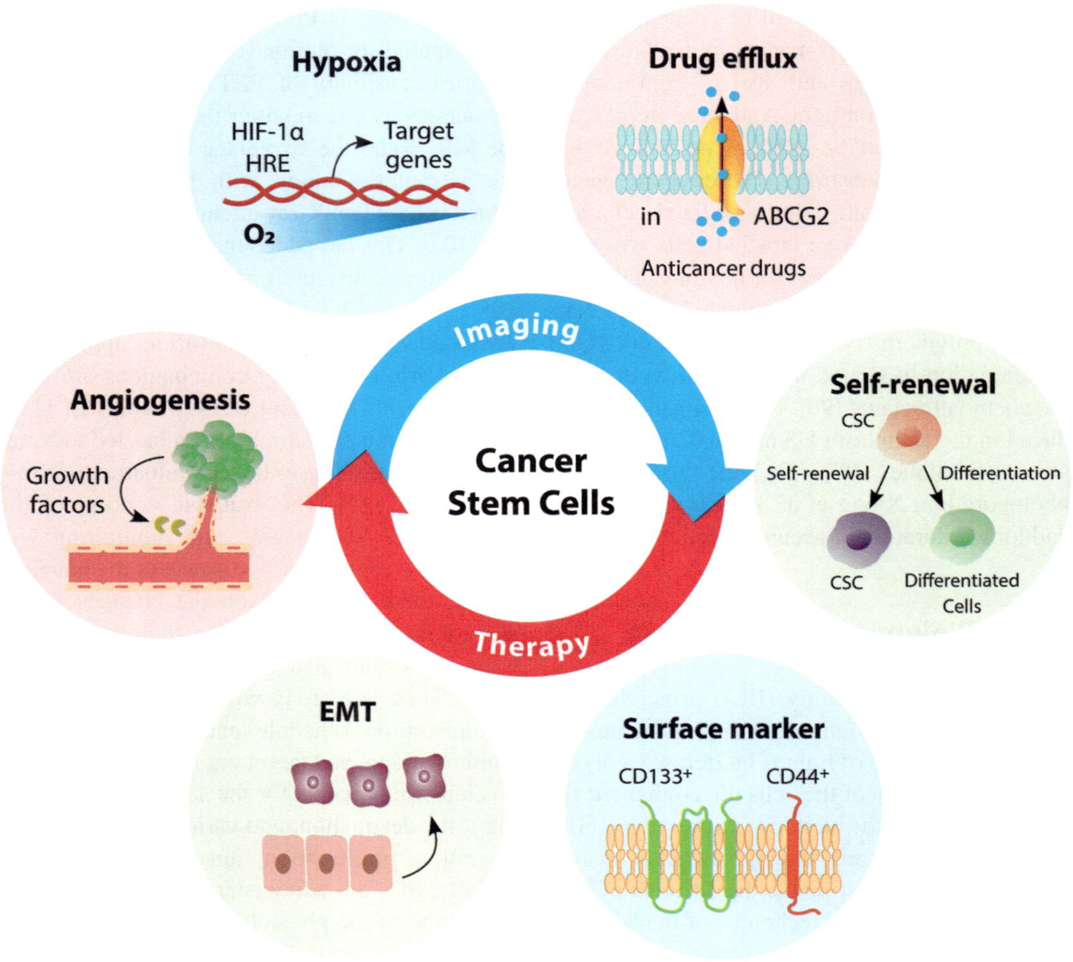

Diagram 20.1 The role of cancer stem cells in the imaging and therapy

tion which will lead to the suitable cancer delivery [133], tumour necrosis agents [134, 135], and tumour tropism for targeted delivery of anticancer agents [136–138] (Diagrams 20.2 and 20.3). Intravenous (IV) injection is the common route for delivering cells which will have the uniform distribution and migration of the tissues [139–141]. Intra-arterially, it will cause the increase in cell uptake and engraftment in target tissues and the localization, retention, and viability status of transplanted cells. Cell labelling can be done by direct cell labelling and reporter gene imaging [142]. Direct cell labelling is done by labelling before the transplantation. Reporter gene imaging is done for the expression of a specific cell surface receptor, transporter, or enzyme used to activate the imaging probe within the cell [142, 143].

Stem cells can be labelled with superparamagnetic iron oxide nanoparticles (SPIONs) for magnetic resonance imaging (MRI) [144–146], for the evaluation of success or failure of stem cell delivery [147–149]. Quantification is challenging due to the dephasing effect SPIONs which is there on the surrounding magnetic spins, leading to "blooming" of the signal leading to overestimation of cell number [150]. Direct labelling method Indium-111 (111In)-oxime for single-photon emission computed tomography (SPECT) imaging, for the white blood cells tracking at the

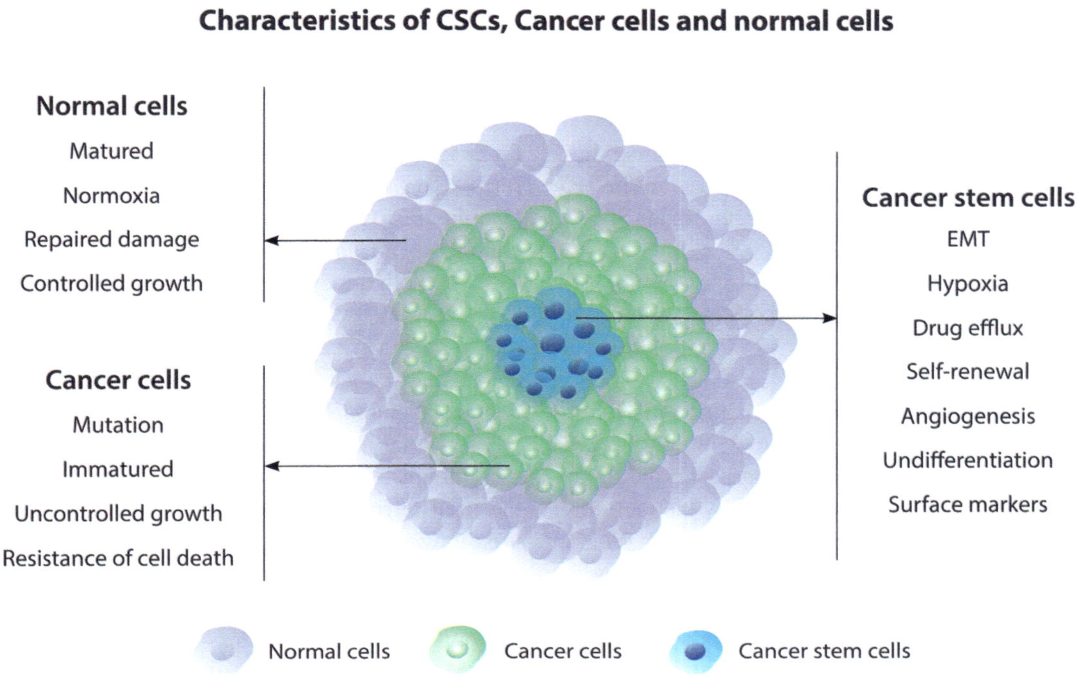

Diagram 20.2 Various aspects involved in cancer stem cells

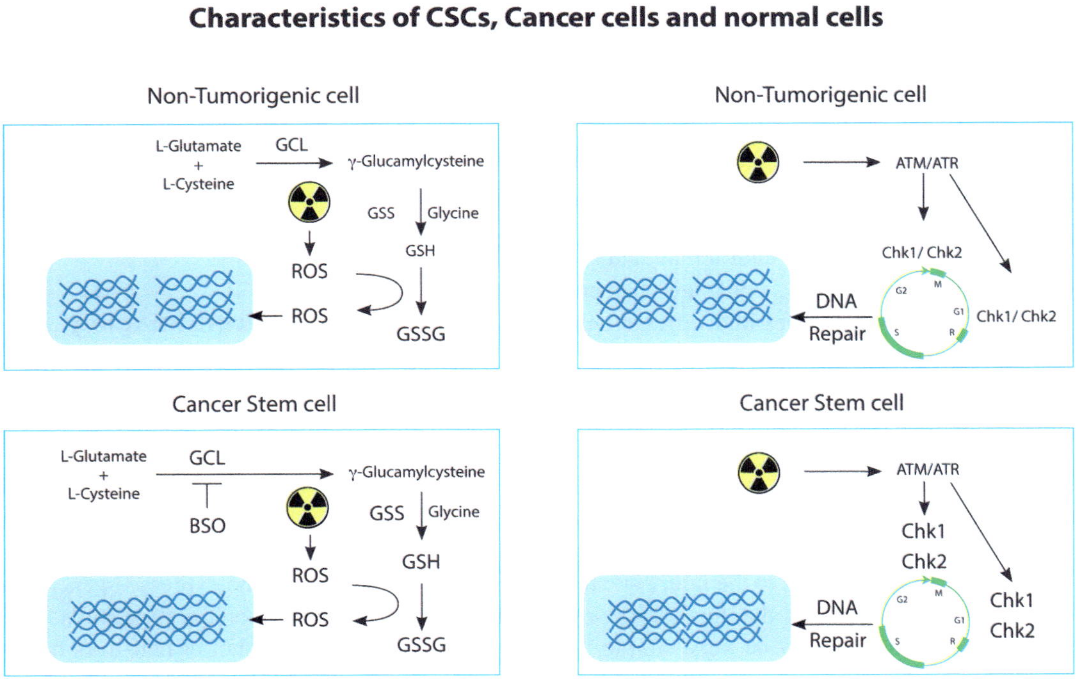

Diagram 20.3 The mechanisms of cancer stem cell, cancer cells, and normal cells

site of the inflammation [151]. This is used for tracking stem cells in both preclinical and clinical studies [140, 149, 152] which is a sensitive method of tracking due to the very low number of the cells [153]. Advantage of SPECT imaging is its ability to semi-quantitatively base on the proportion of cells delivered to target organs [154].

20.12 Bioluminescence Stem Cell Imaging

Bioluminescence stem cell imaging (BLI) commonly used reporter gene for stem cell tracking [155–157]. The principle is based on the oxidation of the substrate D-luciferin by the luciferase enzyme resulting in light emission [158]. With no significant sensitivity for various modalities for cell localization and cell viability, newer multimodal imaging probes for cell tracking need to be evaluated [159]. Some of these are 64Cu-DOTA-SPION as PET/MRI imaging agent for tumour imaging [160]. The fluorescent silica-coated SPIONs with 125Iodine (125I) are a SPECT/MRI/fluorescent imaging agent for stem cell tracking [161]. BLI is to have whole-body distribution for the human adipose-derived stem cell (ADSC) for the two routes IV injection and intracardiac injection versus the venous and arterial routes. Here the ADSCs are being used as cancer drug delivery tools [162].

Stem cells (SCs) are the undifferentiated cells of multicellular organisms, which are characterized multipotent capabilities and differentiation and self-renewal capabilities [163]. We all know the neuro-damage or point of degeneration central nervous system (CNS), in neurons and glial cells. Thus, the role of the SC transplantation occurs in stroke, Parkinson's disease (PD), Alzheimer's disease (AD), spinal cord injury (SCI), etc. [164–169]. The post transplantation, these SCs will be migrating to the injury site thus differentiating and useful the therapeutic role [170]. SC labelling has to be very simple and easy to use, with higher sensitivity and specificity with no obvious toxicity [171, 172].

Magnetic resonance imaging MRI is now an important aspect of molecular and cellular imaging and is developed to have higher spatial resolution for vivo imaging [173]. MRI is very sensitive for excellent cell resolution, and this is important for tracking SCs in neurological disorders [173]. Gadolinium (Gd3+) is the most commonly used contrast agent, and when used with manganese (Mn2+), both are cytotoxic; due to this there will be limitations for their use in vivo [174]. For this reason the superparamagnetic iron-based contrast agents are better than gadolinium-based MRI contrast agents. 19F is also another contrast agent whose signal intensity is directly proportional to the amount of 19F [175]. Newer reporter genes like transferrin gene and ferritin genes are also used nowadays [176]. Superparamagnetic iron oxide (SPIOs) has higher sensitivity in MRI, and due to this reason, they can be used in lower concentrations having very less side effects [177, 178]. As they are coated with organic polymers, they are having better stability and biocompatibility of iron particles [179]. FDA has approved only ferumoxytol SPIO contrast agent [180]. Egawa et al. proposed more specific and fast method for labelling NSCs by using SPIO nanoparticles via DNA hybridization [181]. MRI, even though it is a very good modality for the tracking of the SCs, is still non-specific for imaging, and due to contrast toxicity, further magnetic substances cannot be included [182, 183].

20.13 Nuclear Medicine Imaging

Radionuclide-labelled cell is done by SPECT and positron emission tomography (PET) [184]. PET and SPECT are based on the radioactivity of various tissues and organs [185]. These nuclides can be labelled with the reporter gene having enzymes, receptors, and transporters [186, 187]. PET/SPECT will detect the expressed gene with various probes impacting on the target cells. 18F, 11C, 13N, and 15O and shorter half-lives radiotracers are being used [188]. SPECT uses radionuclides with longer half-lives [189, 190].

20.14 Optical Imaging

Optical imaging will be using the fluorescence imaging and bioluminescence imaging (BLI) [191]. Fluorescent reporter genes are used for fluorescent imaging [192]. Different cell algorithms will be used for bioluminescent imaging recognition and characterization [193]. Imaging of the living cells and tissues can be done by fluorescent reporter genes [194]. Despite of the technological advances, the use of fluorescent and bioluminescence imaging is having many limitations [195].

20.15 Multimodality Imaging

This imaging has a significant advantage in imaging and tracking of SCs. SCs tracking for various neuroimaging applications are having very poor resolution, and this is the limitation [196]. The use of the various ferromagnetic, paramagnetic, or superparamagnetic markers in MRI is less sensitive in comparison with PET and SPECT. And due to higher spatial resolution and the magnetic strength, it can help in evaluating SC migration and differentiation [197–199]. The resolution of optical imaging is 2–5 mm [200], and despite of this SC migration and differentiation is capable of being done by the optical imaging with lower resolution [197, 201]. By using multimodality imaging, there is increase in sensitivity and also the resolution of tissue imaging [202]. Photoacoustic imaging (PAI) is a multimodal combination of optical imaging and ultrasonic imaging.

20.16 SC in Neurological Diseases

A significant role of SC-based therapies for the management of the neurodegenerative and traumatic pathologies is being used [203]. Cellar graft monitoring for the safety assessment of SC-based therapies is being used [204]. Very few clinical trials are there for SC transplantation used for SC tracing [205].

20.16.1 Stroke

Stroke is the commonest cause of death and disability occurring worldwide [206]. SC therapy is forming the basis of various therapies. Various clinical trials are there for chronic stroke but very few for acute and subacute stroke. Most of the various clinical trials for NSCs and MSCs are being done in the primitive stages of the clinical phase I and phase II [207–210]. These uses of phase III clinical trial will have to be validated further [211, 212]. The labelling of the MSCs with SPIO nanoparticles can be done on experimental animals [213]. One of the studies by Walczak et al. validated the use of high-speed MRI to monitor the SPIO-labelled SC to the CNS in real time [213]. Lim et al. developed bicyclic nonyne (BCN) conjugated which will be used as dual-mode SC imaging probes [214]. Chen et al. successfully developed a multifunctional probe, by using the various nanoparticles which are labelled and the endocytosis labelled by endocytosis [215]. With dual modes combining PAI and MRI, MSCs can be successfully monitored [215]. Zhang et al. showed ferritin heavy chain to deliver the reporter gene to NSC [216].

20.16.2 Neurodegenerative Diseases

Neurodegenerative disorders are being increasing diagnosed day by day, and one of the common uses are the loss of neurons and /or myelin sheaths, making it functional PD, AD and amyotrophic lateral sclerosis (ALS) [217]. The role of the SCs therapies in PD is to improve the motor symptoms of stiffness, poor movement, tremors, and instability [218]. Imaging criteria for the NSC and BM-MSC transplantation are being done in phase I/II clinical trial stages [219–221]. American International Stem Cell Corporation showed interim results for the NSC for PD [222]. SC therapy has significantly improved the symptoms in PD [222]. Ramos-Gomez et al. used the tracked magnetic nanoparticle (MNP)-labelled immortalized human NSCs in a rat brain [172].

SC therapy is having significant results in AD [223–225]. Clinical trials of SCs therapies for AD are very less now [226]. Phase I/II clinical trials based on SCs have been conducted and are still in their early stages [227]. No serious adverse effects are seen thus validating the usage [228]. Lee et al. labelled human umbilical cord blood MSCs implanted in hippocampus by stereotactic injection and monitored by MRI [229]. ALS is clinically manifested by progressive degradation of motor neurons (MNs) in the brain and spinal cord, leading to muscle weakness, paralysis, and death. SCs are now important for the treatment of ALS, after being transplanted SCs will release the various neuroprotective nutrition factors protecting the toxic microenvironment of ALS [230]. SC transplantation will improve the functional movements and prevent disease progression [231–233]. Richard et al. used human glial-restricted progenitor cells which are labelled with a perfluorocarbon (PFC) in the spinal cord of mouse models of ALS [234].

20.16.3 Traumatic Brain Injury

Traumatic brain injury (TBI) is the most common cause of neuron injury which is not reversible leading to severe brain injury causing severe impairment of physiological functions. TBI can result in brain injury impairing physiological functions. SC s will play an important role in TBI [235, 236] . TBI research is used for early phase I/II clinical trials of SC therapies [237, 238]. Induced pluripotent SCs (iPS cells) are the most promising cell sources for NSCs [239, 240].

20.16.4 Spinal Cord Injury

Spinal cord injury will result in the severe injury to the injured axons, and stem cell transplantation will result in the building of the synapses between the nerves capable of restoration of the functions of the spinal cord. A lot of the promising results are not seen [241, 242]. So for this reason SC therapies are not validated for the SCI [243, 244]. Available clinical trials for the transplanting SCs into the spinal cord are not used as methods in vivo [245–247].

20.17 Conclusion

With the advent of various stem cells, treatment of the various irreversible and incurable pathologies can be done with the use of the various modalities, markers, and various parameters as described in this article. Still the ongoing research will be giving broader perspective of the application of the stem cells by various methods and cell sources by using various phenotypes and biological characteristics of various cells and tissues which will be involved. Still the future of stem cell application is challenging.

References

1. Mason C, et al. Cell therapy industry: billion-dollar global business with unlimited potential. Regen Med. 2011;6:265–72.
2. Trounson A, DeWitt ND. Pluripotent stem cells progressing to the clinic. Nat Rev Mol Cell Biol. 2016;17:194–200.
3. Boregowda SV, et al. A clinical indications prediction scale based on TWIST1 for human mesenchymal stem cells. EBioMed. 2016;4:62–73.
4. Egawa EY, et al. A DNA hybridization system for labelling of neural stem cells with SPIO nanoparticles for MRI monitoring post-transplantation. Biomaterials. 2015;54:158–67.
5. Wainger BJ, et al. Intrinsic membrane hyperexcitability of amyotrophic lateral sclerosis patient-derived motor neurons. Cell Rep. 2014;7:1–11.
6. Mandai M, et al. Autologous induced stem-cell-derived retinal cells for macular degeneration. N Engl J Med. 2017;376:1038–46.
7. Barker RA, et al. Are stem cell-based therapies for Parkinson's disease ready for the clinic in 2016? J Parkinsons Dis. 2016;6:57–63.
8. Raju R, et al. Cell expansion during directed differentiation of stem cells toward the hepatic lineage. Stem Cells Dev. 2016; https://doi.org/10.1089/scd.2016.0119.
9. Trounson A, McDonald C. Stem cell therapies in clinical trials: progress and challenges. Cell Stem Cell. 2015;17:11–22.
10. Kovacic JC, Fuster V. Cell therapy for patients with acute myocardial infarction. American Heart Association; 2015.

11. Stuckey DW, Shah K. Stem cell-based therapies for cancer treatment: separating hope from hype. Nat Rev Cancer. 2014;14:683–91.
12. Nguyen PK, et al. Stem cell imaging: from bench to bedside. Cell Stem Cell. 2014;14:431–44.
13. Naumova AV, et al. Clinical imaging in regenerative medicine. Nat Biotechnol. 2014;32:804–18.
14. Gu E, et al. Molecular imaging of stem cells: tracking survival, biodistribution, tumorigenicity, and immunogenicity. Theranostics. 2012;2:335–45.
15. Wang Y, et al. Commercial nanoparticles for stem cell labelling and tracking. Theranostics. 2013;3:544–60.
16. Wang J, Jokerst JV. Stem cell imaging: tools to improve cell delivery and viability. Stem Cells Int. 2016;2016:9240652.
17. Gavins FN, Smith HK. Cell tracking technologies for acute ischemic brain injury. J Cereb Blood Flow Metab. 2015;35:1090–9.
18. Tavri S, et al. In vivo transfection and detection of gene expression of stem cells preloaded with DNA-carrying microbubbles. Radiology. 2015;276:518–25.
19. Naumova AV, et al. (2010) Ferritin overexpression for non-invasive magnetic resonance imaging-based tracking of stem cells transplanted into the heart. Mol Imaging. 2010;9(7290):00020.
20. Toyokuni T, et al. Repetitive, non-invasive imaging of the dopamine D2 receptor as a reporter gene in living animals. Gene Ther. 1999;6:785–91.
21. Green LA, et al. A tracer kinetic model for 18F-FHBG for quantitating herpes simplex virus type 1 thymidine kinase reporter gene expression in living animals using PET. J Nucl Med. 2004;45:1560–70.
22. Huang NF, et al. Bioluminescence imaging of stem cell-based therapeutics for vascular regeneration. Differentiation. 2012;41:42.
23. Klibanov AL, et al. Detection of individual microbubbles of ultrasound contrast agents: imaging of free-floating and targeted bubbles. Invest Radiol. 2004;39:187–95.
24. Cui W, et al. Neural progenitor cells labelling with microbubble contrast agent for ultrasound imaging in vivo. Biomaterials. 2013;34:4926–35.
25. Nam SY, et al. In vivo ultrasound and photoacoustic monitoring of mesenchymal stem cells labelled with gold nanotracers. PLoS One. 2012;7:e37267.
26. Ghosh D, et al. Toward optimization of in vivo super-resolution ultrasound imaging using size-selected microbubble contrast agents. Med Phys. 2017;44:6304–13.
27. Tanigaki K, et al. Hyposialylated IgG activates endothelial IgG receptor FcgammaRIIB to promote obesity-induced insulin resistance. J Clin Invest. 2018;128:309–22.
28. Chan AT, Abraham MR. From bench to imaging SPECT and PET to optimize cardiac stem cell therapy. J Nucl Cardiol. 2012;19:118–25.
29. Von der Haar K, et al. Lost signature: progress and failures in in vivo tracking of implanted stem cells. Appl Microbiol Biotechnol. 2015;99:9907–22.
30. Leibacher J, Henschler R. Biodistribution, migration and homing of systemically applied mesenchymal stem/stromal cells. Stem Cell Res Ther. 2016;7:7.
31. Cen P, et al. Noninvasive in-vivo tracing and imaging of transplanted stem cells for liver regeneration. Stem Cell Res Ther. 2016;7:143.
32. Legacz M, et al. Contrast agents and cell labelling strategies for in vivo imaging. Adv Nanoparticles. 2014;3:41–53.
33. Sood V, et al. Biodistribution of 18F-FDG-labeled autologous bone marrow-derived stem cells in patients with type 2 diabetes mellitus: exploring targeted and intravenous routes of delivery. Clin Nucl Med. 2015;40:697–700.
34. Faivre L, et al. 18 F-FDG labelling of hematopoietic stem cells: dynamic study of bone marrow homing by PET–CT imaging and impact on cell functionality. Curr Res Transl Med. 2016;64:141–8.
35. Kircher MF, et al. Non-invasive cell-tracking methods. Nat Rev Clin Oncol. 2011;8:677–88.
36. Guo Z, et al. Simultaneous SPECT imaging of multi-targets to assist in identifying hepatic lesions. Sci Rep. 2016;6:28812.
37. Stojanov K, et al. [18F] FDG labeling of neural stem cells for in vivo cell tracking with positron emission tomography: inhibition of tracer release by phloretin. Mol Imaging. 2012;11(1):1–12.
38. Wolfs E, et al. 18F-FDG labelling of mesenchymal stem cells and multipotent adult progenitor cells for PET imaging: effects on ultrastructure and differentiation capacity. J Nucl Med. 2013;54:447–54.
39. Verma V, et al. In vitro assessment of cytotoxicity and labelling efficiency of 99m TcHMPAO with stromal vascular fraction of adipose tissue. Nucl Med Biol. 2014;41:744–8.
40. Bartelle BB, et al. Divalent metal transporter, DMT1: a novel MRI reporter protein. Magn Reson Med. 2013;70:842–50.
41. Bansal A, et al. Novel 89 Zr cell labelling approach for PET-based cell trafficking studies. EJNMMI Res. 2015;5:19.
42. Holvoet B, et al. Sodium iodide symporter PET and BLI noninvasively reveal mesoangioblast survival in dystrophic mice. Stem Cell Rep. 2015;5:1183–95.
43. Haralampieva D, et al. Noninvasive PET imaging and tracking of engineered human muscle precursor cells for skeletal muscle tissue engineering. J Nucl Med. 2016;57:1467–73.
44. Li L, et al. Superparamagnetic iron oxide nanoparticles as MRI contrast agents for non-invasive stem cell labelling and tracking. Theranostics. 2013;3:595–615.
45. Penheiter AR, et al. The sodium iodide symporter (NIS) as an imaging reporter for gene, viral, and cell-based therapies. Curr Gene Ther. 2012;12:33–47.

46. Liu L, et al. A new method for preparing mesenchymal stem cells and labelling with ferumoxytol for cell tracking by MRI. Sci Rep. 2016;6:26271.
47. Goodfellow FT, et al. Tracking and quantification of magnetically labelled stem cells using magnetic resonance imaging. Adv Funct Mater. 2016;26:3899–915.
48. Yang Y, et al. Superparamagnetic iron oxide is suitable to label tendon stem cells and track them in vivo with MR imaging. Ann Biomed Eng. 2013;41:2109–19.
49. Karussis D, et al. Safety and immunological effects of mesenchymal stem cell transplantation in patients with multiple sclerosis and amyotrophic lateral sclerosis. Arch Neurol. 2010;67:1187–94.
50. Kim SJ, et al. Superparamagnetic iron oxide nanoparticles for direct labelling of stem cells and in vivo MRI tracking. Contrast Media Mol Imaging. 2016;11:55–64.
51. Daldrup-Link HE, et al. Detection of stem cell transplant rejection with ferumoxytol MR imaging: correlation of MR imaging findings with those at intravital microscopy. Radiology. 2017;284(2):495–50.
52. Skelton R, et al. Magnetic resonance imaging of iron oxide-labelled human embryonic stem cell-derived cardiac progenitors. Stem Cells Transl Med. 2016;5:67–74.
53. Shapiro EM, et al. In vivo detection of single cells by MRI. Magn Reson Med. 2006;55:242–9.
54. Boulland J-L, et al. Evaluation of intracellular labelling with micron-sized particles of iron oxide (MPIOs) as a general tool for in vitro and in vivo tracking of human stem and progenitor cells. Cell Transplant. 2012;21:1743–59.
55. Xu C, et al. Tracking mesenchymal stem cells with iron oxide nanoparticle loaded poly (lactide-co-glycolide) microparticles. Nano Lett. 2012;12:4131–9.
56. Faucher L, et al. Rapid synthesis of PEGylated ultrasmall gadolinium oxide nanoparticles for cell labelling and tracking with MRI. ACS Appl Mater Interfaces. 2012;4:4506–15.
57. Rammohan N, et al. Gd(III)-Gold nanoconjugates provide remarkable cell labelling for high field magnetic resonance imaging. Bioconjug Chem. 2016;28:153–60.
58. Randolph LM, et al. Polymeric Gd-DOTA amphiphiles form spherical and fibril-shaped nanoparticle MRI contrast agents. Chem Sci. 2016;7: 4230–6.
59. Zeng Y, et al. Gadolinium hybrid iron oxide nanocomposites for dual T 1- and T 2-weighted MR imaging of cell labeling. Biomater Sci. 2017;5:50–6.
60. Srinivas M, et al. 19 F MRI for quantitative in vivo cell tracking. Trends Biotechnol. 2010;28:363–70.
61. Gaudet JM, et al. Application of dual 19F and iron cellular MRI agents to track the infiltration of immune cells to the site of a rejected stem cell transplant. Magn Reson Med. 2016;78:713–20.
62. Mattrey RF. Perfluorooctylbromide: a new contrast agent for CT, sonography, and MR imaging. Am J Roentgenol. 1989;152:247–52.
63. Riess JG. Reassessment of criteria for the selection of perfluorochemicals for second generation blood substitutes: analysis of structure/property relationships. Artif Organs. 1984;8:44–56.
64. Vu-Quang H, et al. Chitosan-coated poly (lactic-co-glycolic acid) perfluorooctyl bromide nanoparticles for cell labelling in 19 F magnetic resonance imaging. Carbohydr Polym. 2016;136:936–44.
65. Gaudet JM, et al. Tracking the fate of stem cell implants with fluorine-19 MRI. PLoS One. 2015;10:e0118544.
66. Boehm-Sturm P, et al. A multi-modality platform to image stem cell graft survival in the naïve and stroke-damaged mouse brain. Biomaterials. 2014;35:2218–26.
67. Rose LC, et al. Fluorine-19 labelling of stromal vascular fraction cells for clinical imaging applications. Stem Cells Transl Med. 2015;4:1472–81.
68. Ruiz-Cabello J, et al. In vivo "hot spot" MR imaging of neural stem cells using fluorinated nanoparticles. Magn Reson Med. 2008;60:1506–11.
69. Kislukhin AA, et al. Paramagnetic fluorinated nano emulsions for sensitive cellular fluorine-19 magnetic resonance imaging. Nat Mater. 2016;15:662–8.
70. Lee S-W, et al. Magnetic resonance reporter gene imaging. Theranostics. 2012;2:403–12.
71. Patrick PS, et al. Dual-modality gene reporter for in vivo imaging. Proc Natl Acad Sci USA. 2014;111:415–20.
72. Mukherjee A, et al. Non-invasive imaging using reporter genes altering cellular water permeability. Nat Commun. 2016;7:13891.
73. Chan KW, et al. MRI-detectable pH nano sensors incorporated into hydrogels for in vivo sensing of transplanted-cell viability. Nat Mater. 2013;12:268–75.
74. Ziv K, Gambhir SS. Bioengineering and regenerative medicine: keeping track. Nat Mater. 2013;12:180–1.
75. Jin T, et al. Diamagnetic chemical exchange saturation transfer (diaCEST) affords magnetic resonance imaging of extracellular matrix hydrogel implantation in a rat model of stroke. Biomaterials. 2017;113:176–90.
76. Weizenecker J, et al. A simulation study on the resolution and sensitivity of magnetic particle imaging. Phys Med Biol. 2007;52:6363–74.
77. Weizenecker J, et al. Three-dimensional real-time in vivo magnetic particle imaging. Phys Med Biol. 2009;54:L1–10.
78. Zheng B, et al. Magnetic particle imaging tracks the long-term fate of in vivo neural cell implants with high image contrast. Sci Rep. 2015;5:14055.
79. Zheng B, et al. Quantitative magnetic particle imaging monitors the transplantation, biodistribution, and clearance of stem cells in vivo. Theranostics. 2016;6:291–301.

80. Bulte JW, et al. Quantitative "hot spot" imaging of transplanted stem cells using superparamagnetic tracers and magnetic particle imaging (MPI). Tomography. 2015;1:91–7.
81. Behan M, et al. Perfluorooctylbromide as a contrast agent for CT and sonography: preliminary clinical results. Am J Roentgenol. 1993;160:399–405.
82. Hartanto J, Jokerst JV. Nanoparticles for ultrasound-guided imaging of cell implantation. In: Bulte JWM, Modo MMJ, editors. Design and applications of nanoparticles in biomedical imaging. New York: Springer; 2017. p. 299–314.
83. Jokerst JV, et al. Intracellular aggregation of multimodal silica nanoparticles for ultrasound-guided stem cell implantation. Sci Transl Med. 2013;5:177ra35.
84. Kempen PJ, et al. Theranostic mesoporous silica nanoparticles biodegrade after prosurvival drug delivery and ultrasound/magnetic resonance imaging of stem cells. Theranostics. 2015;5:631.
85. Herbst SM, et al. Delivery of stem cells to porcine arterial wall with echogenic liposomes conjugated to antibodies against CD34 and intercellular adhesion molecule-1. Mol Pharm. 2009;7:3–11.
86. Kuliszewski MA, et al. Molecular imaging of endothelial progenitor cell engraftment using contrast-enhanced ultrasound and targeted microbubbles. Cardiovasc Res. 2009;83:653–62.
87. Kaya M, et al. Acoustic radiation force for vascular cell therapy: in vitro validation. Ultrasound Med Biol. 2012;38:1989–97.
88. Toma C, et al. Vascular endoluminal delivery of mesenchymal stem cells using acoustic radiation force. Tissue Eng Part A. 2011;17:1457–64.
89. Wang G, et al. Effects of diagnostic ultrasound-targeted microbubble destruction on the homing ability of bone marrow stromal cells to the kidney parenchyma. Eur Radiol. 2016;26:3006–16.
90. Shapiro MG, et al. Biogenic gas nanostructures as ultrasonic molecular reporters. Nat Nanotechnol. 2014;9:311–6.
91. Maresca D, et al. Nonlinear ultrasound imaging of nanoscale acoustic biomolecules. Appl Phys Lett. 2017;110:073704.
92. Lu GJ, et al. Proteins, air and water: reporter genes for ultrasound and magnetic resonance imaging. Curr Opin Chem Biol. 2018;45:57–63.
93. Kim T, et al. Photoacoustic imaging of human mesenchymal stem cells labelled with Prussian blue-poly(L-lysine) nanocomplexes. ACS Nano. 2017;11:9022–32.
94. Qin X, et al. Photoacoustic imaging of embryonic stem cell-derived cardiomyocytes in living hearts with ultrasensitive semiconducting polymer nanoparticles. Adv Funct Mater. 2018;28:1704939.
95. Hoffman RM. The multiple uses of fluorescent proteins to visualize cancer in vivo. Nat Rev Cancer. 2005;5:796–806.
96. Chen G, et al. In vivo real-time visualization of mesenchymal stem cells tropism for cutaneous regeneration using NIR-II fluorescence imaging. Biomaterials. 2015;53:265–73.
97. Xiong R, et al. Cytosolic delivery of nano labels prevents their asymmetric inheritance and enables extended quantitative in vivo cell imaging. Nano Lett. 2016;16:5975–86.
98. Kang JH, Chung J-K. Molecular-genetic imaging based on reporter gene expression. J Nucl Med. 2008;49:164–179S.
99. Peeters M, et al. Bioluminescence-mediated longitudinal monitoring of adipose-derived stem cells in a large mammal ex vivo organ culture. Sci Rep. 2015;5:13960.
100. Allen AB, et al. In vivo bioluminescent tracking of mesenchymal stem cells within large hydrogel constructs. Tissue Eng Part C Methods. 2014;20:806–16.
101. Janowski M, et al. Survival of neural progenitors allografted into the CNS of immunocompetent recipients is highly dependent on transplantation site. Cell Transplant. 2014;23:253–62.
102. Moriyama EH, et al. The influence of hypoxia on bioluminescence in luciferase-transfected gliosarcoma tumor cells in vitro. Photochem Photobiol Sci. 2008;7:675–80.
103. Ueda I, et al. Molecular mechanism of inhibition of firefly luminescence by local anaesthetics. Proc Natl Acad Sci USA. 1976;73:481–5.
104. Keyaerts M, et al. Plasma protein binding of luciferase substrates influences sensitivity and accuracy of bioluminescence imaging. Mol Imaging Biol. 2011;13:59–66.
105. Iwano S, et al. Single-cell bioluminescence imaging of deep tissue in freely moving animals. Science. 2018;359:935–9.
106. Srinivas M, et al. Cell tracking using multimodal imaging. Contrast Media Mol Imaging. 2013;8:432–8.
107. Kedziorek DA, et al. Using C-arm x-ray imaging to guide local reporter probe delivery for tracking stem cell engraftment. Theranostics. 2013;3:916–26.
108. Guglielmetti C, et al. Multimodal imaging of subventricular zone neural stem/progenitor cells in the cuprizone mouse model reveals increased neurogenic potential for the olfactory bulb pathway, but no contribution to remyelination of the corpus callosum. Neuroimage. 2014;86:99–110.
109. Grossmann U, et al. Double-labelling of stem cells for combined brain PET/MRI. In: Society of Nuclear Medicine annual meeting abstracts. 2014.
110. Lewis CM, et al. 52Mn production for PET/MRI tracking of human stem cells expressing divalent metal transporter 1 (DMT1). Theranostics. 2015;5:227–39.
111. Garikipati VNS, et al. Mesenchymal stem cells from foetal heart attenuate myocardial injury after infarction: an in vivo serial pinhole gated SPECT-CT study in rats. PLoS One. 2014;9:e100982.
112. Rojas SV, et al. Multimodal imaging for in vivo evaluation of induced pluripotent stem cells in a murine model of heart failure. Artif Organs. 2017;41:192–9.

113. Harding J, et al. Large animal models for stem cell therapy. Stem Cell Res Ther. 2013;4:23.
114. Shah S, Heldman AW. Stem cell therapy in heart failure. In: Marin Garcia J, editor. Heart failure. New York: Springer; 2017. p. 727–47.
115. Schrepfer S, et al. Stem cell transplantation: the lung barrier. Transplant Proc. 2007;39:573–6.
116. Kean TJ, et al. MSCs: delivery routes and engraftment, cell-targeting strategies, and immune modulation. Stem Cells Int. 2013;2013:732742.
117. Wei X, et al. Mesenchymal stem cells: a new trend for cell therapy. Acta Pharmacol Sin. 2013;34:747–54.
118. Yin X, et al. Engineering stem cell organoids. Cell Stem Cell. 2016;18:25–38.
119. Quarta M, et al. An artificial niche preserves the quiescence of muscle stem cells and enhances their therapeutic efficacy. Nat Biotechnol. 2016;34:752–9.
120. Bagó JR, et al. Tumor-homing cytotoxic human induced neural stem cells for cancer therapy. Sci Transl Med. 2017;9:eaah6510.
121. Sheng CC, et al. Current stem cell delivery methods for myocardial repair. Biomed Res Int. 2012;2013:547902.
122. Guan J, et al. Transplantation of human mesenchymal stem cells loaded on collagen scaffolds for the treatment of traumatic brain injury in rats. Biomaterials. 2013;34:5937–46.
123. Uchida S, et al. Treatment of spinal cord injury by an advanced cell transplantation technology using brain-derived neurotrophic factor-transfected mesenchymal stem cell spheroids. Biomaterials. 2016;109:1–11.
124. Nicolas CT, et al. Concise review: liver regenerative medicine: from hepatocyte transplantation to bioartificial livers and bioengineered grafts. Stem Cells. 2017;35:42–50.
125. Chen C, Hou J. Mesenchymal stem cell-based therapy in kidney transplantation. Stem Cell Res Ther. 2016;7:16.
126. Sanganalmath SK, Bolli R. Cell therapy for heart failure. Circ Res. 2013;113:810–34.
127. Kumamaru H, et al. Direct isolation and RNA-seq reveal environment-dependent properties of engrafted neural stem/progenitor cells. Nat Commun. 2012;3:1140.
128. Lan F, et al. Safe genetic modification of cardiac stem cells using a site-specific integration technique. Circulation. 2012;126:S20–8.
129. Chandrasekaran AP, et al. Genome editing: a robust technology for human stem cells. Cell Mol Life Sci. 2017;74:3335–46.
130. Wang G, et al. Efficient, footprint-free human iPSC genome editing by consolidation of Cas9/CRISPR and piggyBac technologies. Nat Protoc. 2017;12:88–103.
131. Choi YJ, et al. 3D cell printed tissue analogues: a new platform for theranostics. Theranostics. 2017;7:3118–37.
132. Fung M, Yuan Y, Atkins H, Shi Q, Bubela T. Responsible translation of stem cell research: an assessment of clinical trial registration and publications. Stem Cell Rep. 2017;8(5):1190–201.
133. Park JS, Suryaprakash S, Lao YH, Leong KW. Engineering mesenchymal stem cells for regenerative medicine and drug delivery. Methods. 2015;84:3–16.
134. Sage EK, Kolluri KK, McNulty K, Lourenco SDS, Kalber TL, Ordidge KL, Davies D, Gary Lee YC, Giangreco A, Janes SM. Systemic but not topical TRAIL-expressing mesenchymal stem cells reduce tumour growth in malignant mesothelioma. Thorax. 2014;69(7):638–47.
135. Bagó JR, Alfonso-Pecchio A, Okolie O, Dumitru R, Rinkenbaugh A, Baldwin AS, Miller CR, Magness ST, Hingtgen SD. Therapeutically engineered induced neural stem cells are tumour-homing and inhibit progression of glioblastoma. Nat Commun. 2016;7:10593.
136. Nakamizo A, Marini F, Amano T, Khan A, Studeny M, Gumin J, Chen J, Hentschel S, Vecil G, Dembinski J, Andreeff M, Lang FF. Human bone marrow–derived mesenchymal stem cells in the treatment of gliomas. Cancer Res. 2005;65(8):3307–18.
137. Sasportas LS, Kasmieh R, Wakimoto H, Hingtgen S, van de Water JA, Mohapatra G, Figueiredo JL, Martuza RL, Weissleder R, Shah K. Assessment of therapeutic efficacy and fate of engineered human mesenchymal stem cells for cancer therapy. Proc Natl Acad Sci U S A. 2009;106(12):4822–7.
138. Loebinger MR, Eddaoudi A, Davies D, Janes SM. Mesenchymal stem cell delivery of TRAIL can eliminate metastatic cancer. Cancer Res. 2009;69(10):4134–42.
139. Barbash IM, Chouraqui P, Baron J, Feinberg MS, Etzion S, Tessone A, Miller L, Guetta E, Zipori D, Kedes LH, Kloner RA, Leor J. Systemic delivery of bone marrow-derived mesenchymal stem cells to the infarcted myocardium: feasibility, cell migration, and body distribution. Circulation. 2003;108(7):863–8.
140. Kraitchman DL, Tatsumi M, Gilson WD, Ishimori T, Kedziorek D, Walczak P, Segars WP, Chen HH, Fritzges D, Izbudak I, Young RG, Marcelino M, Pittenger MF, Solaiyappan M, Boston RC, Tsui BM, Wahl RL, Bulte JW. Dynamic imaging of allogeneic mesenchymal stem cells trafficking to myocardial infarction. Circulation. 2005;112(10):1451–61.
141. Gao J, Dennis JE, Muzic RF, Lundberg M, Caplan AI. The dynamic in vivo distribution of bone marrow-derived mesenchymal stem cells after infusion. Cells Tissues Organs. 2001;169(1):12–20.
142. Scarfe L, Brillant N, Kumar JD, Ali N, Alrumayh A, et al. Preclinical imaging methods for assessing the safety and efficacy of regenerative medicine therapies. NPJ Regener Med. 2017;2(1):28.
143. Patrick S, Kalber P. Reporter genes for magnetic resonance. In: Webb GA, editor. Modern magnetic resonance. Cham: Springer; 2017. p. 1–22.
144. Hill JM, Dick AJ, Raman VK, Thompson RB, Yu ZX, Hinds KA, Pessanha BS, Guttman MA, Varney TR, Martin BJ, Dunbar CE, McVeigh ER, Lederman

RJ. Serial cardiac magnetic resonance imaging of injected mesenchymal stem cells. Circulation. 2003;108(8):1009–14.

145. Rogers WJ, Meyer CH, Kramer CM. Technology insight: in vivo cell tracking by use of MRI. Nat Clin Pract Cardiovasc Med. 2006;3(10):554–62.
146. Stuckey DJ, Carr CA, Martin-Rendon E, Tyler DJ, Willmott C, Cassidy PJ, Hale SJ, Schneider JE, Tatton L, Harding SE, Radda GK, Watt S, Clarke K. Iron particles for noninvasive monitoring of bone marrow stromal cell engraftment into, and isolation of viable engrafted donor cells from, the heart. Stem Cells. 2006;24(8):1968–75.
147. de Vries IJ, Lesterhuis WJ, Barentsz JO, Verdijk P, van Krieken JH, Boerman OC, Oyen WJ, Bonenkamp JJ, Boezeman JB, Adema GJ, Bulte JW, Scheenen TW, Punt CJ, Heerschap A, Figdor CG. Magnetic resonance tracking of dendritic cells in melanoma patients for monitoring of cellular therapy. Nat Biotechnol. 2005;23(11):1407–13.
148. Bull E, Madani SY, Sheth R, Seifalian A, Green M, Seifalian AM. Stem cell tracking using iron oxide nanoparticles. Int J Nanomed. 2014;9:1641–53.
149. McColgan P, Sharma P, Bentley P. Stem cell tracking in human trials: a meta-regression. Stem Cell Rev. 2011;7(4):1031–40.
150. Zheng Y, Huang J, Zhu T, Li R, Wang Z, Ma F, Zhu J. Stem cell tracking technologies for neurological regenerative medicine purposes. Stem Cells Int. 2017; https://doi.org/10.1155/2017/2934149.
151. Thakur ML, Segal AW, Louis L, Welch MJ, Hopkins J, Peters TJ. Indium-111-labeled cellular blood components: mechanism of labelling and intracellular location in human neutrophils. J Nucl Med. 1977;18(10):1022–6.
152. Schachinger V, Aicher A, Dobert N, Rover R, Diener J, Fichtlscherer S, Assmus B, Seeger FH, Menzel C, Brenner W, Dimmeler S, Zeiher AM. Pilot trial on determinants of progenitor cell recruitment to the infarcted human myocardium. Circulation. 2008;118(14):1425–32.
153. Gholamrezanezhad A, Mirpour S, Bagheri M, Mohamadnejad M, Alimoghaddam K, Abdolahzadeh L, Saghari M, Malekzadeh R. In vivo tracking of 111Inoxine labelled mesenchymal stem cells following infusion in patients with advanced cirrhosis. Nucl Med Biol. 2011;38(7):961–7.
154. Detante O, Moisan A, Dimastromatteo J, Richard MJ, Riou L, Grillon E, Barbier E, Desruet MD, De Fraipont F, Segebarth C, Jaillard A, Hommel M, Ghezzi C, Remy C. Intravenous administration of 99mTcHMPAO-labeled human mesenchymal stem cells after stroke: in vivo imaging and biodistribution. Cell Transplant. 2009;18(12):1369–79.
155. Chen IY, Greve JM, Gheysens O, Willmann JK, Rodriguez-Porcel M, Chu P, Sheikh AY, Faranesh AZ, Paulmurugan R, Yang PC, Wu JC, Gambhir SS. Comparison of optical bioluminescence reporter gene and superparamagnetic iron oxide MR contrast agent as cell markers for noninvasive imaging of cardiac cell transplantation. Mol Imaging Biol. 2009;11(3):178–87.
156. Wu JC, Chen IY, Sundaresan G, Min JJ, De A, Qiao JH, Fishbein MC, Gambhir SS. Molecular imaging of cardiac cell transplantation in living animals using optical bioluminescence and positron emission tomography. Circulation. 2003;108(11):1302–5.
157. Cao F, Drukker M, Lin S, Sheikh AY, Xie X, Li Z, Connolly AJ, Weissman IL, Wu JC. Molecular imaging of embryonic stem cell misbehaviour and suicide gene ablation. Cloning Stem Cells. 2007;9(1):107–17.
158. Thorne N, Inglese J, Auld DS. Illuminating insights into firefly luciferase and other bioluminescent reporters used in chemical biology. Chem Biol. 2010;17(6):646–57.
159. Patrick PS, Bogart LK, Macdonald TJ, Southern P, Powell MJ, Zaw-Thin M, Voelcker NH, Parkin IP, Pankhurst QA, Lythgoe MF, Kalber TL, Bear JC. Surface radio-mineralisation mediates chelate-free radiolabelling of iron oxide nanoparticles. Chem Sci. 2019;10(9):2592–7.
160. Lee HY, Li Z, Chen K, Hsu AR, Xu C, Xie J, Sun S, Chen X. PET/MRI dual-modality tumor imaging using arginine-glycine-aspartic (RGD)-conjugated radiolabelled iron oxide nanoparticles. J Nucl Med. 2008;49(8):1371–9.
161. Tang Y, Zhang C, Wang J, Lin X, Zhang L, Yang Y, Wang Y, Zhang Z, Bulte JWM, Yang GY. MRI/SPECT/fluorescent tri-modal probe for evaluating the homing and therapeutic efficacy of transplanted mesenchymal stem cells in a rat ischemic stroke model. Adv Funct Mater. 2015;25(7):1024–34.
162. Grisendi G, Bussolari R, Cafarelli L, Petak I, Rasini V, Veronesi E, De Santis G, Spano C, Tagliazzucchi M, Barti-Juhasz H, Scarabelli L, Bambi F, Frassoldati A, Rossi G, Casali C, Morandi U, Horwitz EM, Paolucci P, Conte P, Dominici M. Adipose-derived mesenchymal stem cells as stable source of tumor necrosis factor-related apoptosis-inducing ligand delivery for cancer therapy. Cancer Res. 2010;70(9):3718–29.
163. Shyh-Chang N, Ng H-H. The metabolic programming of stem cells. Genes Dev. 2017;31:336–46.
164. Carletti B, Piemonte F, Rossi F. Neuroprotection: the emerging concept of restorative neural stem cell biology for the treatment of neurodegenerative diseases. Curr Neuropharmacol. 2011;9:313–7.
165. Lee S-T, Chu K, Park J-E, et al. Intravenous administration of human neural stem cells induces functional recovery in Huntington's disease rat model. Neurosci Res. 2005;52:243–9.
166. Lee WC, Arcona S, Thomas SK, et al. Effect of comorbidities on medical care use and cost among refractory patients with partial seizure disorder. Epilepsy Behav. 2005;7:123–6.
167. Lu P, Woodruff G, Wang Y, et al. Long-distance axonal growth from human induced pluripotent stem cells after spinal cord injury. Neuron. 2014;83:789–96.

168. Michelsen KA, Acosta-Verdugo S, Benoit-Marand M, et al. Area specific re-establishment of damaged circuits in the adult cerebral cortex by cortical neurons derived from mouse embryonic stem cells. Neuron. 2015;85:982–97.
169. Napoli E, Borlongan CV. Recent advances in stem cell-based therapeutics for stroke. Transl Stroke Res. 2016;7:452–7.
170. Shah K. Stem cell-based therapies for tumours in the brain: are we there yet? Neuro Oncol. 2016;18:1066–78.
171. Barrow M, Taylor A, Murray P, et al. Design considerations for the synthesis of polymer coated iron oxide nanoparticles for stem cell labelling and tracking using MRI. Chem Soc Rev. 2015;44:6733–48.
172. Ramos-Gómez M, Seiz EG, Martínez-Serrano A. Optimization of the magnetic labelling of human neural stem cells and MRI visualization in the hemi-parkinsonian rat brain. J Nanobiotechnol. 2015;13:20.
173. Hachani R, Lowdell M, Birchall M, et al. Tracking stem cells in tissue-engineered organs using magnetic nanoparticles. Nanoscale. 2013;5:11362–73.
174. Nagaraja TN, Karki K, Ewing JR, et al. The MRI-measured arterial input function resulting from a bolus injection of Gd-DTPA in a rat model of stroke slightly underestimates that of Gd-[14C]DTPA and marginally overestimates the blood-to-brain influx rate constant determined by Patlak plots. Magn Reson Med. 2010;63:1502–9.
175. Srinivas M, Heerschap A, Ahrens ET, et al. (19)F MRI for quantitative in vivo cell tracking. Trends Biotechnol. 2010;28:363–70.
176. Meier S, Gilad AA, Brandon JA, et al. Non-invasive detection of adeno-associated viral gene transfer using a genetically encoded CEST-MRI reporter gene in the murine heart. Sci Rep. 2018;8:4638.
177. Lin MM, Kim DK, El Haj AJ, et al. Development of superparamagnetic iron oxide nanoparticles (SPIONS) for translation to clinical applications. IEEE Trans Nanobiosci. 2008;7:298–305.
178. Gindy ME, Prud'homme RK. Multifunctional nanoparticles for imaging, delivery and targeting in cancer therapy. Expert Opin Drug Deliv. 2009;6:865–78.
179. Patel D, Kell A, Simard B, et al. Cu2+-labeled, SPION loaded porous silica nanoparticles for cell labelling and multifunctional imaging probes. Biomaterials. 2010;31:2866–73.
180. Liu L, Tseng L, Ye Q, et al. A new method for preparing mesenchymal stem cells and labelling with Ferumoxytol for cell tracking by MRI. Sci Rep. 2016;6:26271.
181. Egawa EY, Kitamura N, Nakai R, et al. A DNA hybridization system for labelling of neural stem cells with SPIO nanoparticles for MRI monitoring post-transplantation. Biomaterials. 2015;54:158–67.
182. Thu MS, Bryant LH, Coppola T, et al. Self-assembling nanocomplexes by combining ferumoxytol, heparin and protamine for cell tracking by magnetic resonance imaging. Nat Med. 2012;18:463–7.
183. Liu T, Wang S, Liu H, et al. Detection of vertebral metastases: a meta-analysis comparing MRI, CT, PET, Bs and BS with SPECT. J Cancer Res Clin Oncol. 2017;143:457–65.
184. Sanchez-Catasus CA, Stormezand GN, van Laar PJ, et al. Fdg-PET for prediction of AD dementia in mild cognitive impairment. A review of the state of the art with particular emphasis on the comparison with other neuroimaging modalities (MRI and perfusion SPECT). Curr Alzheimer Res. 2017;14:127–42.
185. Yang C-T, Ghosh KK, Padmanabhan P, et al. Pet-Mr and SPECT-MR multimodality probes: development and challenges. Theranostics. 2018;8:6210–32.
186. Taïeb D, Pacak K. Pet scans with 18F-fluorodeoxyglucose to diagnose adrenal tumours—reply. JAMA. 2017;318:1614–5.
187. Keu KV, Witney TH, Yaghoubi S, et al. Reporter gene imaging of targeted T cell immunotherapy in recurrent glioma. Sci Transl Med. 2017;9
188. Pichler V, Berroteran-Infante N, Philippe C, et al. An overview of PET radiochemistry, part 1: the covalent labels 18 F, 11 C, and 13 N. J Nucl Med. 2018;59:1350–4.
189. Meerwaldt R, Slart RHJA, van Dam GM, et al. PET/SPECT imaging: from carotid vulnerability to brain viability. Eur J Radiol. 2010;74:104–9.
190. Zanzonico P. Principles of nuclear medicine imaging: planar, SPECT, PET, multi-modality, and autoradiography systems. Radiat Res. 2012;177:349–64.
191. Sabapathy V, Mentam J, Jacob PM, et al. Noninvasive optical imaging and in vivo cell tracking of indocyanine green labelled human stem cells transplanted at superficial or in-depth tissue of SCID mice. Stem Cells Int. 2015;2015:1–8.
192. Contag CH. In vivo pathology: seeing with molecular specificity and cellular resolution in the living body. Annu Rev Pathol. 2007;2:277–305.
193. Specht EA, Braselmann E, Palmer AE. A critical and comparative review of fluorescent tools for live-cell imaging. Annu Rev Physiol. 2017;79:93–117.
194. Mezzanotte L, van't Root M, Karatas H, et al. In vivo molecular bioluminescence imaging: new tools and applications. Trends Biotechnol. 2017;35:640–52.
195. Shah K, Weissleder R. Molecular optical imaging: applications leading to the development of present day therapeutics. NeuroRx. 2005;2:215–25.
196. Srivastava AK, Bulte JWM. Seeing stem cells at work in vivo. Stem Cell Rev Rep. 2014;10:127–44.
197. Glover JC, Aswendt M, Boulland J-L, et al. In vivo cell tracking using non-invasive imaging of iron oxide-based particles with particular relevance for stem cell-based treatments of neurological and cardiac disease. Mol Imaging Biol. 2019; https://doi.org/10.1007/s11307-019-01440-4. [Epub ahead of print: 04 Dec 2019]
198. Cromer Berman SM, Walczak P, Bulte JWM. Tracking stem cells using magnetic

nanoparticles. Wiley Interdiscip Rev Nanomed Nanobiotechnol. 2011;3:343–55.
199. Wang S, Chopp M, Nazem-Zadeh M-R, et al. Comparison of neurite density measured by MRI and histology after TBI. PLoS One. 2013;8:e63511.
200. Michonneau D, Bousso P, Negrin RS. In vivo imaging of GVHD and GVL[M]. In: Immune biology of allogeneic hematopoietic stem cell transplantation. 2019. p. 51–68.
201. Aarntzen EHJG, Srinivas M, Walczak P, et al. In vivo tracking techniques for cellular regeneration, replacement, and redirection. J Nucl Med. 2012;53:1825–8.
202. Yang B, Parsha K, Schaar K, et al. Various cell populations within the mononuclear fraction of bone marrow contribute to the beneficial effects of autologous bone marrow cell therapy in a rodent stroke model. Transl Stroke Res. 2016;7:322–30.
203. Alessandrini M, Preynat-Seauve O, De Bruin K, et al. Stem cell therapy for neurological disorders. S Afr Med J. 2019;109:70–7.
204. Bhakoo K. In vivo stem cell tracking in neurodegenerative therapies. Expert Opin Biol Ther. 2011;11:911–20.
205. Zhu J, Wu X, Zhang HL. Adult neural stem cell therapy: expansion in vitro, tracking in vivo and clinical transplantation. Curr Drug Targets. 2005;6:97–110.
206. McIntyre CW, Goldsmith DJ. Ischemic brain injury in hemodialysis patients: which is more dangerous, hypertension or intradialytic hypotension? Kidney Int. 2015;87:1109–15.
207. Kondziolka D, Wechsler L, Goldstein S, et al. Transplantation of cultured human neuronal cells for patients with stroke. Neurology. 2000;55:565–9.
208. Kondziolka D, Steinberg GK, Wechsler L, et al. Neurotransplantation for patients with subcortical motor stroke: a phase 2 randomized trial. J Neurosurg. 2005;103:38–45.
209. Kalladka D, Sinden J, Pollock K, et al. Human neural stem cells in patients with chronic ischaemic stroke (Pisces): a phase 1, first-in-man study. Lancet. 2016;388:787–96.
210. Wechsler LR, Bates D, Stroemer P, et al. Cell therapy for chronic stroke. Stroke. 2018;49:1066–74.
211. Hess DC, Wechsler LR, Clark WM, et al. Safety and efficacy of multipotent adult progenitor cells in acute ischaemic stroke (masters): a randomised, double-blind, placebo-controlled, phase 2 trial. Lancet Neurol. 2017;16:360–8.
212. Mays RW, Savitz SI. Intravenous cellular therapies for acute ischemic stroke. Stroke. 2018;49:1058–65.
213. Walczak P, Wojtkiewicz J, Nowakowski A, et al. Real-Time MRI for precise and predictable intra-arterial stem cell delivery to the central nervous system. J Cereb Blood Flow Metab. 2017;37:2346–58.
214. Lim S, Yoon HY, Jang HJ, et al. Dual-modal imaging-guided precise tracking of bioorthogonally labeled mesenchymal stem cells in mouse brain stroke. ACS Nano. 2019;13:10991–1007.
215. Chen P-J, Kang Y-D, Lin C-H, et al. Multitheragnostic multi-GNRs crystal-seeded magnetic nanoseaurchin for enhanced in vivo mesenchymal-stem-cell homing, multimodal imaging, and stroke therapy. Adv Mater. 2015;27:6488–95.
216. Zhang F, Duan X, Lu L, et al. In vivo long-term tracking of neural stem cells transplanted into an acute ischemic stroke model with reporter gene-based bimodal Mr and optical imaging. Cell Transplant. 2017;26:1648–62.
217. Tang Y, Zhang C, Wang J, et al. MRI/SPECT/Fluorescent TriModal probe for evaluating the homing and therapeutic efficacy of transplanted mesenchymal stem cells in a rat ischemic stroke model. Adv Funct Mater. 2015;25:1024–34.
218. Mani V, Adler E, Briley-Saebo KC, et al. Serial in vivo positive contrast MRI of iron oxide-labeled embryonic stem cell-derived cardiac precursor cells in a mouse model of myocardial infarction. Magn Reson Med. 2008;60:73–81.
219. Venkataramana NK, Pal R, Rao SAV, et al. Bilateral transplantation of allogenic adult human bone marrow-derived mesenchymal stem cells into the subventricular zone of Parkinson's disease: a pilot clinical study. Stem Cells Int. 2012;2012:1–12.
220. Yin F, Tian Z-M, Liu S, et al. Transplantation of human retinal pigment epithelium cells in the treatment for Parkinson disease. CNS Neurosci Ther. 2012;18:1012–20.
221. Brazzini A, Cantella R, De la Cruz A, et al. Intraarterial autologous implantation of adult stem cells for patients with Parkinson disease. J Vasc Interv Radiol. 2010;21:443–51.
222. Garitaonandia I, Gonzalez R, Sherman G, et al. Novel approach to stem cell therapy in Parkinson's disease. Stem Cells Dev. 2018;27:951–7.
223. Bali P, Lahiri DK, Banik A, et al. Potential for stem cells therapy in Alzheimer's disease: do neurotrophic factors play critical role? Curr Alzheimer Res. 2017;14:208–20.
224. Tong LM, Fong H, Huang Y. Stem cell therapy for Alzheimer's disease and related disorders: current status and future perspectives. Exp Mol Med. 2015;47:e151.
225. Hunsberger JG, Rao M, Kurtzberg J, et al. Accelerating stem cell trials for Alzheimer's disease. Lancet Neurol. 2016;15:219–30.
226. Song C-G, Zhang Y-Z, Wu H-N, et al. Stem cells: a promising candidate to treat neurological disorders. Neural Regen Res. 2018;13:1294–304.
227. Kang JM, Yeon BK, Cho S-J, et al. Stem cell therapy for Alzheimer's disease: a review of recent clinical trials. J Alzheimers Dis. 2016;54:879–89.
228. Kim HJ, Seo SW, Chang JW, et al. Stereotactic brain injection of human umbilical cord blood mesenchymal stem cells in patients with Alzheimer's disease dementia: a phase 1 clinical trial. Alzheimers Dement. 2015;1:95–102.

229. Lee NK, Kim HS, Yoo D, et al. Magnetic resonance imaging of Ferumoxytol-Labeled human mesenchymal stem cells in the mouse brain. Stem Cell Rev Rep. 2017;13:127–38.
230. Bonafede R, Mariotti R. ALS pathogenesis and therapeutic approaches: the role of mesenchymal stem cells and extracellular vesicles. Front Cell Neurosci. 2017;11:80.
231. Abdul Wahid SF, Law ZK, Ismail NA, et al. Cell-Based therapies for amyotrophic lateral sclerosis/motor neuron disease. Cochrane Database Syst Rev. 2016;11:CD011742.
232. Petrou P, Gothelf Y, Argov Z, et al. Safety and clinical effects of mesenchymal stem cells secreting neurotrophic factor transplantation in patients with amyotrophic lateral sclerosis: results of phase 1/2 and 2A clinical trials. JAMA Neurol. 2016;73:337–44.
233. Mazzini L, Mareschi K, Ferrero I, et al. Mesenchymal stromal cell transplantation in amyotrophic lateral sclerosis: a long-term safety study. Cytotherapy. 2012;14:56–60.
234. Richard J-P, Hussain U, Gross S, et al. Perfluorocarbon labeling of human glial-restricted progenitors for 19 F magnetic resonance imaging. Stem Cells Transl Med. 2019;8:355–65.
235. Hess DC, Borlongan CV. Stem cells and neurological diseases. Cell Prolif. 2008;41:94–114.
236. Chen Z, Palmer TD. Cellular repair of CNS disorders: an immunological perspective. Hum Mol Genet. 2008;17:R84–92.
237. Tian C, Wang X, Wang X, et al. Autologous bone marrow mesenchymal stem cell therapy in the subacute stage of traumatic brain injury by lumbar puncture. Exp Clin Transplant. 2013;11:176–81.
238. Gennai S, Monsel A, Hao Q, et al. Cell-based therapy for traumatic brain injury. Br J Anaesth. 2015;115:203–12.
239. Wang P, Zhang HL, Li W, et al. Generation of patient-specific induced neuronal cells using a direct reprogramming strategy. Stem Cells Dev. 2014;23:16–23.
240. Jiang L, Li R, Tang H, et al. MRI tracking of iPS cells-induced neural stem cells in traumatic brain injury rats. Cell Transplant. 2019;28:747–55.
241. Saxena T, Loomis KH, Pai SB, et al. Nanocarrier-mediated inhibition of macrophage migration inhibitory factor attenuates secondary injury after spinal cord injury. ACS Nano. 2015;9:1492–505.
242. Donnelly EM, Lamanna J, Boulis NM. Stem cell therapy for the spinal cord. Stem Cell Res Ther. 2012;3:24.
243. Sahni V, Kessler JA. Stem cell therapies for spinal cord injury. Nat Rev Neurol. 2010;6:363–72.
244. Lindvall O, Kokaia Z. Stem cells in human neurodegenerative disorders—time for clinical translation? J Clin Invest. 2010;120:29–40.
245. Satti HS, Waheed A, Ahmed P, et al. Autologous mesenchymal stromal cell transplantation for spinal cord injury: a phase I pilot study. Cytotherapy. 2016;18:518–22.
246. Cheng H, Liu X, Hua R, et al. Clinical observation of umbilical cord mesenchymal stem cell transplantation in treatment for sequelae of thoracolumbar spinal cord injury. J Transl Med. 2014;12:253.
247. Mendonça MVP, Larocca TF, de Freitas Souza BS, et al. Safety and neurological assessments after autologous transplantation of bone marrow mesenchymal stem cells in subjects with chronic spinal cord injury. Stem Cell Res Ther. 2014;5:126.

Molecular Imaging and Theranostics

21

Key Points (Abstract)

Theranostics is the newer exciting modality which is a combination of the terms diagnostics and therapeutics in which diagnostic biomarkers and therapeutic agents are used for a specific target in various diseased cells or tissues. Theranostics imaging is different from the routine imaging modalities which has the capability to diagnose lesions and acts like therapeutic agents. There is significant interest which is being developed for the concept of the personalized medicine which will be precise in customising the management for various diseases. This will ultimately lead to the focussed selection of the patients for the prediction of the response of the therapy and toxicity, for determining the exact prognosis, preventing multiple investigations, and providing the single platform for the management of various diseases. This advantage will significantly increase the efficacy of preventing the therapy side effects leading to the significant increase of patient outcome and lowering the costs.

Drugs having the diagnostic and therapeutic properties are known as theranostics. These drugs are the small therapeutic molecular components which will be tagged to a contrast dye or radioactive tracer and also to the radioimmune therapeutic agents. Commonly used are liposomes, polymers, and nanoparticles, which have very high sensitivity that are used as therapeutic drugs and diagnostic markers.

Keywords

Molecular imaging · Metaiodobenzylguanidine (MIBG) · PET-CT · DOTATAC · DOTANAC · PSMA · MRI

21.1 Introduction

In 1900, a German researcher together with the Nobel Prize laureate Paul Ehrlich developed a scientific concept called "magic bullet" [1]. The magic bullets are special drugs with varied chemical and biologic properties and will be used in the near future for the diagnosis and treatment of particular disease with no impact on the adjacent normal tissues. Ehrlich's research involves the use of the new dyes, design of drugs, and newer chemotherapeutic and targeted agents [2]. Nowadays, the concept of personalized medicine or targeted medicine and precision medicine continues to evolve due to the discoveries of various newer drugs and newer management protocols. This will help for the better characterization, patient selection, outcome of the treatment responses, as well as tissue toxicity and thus can quantify the prognosis to some extent [3, 4]. This is the hybrid word, which is the amalgamation of the therapy and diagnostics, first proposed in

S. Shaikh, *Advances in Imaging*, https://doi.org/10.1007/978-981-16-9535-3_21

2002 [5]. Being the newer concept, this theranostics has not evolved in many years [6]. Human epidermal growth factor receptor 2 (HER2) receptors in a breast cancer for the specific treatment with anti-HER2 receptor antibodies like (e.g., trastuzumab) by immunohistochemical methods is now routinely used [7].

As already mentioned, theranostics is a combination of "therapeutics" and "diagnostics" where diagnosis and therapeutic options can be done [8]. Here the diagnostic biomarkers are combined with the therapeutic agents for a very specific target for diseased cells or tissues. This is again based on the molecular heterogeneity of cells in the tumor, which can be of same cancer type, and also between primary tumor and its metastases [9]. The best example is the theranostics with radioiodine in thyroid disease. Various forms of theranostics are nanotheranostics, optotheranostics, and magneto-theranostics where no radioactivity is present [10, 11] (Diagram 21.1).

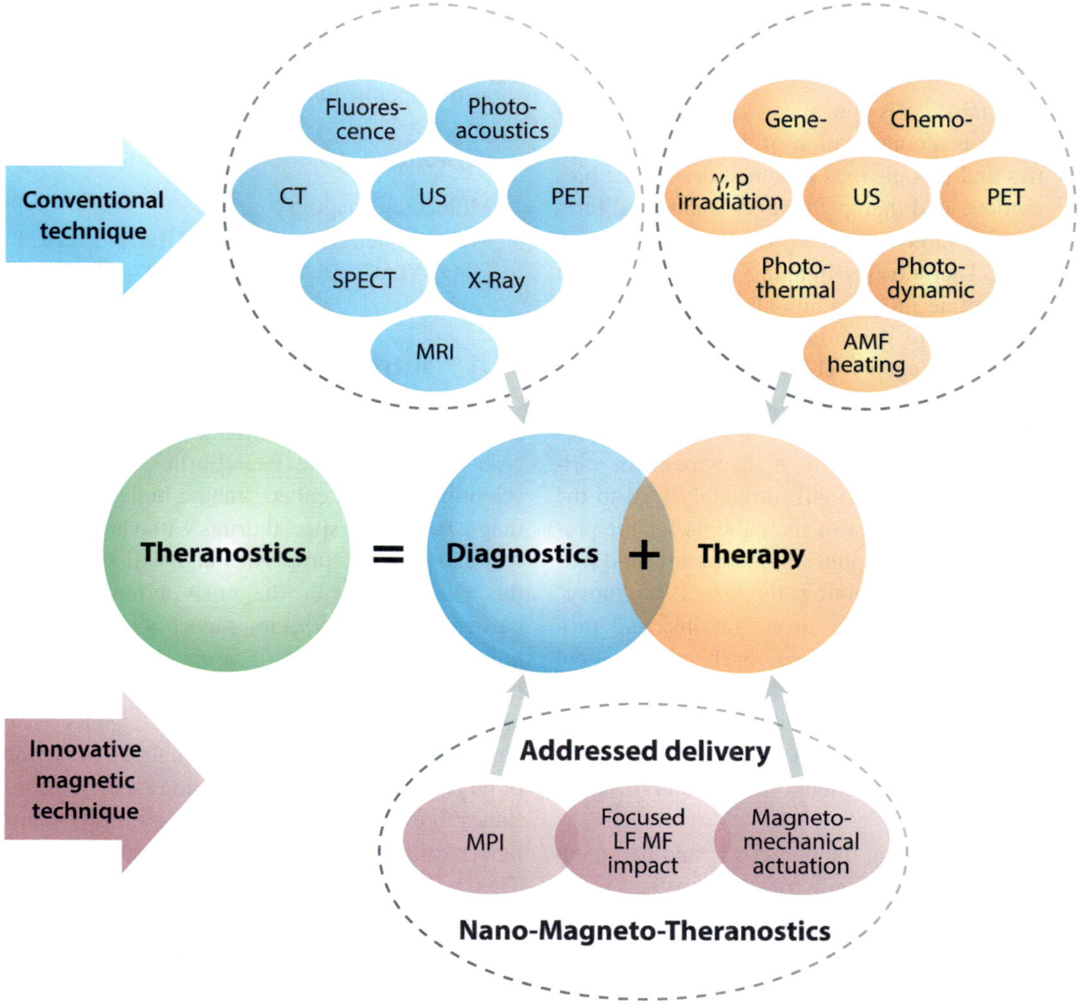

Diagram 21.1 Various modalities and theranostic applications

21.2 Molecular Imaging and Theranostics

Theranostics is the important modality of the characterisation of the various physiological aspects based on the anatomical, biochemical, and functional changes. Molecular imaging by theranostics system will give the important information of the anatomical site of the cellular targets by which the therapeutic agent can be used. 123I (a γ-emitter) is used for the imaging along with the 131I (β and γ emitter) for the various thyroid cancers and 131I ablative therapy.

Metaiodobenzylguanidine (MIBG) combined with the 131I can be used in diagnosis and therapy [12, 13]. Various somatostatin peptide analogs are in various stages of trial for the various aspects of radionuclides [14–16]. PET is also the established imaging modality for various cancer staging, restaging, and monitoring therapy response [17]. Despite of this, PET cannot give the specific cellular target. Molecular imaging therapy is also associated with cellular proliferation, steroid synthesis, growth factor receptor expression, catecholamine production, hypoxia-induced gene expression, or apoptosis. 18F-labeled oestradiol is the imaging modality, used to diagnose the estrogenic receptor-positive lesions [18, 19]. By the same probe, PET is more accurate in predicting the response to hormonal therapy by tamoxifen [20]. If the decision for hormonal therapy is directly dependent on the imaging findings, then it is the true theranostics system. Some of the findings are the presence of various radio immunotherapies for B-cell lymphoma imaging. This is done before with the administration to specific agents for screening the abnormal biodistribution; tumor targeting or quantification is not required to proceed with therapy [21]. It has now become the analytical tool identifying the various neoplastic targets of very high sensitivity and relatively high specificity. Newer biological targets are also used which will have the more predictivity for monitoring response to therapy. Various promising cellular combinations with the various imaging radionuclides can be done by using the various paramagnetic and superparamagnetic metals and optically active compounds. Due to the better modular construction, the nanoparticles are used for another reason: due to their very small size, they cannot come out of the intravascular compartment. Another important aspect is the enhanced permeability effect which will cause the passive accumulation of nanoparticles at the various tumor sites due to leaking neovascularity. Nanomedicines are having the nanoparticle-based therapeutics, of very small size 10 and 200 nm and made up of various lipids, polymers, metals, and semiconductors. It has another advantage to carrying various targeting agents, various imaging moieties, and different drugs and can have variety of the drug compositions. The various targeted medicines are also being used along with the EPR effect. This targeted imaging and therapeutic options by using the various specific disease focussed receptors which have tumor-induced angiogenesis [22–24]. By the action of an enzyme overexpressed by tumours, such as proteases this has shown significant change in the optical imaging [25–29]. Various newer biomarkers development has resulted in the possible use in the immunology, cardiology, and infectious diseases (Diagram 21.2).

21.3 Radiotheranostics

The use of radioactive material in the theranostics is known as radiotheranostics. Radio iodine and MIBG scan is also important for the diagnostic imaging and treatment of patients with neuroblastoma, paraganglioma, and pheochromocytoma [30]. Various newer agents like somatostatin receptors (SSTRs) for the neuroendocrine tumours, prostate-specific membrane antigen [PSMA] in prostate cancer, and chemokine receptors in multiple myeloma are few of the newer ones with very high potential. Radioiodine is the first theranostics agent in use [31] (Diagram 21.3).

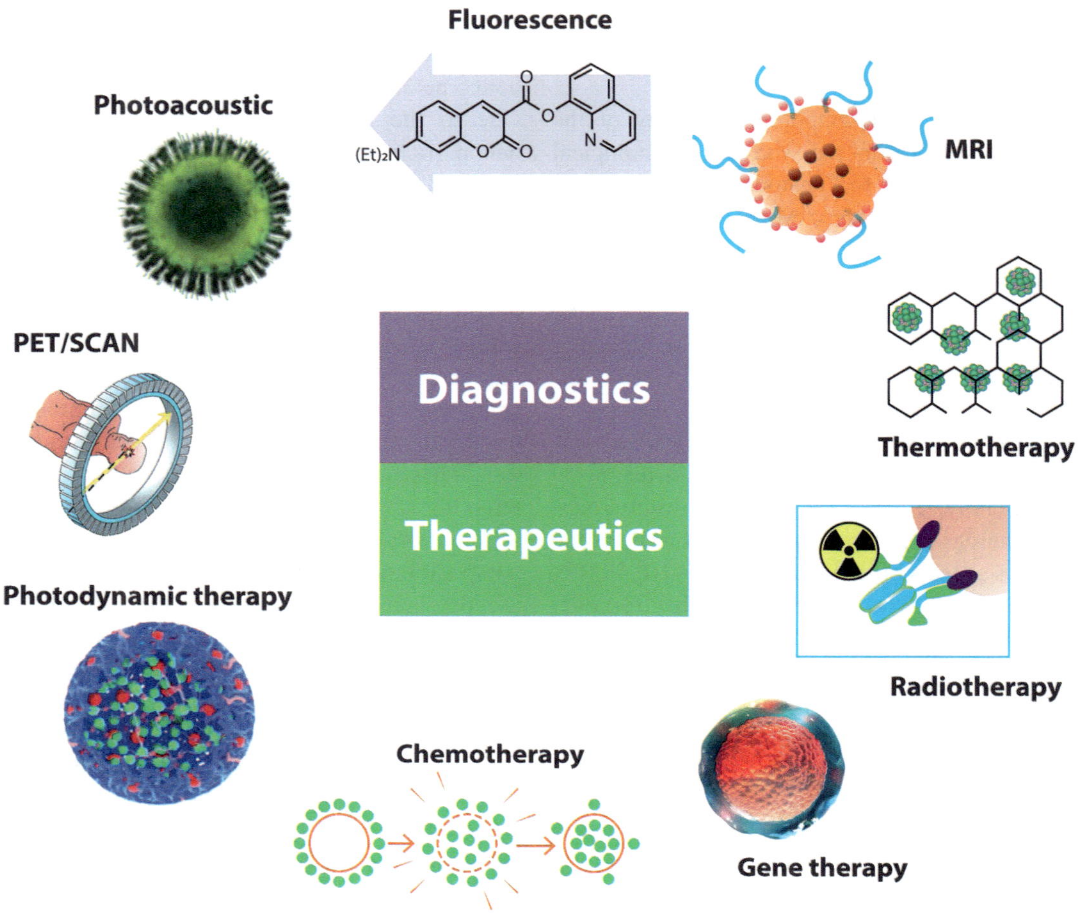

Diagram 21.2 Different modalities and various therapeutic options

21.3.1 Peptide Receptor Radionuclide Therapy

Neuroendocrine tumor therapy is used in tumours which are forming, the neuroendocrine tumours arising from small bowel, pancreas, lung, and paediatric brain will be showing higher level of SSTR, and around 80% of gastroenteropancreatic neuroendocrine tumours express SSTR [32]. The hallmark of the neuroendocrine tumours is that they secrete peptides and amines, and these agonists and antagonists will define the amount of the clinical symptoms. Imaging of the SSTR expression, 68Ga which is the radiometal, has been significantly used in the last couple of years [33, 34]. 68Ga can also be chelated with DOTA for STTR imaging.

For the evaluation of neuroendocrine tumor, imaging and DOTATOC and DOTATATE are used and are widely used worldwide [35].

PSMA radiotheranostics is also based on the same principle of the optimal imaging and therapy protocols and also uses the response to PSMA-based radionuclide therapy and neuroendocrine differentiation along with the utility of SSTR theranostics [36]

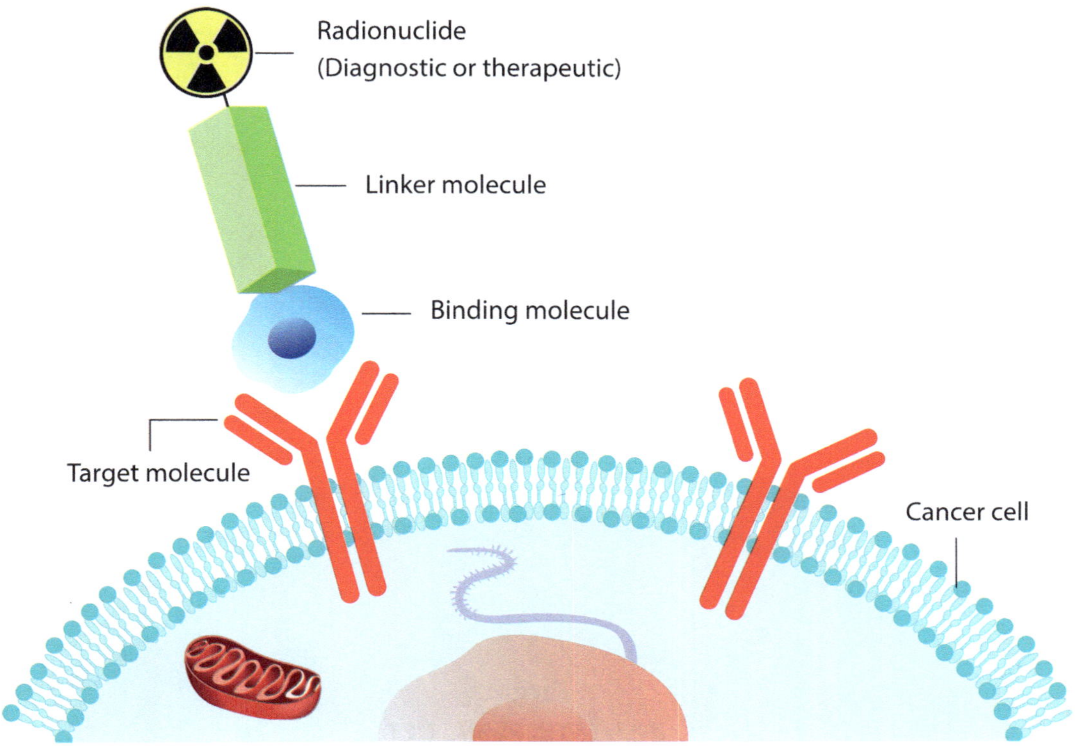

Diagram 21.3 The general concept of radiopharmaceuticals

21.3.2 Chemokine Receptor-Targeted Radiotheranostics

Chemokine receptors and their ligands play an important role in the initiation, progression, and metastasis of various cancer types [37], human immunodeficiency virus infection [38, 39] atherosclerosis [40], autoimmune disorders [41], and many others. CXCR4 is the commonest chemokine used in various cancers [42–45]. As many tumor types are there, then CXCR4 expression can be established for the tumor development and/or metastasis [46, 47], and most important is the poor prognosis of the tumours and therapeutic resistance of the tumours [48, 49]. Thus, the concept of "see and treat" with various radiotracers radionuclides has led to the study of cancer biology, radiochemistry, and imaging science. This is very important in cancer management. With radioiodine in thyroid diseases, neuroendocrine tumours, and prostate cancer, many new indications will come up in the near future (Diagram 21.4).

21.3.3 Theranostics Nuclear Oncology

There is the use of precise molecular imaging components for identifying the specific pathology of tumour cells. "We see what we treat, and we treat what we see" (Richard Baum). Here the theranostics will be used to predict the radiation dose which will be absorbed in the radiotherapy [50].

Modern theranostics radionuclide for the neuroendocrine tumours (NETs) was established by Professor Eric Krenning at the Erasmus Medical Centre Rotterdam for the clinical development DOTA—octreotide for peptide receptor radionuclide therapy (PRRT) of gastroenteropancreatic (GEP) NETs [51, 52].

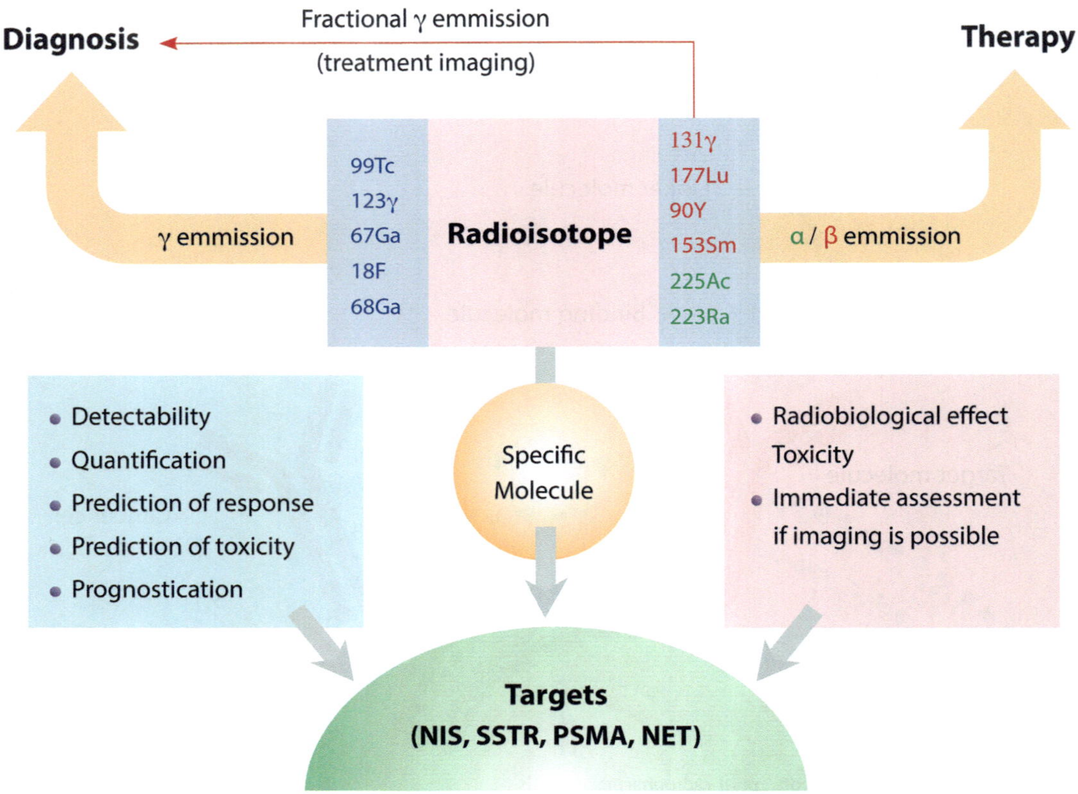

Diagram 21.4 Specific molecule and radio isotopes in the theranostics

Prostate cancer is the most common cancer and second-most common cancer in the USA [53]. 68-gallium-PSMA PET/CT imaging has become the hallmark for the diagnosis and treatment of prostate cancer based on the multicentre Australian study of 431 patients imaged for primary staging (25%), or for restaging/biochemical recurrence (75%) [54]. Another retrospective study showed the impact of the PSMA on the overall management in 39% of patients with biochemically recurrent prostate cancer [55].

21.4 Theranostic Imaging in Cancer

Theranostics have become more specific and focussed for the imaging of the cancer, based on the various targets to see their delivery and monitor response to treatment and also the associated damage to normal tissues. Theranostics imaging is also based on the complexity of the cancer.

There are various challenges in theranostics imaging like quantitative image analyses, cost of synthesizing theranostics agents, other contraindications associated with these agents, and other challenges.

Theranostics imaging needs cancer-specific targets for non-invasive visualisation of the structures. Receptors and antigens of various cancers will be used for the non-invasive imaging, for example, breast cancers expressing the human epidermal growth factor receptor (Her-2) and the use of Trastuzumab, for metastatic breast cancer [56, 57]; prostate-specific membrane antigen (PSMA) expression on the surface of prostate carcinomas, especially in the advanced and metastatic disease [58, 59]; and ideal target for immunotherapy, which is associated with the cell surface and relation to the enzymatic or signalling activity [58, 60]. Abnormal glucose and choline metabolism, angiogenesis, are some of the things to be seen in cancer [61]. As we know physiologically, there will be hypoxia, acidic extracellular pH, and substrate deprivation. The tumour microenvironment is also important for theranostics imaging [62]. Nanoplatforms which are comprised of the various liposomes, nanoparticles, micelles, and viral vectors which can be molecular targeted with DNA (cDNA) or small interfering RNA (siRNA). Drug-activating enzyme is used in prodrug therapy to minimize the side effects. Various prototype agents made up of cytosine deaminase (CD) labelled with multimodal MR as well as by different optical imaging reporters can be used for evaluation [63]. Like the PSMA binding agent [64] to target the nanoplex to PCa cells. Along with the choline kinase (Chk) to see the aggression of the tumours [65]. Furthermore, these will have capacity to deliver multiple siRNA.

21.5 PET Tracers for Theranostics Imaging of CNS Tumours

PRRT is used to target the various peptide receptors. The expression and accessibility of a target peptide receptor is studied using an analog of somatostatin, octreotide, and labelled gallium-68 DOTA chelator [66]. DOTA-TOC in GBM will also show the therapeutic efficacy [67]. Other forms of the PRRT for treatment of CNS tumours like meningioma can be used [68–70].

Theranostics nanocarriers with MRI is based on the theranostics imaging which will be a combination of the molecular biology, synthetic chemistry, and nanotechnology. Organic and inorganic materials are the two most commonly used nanoparticles. Organic nanoparticles are polymers, polymeric micelles, and dendrimers and are for primarily drug delivery [71]. Inorganic is based on the physical features and their size and composition. The synthesis of magnetic nanoparticles will show the additional therapeutic and targeting functionalities along with these systems to make the smart platform for the MRI. Different cell-specific imaging, targeting, and therapeutic moieties can be incorporated into a single magnetic nanoparticle that is designed for theranostics MRI [11, 72].

21.6 Theranostics Reagents of MRI

MRI probes which will be used for theranostics should have the following characteristic features:

- They should accumulate in the specific target tissues.
- Deliver effectively.
- It should have structural and functional information of the region of interest.
- It should be safe.

The various probes which will be used in the theranostics MRI will be having affinity to iron oxide nanoparticles, gadolinium (Gd)-loaded nanoparticles, and manganese (Mn)-based nanoparticles. The theranostics MRI should have three important components which are as follows:

- Biodegradable superparamagnetic iron core for MRI
- Polymer surface coating having protective and functional properties
- Capable of getting attached various functional moieties [71, 73]

Iron oxide core has an impact on the relaxation time causing the darkening in T2-weighted sequences. Different coating materials will stabilize the particle size converting it into multifunctional drugs [73]. Theranostic nanogel can be imaged by MRI [74]. The important characteristic features are the particle size, surface coating, and surface charge which are important components to identify the biodistribution and pharmacokinetics of SPIO nanoparticles [75]. SPIO nanoparticles are the negative contrast agents, which are difficult to differentiate between the small haemorrhagic components in the spleen and liver [76, 77]. Gd-loaded nanoparticles are

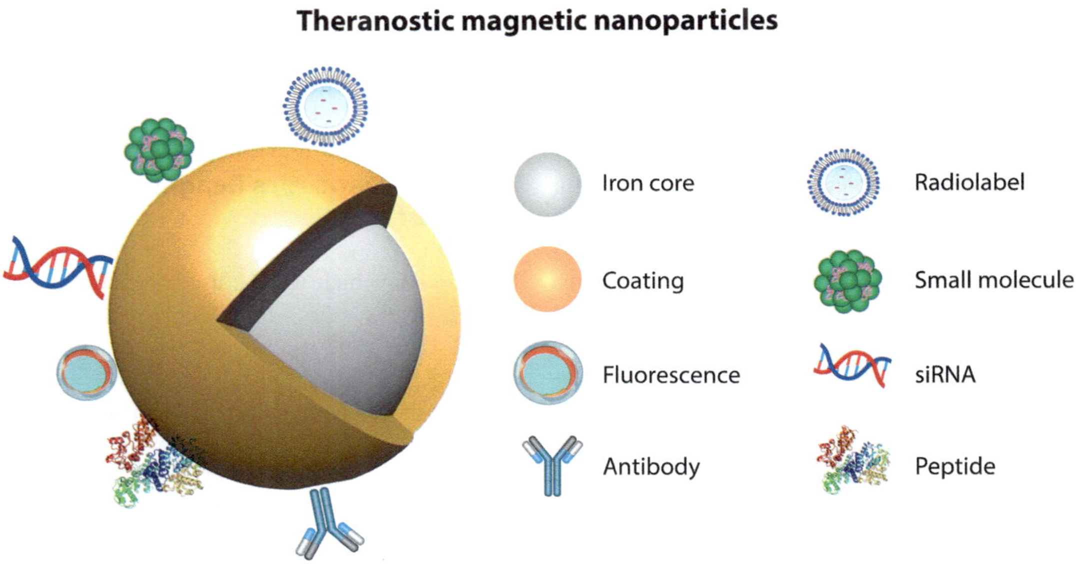

Diagram 21.5 Various theranostic nanoparticles

paramagnetic contrast agents that will have brighter contrast on T1-weighted images [78, 79]. Various gadolinium nanoparticles are lipid-based nanoparticles, polymeric nanoparticles, micelles, dendrimers, and Gd–silica nanoparticles [80, 81] (Diagram 21.5).

21.7 Mn-Based Nanoparticles for Theranostic Imaging

Mn is having the paramagnetic properties, that is, the high spin number, very long electronic relaxation times, and labile water exchange [82]. These agents are of two types: small molecule agents and macromolecular agents. Small Mn agents are similar to Gd chelates; macromolecular agents are MnO, MnO2, and Mn3 O4 manganese oxides [83]. These oxides be added to nanoparticles and form the component of the theranostics [80, 84]. MnO nanoparticles can be used as adhesive component for specific targeted delivery [85]. Oleic acid-coated MnO nanoparticles when attached with the micelles can be taken up by target cells in vivo as the theranostic approach of the MRI [82]. Mn can have some Parkinson's disease-like symptoms [84]. Nanoparticle transport can have the significant solubility of small molecules, which can be delivered as effective platforms [11, 71]. siRNAs are the important component for the nonspecific distribution, poor cellular uptake, and the failure of endosomal escape [86]. Nanoparticles are having major advantages like they have similar size and better biocompatibility.

21.8 DNA

DNA is the genetic material having the hereditary information and reproduced in most cells of living organisms [87]. DNA is the double helical structure for replacement of the mutated gene which will be causing the changes in the genetic information.

Nanoparticle surface will have the plasmin particles which are paramagnetic with high transfection efficiencies in cells in vitro [88]. The reporter gene assay will have nanoplatform which will be producing the gene transfection in a T-lymphocyte cell line and can be seen by MRI [89]. Here the nanoparticle will bind with mcDNA and protect its enzymatic degradation [90]. Targeting agents like mRNAs can be seen for the cleavage or translational repression [91]. Various other biological processes will be happening: cellular differentiation, proliferation, and apoptosis [92–94]. These theranostic imaging techniques will help in the correction of the level of miRNAs in known diabetic patients and also for the newer treatment options for T1D [95]. T1D is an autoimmune disease comprising of the complex lymphocytic infiltration with microvasculature alterations, resulting in the significant loss of the insulin-producing β cells [96]. Inflammation causes changes in pancreatic vascularity with significant dysfunction resulting in the extravasation through the walls of the damaged vessel into the surrounding tissue. By this effect, the nanoparticles accumulation at this site will result in the enhanced permeability and retention effect [11]. SPIO nanoparticles are commonly used for the detection of vascular leakage causing the better visualization of these inflammatory lesions in real time [97, 98]. Theranostic imaging of the lymphocyte will result in the destruction of insulin-producing β cells, causing the T1D [99]. Various potential studies for the MRI tracking of the labelled cytotoxic T lymphocytes which will be infiltrating pancreatic islet in different animal models can be used [100–103]. Autoantigen recognition, antigen-specific SPIO nanoparticles which were synthesized by Medarova et al. can be done [104]. They are made up of the nanoparticles which are conjugated with NRP-V7 peptide (a high-avidity mimotope of IGRP) [96, 105]) (Diagrams 21.6 and 21.7).

Theranostic MRI for graft rescue can be the important modality for the diagnostic imaging of islet grafts, where the contrast agents will deliver

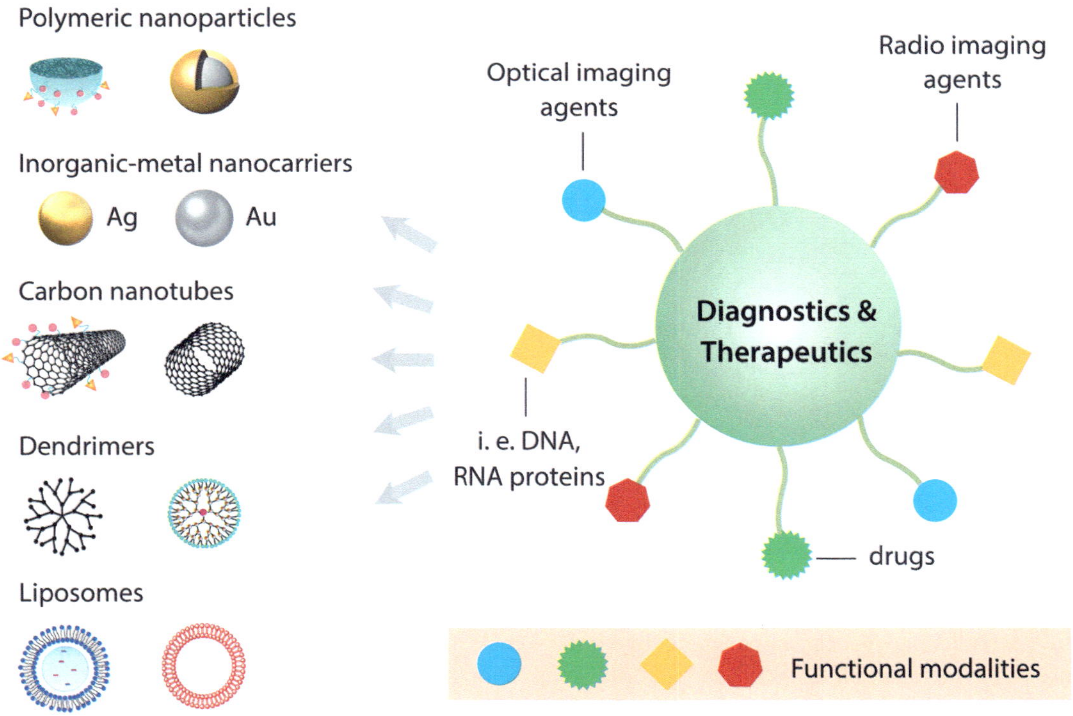

Diagram 21.6 Various particles in nanotheranostics

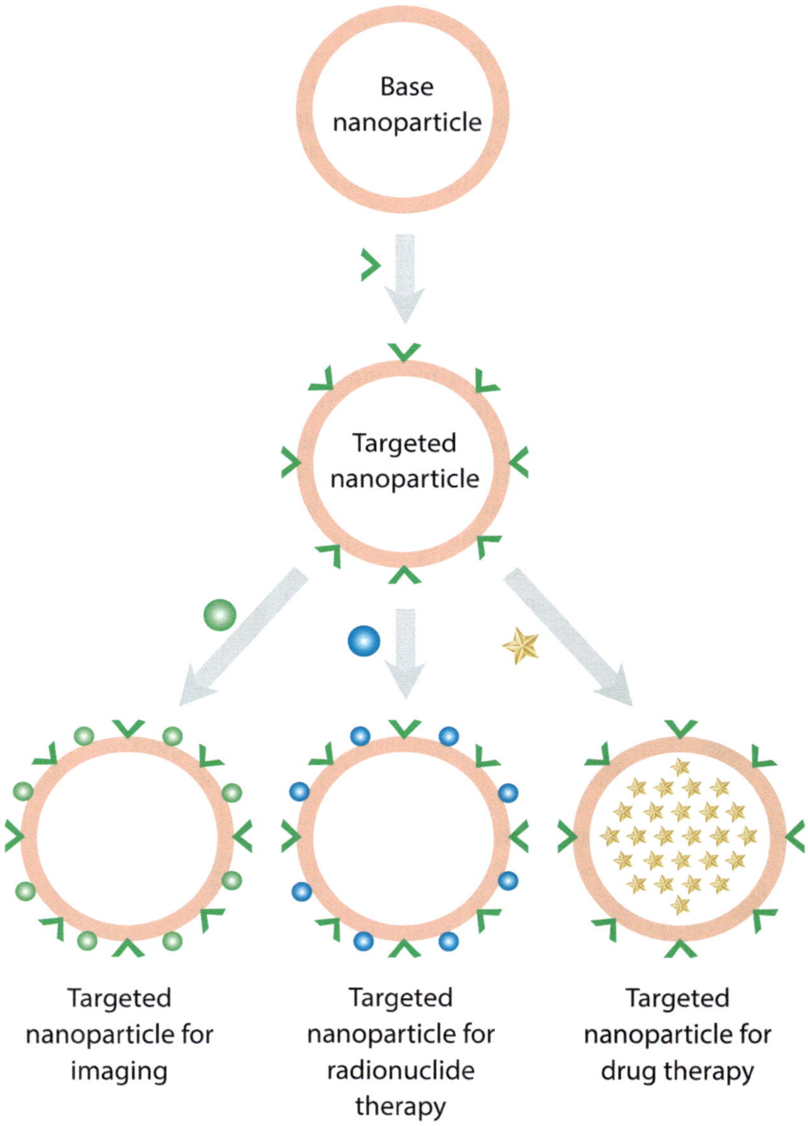

Diagram 21.7 Various targeted nanoparticles in various therapies

the therapeutic options. siRNAs will silence the gene expression of choice [106]. These theranostic probes can cause significant clinical translation; islet damage genes can be targeted with the use of the nanoparticles.

Theranostic imaging is of significance for the encapsulated islet grafts and for transplanted islets is graft encapsulation with magneto capsules.

21.9 Hepatic Radioembolization

Hepatic radioembolization for various primary or metastatic secondary by using the multi-modality scintigraphy, SPECT/CT, CT, MRI, PET/CT/MRI, arteriography, and associated with the clinical evaluation. In radioembolization, therapeutic radioisotopes will be useful by using the microspheres to tumours for the neoplastic microarterial vasculature. Hepatic lesions are supplied by the arterial tumours, so the hepatic arterial route is the option for the delivery of the agents. Various radioactive microspheres are made up of the glass or resin with high-energy β- and γ-particle-emitting radioisotopes. Placing this microsphere in the tumor is important for the delivery of required high-radiation doses to the tumor lower dose to the surrounding tissues. There should not be any leakage of these radioactive substances into the systemic circulation causing the microvascular embolization of the lung parenchyma. The possibility of the pulmonary embolization from the intrahepatic arteriovenous shunt and the embolization due to anatomic variations in arterial supply of the various abdominal can be seen by using the scintigraphy planar and hybrid (SPECT/CT) techniques, thus enhancing the safety of the procedure [107]. Thus, with the modern theranostic procedures, hepatic radioembolization is used primary for hepatocellular carcinoma and secondarily for colorectal cancer and neuroendocrine tumours [108].

18F-fluorodeoxyglucose (FDG) PET and PET/CT are being widely used for the cancer, inflammatory and infectious conditions, and neurologic diseases [99–102]. Glycolysis is the main metabolic activity leading to carcinogenesis, overall cancer cell survival, progression of the cancers and will define the aggressiveness of the cancer and its antitumoral therapy effectiveness [103]. Thus, the significant changes in the normal glucose metabolism into aerobic glycolysis occurring in neoplastic cells are known as the Warburg effect [104]. Due to this, FDG PET-CT has significantly evolved as an important modality for the identification, quantification of neoplastic cells, prognosis, and various follow-up options which will define the activity in the particular tumour tissue.

References

1. Valent P, Groner B, Schumacher U, et al. Paul Ehrlich (1854-1915) and his contributions to the foundation and birth of translational medicine. J Innate Immun. 2016;8(2):111–20.
2. Strebhardt K, Ullrich A. Paul Ehrlich's magic bullet concept: 100 years of progress. Nat Rev Cancer. 2008;8(6):473–80.
3. Hricak H. Oncologic imaging: a guiding hand of personalized cancer care. Radiology. 2011;259(3):633–40.
4. Jadvar H, Chen X, Cai W, Mahmood U. Radiotheranostics in cancer diagnosis and management. Radiology. 2018;286(2):388–400.
5. Funkhouser J. Reinventing pharma: the theranostic revolution. Curr Drug Discov. 2002;2:17–9.
6. DeNardo GL, DeNardo SJ. Concepts, consequences, and implications of theranosis. Semin Nucl Med. 2012;42(3):147–50.
7. European Society of Radiology. Medical imaging in personalised medicine: a white paper of the research committee of the European Society of Radiology (ESR). Insights Imaging. 2015;6(2):141–55.
8. Warner S. Diagnostics + therapy = theranostics. Scientist. 2004;18:38–9.
9. Sumer B, Gao J. Theranostic nanomedicine for cancer. Nanomedicine (Lond). 2008;3(2):137–40.
10. Xie J, Lee S, Chen X. Nanoparticle-based theranostic agents. Adv Drug Deliv Rev. 2010;62(11):1064–79.
11. Lee DY, Li KCP. Molecular theranostics: a primer for the imaging professional. AJR Am J Roentgenol. 2011;197(2):318–24.
12. Sisson JC, Shapiro B, Beierwaltes WH, Copp JE. Locating pheochromocytomas by scintigraphy using 131I-metaiodobenzylguanidine. CA Cancer J Clin. 1984;34:86–92.
13. Sisson JC, Shapiro B, Beierwaltes WH, et al. Radiopharmaceutical treatment of malignant pheochromocytoma. J Nucl Med. 1984;25:197–206.
14. Kwekkeboom DJ, de Herder WW, van Eijck CH, et al. Peptide receptor radionuclide therapy in patients with gastroenteropancreatic neuroendocrine tumours. Semin Nucl Med. 2010;40:78–88.
15. Nisa L, Savelli G, Giubbini R. Yttrium-90 DOTATOC therapy in GEP-NET and other SST2 expressing tumours: a selected review. Ann Nucl Med. 2011;25:75–85.
16. van Essen M, Krenning EP, Kam BL, de Jong M, Valkema R, Kwekkeboom DJ. Peptide-receptor radionuclide therapy for endocrine tumours. Nat Rev Endocrinol. 2009;5:382–93.
17. Czernin J, Benz MR, Allen-Auerbach MS. PET/ CT imaging: the incremental value of assessing the glucose metabolic phenotype and the structure of cancers in a single examination. Eur J Radiol. 2010;73:470–80.
18. Peterson LM, Mankoff DA, Lawton T, et al. Quantitative imaging of oestrogen receptor expression in breast cancer with PET and 18F-fluoroestradiol. J Nucl Med. 2008;49:367–74.
19. Mintun MA, Welch MJ, Siegel BA, et al. Breast cancer: PET imaging of oestrogen receptors. Radiology. 1988;169:45–8.
20. Linden HM, Stekhova SA, Link JM, et al. Quantitative fluoroestradiol positron emission tomography imag-

ing predicts response to endocrine treatment in breast cancer. J Clin Oncol. 2006;24:2793–9.
21. Spies SM. Imaging and dosing in radioimmunotherapy with yttrium 90 ibritumomab tiuxetan (Zevalin). Semin Nucl Med. 2004;34:10–3.
22. Sipkins DA, Cheresh DA, Kazemi MR, Nevin LM, Bednarski MD, Li KC. Detection of tumor angiogenesis in vivo by alphaVbeta3-targeted magnetic resonance imaging. Nat Med. 1998;4:623–6.
23. Li L, Wartchow CA, Danthi SN, et al. A novel antiangiogenesis therapy using an integrin antagonist or anti-Flk-1 antibody coated 90Y-labeled nanoparticles. Int J Radiat Oncol Biol Phys. 2004;58:1215–27.
24. Hood JD, Bednarski M, Frausto R, et al. Tumor regression by targeted gene delivery to the neo vasculature. Science. 2002;296:2404–7.
25. Bremer C, Bredow S, Mahmood U, Weissleder R, Tung CH. Optical imaging of matrix metalloproteinase-2 activity in tumours: feasibility study in a mouse model. Radiology. 2001;221:523–9.
26. Galande AK, Hilderbrand SA, Weissleder R, Tung CH. Enzyme-targeted fluorescent imaging probes on a multiple antigenic peptide core. J Med Chem. 2006;49:4715–20.
27. Mahmood U, Tung CH, Bogdanov A Jr, Weissleder R. Near-infrared optical imaging of protease activity for tumor detection. Radiology. 1999;213:866–70.
28. Tung CH, Mahmood U, Bredow S, Weissleder R. In vivo imaging of proteolytic enzyme activity using a novel molecular reporter. Cancer Res. 2000;60:4953–8.
29. Feng X, Lv F, Liu L, et al. Conjugated polymer nanoparticles for drug delivery and imaging. ACS Appl Mater Interfaces. 2010;2:2429–35.
30. Parisi MT, Eslamy H, Park JR, Shulkin BL, Yanik GA. ^{131}I-metaiodobenzylguanidine theranostics in neuroblastoma: historical perspectives; practical applications. Semin Nucl Med. 2016;46(3):184–202.
31. Silberstein EB. Radioiodine: the classic theranostic agent. Semin Nucl Med. 2012;42(3):164–70.
32. Baldelli R, Barnabei A, Rizza L, et al. Somatostatin analogs therapy in gastroenteropancreatic neuroendocrine tumours: current aspects and new perspectives. Front Endocrinol (Lausanne). 2014;5:7.
33. Buchmann I, Henze M, Engelbrecht S, et al. Comparison of 68Ga-DOTATOC PET and 111In-DTPAOC (Octreoscan) SPECT in patients with neuroendocrine tumours. Eur J Nucl Med Mol Imaging. 2007;34(10):1617–26.
34. Hofmann M, Maecke H, Börner R, et al. Biokinetics and imaging with the somatostatin receptor PET radioligand (68)GaDOTATOC: preliminary data. Eur J Nucl Med. 2001;28(12):1751–7.
35. Virgolini I, Ambrosini V, Bomanji JB, et al. Procedure guidelines for PET/CT tumour imaging with 68Ga-DOTA-conjugated peptides: 68Ga-DOTA-TOC, 68Ga-DOTA-NOC, 68Ga-DOTA-TATE. Eur J Nucl Med Mol Imaging. 2010;37(10):2004–10.
36. Jadvar H. PSMA PET in prostate cancer. J Nucl Med. 2015;56(8):1131–2.
37. Vandercappellen J, Van Damme J, Struyf S. The role of CXC chemokines and their receptors in cancer. Cancer Lett. 2008;267(2):226–44.
38. De Clercq E. Inhibition of HIV infection by bicyclams, highly potent and specific CXCR4 antagonists. Mol Pharmacol. 2000;57(5):833–9.
39. Fujii N, Nakashima H, Tamamura H. The therapeutic potential of CXCR4 antagonists in the treatment of HIV. Expert OpinInvestig Drugs. 2003;12(2):185–95.
40. Braunersreuther V, Mach F, Steffens S. The specific role of chemokines in atherosclerosis. ThrombHaemost. 2007;97(5):714–21.
41. Iwamoto T, Okamoto H, Toyama Y, Momohara S. Molecular aspects of rheumatoid arthritis: chemokines in the joints of patients. FEBS J. 2008;275(18):4448–55.
42. Müller A, Homey B, Soto H, et al. Involvement of chemokine receptors in breast cancer metastasis. Nature. 2001;410(6824):50–6.
43. Kang H, Watkins G, Douglas-Jones A, Mansel RE, Jiang WG. The elevated level of CXCR4 is correlated with nodal metastasis of human breast cancer. Breast. 2005;14(5):360–7.
44. Balkwill F. The significance of cancer cell expression of the chemokine receptor CXCR4. Semin Cancer Biol. 2004;14(3):171–9.
45. Kulbe H, Levinson NR, Balkwill F, Wilson JL. The chemokine network in cancer: much more than directing cell movement. Int J Dev Biol. 2004;48(5-6):489–96.
46. Yoon Y, Liang Z, Zhang X, et al. CXC chemokine receptor-4 antagonist blocks both growth of primary tumor and metastasis of head and neck cancer in xenograft mouse models. Cancer Res. 2007;67(15):7518–24.
47. Li JK, Yu L, Shen Y, Zhou LS, Wang YC, Zhang JH. Inhibition of CXCR4 activity with AMD3100 decreases invasion of human colorectal cancer cells in vitro. World J Gastroenterol. 2008;14(15):2308–13.
48. Zeng Z, Samudio IJ, Munsell M, et al. Inhibition of CXCR4 with the novel RCP168 peptide overcomes stroma-mediated chemoresistance in chronic and acute leukemias. Mol Cancer Ther. 2006;5(12):3113–21.
49. Oda Y, Tateishi N, Matono H, et al. Chemokine receptor CXCR4 expression is correlated with VEGF expression and poor survival in soft-tissue sarcoma. Int J Cancer. 2009;124(8):1852–9.
50. Eberlein U, Cremonesi M, Lassmann M. Individualized dosimetry for theranostics: necessary, nice to have, or counterproductive? J Nucl Med. 2017;58:97S–103S.
51. Levine R, Krenning EP. Clinical history of the theranostic radionuclide approach to neuroendocrine

tumors and other types of cancer: historical review based on an interview of Eric P Krenning. J Nucl Med. 2017;58:3S–9S.
52. Strosberg J, El-Haddad G, Wolin E, et al. Phase 3 trial of 177-Lu-dotatate for midgut neuroendocrine tumors. N Engl J Med. 2017;376:125–35.
53. Torre LA, Bray F, Siegel RL, et al. Global cancer statistics 2012. CA Cancer J Clin. 2015;65:87–108.
54. Roach PJ, Francis R, Emmett L, et al. The impact of 68-Ga-PSMA PET/CT on management intent in prostate cancer; Results of an Australian prospective multicentre study. J Nucl Med. 2018;59:82–8.
55. Afaq A, Alahmed S, Chen S-H, et al. Impact of ^{68}Ga-prostate-specific membrane antigen PET/CT on prostate cancer management. J Nucl Med. 2018;59(1):89–92.
56. Metro G, Mottolese M, Fabi A. HER-2-positive metastatic breast cancer: trastuzumab and beyond. Expert Opin Pharmacother. 2008;9(15):2583–601. [PubMed: 18803447]
57. Freudenberg JA, Wang Q, Katsumata M, Drebin J, Nagatomo I, Greene MI. The role of HER2 in early breast cancer metastasis and the origins of resistance to HER2-targeted therapies. Exp Mol Pathol. 2009;87(1):1–11. [PubMed: 19450579]
58. Schulke N, Varlamova OA, Donovan GP, et al. The homodimer of prostate-specific membrane antigen is a functional target for cancer therapy. Proc Natl Acad Sci U S A. 2003;100(22):12590–5. [PubMed: 14583590]
59. Huang X, Bennett M, Thorpe PE. Anti-tumor effects and lack of side effects in mice of an immunotoxin directed against human and mouse prostate-specific membrane antigen. Prostate. 2004;61(1):1–11. [PubMed: 15287089]
60. Tasch J, Gong M, Sadelain M, Heston WD. A unique folate hydrolase, prostate-specific membrane antigen (PSMA): a target for immunotherapy? Crit Rev Immunol. 2001;21(1–3):249–61. [PubMed: 11642607]
61. Penet MF, Mikhaylova M, Li C, et al. Applications of molecular MRI and optical imaging in cancer. Future Med Chem. 2010;2(6):975–88. [PubMed: 20634999]
62. Stasinopoulos I, Penet MF, Chen Z, Kakkad S, Glunde K, Bhujwalla ZM. Exploiting the tumor microenvironment for theranostic imaging. NMR Biomed. 2011;24(6):636–47. [PubMed: 21793072]
63. Li C, Penet MF, Winnard P Jr, Artemov D, Bhujwalla ZM. Image-guided enzyme/prodrug cancer therapy. Clin Cancer Res. 2008;14(2):515–22. [PubMed: 18223227]
64. Wang H, Byun Y, Barinka C, et al. Bioisosterism of urea-based GCPII inhibitors: synthesis and structure-activity relationship studies. Bioorg Med Chem Lett. 2010;20(1):392–7. [PubMed: 19897367]
65. Glunde K, Bhujwalla ZM, Ronen SM. Choline metabolism in malignant transformation. Nat Rev Cancer. 2011;11(12):835–48. [PubMed: 22089420]
66. Breeman WA, de Blois E, Sze Chan H, Konijnenberg M, Kwekkeboom DJ, Krenning EP. (68)Ga-labeled DOTA-peptides and (68) Ga-labeled radiopharmaceuticals for positron emission tomography: current status of research, clinical applications, and future perspectives. Semin Nucl Med. 2011;41:314–21.
67. Heute D, Kostron H, von Guggenberg E, Ingorokva S, Gabriel M, Dobrozemsky G, Stockhammer G, Virgolini IJ. Response of recurrent high-grade glioma to treatment with (90)Y-DOTATOC. J Nucl Med. 2010;51:397–400.
68. Seystahl K, Stoecklein V, Schuller U, Rushing E, Nicolas G, Schafer N, Ilhan H, Pangalu A, Weller M, Tonn JC, et al. Somatostatin receptor-targeted radionuclide therapy for progressive meningioma: benefit linked to 68Ga-DOTATATE/-TOC uptake. Neuro Oncol. 2016;18:1538–47.
69. Collamati F, Pepe A, Bellini F, Bocci V, Chiodi G, Cremonesi M, De Lucia E, Ferrari ME, Frallicciardi PM, Grana CM, et al. Toward radioguided surgery with beta-decays: uptake of a somatostatin analogue, DOTATOC, in meningioma and high-grade glioma. J Nucl Med. 2015;56:3–8.
70. Parghane R, Talole S, Basu S. Prevalence of hitherto unknown brain meningioma detected on 68 Ga-DOTATATE positron-emission tomography/computed tomography in patients with metastatic neuroendocrine tumor and exploring potential of 177 Lu-DOTATATE peptide receptor radionuclide therapy as single-shot treatment approach targeting both tumors. World. J Nucl Med. 2019;18:160.
71. Yoo D, Lee JH, Shin TH, Cheon J. Theranostic magnetic nanoparticles. Acc Chem Res. 2011;44(10):863–74.
72. Lee JH, Lee K, Moon SH, Lee Y, Park TG, Cheon J. All-in-one target-cell-specific magnetic nanoparticles for simultaneous molecular imaging and siRNA delivery. Angew Chem Int Ed Engl. 2009;48(23):4174–9.
73. Yigit MV, Moore A, Medarova Z. Magnetic nanoparticles for cancer diagnosis and therapy. Pharm Res. 2012;29(5):1180–8.
74. Zhang L, Xue H, Cao Z, Keefe A, Wang J, Jiang S. Multifunctional and degradable zwitterionic nanogels for targeted delivery, enhanced MR imaging, reduction-sensitive drug release, and renal clearance. Biomaterials. 2011;32(20):4604–8.
75. Wahajuddin, Arora S. Superparamagnetic iron oxide nanoparticles: magnetic nanoplatforms as drug carriers. Int J Nanomed. 2012;7:3445–71.
76. Muja N, Bulte JW. Magnetic resonance imaging of cells in experimental disease models. Prog Nucl Magn Reson Spectrosc. 2009;55(1):61–77.
77. Wang P, Moore A. Molecular imaging of stem cell transplantation for neurodegenerative diseases. Curr Pharm Des. 2012;18(28):4426–40.

78. Baumann D, Rudin M. Quantitative assessment of rat kidney function by measuring the clearance of the contrast agent Gd(DOTA) using dynamic MRI. Magn Reson Imaging. 2000;18(5):587–95.
79. Ai H. Layer-by-layer capsules for magnetic resonance imaging and drug delivery. Adv Drug Deliv Rev. 2011;63(9):772–88.
80. Rumenapp C, Gleich B, Haase A. Magnetic nanoparticles in magnetic resonance imaging and diagnostics. Pharm Res. 2012;29(5):1165–79.
81. Zhao Y, Vivero-Escoto JL, Slowing II, Trewyn BG, Lin VS. Capped mesoporous silica nanoparticles as stimuli-responsive controlled release systems for intracellular drug/gene delivery. Expert Opin Drug Deliv. 2010;7(9):1013–29.
82. Howell M, Mallela J, Wang C, et al. Manganese-loaded lipid-micellar theranostics for simultaneous drug and gene delivery to lungs. J Control Release. 2013;167(2):210–8.
83. Kim T, Momin E, Choi J, et al. Mesoporous silica-coated hollow manganese oxide nanoparticles as positive T1 contrast agents for labeling and MRI tracking of adipose-derived mesenchymal stem cells. J Am Chem Soc. 2011;133(9):2955–61.
84. Pan D, Caruthers SD, Senpan A, Schmieder AH, Wickline SA, Lanza GM. Revisiting an old friend: manganese-based MRI contrast agents. Wiley Interdiscip Rev Nanomed Nanobiotechnol. 2011;3(2):162–73.
85. Bae KH, Lee K, Kim C, Park TG. Surface functionalized hollow manganese oxide nanoparticles for cancer targeted siRNA delivery and magnetic resonance imaging. Biomaterials. 2011;32(1):176–84.
86. Prabhu P, Patravale V. The upcoming field of theranostic nanomedicine: an overview. J Biomed Nanotechnol. 2012;8(6):859–82.
87. Abu-Salah KM, Ansari AA, Alrokayan SA. DNA-based applications in nanobiotechnology. J Biomed Biotechnol. 2010;2010:715295.
88. Bhakta G, Sharma RK, Gupta N, Cool S, Nurcombe V, Maitra A. Multifunctional silica nanoparticles with potentials of imaging and gene delivery. Nanomedicine. 2011;7(4):472–9.
89. Chen G, Chen W, Wu Z, et al. MRI-visible polymeric vector bearing CD3 single chain antibody for gene delivery to T cells for immunosuppression. Biomaterials. 2009;30(10):1962–70. Future Science Group Perspective Wang & Moore. www.future-medicine.com, 37.
90. Wan Q, Xie L, Gao L, et al. Self-assembled magnetic theranostic nanoparticles for highly sensitive MRI of minicircle DNA delivery. Nanoscale. 2013;5(2):744–52.
91. Guo H, Ingolia NT, Weissman JS, Bartel DP. Mammalian microRNAs predominantly act to decrease target mRNA levels. Nature. 2010;466(7308):835–40.
92. Bartel D. MicroRNAs: genomics, biogenesis, mechanism, and function. Cell. 2004;116:281–97.
93. Krek A, Grun D, Poy MN, et al. Combinatorial microRNA target predictions. Nat Genet. 2005;37(5):495–500.
94. Lewis B, Burge C, Bartel D. Conserved seed pairing, often flanked by adenosines, indicates that thousands of human genes are microRNA targets. Cell. 2005;120:15–20.
95. Guay C, Roggli E, Nesca V, Jacovetti C, Regazzi R. Diabetes mellitus, a microRNA-related disease? Transl Res. 2011;157(4):253–64.
96. Amrani A, Verdaguer J, Serra P, Tafuro S, Tan R, Santamaria P. Progression of autoimmune diabetes driven by avidity maturation of a T-cell population. Nature. 2000;406(6797):739–42.
97. Denis MC, Mahmood U, Benoist C, Mathis D, Weissleder R. Imaging inflammation of the pancreatic islets in Type 1 diabetes. Proc Natl Acad Sci USA. 2004;101(34):12634–9.
98. Turvey SE, Swart E, Denis MC, et al. Noninvasive imaging of pancreatic inflammation and its reversal in Type 1 diabetes. J Clin Invest. 2005;115(9):2454–61.
99. Lernmark A, Larsson HE. Immune therapy in Type 1 diabetes mellitus. Nat Rev Endocrinol. 2013;9(2):92–103.
100. Moore A, Grimm J, Han B, Santamaria P. Tracking the recruitment of diabetogenic CD8+ T-cells to the pancreas in real time. Diabetes. 2004;53(6):1459–66. 11 Demonstrated that inflammation of pancreatic islets by autoreactive T cells could be detected in real-time by MRI. The labeled T cell could be potentially used for visualizing the presence of ongoing autoimmune responses and further for the drug delivery.
101. Moore A, Sun PZ, Cory D, Hogemann D, Weissleder R, Lipes MA. MRI of insulitis in autoimmune diabetes. Magn Reson Med. 2002;47(4):751–8.
102. Billotey C, Aspord C, Beuf O, et al. T-cell homing to the pancreas in autoimmune mouse models of diabetes: in vivo MR imaging. Radiology. 2005;236(2):579–87.
103. Srinivas M, Morel PA, Ernst LA, Laidlaw DH, Ahrens ET. Fluorine-19 MRI for visualization and quantification of cell migration in a diabetes model. Magn Reson Med. 2007;58(4):725–34.
104. Medarova Z, Tsai S, Evgenov N, Santamaria P, Moore A. In vivo imaging of a diabetogenic CD8+ T cell response during Type 1 diabetes progression. Magn Reson Med. 2008;59(4):712–20.
105. Amrani A, Serra P, Yamanouchi J, et al. Expansion of the antigenic repertoire of a single T cell receptor upon T cell activation. J Immunol. 2001;167(2):655–66.

106. Elbashir SM, Harborth J, Lendeckel W, Yalcin A, Weber K, Tuschl T. Duplexes of 21-nucleotide RNAs mediate RNA interference in cultured mammalian cells. Nature. 2001;411(6836):494–8.
107. Brown KT, Do RK, Gonen M, Covey AM, Getrajdman GI, Sofocleous CT, et al. Randomized trial of hepatic artery embolization for hepatocellular carcinoma using doxorubicin-eluting microspheres compared with embolization with microspheres alone. J Clin Oncol. 2016;34:2046–53. https://doi.org/10.1200/JCO.2015.64.0821.
108. Caine M, Zhang X, Hill M, Guo W, Ashrafi K, Bascal Z, et al. Comparison of microsphere penetration with LC Bead LUMI versus other commercial microspheres. J Mech Behav Biomed Mater. 2018;78:46–55. https://doi.org/10.1016/j.jmbbm.2017.10.034.

Molecular Imaging and Radiobiology

22

Key Points (Abstract)

Radiobiology which is also known as radiation biology is a combination of the field of clinical and basic medical sciences which studies the effects of the ionizing radiation on living things. This radiobiological research is based on the various clinical trials which has capabilities to evaluate the radiation therapy's role in combining with various inhibitor substrates like kinases DNA-dependent protein kinase (DNA-PK), ataxia telangiectasia mutated (ATM), ataxia telangiectasia related (ATR), and immune or cell cycle checkpoint inhibitors. The advancements in the radiation oncology research along with the radiation sciences have been studied with the concept of the radiobiology to radiation oncology.

Keywords

DNA · Cancer stem cells · ATP · Hypoxia · Radiotherapy · Biomarkers · Ligands

22.1 Introduction

22.1.1 Radiation Biology

The study of the radiation biology is not new, but with the recent advances, there is more focus on the effects of the ionizing radiation on living organisms. This study is the combination of the broad specialities of physics, chemistry, and biology, and again it is based on the various types of ionizing radiation and their effects. The concept established here is that the energy absorption in the cells will lead to biological damage.

There will be some amount of the damage to the adjacent cancer cells when the radiation is given to the cancer cells. Here the concept will be to have minimal damage to the cells because of the radiation induced.

22.1.2 Evolution of the Radiobiology

Whether there is cellular response to the amount of the radiation in some way or another is a well-established concept. This will be based on the fundamental insights to demonstrate the presence of the stem/progenitor cells and also to see the DNA damage response pathway [1, 2]. Radiobiology has significant impact by various factors like improving the response of the cancer patient's outcomes in all possible way by reducing the various morbid changes due to radiation. With this, the potential of possible carcinogenesis risk can also be evaluated and quantified to a great possible extent where the chances of the radiation will be present [3].

Various forms of radiation therapies are used for management of many cancers resulting in radiation injury [4]. With this all-various possibilities, radiation biology is very important and plays

S. Shaikh, *Advances in Imaging*, https://doi.org/10.1007/978-981-16-9535-3_22

a significant role for further research in radiation biology, cancer biology, and immunologists.

This comprises of radiation aspects where many studies are there to find out possible impact on the cells like DNA repair and also the cancer stem cell due to radiation (Diagram 22.1). With these available resources, much has to be changed in radiation research approaches and focussed scientific approach. A lot of research continues on the various fronts to assess the radiation sensitivity, and various agents impact for better radiation survival. The radiation doses are sensitive to the various clonogenic assays, and the medium-/high-throughput-adapted colony assays will give better results in quantifying the impact [5]. Newer drugs can be produced by the radio sensitization with better efficacy, selectivity, and drug development programs [6].

There is increased viability seen in various radiation-induced areas (e.g., cH2AX) [6, 7], by adenosine triphosphate (ATP), or luciferase-based reporters [8, 9]. This can be done by clonogenic assays and xenograft (PDX) models used for the evaluation in radiation research. The radiation responses can be measured by the orthotopic models which will validate the tumour microenvironment. Radiosensitizing agents are having very good therapeutic options against tumour cells. The tumour tissue toxicity needs also to be monitored especially in more prone regions like oral mucosa and mucosa in the small intestine. The anatomical and physiologic impact of the tumour in relation to the cell-matrix interactions and hypoxia is also to be studied. The molecular response to the radiation injury can also be done by using the selective molecular targets and radiosensitization of cancer. Modular pathways like ataxia-telangiectasia mutated (ATM) and ataxia-telangiectasia and Rad3-related (ATR) protein are important proteins in the DNA damage response pathways [10]. The regulation of the DNA repair, RNA posttransla-

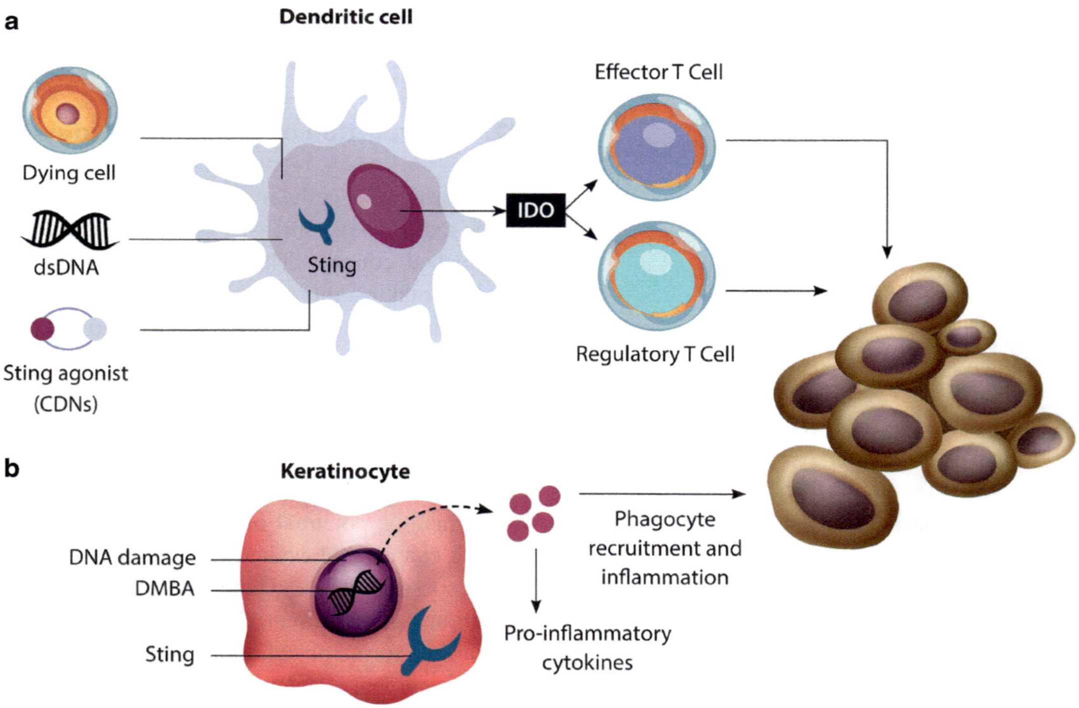

Diagram 22.1 The dendritic cell and the keratocyte in relation with the biological process of the T cell for the defensive mechanism of the body. (**a**) showing the Dendritic cell and (**b**) showing keratinocyte

tional modification, and cell morphology can be done by various proteins by increasing the possibility of the tumour radiosensitivity by modulating ATM or ATR pathways.

ATR inhibitor like VE-822 is used as single-agent radiosensitizing the pancreatic cancer cells in vitro and in xenograft models and similarly cisplatin for the lung cancers [11, 12]. Various extracellular factors can modulate by impacting the various factors like transforming growth factor-beta, tumour necrosis factor alpha, and platelet-derived growth factor, or transcription factors [13]. Warburg's phenomenon is used by the tumours which consume significant amount of glucose and secrete lactate in high levels without any change in the oxygen concentration; thus "aerobic glycolysis" is helping the tumour growth by fast growth of the cells [14]. RAS cancers will cause significant tumour alterations in both extracellular and intracellular cell providing the tricarboxylic acid (TCA) cycle. Redox balance is needed for the radiation therapy, and its connection with glucose is also important between glucose metabolism and redox stress. Ribose is generated by the consumption of glucose via the pentose phosphate pathway which can be used to generate nucleotides for DNA replication and repair. Radiation therapy will result in increased intracellular redox stress. Thus, the metabolic pathways which will be balancing the redox pathways will help in stabilizing the effects of the radiation [15, 16]. Tumours also use many other metabolic pathways as fuel which are very good therapeutic targets. By studying the tumour metabolic phenotypes, the association of the radiation and drugs having impact on the target tumour metabolism can be evaluated. Tumours have different metabolism and phenotypes and thus are diverse in gene mutations; also this is not easy for the critical evaluation of the genetic context. The interaction between the tumour and stroma needs to precisely understand the treatment-associated changes in tumour metabolism after radiation using various drugs and combination of both the treatment options.

22.2 Cancer Stem Cells

Cancer stem cells (CSCs) have affinity towards tumour regeneration. CSCs are capable of easily converting the aerobic glycolysis and oxidative phosphorylation which is affected and dependent on the local microenvironment. This will also cause the significant increase in the expression of enzymes which are regulating the redox metabolism and activation of DNA repair mechanisms within the cell [17] (Diagram 22.2). Glioblastoma multiforme (GBM) in these CSCs is capable of the migration to the subventricular zone (SVZ) within the brain and escaping into the regions where there is high radiation dose [18, 19]. This is based on the various factors which will be having environmental stress based on radiotherapy, chemotherapy, hypoxia, and pH variations especially low pH which can increase the CSC and increase the radiation sensitivity. In this, some of the normal and non-neoplastic cells will be spontaneously converted into the stem-like state. With the amount of the radiation toxicity to normal tissues and stem cells following ionizing radiation, the cell death will start when cells with chromosomal aberrations will divide. Radiation toxicity in normal tissues often correlates with the cell cycle rate in particular organ [20]. The amount of the radiation toxicity is based on the cells which have very high proliferation rate as compared to the slow proliferating cells; again, the radiation response is also based on these factors. The exception to this rule is the salivary gland which has very slow cell proliferation but very high radiation toxicity. The first stage in this toxicity is the involvement of the secretory cells in which the water secretion is affected and lost followed by the cell death. Cell loss is the important component of the acute cell toxicity. Other features like endothelial cell function loss [21], inflammation and followed by cell loss and also the neural cell involvement leading to the dysregulation [22]. Every organ cell has radiation tolerance limit above which will result to cell loss and ultimately organ dysfunction. The number of the

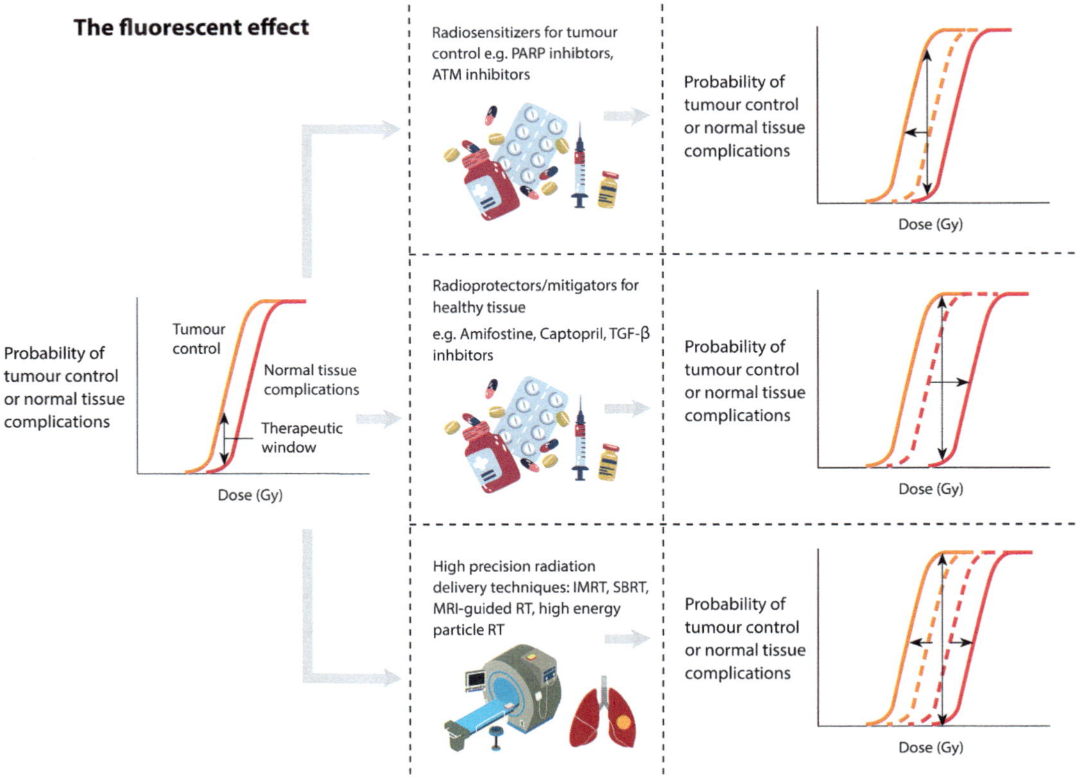

Diagram 22.2 Explains the fluorescent effects for the various factors affecting the radiobiology

survival cells and functional stem and progenitor cells [23] after radiation will determine the amount of the radiation effects. These epithelial stem/progenitor cells are important for balancing the haemostasis by forming the peripheral cells in the surroundings [24], and these are in the form of the stroma, endothelial, and neuronal cells. The impact of the radiation is based on the internal communication network of the cells in their surroundings to prevent damage and also for the repair process. The prevention of radiation effects is important, and the role of radioprotectors appears to prevent the side effects of tumour radiation. The amount of radiation to the surrounding tissues is of concern, and this has to be planned in such a way that the optimal radiation should be present for the surrounding normal tissues. This can be done with the novel radioprotectors to have specific local delivery of organ-specific radiation mitigators [25, 26]. The use of these radioprotectors should be planned in such a way that the other important agents like antioxidants, prosurvival, pro-proliferation, and/or anti-inflammatory agents should be delivered timely; any plans of delivering at the wrong time will lead to more toxicity rather than reducing the radiation effects. The classical example is the planning of radiation delivery to structures or tissues adjacent to the salivary glands by using newer techniques where the radiation dose to the salivary gland is minimized and toxicity is prevented [27]. The various other aspects of the regenerative therapies are newer and novel techniques like cell transplantation, gene transfer, and tissue engineering; these are some of the avenues which can be helpful in repairing the radiation-damaged organs or cells. The combination of radiotherapy with immunotherapy can be used for the local control of the disease. Some of the studies has also shown that the radiation therapy itself can increase the systemic immune response to the tumour cells by using various newer drugs like immunomodulatory drugs [28]. Some of the animal studies which are having two synchronous tumours where radiation is delivered to one tumour and to see the out-field response of this radiation into another tumour (abscopal effect). When radiation is combined with immunotherapies, then this will result in the formation of the antitumour T cells like anti-CTLA4 or anti-PD-1 antibodies [29–31]. Various case studies, retrospective series, and a recent prospective trial will result in the support of the clinical aspects. Some of the studies showing the various trials of the combination radiotherapy with granulocyte-macrophage colony-stimulating factor for double tumours have shown the abscopal response in more than 25% of patients in the known cases of the metastatic solid tumours, which has resulted in establishing the role of the radiotherapy as a potential in situ antitumour vaccine [32]. The tumour immune response which is developed by radiotherapy is multifactorial [33–35]. Thus, with this radiation there will be the release of the danger signals and tumour-specific antigens, causing the development of the T-cell-mediated immune response [36–38]. By developing the immune inhibitory pathways along with the immune stimulatory pathways by the radiation, ultimately it will be decided whether this will be useful or harmful to the patients based on the actions of these two entities [39]. These immunosuppressive pathways which are induced by radiation also have the exacerbation, and these effects need to be evaluated [40]. The successful radiotherapy is based on the healthy immune system [41]; along with this, the combination of radiation and immunotherapy is important [42]. The newer immune-targeting agents are important as the radiation can convert the immune-privileged tumour into T cell inflamed. Radiation in immuno-oncology is the important concept, and this needs to be validated by various studies [43]. The amount of the radiation dose in combination with the immunotherapy should provide the optimal effect based on the dose selection [44, 45].

Tumour pathophysiology shows a lot of the changes in form of the increased interstitial fluid pressure, hypoxia, excess lactate accumulation, and changed pH which is lower, all these causing the environment to alter. The presence of hypoxia in cancers is an indicator of poor prognosis [46–48]. Hypoxic cells are more resistant to radiotherapy and chemotherapies due to the impact of the O2 which will participate in various chemical reactions which will enhance initial DNA damage, and here without O2, there is less DNA damage [48]. The biological signalling pathways is impacted by the hypoxia where there will be activation of the transcription factor hypoxia-inducible factor 1 (HIF-1), promoting the cellular metabolism [49–52]. The impact of the hypoxia-induced changes will cause increase in the generation of the cancer stem cells in the tumour region [53]; this is resistant to DNA damage by causing the genomic instability and metastatic potential, thus promoting the malignant progression by changing the microenvironment of the tumour [54]. Along with the hypoxia and radiation therapy, the various hypoxic cell radiosensitizers will be acting to reduce the amount of the radiation damage [55]. Various trials are being done to verify the Bioreductive prodrugs seen as hypoxic cytotoxin [56]. Using hyperbaric oxygen during radiotherapy or using higher levels of O2 along with the various vasodilators has shown significant changes [57]. Reduction of hypoxia can be done by reducing the amount of the tumour O2 consumption. One of the studies by Secomb et al. showed that 30% decrease in O2 consumption will cause the fall of the hypoxic fraction from 37 to 11% [58]. Some of the studies also confirmed that by reducing O2 consumption and tumour hypoxia this will cause significant increase in the radiation sensitivity more selectively for the hypoxic tumours [55, 59]. Another therapeutic option is the use of the aberrant vasculature by reducing the tumour supply by collapsing the vessels by using the vascular disrupting agents, thus significantly reducing hypoxia [60]. Another concept is to disrupt the CXCR4/CXCL12 interaction by myeloid cells to reduce the vasculogenesis and metastasis after therapy [61, 62]. These patterns will improve treatment outcomes. However, the biggest advantage is the hypoxia status of the tumour which can easily identify the chances of recurrence or metastasis after primary therapy [63, 64]. The role of the nanomedicine by development and use of multifunctional agents acting on the tumour microvasculature, which will be useful for both imaging for and therapy with radiation [65–67]. By using higher radiation, there will be vascular [68–70]. These increased doses are being widely used in stereotactic body radiotherapy (SBRT). This SBRT is increasingly used with better efficacy by tumour cell killing by vascular ablation. The killing of blood vessels will impact on the growth delay, not by SBRT [49–52]. The presence of hypoxia within tumours also shows the failure after SBRT. With other available options of adjuvant therapies, vascular-targeted nanoparticles, or high-frequency ultrasound ablation (HiFU), the tumour debulking can be done and will lead to increase in local of the tumour.

22.3 Extracellular Matrix and Physical-Mechanical Properties of the Tumour Microenvironment and Radiotherapy

The extracellular matrix (ECM) is important for the tumour microenvironment evaluation which will have an impact on the cancer cell survival after radiation. This matrix is composed of the structural, cellular, and molecular components along with the basement membrane which usually separates the epithelial compartment from the stroma [71]. Adhesion-mediated signalling also acts between the epithelial and stromal compartments. The integrin-mediated cell interactions will cause more increased radiation and chemoresistance on many tumours by activating prosurvival signalling [72–75]. The adhesion of tumour cells to ECM proteins will also signify the amount of the efficacy of molecularly targeted therapy [76, 77]. By studying the various mechanical signals which will cause cell survival is now can be done by various advancements of biophysical mechanics and its applications in cell biology [78]. Direct binding to combination of ECM ligands has a significant impact by facilitating increased ligand-receptor binding [79]. Thus, the various properties of ECM and the associated tissues have important role in the monitoring of the cellular function and signalling [80]. We all know that by elastic property of tissues, tumours will have more stiffness as compared to normal tissues, and thus increased stiffness will result in the tumour progression [81].

22.4 Predictive Biomarkers for Radiotherapy

Predictive biomarkers are important in the concept of precision cancer medicine revolution [82]. Biomarkers have changed the impact of the cancer treatment and along with the couple of biomarkers which are used for radiotherapy [83, 84]. With these available resources, there is more heterogeneity in evaluation, prognosis, and possible outcomes in relation to the tumour control and treatment toxicity. Thus, with the advent of the various biomarkers which will predict tumour impact and also on the surrounding tissues will be able to analyse the care in the individual patients [85] (Diagram 22.3).

The bigger research in the coming days will be more focussed on the biomarker's predictivity of radiation response impacting the genes which are involved in DNA repair. Mutations in single genes are rare, and as we know, the quantum of the DNA damage response and repair networks is complex so the combination of the radiotherapy and DNA repair inhibitors can be more precise [86]. Some of the studies showed the proactive nature of the radiation therapy for some of the tumours like prostate cancer studies [87]. The Cancer Genome Atlas and the International Cancer Genome Consortium showed (1) the liquid biopsy concept for the non-invasive and can be done for radiation therapy, (2) tumoural heterogeneity to be quantified as a biomarker, and (3) radiation therapy assessment and (4) to identify the residual disease. Biomarkers play an important role in analysing

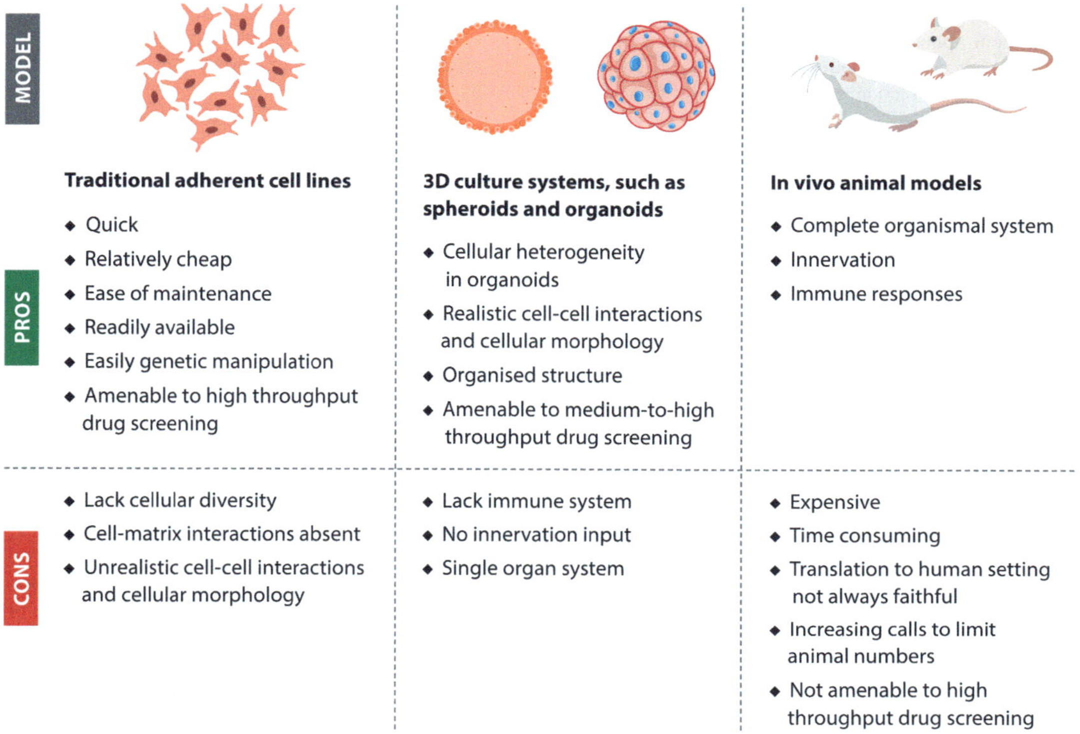

Diagram 22.3 Various mechanisms which will have the impact on the various models of the radiobiology and its pros and cons

the impact of the radiation therapy; still there is no single biomarker which can be used. Due to this various combination, biomarkers can be used; one of the combinations is the genomic-adjusted radiation dose (GARD) [88] and Postoperative Radiation Therapy Outcomes Score (PORTOS) [89].

22.5 Conclusions

Radiobiology has made an important impact on the advancement of the human biology. This is possible due to the various advances in radiation research, new model systems, and genome tools. Many studies involving the combination of radiotherapy and immunotherapy have shown a very big potential for revolutionizing the current knowledge with future advantages for overall improvement of the outcomes for the cancer patients.

References

1. Till JE, Mc CE. A direct measurement of the radiation sensitivity of normal mouse bone marrow cells. Radiat Res. 1961;14:213–22.
2. Kastan MB, Zhan Q, el-Deiry WS, et al. A mammalian cell cycle checkpoint pathway utilizing p53 and GADD45 is defective in ataxia-telangiectasia. Cell. 1992;71(4):587–97.
3. Durante M, Cucinotta FA. Heavy ion carcinogenesis and human space exploration. Nat Rev Cancer. 2008;8(6):465–72.
4. Williams JP, Brown SL, Georges GE, et al. Animal models for medical countermeasures to radiation exposure. Radiat Res. 2010;173(4):557–78.
5. Tiwana GS, Prevo R, Buffa FM, et al. Identification of vitamin B1 metabolism as a tumor-specific radiosensitizing pathway using a high-throughput colony formation screen. Oncotarget. 2015;6(8):5978–89.
6. Higgins GS, Prevo R, Lee YF, et al. A small interfering RNA screen of genes involved in DNA repair identifies tumor-specific radiosensitization by POLQ knockdown. Cancer Res. 2010;70(7):2984–93.
7. Labay E, Mauceri HJ, Efimova EV, et al. Repurposing cephalosporin antibiotics as pro-senescent radiosensitizers. Oncotarget. 2016;7(23):33919–33.

8. Wei D, Parsels LA, Karnak D, et al. Inhibition of protein phosphatase 2A radiosensitizes pancreatic cancers by modulating CDC25C/CDK1 and homologous recombination repair. Clin Cancer Res. 2013;19(16):4422–32.
9. Hatano K, Kumar B, Zhang Y, et al. A functional screen identifies miRNAs that inhibit DNA repair and sensitize prostate cancer cells to ionizing radiation. Nucleic Acids Res. 2015;43(8):4075–86.
10. Zhou BB, Bartek J. Targeting the checkpoint kinases: chemo sensitization versus chemoprotection. Nat Rev Cancer. 2004;4(3):216–25.
11. Fokas E, Prevo R, Pollard JR, et al. Targeting ATR in vivo using the novel inhibitor VE-822 results in selective sensitization of pancreatic tumours to radiation. Cell Death Dis. 2012;3:e441.
12. Hall AB, Newsome D, Wang Y, et al. Potentiation of tumor responses to DNA damaging therapy by the selective ATR inhibitor VX-970. Oncotarget. 2014;5(14):5674–85.
13. De Craene B, Berx G. Regulatory networks defining EMT during cancer initiation and progression. Nat Rev Cancer. 2013;13(2):97–110.
14. Feron O. Pyruvate into lactate and back: from the Warburg effect to symbiotic energy fuel exchange in cancer cells. Radiother Oncol. 2009;92(3):329–33.
15. Cairns RA, Harris IS, Mak TW. Regulation of cancer cell metabolism. Nat Rev Cancer. 2011;11(2):85–95.
16. Menon SS, Uppal M, Randhawa S, et al. Radiation metabolomics: current status and future directions. Front Oncol. 2016;6:20.
17. Bao S, Wu Q, McLendon RE, et al. Glioma stem cells promote radioresistance by preferential activation of the DNA damage response. Nature. 2006;444(7120):756–60.
18. Kroonen J, Nassen J, Boulanger YG, et al. Human glioblastoma-initiating cells invade specifically the subventricular zones and olfactory bulbs of mice after striatal injection. Int J Cancer. 2011;129(3):574–85.
19. Evers P, Lee PP, DeMarco J, et al. Irradiation of the potential cancer stem cell niches in the adult brain improves progression-free survival of patients with malignant glioma. BMC Cancer. 2010;10:384.
20. Vissink A, Mitchell JB, Baum BJ, et al. Clinical management of salivary gland hypofunction and xerostomia in head-and-neck cancer patients: successes and barriers. Int J Radiat Oncol Biol Phys. 2010;78(4):983–91.
21. Lombaert IM, Brunsting JF, Wierenga PK, et al. Cytokine treatment improves parenchymal and vascular damage of salivary glands after irradiation. Clin Cancer Res. 2008;14(23):7741–50.
22. Knox SM, Lombaert IM, Haddox CL, et al. Parasympathetic stimulation improves epithelial organ regeneration. Nat Commun. 2013;4:1494.
23. Lombaert IM, Brunsting JF, Wierenga PK, et al. Keratinocyte growth factor prevents radiation damage to salivary glands by expansion of the stem/progenitor pool. Stem Cells. 2008;26(10):2595–601.
24. Lombaert IM, Abrams SR, Li L, et al. Combined KIT and FGFR2b signaling regulates epithelial progenitor expansion during organogenesis. Stem Cell Rep. 2013;1(6):604–19.
25. Xiao N, Lin Y, Cao H, et al. Neurotrophic factor GDNF promotes survival of salivary stem cells. J Clin Invest. 2014;124(8):3364–77.
26. Zeidan YH, Xiao N, Cao H, et al. Botulinum toxin confers radioprotection in murine salivary glands. Int J Radiat Oncol Biol Phys. 2016;94(5):1190–7.
27. van Luijk P, Pringle S, Deasy JO, et al. Sparing the region of the salivary gland containing stem cells preserves saliva production after radiotherapy for head and neck cancer. Sci Transl Med. 2015;7(305):305ra147.
28. Formenti SC, Demaria S. Combining radiotherapy and cancer immunotherapy: a paradigm shift. J Natl Cancer Inst. 2013;105(4):256–65.
29. Demaria S, Ng B, Devitt ML, et al. Ionizing radiation inhibition of distant untreated tumours (abscopal effect) is immune mediated. Int J Radiat Oncol Biol Phys. 2004;58(3):862–70.
30. Dewan MZ, Galloway AE, Kawashima N, et al. Fractionated but no single dose radiotherapy induces an immune-mediated abscopal effect when combined with anti-CTLA-4 antibody. Clin Cancer Res. 2009;15(17):5379–88.
31. Twyman-Saint Victor C, Rech AJ, Maity A, et al. Radiation and dual checkpoint blockade activate nonredundant immune mechanisms in cancer. Nature. 2015;520(7547):373–7.
32. Golden EB, Chhabra A, Chachoua A, et al. Local radiotherapy, and granulocyte-macrophage colony-stimulating factor to generate abscopal responses in patients with metastatic solid tumours: a proof-of-principle trial. Lancet Oncol. 2015;16(7):795–803.
33. Kwilas AR, Donahue RN, Bernstein MB, et al. In the field: exploiting the untapped potential of immunogenic modulation by radiation in combination with immunotherapy for the treatment of cancer. Front Oncol. 2012;2:104.
34. Burnette B, Fu YX, Weichselbaum RR. The confluence of radiotherapy and immunotherapy. Front Oncol. 2012;2:143. Review 338 | JNCI J Natl Cancer Inst. 2018;110(4). Downloaded from https://academic.oup.com/jnci/article/110/4/329/4590265 by guest on 3 Jan 2021.
35. Schaue D, Micewicz ED, Ratikan JA, et al. Radiation and inflammation. Semin Radiat Oncol. 2015;25(1):4–10.
36. McBride WH, Chiang CS, Olson JL, et al. A sense of danger from radiation. Radiat Res. 2004;162(1):1–19.
37. Reits EA, Hodge JW, Herberts CA, et al. Radiation modulates the peptide repertoire, enhances MHC class I expression, and induces successful antitumor immunotherapy. J Exp Med. 2006;203(5):1259–71.
38. Ratikan JA, Micewicz ED, Xie MW, et al. Radiation takes its toll. Cancer Lett. 2015;368(2):238–45.
39. Schaue D, Comin-Anduix B, Ribas A, et al. T-cell responses to surviving in cancer patients

undergoing radiation therapy. Clin Cancer Res. 2008;14(15):4883–90.
40. Vanpouille-Box C, Diamond JM, Pilones KA, et al. TGFbeta is a master regulator of radiation therapy-induced antitumor immunity. Cancer Res. 2015;75(11):2232–42.
41. Stone HB, Peters LJ, Milas L. Effect of host immune capability on radio curability and subsequent transplatability of a murine fibrosarcoma. J Natl Cancer Inst. 1979;63(5):1229–35.
42. Haddow A, Alexander P. An immunological method of increasing the sensitivity of primary sarcomas to local irradiation with x rays. Lancet. 1964;1(7331):452–7.
43. Demaria S, Coleman CN, Formenti SC. Radiotherapy: changing the game in immunotherapy. Trends Cancer. 2016;2(6):286–94.
44. Gandhi SJ, Minn AJ, Vonderheide RH, et al. Awakening the immune system with radiation: optimal dose and fractionation. Cancer Lett. 2015;368(2):185–90.
45. Vanpouille-Box C, Alard A, Aryankalayil MJ, et al. DNA exonuclease Trex1 regulates radiotherapy-induced tumour immunogenicity. Nat Commun. 2017;8:15618.
46. Horsman MR, Vaupel P. Pathophysiological basis for the formation of the tumor microenvironment. Front Oncol. 2016;6:66.
47. Vaupel P, Hoeckel M. Predictive power of the tumor oxygenation status. Adv Exp Med Biol. 1999;471:533–9.
48. Hall EJ, Giaccia AJ. Chapter 6: Oxygen effect and reoxygenation. In: Radiobiology for the radiologist. Philadelphia: Lippincott Williams & Wolters Kluwer; 2012.
49. Perez BA, Ghafoori AP, Lee CL, et al. Assessing the radiation response of lung cancer with different gene mutations using genetically engineered mice. Front Oncol. 2013;3:72. Review D. G. Kirsch et al. | 337.
50. Moding EJ, Lee CL, Castle KD, et al. Atm deletion with dual recombinase technology preferentially radiosensitizes tumor endothelium. J Clin Invest. 2014;124(8):3325–38.
51. Moding EJ, Castle KD, Perez BA, et al. Tumor cells, but not endothelial cells, mediate eradication of primary sarcomas by stereotactic body radiation therapy. Sci Transl Med. 2015;7(278):278ra34.
52. Zhang M, Qiu Q, Li Z, et al. HIF-1 alpha regulates the response of primary sarcomas to radiation therapy through a cell autonomous mechanism. Radiat Res. 2015;183(6):594–609.
53. Baumann M, Krause M, Hill R. Exploring the role of cancer stem cells in radio resistance. Nat Rev Cancer. 2008;8(7):545–54.
54. Vaupel P. Metabolic microenvironment of tumor cells: a key factor in malignant progression. Exp Oncol. 2010;32(3):125–7.
55. Lin A, Maity A. Molecular pathways: a novel approach to targeting hypoxia and improving radiotherapy efficacy via reduction in oxygen demand. Clin Cancer Res. 2015;21(9):1995–2000.
56. Wilson WR, Hay MP. Targeting hypoxia in cancer therapy. Nat Rev Cancer. 2011;11(6):393–410.
57. Janssens GO, Rademakers SE, Terhaard CH, et al. Improved recurrence-free survival with ARCON for anemic patients with laryngeal cancer. Clin Cancer Res. 2014;20(5):1345–54.
58. Secomb TW, Hsu R, Dewhirst MW. Synergistic effects of hyperoxic gas breathing and reduced oxygen consumption on tumor oxygenation: a theoretical model. Int J Radiat Oncol Biol Phys. 2004;59(2):572–8.
59. Koritzinsky M. Metformin: a novel biological modifier of tumor response to radiation therapy. Int J Radiat Oncol Biol Phys. 2015;93(2):454–64.
60. Jain RK. Anti-angiogenesis strategies revisited: from starving tumours to alleviating hypoxia. Cancer Cell. 2014;26(5):605–22.
61. Kioi M, Vogel H, Schultz G, et al. Inhibition of vasculogenesis, but not angiogenesis, prevents the recurrence of glioblastoma after irradiation in mice. J Clin Invest. 2010;120(3):694–705.
62. Chaudary N, Pintilie M, Jelveh S, et al. Plerixafor improves primary tumor response and reduces metastases in cervical cancer treated with radio-chemotherapy. Clin Cancer Res. 2017;23(5):1242–9.
63. Koonce NA, Levy J, Hardee ME, et al. Targeting artificial tumor stromal targets for molecular imaging of tumor vascular hypoxia. PLoS One. 2015;10(8):e0135607.
64. Terman DS, Viglianti BL, Zennadi R, et al. Sickle erythrocytes target cytotoxics to hypoxic tumor micro vessels and potentiate a tumoricidal response. PLoS One. 2013;8(1):e52543.
65. Kotb S, Detappe A, Lux F, et al. Gadolinium-based nanoparticles and radiation therapy for multiple brain melanoma metastases: proof of concept before phase I trial. Theranostics. 2016;6(3):418–27.
66. Dorsey JF, Sun L, Joh DY, et al. Gold nanoparticles in radiation research: potential applications for imaging and radiosensitization. Transl Cancer Res. 2013;2(4):280–91.
67. Koonce NA, Quick CM, Hardee ME, et al. Combination of gold nanoparticle conjugated tumor necrosis factor-alpha and radiation therapy results in a synergistic antitumor response in murine carcinoma models. Int J Radiat Oncol Biol Phys. 2015;93(3):588–96.
68. Song CW, Lee YJ, Griffin RJ, et al. Indirect tumor cell death after high-dose hypofractionated irradiation: implications for stereotactic body radiation therapy and stereotactic radiation surgery. Int J Radiat Oncol Biol Phys. 2015;93(1):166–72.
69. Maeda A, Leung MK, Conroy L, et al. In vivo optical imaging of tumor and microvascular response to ionizing radiation. PLoS One. 2012;7(8):e42133.
70. Jani A, Shaikh F, Barton S, et al. High-dose, single-fraction irradiation rapidly reduces tumor vasculature and perfusion in a xenograft model of neuroblastoma. Int J Radiat Oncol Biol Phys. 2016;94(5):1173–80.

71. Malik R, Lelkes PI, Cukierman E. Biomechanical and biochemical remodelling of stromal extracellular matrix in cancer. Trends Biotechnol. 2015;33(4):230–6.
72. Park CC, Zhang HJ, Yao ES, et al. Beta1 integrin inhibition dramatically enhances radiotherapy efficacy in human breast cancer xenografts. Cancer Res. 2008;68(11):4398–405.
73. Nam JM, Onodera Y, Bissell MJ, et al. Breast cancer cells in three-dimensional culture display an enhanced radio response after coordinate targeting of integrin alpha5beta1 and fibronectin. Cancer Res. 2010;70(13):5238–48.
74. Eke I, Zscheppang K, Dickreuter E, et al. Simultaneous beta1 integrin-EGFR targeting and radio sensitization of human head and neck cancer. J Natl Cancer Inst. 2015;107(2):dju419.
75. Sethi T, Rintoul RC, Moore SM, et al. Extracellular matrix proteins protect small cell lung cancer cells against apoptosis: a mechanism for small cell lung cancer growth and drug resistance in vivo. Nat Med. 1999;5(6):662–8.
76. Lin CH, Pelissier FA, Zhang H, et al. Microenvironment rigidity modulates responses to the HER2 receptor tyrosine kinase inhibitor lapatinib via YAP and TAZ transcription factors. Mol Biol Cell. 2015;26(22):3946–53.
77. Eke I, Schneider L, Forster C, et al. EGFR/JIP-4/JNK2 signalling attenuates cetuximab-mediated radio sensitization of squamous cell carcinoma cells. Cancer Res. 2013;73(1):297–306.
78. Halder G, Dupont S, Piccolo S. Transduction of mechanical and cytoskeletal cues by YAP and TAZ. Nat Rev Mol Cell Biol. 2012;13(9):591–600.
79. Friedland JC, Lee MH, Boettiger D. Mechanically activated integrin switch controls alpha5beta1 function. Science. 2009;323(5914):642–4.
80. Kai F, Laklai H, Weaver VM. Force matters: biomechanical regulation of cell invasion and migration in disease. Trends Cell Biol. 2016;26(7):486–97.
81. Levental KR, Yu H, Kass L, et al. Matrix crosslinking forces tumor progression by enhancing integrin signalling. Cell. 2009;139(5):891–906.
82. La Thangue NB, Kerr DJ. Predictive biomarkers: a paradigm shift towards personalized cancer medicine. Nat Rev Clin Oncol. 2011;8(10):587–96.
83. Baumann M, Krause M, Overgaard J, et al. Radiation oncology in the era of precision medicine. Nat Rev Cancer. 2016;16(4):234–49.
84. Yard B, Chie EK, Adams DJ, et al. Radiotherapy in the era of precision medicine. Semin Radiat Oncol. 2015;25(4):227–36.
85. Willers H, Held KD. Introduction to clinical radiation biology. Hematol Oncol Clin North Am. 2006;20(1):1–24.
86. Jackson SP, Helleday T. DNA REPAIR. Drugging DNA repair. Science. 2016;352(6290):1178–9.
87. Lalonde E, Ishkanian AS, Sykes J, et al. Tumour genomic and microenvironmental heterogeneity for integrated prediction of 5-year biochemical recurrence of prostate cancer: a retrospective cohort study. Lancet Oncol. 2014;15(13):1521–32.
88. Scott JG, Berglund A, Schell MJ, et al. A genome-based model for adjusting radiotherapy dose (GARD): a retrospective, cohort-based study. Lancet Oncol. 2017;18(2):202–11.
89. Zhao SG, Chang SL, Spratt DE, et al. Development and validation of a 24-gene predictor of response to postoperative radiotherapy in prostate cancer: a matched, retrospective analysis. Lancet Oncol. 2016;17(11):1612–20.

Robotic Imaging

23

Key Points (Abstract)

Medicine has undergone the helm of revolution with the various procedures and surgeries becoming minimally invasive and more precise and more sensitive. In the imaging also with the multimodality technological revolution and hybrid functional imaging modalities, it has led to the significant revolution in the diagnosis and prognostication of the various pathologies based on the molecular level. One of the important areas is the significant advancement and growth in the use of the medical robotics based on the advancements in all the aspects of the robotic applications. The technological advances in medical imaging of all the modalities based on the techniques, software applications, and ease to diagnose have led to more and more use of the robotics in the imaging which is ultimately driven by the technology.

Keywords

Robotics · Magnetic particle imaging · Optical imaging · Magneto-acoustic imaging · Mini robots · Nanoparticles

23.1 Introduction

As per the definition, a robot is "a reprogrammable, multifunctional manipulator designed to move materials, parts, tools, or other specialised devices by the various programmed motions for the performance of a variety of tasks" [1]. ROBODOC is the first medically used robot in 1992. This robot was used in the orthopaedics for the drilling of the implants by the robots [2]. Butit took very long for getting this robot to be approved by the Food and Drug Administration (FDA) in 2008. With this, there is significant revolution in the various surgical and other fields of the medicine like laparoscopy, neurosurgery, orthopaedic surgery, emergency response, and other medical conditions. It was long back the concept of the robot was invented and was defined for various purposes in 1979, at the Robot Institute of America, and the robot was defined as "a reprogrammable, multifunctional manipulator designed to move the various materials, parts, tools, or other by the use of the specialized devices by the programmed motions for the performance of a variety of tasks". However, this definition is not of much relevance as many doubts were not cleared. Now with this, the robots are used for the various tasks which are especially the requirement is more specific, strong, accurate, untiring, and needing complex manoeuvring where the human efficiency is very less. With this, the other aspect is the very high cost, more space requirement, and extensive training. In the medicine, the greatest impact of medical robots is on surgeries especially both radiosurgery and tissue manipulation surgeries where more precise and accurate motions are required.

S. Shaikh, *Advances in Imaging*, https://doi.org/10.1007/978-981-16-9535-3_23

23.2 Interventional Radiology Role of Robotics

Interventional radiology is the newer specialities where the robotic imaging is playing an important role as an alternative to the minimal invasive surgeries. The use of the robotics in the pre- and intraoperative imaging for the various minimally or non-invasive interventions is due to the various technological advances in the imaging modalities, and each of these modalities offering various diagnostic and therapeutic options and robotics is one of them. Robot is used to do the various complex interventional procedures as a lot of the radiation is involved in this. With the availability of the various flexible robotic instruments for navigation, it has become easier to do many procedures where the complex anatomy is involved. With the advent of the technology, the newer robotic instruments are MRI compatible making it more widely used for the interventions which will be faster and more precise. Robotics in the cavities will need stable continuous power supply which can be by wireless technology. With the ongoing research, the availability of the wireless power supplies is available by MR scanner [3]. Most commonly used guided interventions are CT and MRI guided which are having biggest advantage that they are three. The CT-guided interventions are the commonest used for interventions, but there is big challenge due to the radiation exposure, smaller CT gantry, and difficulties in proper positioning of the needle in the scan room. However, with the robotic instruments, there is flexibility as well as significantly increased accuracy and efficiency for this CT-guided procedures. The more commonly used robotic CT and MRI procedures are the various types of biopsies, radiofrequency ablation, and cryoablation [4]. Due to technological advancements, there is the bigger advantage of real-time three-dimensional functional imaging with functional and hybrid imaging modalities involving the CT and MRI.

The use of the MRI-guided interventions had an advantage because of the various multiparametric parameters involved like tissue blood flow, blood volume, tissue temperature, and tissue oxygenation [5]. These MR-guided various interventions are also possible in the real-time MR imaging along with the live tracking of the catheters and various instruments. Due to the live imaging, the imaging will be faster and reducing the time of these procedures. These robot ultrasound-guided procedures are still operator dependent with a lot of developments to be done. However, due to the compatibility issues of the MR materials, still there is limitation for the development of a versatile and robust robotic system. The use of the ultrasound will have an advantage of manoeuvring the needles into a planned way by using the use of the tissue motion [6]. The use of the transrectal ultrasound (TRUS) will allow the use of the various instrument tips, dissection planes, bladder neck, and neurovascular bundle to reduce the complications arising from these procedures [7]. Ultrasound is used as an alternative to the surgical robots. Robotics in ultrasound will be useful to provide the diagnostic ultrasound where no radiologist is available. Other procedures which are not used widely are the robot fluoroscopy guided procedures and biplanar fluoroscopy due to availability of the CT and MRI. AcuBot is a newer concept of the robot which is capable of doing the fluoroscopic interventions like paraspinal nerve and facet joint injections with significant amount of accuracy [8].

23.3 Robotic Endovascular Procedures

The advantage of the robotic catheter steering systems for the correct placement of the catheter in conditions like cardiac ablations is being used in percutaneous coronary intervention (PCI). With the availability of the endovascular robots, they are capable of moulding the tips of catheter more precisely even in the MRI. By using the robots for the vascular network, there is significant reduction in the cost, and another advantage is the human limitations of these procedures due to excessive radiation [9].

23.4 Ultrasound in Robotics

Ultrasound is the most commonly used form of the imaging due to many reasons like it is inexpensive and no radiation, and therefore, it is being used in various interventional procedures. In various abdominal procedures, the ultrasound probe has to be manipulated and kept steady for various procedures especially during the respiration. In the ultrasound, three different approaches are available for the use of the ultrasound. Autonomous robotic ultrasound where ultrasound can be done without the operator like Teleoperated ultrasound imaging and Human-robot for the ultrasound imaging [2, 10, 11].

The different components of the various autonomous robotic ultrasound imaging are as follows:

1. Robotic arm for placing and manipulating the US probe
2. Robot controller
3. Tracking system see the movement of the probe. The use of the tracking systems is to provide the information in the 2D and 3D planes

The type of the devices used for the navigation is based on the optical tracking systems, electromagnetic (EM) tracking systems, and passive encoded mechanical systems. Dual components comprising of the preoperative MRI/CT imaging and intraoperative ultrasound imaging are being used for more precise location and efficiency. This dual-armed robotic system can be used for the placement and manipulation of the devices by robot arms. 3D ultrasound images will be giving better volumetric information of the various aspects like needle entry and specific target areas of interest.

23.5 Teleoperated Ultrasound Imaging

Here the robot is designed to manoeuvre the ultrasound probe where no radiologist is present, but still it is dependent on the skill of the radiologist [12–14]. The European Space Agency (ESA) has sponsored the project titled "Advanced Robotised Tele-Sonography Integrated Service (ARTIS)". The teleoperated system has the remote site and local site. The remote site will manipulate the robotic system, and this remote site will have force feedback which will be applied to the probe. When these forces are in excess, this will be alerted to the operator.

23.5.1 Human-Robot Cooperation for Ultrasound Imaging

In these robotic systems, the human operator will be controlling the operating system. The robot-held ultrasound probes will be positioned for the automated alignment of the two probes which is programmed by the radiologist [15, 16]. The remote operation of the systems will require the control of the various functions and prevent the remote system to be overloaded.

Thus, these three approaches of robot-assisted US imaging systems which are autonomous US imaging, teleoperated US imaging, and human-robot cooperative US imaging are used for the imaging.

23.6 Neurological Applications

Various newer applications are seen evolving in the neurological imaging like evaluation of the mental intent which can be done by the external devices by the brain-computer interface (BCI) technology. This is significantly helpful in the evaluation of the various neurological disorders, like amyotrophic lateral sclerosis and spinal cord injury [1–5, 10–13, 17–21]. With this, the patients can communicate by using the various actions of the different body parts to the clinicians as well as researchers [22, 23]. Thus, BCIs are the non-invasive systems, where the BCIs are independent of the ambulation [24], functional manipulations of the hands [19, 20], and also the linguistic communication [25, 26]. Due to these systems, it will be possible for the patients to interact by the autonomous neural control in their environment. [18, 24, 27]. Here, the use of the robotic technology is for the restoration and augmentation of arm and hand control and also by the use of the electroencephalography (EEG)-based BCIs targeting techniques [28, 29]. These robotic- or orthosis-assisted controlling of the hand [20] and better coordination are also needed for the navigation of a robotic arm [30]. Thus, the non-invasive based on the user's motivation and cognitive motivation which will play an important role in the skill acquisition ultimately leads to better performance [31–33]. Based on the Yerkes-Dodson law, there will be stronger behavioural and physiological learning effects [34]. One of the important disadvantages is the very poor signal quality which will have an impact on the neuronal signals like EEG [35]. The filtering effect can also have a non-invasive BCI signal [36, 37]; thus, it will be helpful in identifying the various diverse signal commands [26, 38, 39]. Electrical source imaging (ESI) is the entity where electrical properties along with the geometry of the structure like head have the precise identification of the signals. Significant increase in the neural decoding is being seen in ESI in comparison with the traditional techniques [38].

23.7 Artificial Intelligence (AI)

Artificial Intelligence is defined by Alan Turing, the founding father of AI, as "the science and engineering of making intelligent machines, especially intelligent computer programs" [40]. AI in our health systems is based on the significant use of the various algorithms and software to analyse the various aspects of the varied medical data. AI research is further categorized into the machine learning or deep learning and also based on the various tools like neural networks, which is part of the machine learning [41]. With this available research, the AI has significantly revolutionized for the practice of medicine, doctors, and leadership positions for making the potential changes, which will have a significant impact on the medium- and long-term goals of the healthcare systems.

23.8 Medical Microrobots

Medical microrobots (MRs) are being used in various newer applications like tissue engineering, drug delivery, and assisted fertilization. They are being used in majority of the in vitro settings like optical microscopy, which are different from our routine clinical indications.

Here the requirement of the imaging modalities are localizing and tracking for various applications. The principle behind these various imaging strategies is the spatiotemporal resolution and also the penetration depth of the targeted tissues.

The miniaturized robots are also called MRs which are tiny structures of various shapes like rods, tubes, spheres, and helices; by various chemical reactions, physical fields, motile cells, or microorganism inclusion, they are capable of performing various functions like focussed targeted drug deliveries and also for the diagnosis [42–45]. Thus, the efficient movement and control of these MRs is important for the focussed targeting and for execution of the specific functions. It is very important to have a precise idea of the various vascular routes for therapy targeting and for the location of the MRs in biological environment. The microrobot's exact localization is not only an issue but also the resolution, field of view (FoV), depth, and invasiveness of the imaging technique. Some of the components need deep tissue imaging in cancer management or in the assisted in vivo fertilization. Various imaging modalities are also being more useful for analysing the potentialities to evaluate the microscale structures in biological environment, further consolidating the evaluation of the microcirculation, implanted materials evaluation, cell migration, and any process occurring at the micro- and nanoscale [46–48].

Already existing techniques are "optical, ultrasound, magnetic and radiation-based imaging techniques to evaluate medical MRs". Newer imaging "hybrid techniques" like photoacoustic (PA) and magnetomotive ultrasound (MMUS) are also being evolved. It explores the sources of light, magnetic field, and ultrasound using the various photo acousto-mechanics, light reflection, etc. from current diagnostic techniques to future MR-assisted theranostics applications.

23.9 Conventional Imaging Techniques

All conventional imaging techniques are based on the same principles like physical signal passing in the body and causing the interaction by various processes like transmission or reflection which is being detected easily, various energy sources like electromagnetic fields and ultrasound energy, and magnetic resonance imaging (MRI), ultrasound (US), and optical- and ionizing radiation-based techniques which are defined as "conventional techniques". Various systems are based on magnetic field, ultrasound, and optical- and ionizing radiation-based ones. MRI and magnetic particle imaging (MPI) are magnetic field-based techniques and pulse-echo like B-mode and Doppler mode are the US-based imaging techniques. The optical-based imaging techniques are to visualize MRs by reflection-based imaging (RI) and fluorescence-based imaging (FI). Radiation-based computed tomography (CT), X-rays, fluoroscopy, positron emission tomography (PET), and single photon emission computed tomography (SPECT) are also used.

23.10 Magnetic Field-Based Techniques

Magnetic field-based techniques are the well-established imaging techniques for the evaluation of the anatomy, physiology, and various pathologies like tumours, inflammation, strokes, etc. These magnetic fields will penetrate into the deeper tissues as non-destructive radio waves. With this electrodynamic phenomenon, the generation of mechanical forces and torques will be translated into the detectable electrical signals. MR techniques are based on the functional and anatomical imaging by quantifying the specific materials, for MPI. Thus, it will be an expensive coil-based equipment which will need the dedicated powering and cooling systems. There will be very high penetration depth in MRI because of the low attenuation of magnetic fields across tissues, which will have diagnostic imaging, and manipulation of MRs by the size of a voxel in a standard 3T MRI scanner is about 500 μm. Single microrobot imaging is an agent of at least 10 μm in size provided there are suitable magnetic fields like swarm imaging appearing as more realistic for the magnetic microrobots which are small and weak [49–52]. In the MRI robotic systems, the important aspect is the safety issues like the material compatibility and effect of magnetic and electric fields which are generated associated with the specific procedures and parts of the body. These aspects need to be ascertained before any use.

Magnetic particle imaging (MPI) was proposed in 2001 by Bernhard Gleich and Jürgen Weizenecker. This is the new imaging modality for the use of the magnetic devices with the use of the gradient between field free point (FFP) regions and the adjacent magnetic sources.

Quantification of the paramagnetic materials, in particular, FoV, is the principle behind it which is based on the saturation of their magnetization. MPI can be used to quantify the presence and the amount of the paramagnetic substances. For the construction of the MPI scanner, two permanent magnets are opposing each other having the identical poles in such a way that the magnetic field is nullified by the field-free point (FFP). The magnetic field is produced in the presence of the electromagnetic field to visualize the changes in the magnetization. These magnetization saturations will generate the harmonics which is directly proportional to the gradient field. These FFP points can be focussed through the various time varying by the drive coils. MPI has speciality to cover the volume like that of the single organ heart or brain. MPI spatial resolution is directly proportional to the magnetic field gradient and the magnetic susceptibility of the particle, and the resolution can be as small as one to few millimetres for currently developed MPI scanners [53]. Significant promising results are there for the MPI for the visualization and navigation of small magnetic devices. In 2019, Bakenecker and co-workers showed the 3D-printed helical swimmer (2 mm in length) and navigated it through a vessel phantom with an MPI scanner. This swimmer is coated with the paramagnetic NPs used for the imaging and navigation. In 2020, Griese and co-workers studied different NPs which were navigated in bifurcation flow by an MPI scanner. Dextran-coated iron oxide NPs with 250 nm diameter are the best for the magnetic manipulability and imaging performance [54]. These emitted signals can be recorded by placing the antenna over the body. Few of the ultrasonic signals will travel through the media once but will need sufficient energy for ultrasound emission for the microrobot location. Ultrasound localization microscopy (ULM) technique is another promising approach for the super resolution. Yu and co-workers had invented the technique by which the acquisition time for each ULM image is about 6 s, and other groups are working in the same direction [55]; still a lot of the efforts are needed for making this method real time.

23.10.1 Optical-Based Techniques

Optical imaging is done by the non-ionizing radiation lasers or LED sources. These techniques are very fast, safe, and low cost with the very high spatial and temporal resolutions.

23.10.2 Magneto-Optic Imaging

Magneto-optic imaging (MOI) is also the hybrid imaging technique which combines the electromagnetic effect and the Faraday effect for generating the images [56]. Here the propagation of light in the magnetic field is used to image the target objects.

23.10.3 Magneto-Acoustic Imaging

Magneto-acoustic tomography (MAI) uses the very high-frequency (MHz range) pulsed magnetic fields producing the vibrations within the tissues which are to be loaded with magnetic NPs [57]. This is based on the principle of the continuous low-frequency magnetic fields which are being detected for the pulse-echo US sequencing. However, in the MAI, the receiver is the transducer [58].

23.10.4 Microrobots

The future of the robotic systems will be smart and intelligent microscale mobile robots which can be controlled by the external source. The small size of these microrobots when present in the human tissue will be the biggest limitation to get identified and also for the use in the various clinical applications. These microrobots can be identified by the non-invasive, real-time imaging modalities ultrasound (US) and photoacoustic (PA) imaging combined for detection and the motion of a single microrobot especially in the deeper tissues in the body. These microrobots are being used by the photoresist mixed with nickel (Ni) particles, and these are being controlled by the externally applied magnetic field. The PA imaging is capable of the detection which is not being detected by the ultrasound down to 50 μm. Thus, the US and PA imaging will be used for the various microrobot into translational applications [59–62].

A mobile device several millimetres down to few micrometres in all dimensions appointed to perform specific tasks in a controllable fashion. The MRI microrobotics like our routine spatial and temporal resolutions and these are the important components for single microrobot visualization, the detection of the targets, and the transformation of the shape along with the activation of various mechanisms including the drug delivery. Here in the MRI, we know that the spatial resolution is directly proportional to the relaxation signal and also inversely related to the FoV and slice thickness. By increasing the acquisition time, we can increase the resolution especially spatial, but here the temporal resolution will be reduced [63, 64].

23.11 Conclusion

The faster pace changes in the technology have revolutionized in the use of the robots in the imaging in all the modalities. There are many changes in the robotic technologies which along with the different modalities are having the advantage of each other based on the various imaging perspectives in the diagnostic and the therapeutic options. Thus, the role of both diagnostic and therapeutic options is being explored more and more, and this will revolutionize the future of the imaging

References

1. Birkfellner W, Watzinger F, Wanschitz F, Ewers R. Calibration of tracking systems in a surgical environment. IEEE Trans Med Imaging. 1998;17(5):737–42.
2. Boctor EM, Fisher G, Choti MA, Fichtinger G, Taylor RH. A dual-armed robotic system for intraoperative ultrasound guided hepatic ablative therapy: a prospective study. In: IEEE international conference on robotics and automation, New Orleans, LA; 2004. p. 2517–22.
3. Rousseau F. Méthodes d'analyse d'image et de calibration pour l'échographie 3D en mode main-libre. PhD. Thesis, Institut de Formation Supérieureen Informatiqueet Communication VISTA (IRISA, RENNES). 15 Dec 2003.
4. Wojcinski S, Farrokh A, Hille U, Wiskirchen J, Gyapong S, Soliman AA, Degenhardt F, Hillemanns P. The automated breast volume scanner (ABVS): initial experiences in lesion detection compared with conventional handheld b mode ultrasound: a pilot study of 50 cases. Int J Womens Health. 2011;3:337–46.
5. Chen TK, Leung C, Azar RZ, Chan K, Bo Zhuang K, Dickie J, Dixon L, Pendziwol L, Pelissier L. Importance of transducer position tracking for automated breast ultrasound: initial assessments. In: Ultrasonics symposium (IUS), Dresden, Germany, 2012. p. 2623–6.
6. Vilchis A, Troccaz J, Cinquin P, Masuda K, Pellissier F. A new robot architecture for tele-echography. IEEE Trans Robot Autom. 2003;19(5):922–6. Special issue on Medical Robotics
7. Martinelli T, Bosson J, Bressollette L, Pelissier F, Boidard E, Troccaz J, Cinquin P. Robot-based teleechography clinical evaluation of the TER system in abdominal aortic exploration. J Ultrasound Med. 2007;26:1611–6.
8. Nouaille L, Smith-Guerin N, Poisson G, Arbeille P. Optimization of a 4 DOF tele-echography robot. In: IEEE/RSJ international conference on intelligent robots and systems, Taipei. 2010. p. 3501–6.
9. Salcudean SE, Zhu WH, Abolmaesumi P, Bachmann S, Lawrence PD. A robot system for medical ultrasound. In: 9th international symposium of robotics research (ISRR). Snowbird; 1999. p. 152–9.
10. Krupa A. Automatic calibration of a robotized 3D ultrasound imaging system by visual servoing. In: IEEE international conference on robotics and automation, Florida. 2006. p. 4136–41.
11. Mebarki R, Krupa A, Chaumette F. 2-D ultrasound probe complete guidance by visual servoing using image moments. IEEE Trans Robot. 2010;26(2):296–306.
12. Janvier M, Durand L, Cardinal M, Renaud I, Chayer B, Bigras P, Guise J, Soulez G, Cloutier G. Performance evaluation of a medical robotic 3D-ultrasound imaging system. Med Image Anal. 2008;12:275–90.
13. Martinelli T, Bosson J, Bressollette L, Pelissier F, Boidard E, Troccaz J, Cinquin P. Robot-based tele-echography clinical evaluation of the TER system in abdominal aortic exploration. J Ultrasound Med. 2007;26:1611–6.
14. Najafi F, Sepehri N. A robotic wrist for remote ultrasound imaging. J Mech Mach Theory. 2011;46(8):1153–70.
15. Vieyres P, Poisson G, Courreges F, Merigeaux O, Arbeille P. The TERESA project: from space research to ground tele-echography. Int J Ind Robot. 2003;30(1):77–82.
16. Arbeille P, Capri A, Ayoub J, Kieffer V, Georgescu M, Poisson G. Use of a robotic arm to perform remote abdominal telesonography. Am J Roentgenol. 2007;188(4):317–22.
17. Pandarinath C, Nuyujukian P, Blabe CH, Sorice BL, Saab J, Willett FR, Hochberg LR, Shenoy KV, Henderson JM. High performance communication by people with paralysis using an intracortical brain-computer interface. eLife. 2017;6:e18554.
18. Vansteensel MJ, Pels EGM, Bleichner MG, Branco MP, Denison T, Freudenburg ZV, Gosselaar P, Leinders S, Ottens TH, van den Boom MA, Van Rijen PC, Aarnoutse EJ, Ramsey NF. Fully implanted brain–computer interface in a locked-in patient with ALS. N Engl J Med. 2016;375:2060–6.
19. Bouton CE, Shaikhouni A, Annetta NV, Bockbrader MA, Friedenberg DA, Nielson DM, Sharma G, Sederberg PB, Glenn BC, Mysiw WJ, Morgan AG, Deogaonkar M, Rezai AR. Restoring cortical control of functional movement in a human with quadriplegia. Nature. 2016;533:247–50.
20. Soekadar SR, Witkowski M, Gómez C, Opisso E, Medina J, Cortese M, Cempini M, Carrozza MC, Cohen LG, Birbaumer N, Vitiello N. Hybrid EEG/EOG-based brain-neural hand exoskeleton restores fully independent living activities after quadriplegia. Sci Robot. 2016;1:eeag3296.
21. Chaudhary U, Xia B, Silvoni S, Cohen LG, Birbaumer N. Brain–computer interface-based communication

in the completely locked-in State. PLoS Biol. 2017;15:e1002593.
22. He B, Baxter B, Edelman BJ, Cline CC, Ye W. Noninvasive brain-computer interfaces based on sensorimotor rhythms. Proc IEEE. 2015;103:907–25.
23. Millán JDR, Rupp R, Müller-Putz GR, Murray-Smith R, Giugliemma C, Tangermann M, Vidaurre C, Cincotti F, Kübler A, Leeb R, Neuper C, Müller K-R, Mattia D. Combining brain-computer interfaces and assistive technologies: state-of-the-art and challenges. Front Neurosci. 2010;4:161.
24. Leeb BR, Tonin L, Rohm M, Desideri L, Carlson T, Millán JDR. Towards independence: a BCI telepresence robot for people with severe motor disabilities. Proc IEEE. 2015;103:969–82.
25. Gilja V, Pandarinath C, Blabe CH, Nuyujukian P, Simeral JD, Sarma AA, Sorice BL, Perge JA, Jarosiewicz B, Hochberg LR, Shenoy KV, Henderson JM. Clinical translation of a high-performance neural prosthesis. Nat Med. 2015;21:1142–5.
26. Chen X, Wang Y, Nakanishi M, Gao X, Jung T-P, Gao S. High-speed spelling with a noninvasive brain–computer interface. Proc Natl Acad Sci USA. 2015;112:E6058–67.
27. Holz EM, Botrel L, Kaufmann T, Kübler A. Long-term independent brain-computer interface home use improves quality of life of a patient in the locked-in state: a case study. Arch Phys Med Rehabil. 2015;96:S16–26.
28. Collinger JL, Kryger MA, Barbara R, Betler T, Bowsher K, Brown EHP, et al. Collaborative approach in the development of high-performance brain-computer interfaces for a neuroprosthetic arm: translation from animal models to human control. Clin Transl Sci. 2014;7:52–9.
29. Anderson KD. Targeting recovery: priorities of the spinal cord-injured population. J Neurotrauma. 2004;21:1371–83.
30. Chaudhary U, Birbaumer N, Ramos-Murguialday A. Brain–computer interfaces for communication and rehabilitation. Nat Rev Neurol. 2016;12:513–25.
31. Lotze M, Braun C, Birbaumer N, Anders S, Cohen LG. Motor learning elicited by voluntary drive. Brain. 2003;126:866–72.
32. Musallam S, Corneil BD, Greger B, Scherberger H, Andersen RA. Cognitive control signals for neural prosthetics. Science. 2004;305:258–62.
33. Daly JJ, Wolpaw JR. Brain-computer interfaces in neurological rehabilitation. Lancet Neurol. 2008;7:1032–43.
34. Yerkes RM, Dodson JD. The relation of strength of stimulus to rapidity of habit formation. J Comp Neurol Psychol. 1908;18:459–82.
35. Ball T, Kern M, Mutschler I, Aertsen A, Schulze-Bonhage A. Signal quality of simultaneously recorded invasive and non-invasive EEG. Neuroimage. 2009;46:708–16.
36. Ramoser H, Müller-Gerking J, Pfurtscheller G. Optimal spatial filtering of single trial EEG during imagined hand movement. IEEE Trans Rehabil Eng. 2000;8:441–6.
37. Qin L, Ding L, He B. Motor imagery classification by means of source analysis for brain computer interface applications. J Neural Eng. 2004;1:135–41.
38. Edelman BJ, Baxter B, He B. EEG source imaging enhances the decoding of complex right-hand motor imagery tasks. IEEE Trans Biomed Eng. 2016;63:4–14.
39. Ang KK, Chin ZY, Wang C, Guan C, Zhang H. Filter bank common spatial pattern algorithm on BCI competition IV datasets 2a and 2b. Front Neurosci. 2012;6:39.
40. Turing AM. I.—Computing machinery and intelligence. Mind. 1950;LIX:433–60.
41. Acemoglu D, Restrepo P. Robots and jobs: evidence from US labor markets, 2017. NBER Working Paper No. 23285.
42. Solovev AA, Mei Y, Ureña EB, Huang G, Schmidt OG. Catalytic microtubular jet engines self-propelled by accumulated gas bubbles. Small. 2009;5:1688–92.
43. Sanchez S, Soler L, Katuri J. Chemically powered micro- and nanomotors. Angew Chem Int Ed. 2015;54:1414–44.
44. Sun J, Mathesh M, Li W, Wilson DA. Enzyme-powered nanomotors with controlled size for biomedical applications. ACS Nano. 2019;13:10191–200.
45. Villa K, Krejčová L, Novotný F, Heger Z, Sofer Z, Pumera M. Cooperative multifunctional self-propelled paramagnetic microrobots with chemical handles for cell manipulation and drug delivery. Adv Funct Mater. 2018;28:1804343.
46. Zhou M, Hou T, Li J, Yu S, Xu Z, Yin M, Wang J, Wang X. Self-propelled and targeted drug delivery of poly(aspartic acid)/iron–zinc microrocket in the stomach. ACS Nano. 2019;13:1324–32.
47. Chen C, Soto F, Karshalev E, Li J, Wang J. Hybrid nanovehicles: one machine, two engines. Adv Funct Mater. 2019;29:1806290.
48. Llopis-Lorente A, García-Fernández A, Murillo-Cremaes N, Hortelão AC, Patiño T, Villalonga R, Sancenón F, Martínez-Máñez R, Sánchez S. Enzyme-powered gated mesoporous silica nanomotors for on-command intracellular payload delivery. ACS Nano. 2019;13:12171–83.
49. Yan X, Zhou Q, Vincent M, Deng Y, Yu J, Xu J, Xu T, Tang T, Bian L, Wang Y-XXJ, Kostarelos K, Zhang L. Multifunctional biohybrid magnetite microrobots for imaging-guided therapy. Sci Robot. 2017;2:eaaq1155.
50. Gao W, Dong R, Thamphiwatana S, Li J, Gao W, Zhang L, Wang J. Artificial micromotors in the mouse's stomach: a step toward in vivo use of synthetic motors. ACS Nano. 2015;9:117–23.
51. Xie L, Pang X, Yan X, Dai Q, Lin H, Ye J, Cheng Y, Zhao Q, Ma X, Zhang X, Liu G, Chen X. Photoacoustic imaging-trackable magnetic microswimmers for pathogenic bacterial infection treatment. ACS Nano. 2020;14:2880–93.

52. Chatzipirpiridis G, Ergeneman O, Pokki J, Ullrich F, Fusco S, Ortega JA, Sivaraman KM, Nelson BJ, Pané S. Electroforming of implantable tubular magnetic microrobots for wireless ophthalmologic applications. Adv Healthc Mater. 2015;4:209–14.
53. Kruk D, Masiewicz E, Umut E, Petrovic A, Kargl R, Scharfetter H. Estimation of the magnitude of quadrupole relaxation enhancement in the context of magnetic resonance imaging contrast. J Chem Phys. 2019;150:184306.
54. Tay ZW, Hensley DW, Vreeland EC, Zheng B, Conolly SM. The relaxation wall: experimental limits to improving MPI spatial resolution by increasing nanoparticle core size. Biomed Phys Eng Express. 2017;3:35003.
55. Tay ZW, Hensley DW, Chandrasekharan P, Zheng B, Conolly SM. Optimization of drive parameters for resolution, sensitivity and safety in magnetic particle imaging. Page 92 of 100 ACS Paragon Plus Environment ACS Nano. IEEE Trans Med Imaging. 2019;39:1724–34.
56. Radtke U, Zielke R, Rademacher H-G, Crostack H-A, Hergt R. Application of magneto-optical method for real-time visualization of Eddy currents with high spatial resolution for nondestructive testing. Opt Lasers Eng. 2001;36:251–68.
57. Zhou Z-F, Cheng Y-H. Magneto-optic microscope for visually detecting subsurface defects. Appl Opt. 2008;47:3463–6.
58. Cheng Y, Deng Y, Bai L, Chen K. Enhanced laser-based magneto-optic imaging system for nondestructive evaluation applications. IEEE Trans Instrum Meas. 2013;62:1192–8.
59. Palagi S, Fischer P. Bioinspired microrobots. Nat Rev Mater. 2018;3:113.
60. Chautems C, Zeydan B, Charreyron S, Chatzipirpiridis G, Pane S, Nelson BJ. Magnetically powered microrobots: a medical revolution underway? Eur J Cardio-Thorac Surg. 2017;51:405–7.
61. Sitti M, Ceylan H, Hu W, Giltinan J, Turan M, Yim S, Diller ED. Biomedical applications of untethered mobile milli/microrobots. Proc IEEE. 2015;103:205–24.
62. Wang Q, Yang L, Yu J, Vong C-I, Chiu PWY, Zhang L. Magnetic navigation of a rotating colloidal swarm using ultrasound images. In: Proceedings of the 2018 IEEE/RSJ international conference on intelligent robots and systems (IROS), Madrid, Spain, 1–5 Oct 2018. p. 5380–5.
63. Cappelleri D, Efthymiou D, Goswami A, Vitoroulis N, Zavlanos M. Towards mobile microrobot swarms for additive micromanufacturing. Int J Adv Robot Syst. 2014;11:150.
64. Xu T, Zhang J, Salehizadeh M, Onaizah O, Diller E. Millimeter-scale flexible robots with programmable three-dimensional magnetization and motions. Sci Robot. 2019;4:eaav4494.

Molecular Imaging and Artificial Intelligence

24

Key Points (Abstract)

Artificial intelligence (AI) in the medicine is now becoming the well-established entity and is being rapidly evolving in the radiology. AI is one of the most sought topics for research in our medical field and also had the great impact on the various newer innovations in recent years. With these advancements in the technologies, there is significant demand for the use of the artificial intelligence for the interpretation of various information's by allowing machines to evaluate the complex data. Many apprehensions are present despite the various risks and quality issues in it. AI has demonstrated the more precise way of the radiological services rendered. A lot of debate is going on whether the radiologist will have impact on his profession, or it is more of like complimentary and assisting to the radiologist. Artificial intelligence (AI) is one of the fastest growing technology in medical imaging. The applications are of many activities which are based on the radiomics, various artificial neural networks, and various machine learning techniques. This deep learning is now based on the various protocols and algorithms in imaging leading to the significant impact on the outcomes, especially in relation to the quality and efficiency.

Keywords

Artificial intelligence · Deep learning · Machine learning · Artificial neural network · Convolutional neural network · Radiomics

24.1 Introduction

Artificial intelligence (AI) is defined as computer systems which are able to perform various tasks normally requiring human intelligence, e.g., visual perception, speech recognition, decision making, and language translating [1] (Diagram 24.1). Other way to describe AI is the ability of a computer program or a machine for thinking and learning. The study involves that the computer is "smart", by making them, by encoding, and by their commands [2]. AI is made up of two components: machine learning (ML) and the brain-inspired deep learning convolutional neural networks (CNN). AI in radiology is made up of the more advanced components of deep learning/CNN. AI working is based on the automatically recognizing complex imaging data showing the quantitative assessment of image characteristics [3]. Deep learning CNN networks are based on the similar pattern of the functioning of the intelligent human brain which will mimic human neural networks in the functioning pattern. The input

S. Shaikh, *Advances in Imaging*, https://doi.org/10.1007/978-981-16-9535-3_24

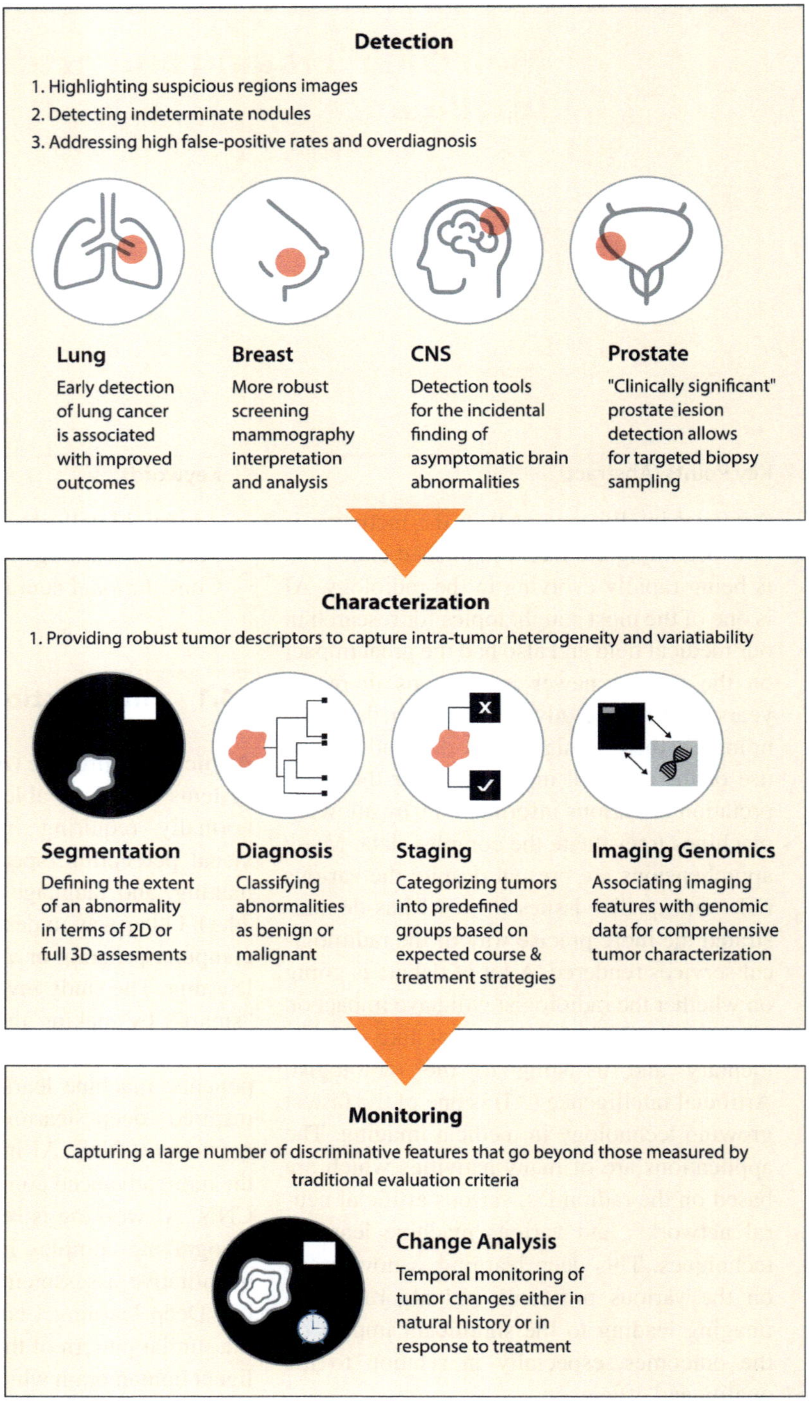

Diagram 24.1 Various algorithms for the detection, characterization, and monitoring of the various AI algorithms

is given by the data which is entered in many layers of neural rows, and the final neural layer will be made of the output layer. The language for programming which is used in AI is Python, and radiology has evolved as the speciality in such a way that it is mostly technology driven and continuously evolving in comparison to the other medical specialities (Diagram 24.2).

The important reason for the emergence of AI in medical imaging is for the faster, better workflow of the images with greater efficacy. One of the major reasons is that radiological imaging data is growing at the very faster pace as compared to the analysing data by the radiologists which is becoming overloaded. To overcome this, the increasing role of the AI is seen which will have significant increase in efficiency, by reducing the errors and helping the radiologists with pre-screened images which have features added for early interpretation.

With the emergence of the artificial intelligence (AI) in medical imaging, it is the most important invention after the Roentgen, Becquerel, and Curie Hounsfield and Anger. The Artificial intelligence in the form of the artificial neural network (ANN) is the important component of the machine learning (ML) and deep learning (DL). In ANN, various algorithms of different layers of connected nodes are present. The various types of the inputs can be radiomic features from the image files or convolutional neural network (CNN) which can be the images themselves. AI in medical imaging will help enhance visual recognition in radiology resulting in less error as compared with human errors (2015) [1, 2]. ML can do a lot of things in medical imaging including detecting and classifying the lesions by automated image segmentation, various data analysis, the extraction of the various radiomic features, image reconstruction, and prioritizing the studies [1, 3–5]. ANN will also be helpful along the conventional statistical analysis thus providing the in-depth knowledge of the research data [6]. The ANN nodes will be having the huge number from thousands to millions which will be configured in depth (depth) [7]. DL uses an ANN comprised of the various layers thus making the implementation of ML easier to perform the information as received their nodes and the outputs. The best outcomes with a large data set can have the larger iteration, causing the significant increase of the differences will be getting the marginally smaller [7] (Diagram 24.3). Another data set will be used for large reliable training data for ML and DL algorithms. DL is programmed to describe the exact number of the layers in the ANN. It is based on CNNs whether to identify and correctly extract features directly from images [8]. The activation function (A), along with the linear or logistic (sigmoidal) activation then combining the shapes for the output of the node [8–13]. Each node is having only one, but this single output will become the input for multiple nodes in the next perception layer. The ANN is having the probable output function for the upscaling layer [10–13]. Thus, to train and optimize the ANN, the error team will measure the loss index along with the size of change in outputs in response to change in inputs [8, 9, 11–14]. The regularization of the various errors is from the output layers towards the input layers [10, 11]. Small data set will have iterations, and the larger data sets cannot pass through the inn in one batch. Thus, the larger data is split into the smaller ones, and sometimes these data will be lost. Various convolutions will be applied to the kernels to the input tensor [8–10, 12–15]. These kernels will be placed in such a way that they will be superimposed on various pixels, and thus, the distance between these kernels will be striding [8, 9, 11–13, 16]. Multiple convolution layers will be produced by applying various multiple kernel data. This will be activated once after passing through the rectified linear unit [8–10, 12–15].

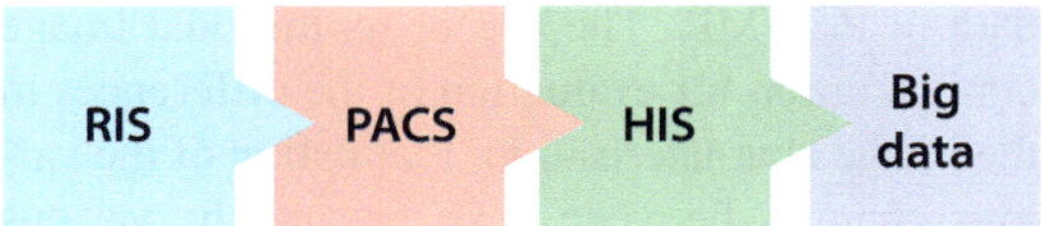

Diagram 24.2 Correlation of the bigger data samples to be taken cared

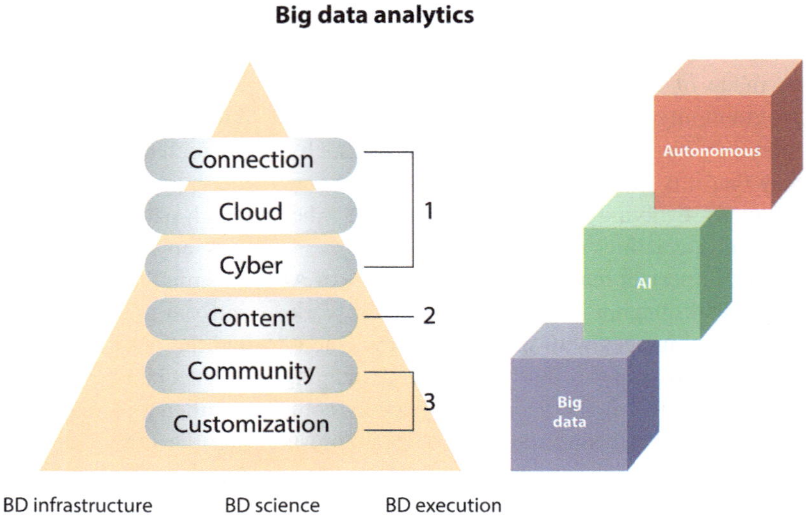

Diagram 24.3 Bigger data analysis in various steps

24.2 The Role of the AI in Radiomic Feature Extraction and Selection

The tern radiomics is coined by Lambin et al. [17] in which the useful imaging data will be extracted from the available radiological data. This important component and process of extracting the data will result in the better outcomes of the precision medicine [18]. In the oncological set up, this process of collecting and processing the medical images data, focussing on the lesion of interest, radiomic features which can be extracted, and along with the conventional methods to predict outcomes related with the response to therapy is the basis of radiomic AI (Diagram 24.4). The various radiomic features will define the complete three-dimensional (3D) tumour volume by using the pixel-based features [19]. For identifying and extracting the various radiomic features, the CNN is very important.

24.3 Deep Learning (DL) in Diagnosis and Therapy

Deep learning is a part of the of machine learning which functions on the basis of the neural network structures, and these structures learn from the programmed data, which is feeded automatically, by which the complex data can be evaluated with various nonlinear relationships. With the recent research advances, there are many newer protocols and algorithms which are not defined but will be the fundamental shift in the paradigm in machine learning. DL is mostly used for the location of a lesion, segmentation for contouring, and for characterisation between the malignant vs. benign lesion [20]. One of the most common application of the object detection is the diagnosis of mammograms and suspected lesions in the lung and liver. Object segmentation is mostly used in the areas where automated segmentation is needed in the radiation treatment for precise planning to reduce the radiation dose to the surrounding areas of the main tumour. Various uses of these techniques are possible with the use of the AI; one of the examples is the segmentation of the spleen.

Triaging gestalt classification which is based on the normal versus abnormal anatomy and used to validate the degree of severity of the cases. Attenuation correction can be done from MR with the attenuation correction maps from MR data in PET/MR. The use of multimodal image coregistration for evaluation of the differences in the image characterisation. Evaluation of the various changes between baseline and the various stages of the disease will determine the status of the disease progression or response to therapy.

The concept of machine learning in computer science and engineering has revolutionized the

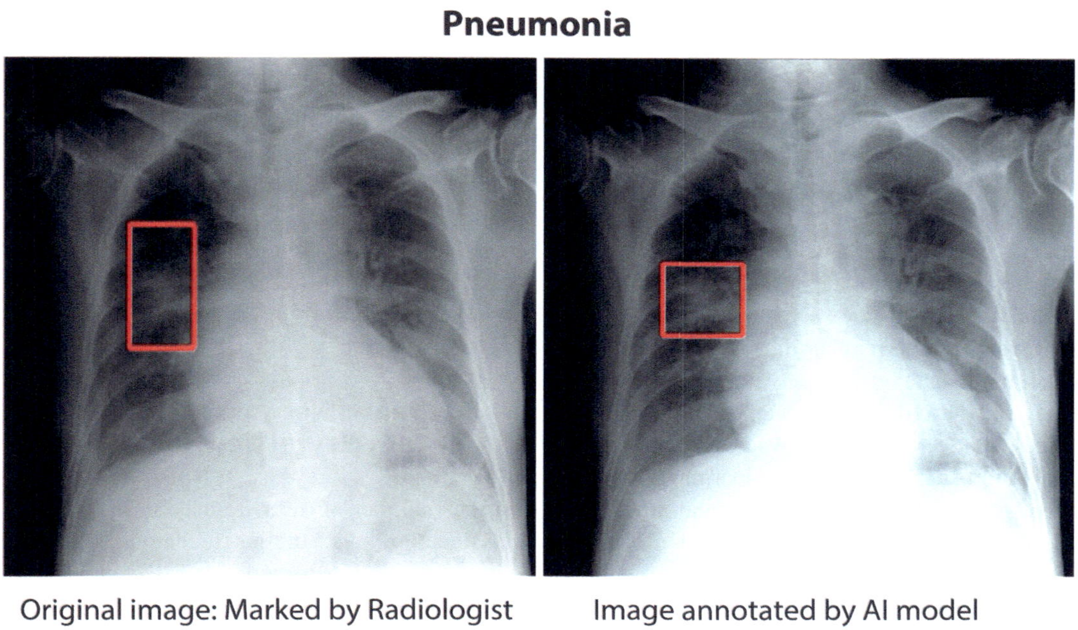

Diagram 24.4 Difference between the annotation of the radiologist and AI

concept of imaging. It is an important branch as it helps in the extraction of significant data similar to the component of human intelligence. Recent research has shown the capability of the machines to learn by various learning algorithms for better computer-aided diagnosis and various decision support systems. Thus, there is significant increase in the interest and research in the field of machine learning which is being applied to the medical images [21]. By using the computer-aided detection and diagnosis used for the various machine learning algorithms, this will help in reducing the interpretation times [22]. Some of the important tasks being done by this algorithm are evaluation of the pulmonary embolism segmentation and the computed tomographic (CT) angiography [23, 24], use of the virtual colonoscopy in suspicion of the cancer [25, 26], mammography evaluation of the cancers [27], segmentation of the intracranial neoplasms with MR imaging [28], and functional MR imaging for the quantification of the neurologic disease pathologies [29–31].

Machine learning is also being used widely for the evaluation of the various other functional entities like speech therapy and recognition and conversion between the different languages and many more. Classification: The different labels based on the various group of pixels can be done with the segmentation to determine the normal and abnormal brain and even for the differentiation with the benign or malignant tissue.

24.4 The Different Aspects of Machine Learning

Training: Machine learning algorithm system for various data sets. These different sets of weights or different models will lead to better advancement in the final improvement of the various algorithms.

Validation Set: The different algorithms for the various systems are to significantly improve the various sets of the validation.

Layer: The final computation of the nodes will increase the various outputs from one or more inputs.

Weights: Some value or weight is added to the input feature. This will involve the usage of the various images of brain tumor for more specific differentiation of the "benign" and "malignant" labels and also to differentiate between the benign and malignant entities (test data).

Segmentation: This is simply dividing the images in various parts. It is the process of defining tumor limits where it starts and ends. This will have the different segmentations for the differentiation of the enhancing tumor in one segment and another which is showing the nonenhancing tumor or necrotic area or perilesional oedema.

Overfitting: The classifier is too specific for the training data set. As we see that in the medical images, where the actual pixel values, the lesion edges, changes in the pixel values.

Computation: Machine learning is completely based on the source information which is basic and important to make various decisions. The features can be extracted in different ways as seen in various aspects [32, 33]. The various imaging features are different in relation to the various aspects of the noise, intensity, and rotation angles.

Feature Selection: Computing the various features of an image, it can be based on the decision [34]. The best predictions are known as the more specific features of the selection [35, 36]. Various feature selection is based on the various features without the relevant information being maintained. Some of the feature evaluation may have complex relationship.

Training and Testing: The learning process and the supervised machine seen as various sort of the learnings are required. Some of the examples need to be identified based on the features of that objects which will differentiate from each other [34]. Cross-validation technique is one of the important techniques for the accuracy [37, 38]. In cross-validation, the one part is selected for training and the rest for validation. In some cases, one entity for the testing and all remaining for the training are known as leave-one-out cross-validation [39].

Machine Learning with Use of Cross-Validation. One of the best examples is the differentiation of the brain tumor from adjacent normal brain parenchyma with or without CT images. Thus, the attenuation value of non-contrast CT is less and for the contrast study is more. Here the patterns of enhancements will vary, for example, the vessels will enhance, while necrotic areas of the tumour will not enhance. In non-enhanced images, the tumour will be darker, whereas haemorrhage and calcifications will be brighter. The various neural networks are also seen like k-nearest neighbours, support vector machines, decision trees, the naive Bayes algorithm, and deep learning.

24.5 Neural Networks Learning with Neural Networks

Various number of trees are used to improve the classification rate. In this technique, the total number of features is randomly selected, and further each subset is used to split like a splitting node.

24.5.1 Deep Learning

Deep learning, which is known as deep neural network learning, is the newer area of research with significantly increased research and results. The initial networks are the deep and largely and single as many layers cannot be hold together due to some of the weight-bearing challenges. Again, the concept of deep learning is the use of neural networks of more than 20. Various deep learning networks are being used for the various purposes like automatic detection of the objects [40] and segmentation of the images [41], automatic speech recognition [42], and various detection of the subsets of the genotypes and phenotypes by the bioinformatics for the better identification and classification of various diseases. The important step here is to identify the various training deep networks for the regularization [43].

These networks need to be regularized in the better way for the proper scaling of the weights which will be connecting the various pairs of layers. Many different combinations of the various layers and the layer sizes can be done, and there is no specific criteria established for evaluation.

24.5.2 An Introduction to Deep Learning Terminology

The concept of deep learning can be understood better by understanding the various principles and applications of the artificial intelligence and machine learning. Artificial intelligence is the foremost of all the three sets which is capable of performing the varied tasks of high intelligence if similar tasks are performed by human.

Machine learning is a part of the artificial intelligence algorithms to perform the various complicated tasks, which can be done from the available preset data and do not need proper programming. With this concept, machine learning is capable of doing the various applications in medical imaging [44]. The different layers are the input layer, functioning to receive the input data; the output layer, which has data processing; and the hidden layer(s), whose function is to extract the different information from the data. The DL approach was developed to improve the performance of conventional ANN when using deep architectures. Deep learning is part of machine learning having simple interconnected network units. Here the various units are interconnected to provide inputs like the various images. The deep learning model architecture can be defined by the use of the various artificial neural networks in specific and general.

24.5.3 Artificial Neural Networks

Artificial neural networks (ANNs) are the older form of the concept dated in the 1940s. This networking is similar to the artificial neuron like nerve cell. The neuron input by the various neurons will add all inputs, and the mathematical function is applied for the activation function for the single-output value. Deep convolutional neural network (CNN) is the common form of neural network. Deep convolutional neural networks having the word "deep" are comprised of 10–30 layer, and also it could be 1000 layers. These neurons which they are connected are sharing the multiple neuron's weights. Thus, the network performing the (or template matching) of the input image with the filters (defined by the weights) within the CNN can be connected. These layers comprising of the convolutional layers, pooling layers, and fully connected layers will form the convolutional neural network. Thus, the convolutional neural network is made up of changing the weights of the individual neurons based on input data. One of the learning processes is supervised learning based on the particular characteristics of the tumour. Transfer learning [45] and off-the-shelf features are the features seen in these techniques [46]. Pretraining uses the data set for the various aspects of the images, like the size of data after this data is fine-tuned. This data will be helpful in prediction of the possible outcomes of the various pathologies like glioblastoma [47] or various skin lesion classification [48]. Deep learning vs. "traditional" machine learning. In deep learning, the process of extraction of data and decision making can be combined and merged.

24.5.4 Deep Learning in Radiology

24.5.4.1 Classification

Various classifications are based on radiology like the classification of an image, to identify the presence or absence of an abnormality; benign or malignant; cancerous lesions classifications based on the histopathological and genomic features; prognosis of the lesion; and to organise the radiological data. The deep learning classifiers use various convolutional neural networks having convolutional layers and fully connected layers. With the use of this technology [49], long-term and short-term survival based on 29% accuracy for lung carcinoma was predicted. Transfer learning, for example, is used in differentiating prostate cancer vs benign prostate conditions in prostate MRI [50]. An ensemble of fine-tuned CNN classifiers was shown to outperform traditional CNNs in predicting radiological image modality on a test set of 4166 images [51]. Deep features and transfer learning are being more useful for identifying the radiogenomic relationships in breast cancer MRI [52]. The deep learning features are better compared to transfer learning, but the drawback is the smaller data set. With enough data, the entire deep neural network can be trained. One of the studies in differentiating Alzheimer's disease versus normal controls shows better results, due to better designs of the CNN architectures which can train better. Autoencoder is being used [53] to diagnose the possibility of Alzheimer's disease. The two encoders are auto-encoders and stacked auto-encoders which are used to identify the data from the hidden layers the same as used to identify the multiple sclerosis lesions when using MRI along with the myelin maps jointly [54]. The various applications are the segmentation of various organs, substructures, or lesions, along with the property to do the extraction and classification [55, 56]. For image segmentation, the various individual voxels are used in the form of patches to identify and extract the details of the voxel. This technique is being used for brain tumor segmentation in various conditions [57–59], to segment the white matter in multiple sclerosis patients [60], to evaluate the normal anatomy of the brain [61], and to segment the rectal cancer [62]. Convolutional neural network (CNN) is better used for this evaluation [63]. These are important advantages of the various CNN networks. Recurrent neural networks are one of the deep learning approaches used. In [64], the use of CNN which is based on the convolutional neural network segmentation of the left ventricular segmentation in cardiac MRI. Similarly, [65] long short-term memory (LSTM) [66] is a recurrent neural network which is trained for the advantage of 3D contextual information like pancreatic segmentation in MR images. Novel loss function can be identified by the use of Jaccard index [67].

24.5.4.2 Detection

In the routine, radiologists practise identifying any abnormality or if the lesion is based on the perceptive skills, experience, knowledge, and technical aspects of the window width and other technical parameters of the image visualisation, of which many are subjective. Thus, the concept of localizing and identifying the object in an image is known as detection. Detection in radiology imaging is an important step as it identifies the abnormality first. This abnormality can be in various forms like the tissue, lesion, mass, and nodularity in the region of interest which will be further characterized by the segmentation as well [68, 69]. The initial stage will be the identification of all these structures which are suspicious for abnormality [70], and in the absence of this, the precise location cannot be ascertained, so many false positives will be present. One of the applicatisons is the evaluation of the cerebral microhaemorrhages which are used for detection of a single data set with 93% sensitivity [71] (Diagram 24.4). Transfer learning can be used for classification. Thoracoabdominal lymph node detection can be done with the pre-trained evaluation [72] and in the pulmonary embolism detection with CT pulmonary angiogram data sets [73]. Can be also used for the intervertebral disc detection in X-ray images [74] and for the diagnosis of the colitis in CT images [75]. Single-phase detector is also being used in the first line of approach and then apply the you only look once (YOLO) approach [76]. Breast tumor identification in ultrasound images can be performed with the various deep learning methods which are available at the time [77]. The use of two-dimensional data, that is, the CT and MRI 3D data, provides very good results. One of the classical examples, in [78], is the detection of 3D anatomy in chest CT images with the slice-by-slice detection of the data in one direction (Diagram 24.5). The data is compiled in this fashion and is being used [79–81] in various planes of the MRI and CT. The final results can be quantified by the algorithms with various output probabilities [78] or by another machine learning protocols [82].

24.5.4.3 Image Registration

The registration of the two set of images which are different like T1-weighted and T2-weighted images or their set of data so that same location will show the same pathology in different presentations [83]. Here deep learning will be used to measure the T1–T2 MRI images from the brain and can co-register with the neonatal brain images. The basis of this is the mutual information used for the registration [84].

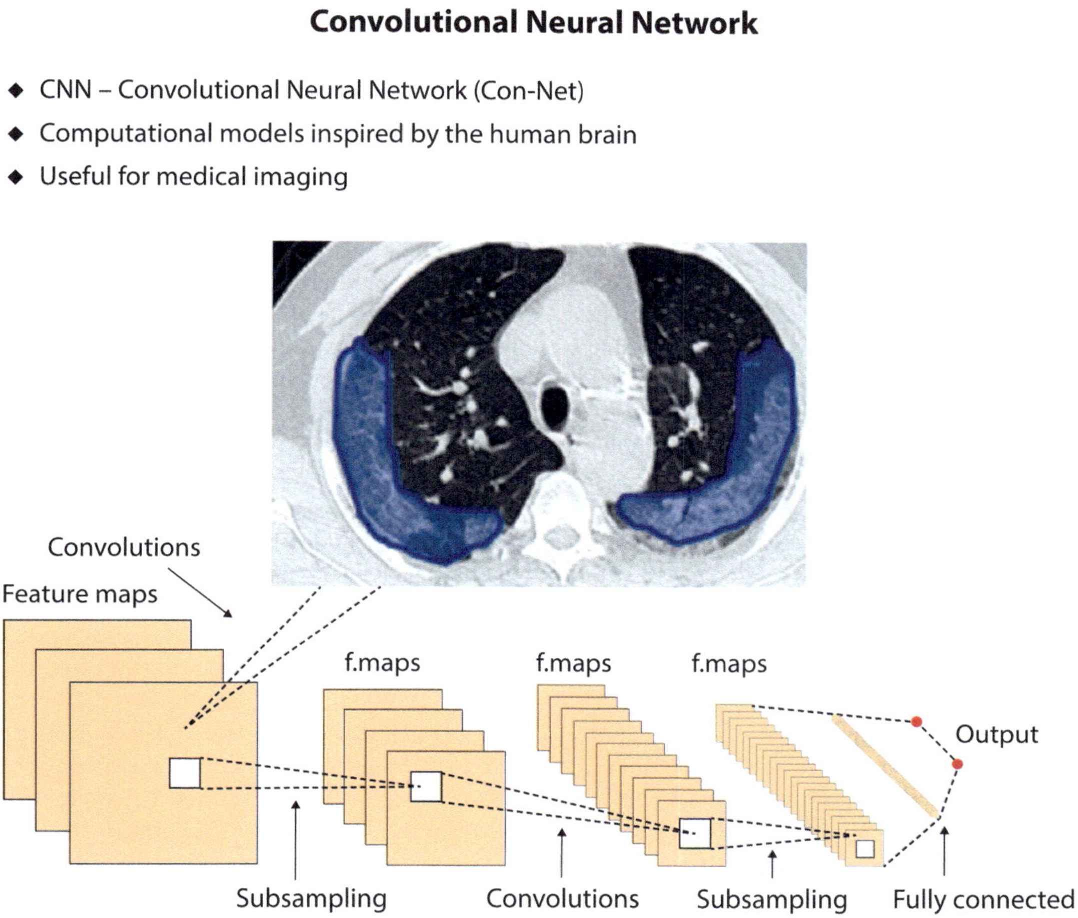

Diagram 24.5 CNN computational models

24.5.4.4 Image Generation/Reconstruction

The image acquisition and the hardware parameters are also based on the visual and the quality of the images like the TE and TR in the MRI. In [85], even the difference in technology can be useful for the image formation of one type of the technology with the other, for example, the 7T images which will be generated by the 3T MR images by CNN. K-space cardiac MRIs are being generated by the use of the deep cascade of CNNs in [86]. Sometimes with the advancement of technology, the images reconstructed like the low radiation acquired images in CT by using the CNN [87]. Deep CNN can also acquire the low-dose CT images for reconstruction of normal-dose CT [88]. Deep learning can also be used for synthesizing images of different modalities. CT images ca be generated by using the MR images by end-to-end non-linear mapping between pelvic CT and MR images [89]. Synthetic CT images of the brain also can be generated from T1-weighted MR image set [90]. Alzheimer's disease diagnosis without PET images can be constructed from the RI using CNN [91].

24.5.4.5 Image Enhancement

Image enhancement will be having the different features of the image such as resolution, signal-to-noise-ratio, and anatomical structures by the super-resolution and denoising. These super-resolutions of images are being used in the cardiac and lung imaging. The various subsets of the comparison can also be able to hold his or her breath. The use of the synthetic 3D MR images by deep convolutional neural network will be helpful for the evaluation of the residual learning which can be done by the evaluation of the various noise level parameters [92].

24.5.4.6 Content-Based Image Retrieval

The task which will be given as query image finds the most similar images in a given database. To accomplish this task, a deep CNN can first be trained to distinguish between different organs [93]. The various connected layers in the network are being extracted for the images from the retrieved data sets.

24.5.4.7 Objective Image Quality Assessment

Quality assessment of the images to be done to evaluate the images is satisfactory or unsatisfactory. This will definitely help in providing more information from the optimal images leading to better treatment [94]. Fatal ultrasound quality of the images can be done by CNN [95]. These are the main challenges and also the fallacies for the use of deep learning algorithms. Better sensitivity can be evaluated by the pre-training of the models by using the various data sets and different models and also the augmentation of the data by changing the various data sets. This imbalance will also have an impact on the low performance [96].

24.5.4.8 Future of Deep Learning in Radiology

Deep learning is having the very important role for the evaluation of future roles of radiology and mostly the MRI specifically. The basis here is the evaluation of the various skilled tasks for deep learning, while more intellectual things can be done for the radiologists. Still with these aspects kept in the mind, the work of the radiologists as well as the deep learning algorithms will be complementary to each other rather than replacing each other. Deep learning again are challenging aspects. The various alignments with the reproducibility of the data sets, various performance metrics, and newer imaging protocols which are standardized along with the reporting formats will become the various unbiased indicators which are to be aligned as per the specific disease protocols. Despite of the significant advances, they are crucial for accurate patient outcome; it is still in the infancy which needs to be validated more.

This will also be having many legal and ethical issues.

The most important is that who is responsible for the mistakes done by the programmed computer artificial intelligence will be penetrating the various human activities in the coming years. Another most important is the acceptance or non-acceptance for interpreting their images (regardless of the performance) as well as regulatory issues. Finally, an important practical issue is how to incorporate deep learning algorithms into the radiology workflow in order to improve, rather than disrupt, the radiology practice. Moreover, the role of the radiologists will not be reduced; in fact it will be added as the basic programming and foreseeing the overall outcome are done by radiologist alone.

24.6 AI Challenges in Medical Imaging

The important concern is that to what extent this newer deep learning will be implemented and can be used for various tasks in radiology [88], of which the tasks can be varying from months and fully also the automatic clinical tasks ranging from a few years to decades. Thus, the development of deep learning-based automated protocols can be used for the best clinical problems where sufficient data are available, such as the use of the human images like lung pathologies, mammograms, and images from virtual colonoscopy. The disadvantage is that the current AI tools available can be only used for one task and also variable for the general and narrow AI (Diagram 24.6). A comprehensive AI system which can detect multiple abnormalities is not developed. One out of four Americans undergoing the CT examination [97] and one out of ten who is receiving MRI [98]. Segmentation of the brain MRI, for the accuracy similar to these learning methods [99]. "Cryptonets" are deep learning networks which are programmed based on the encrypted data, which can be decrypted by those who had encrypted it, and thence, it has become very much confidential [100]. With the advances in technology in relation to the quality, sensitivity, and resolution, still these techniques are not on par with the precise diagnosis and localization. Deep learning algorithms will play a significant role in the improvement of the performance. AI is based on one task which is programmed, and here the human intelligence is far better. Still the radiologists will play major role for the better use of the technology tools. Thus, the AI should be trained on more options for the robust AI which will have the blend of the various details like various patient demographics, different geographic regions, various diseases, and standards of care. Thus, the use of AI will benefit the larger community in terms of the enhancement of the various technical protocols, image quality significantly improved, radiation dose optimization, decreasing the scan time for various studies, and reducing the costs of the examinations along with reducing the reporting time, thus improving the overall efficiency and standard of the patient care (Diagram 24.7).

Narrow AI

Narrow AI is a term used to describe artificial intelligence systems that are specified to handle singular or limited task.

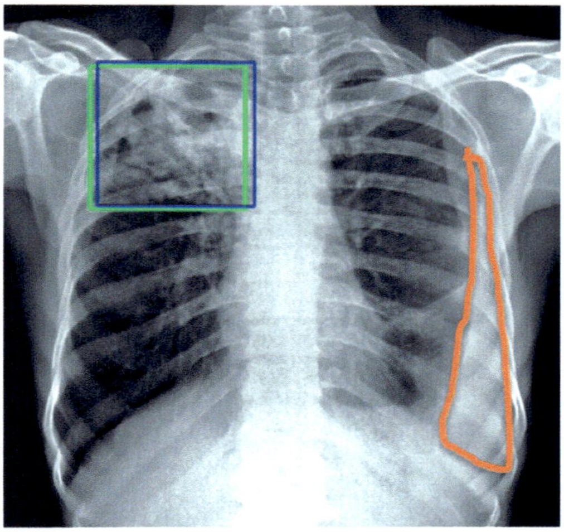

General AI

General AI is capable of handling a wide range of tasks rather than one particular task or problem.

The variation of artificial intelligence can be roughly conceptualized as a foundation for neural networks emulating sentience or consciousness.

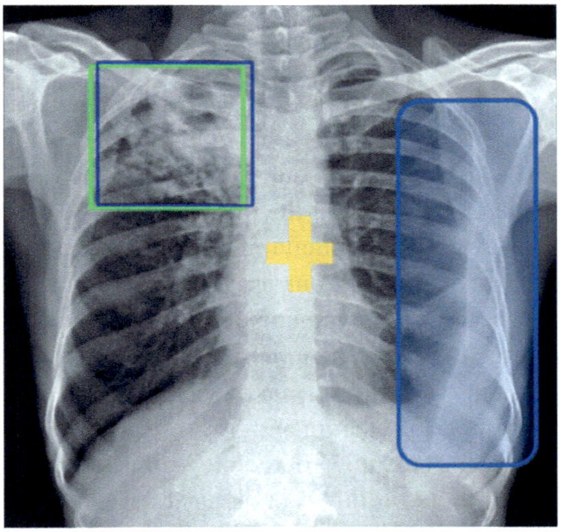

Diagram 24.6 Difference between narrow AI and general AI

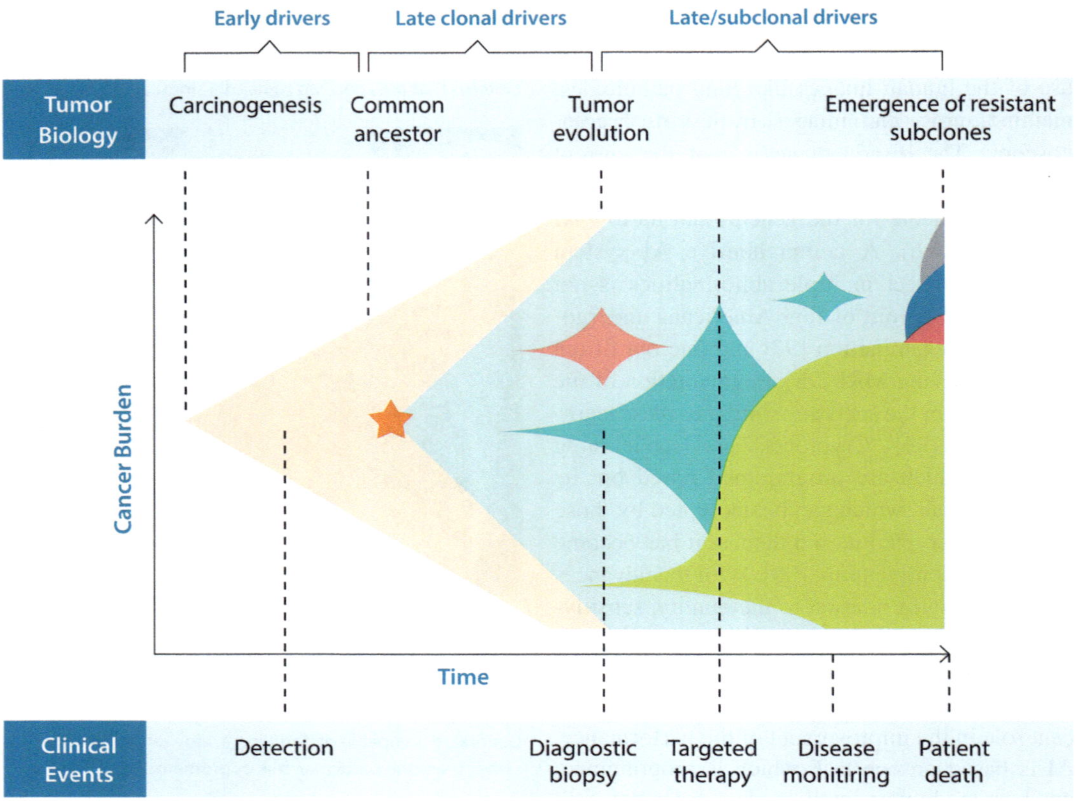

Diagram 24.7 Various clinical events and the role of AI

24.7 Conclusion

AI, ML, and DL are being used in our medical imaging without much impact. ANN and CNN will be significantly used to enhance the diverse use. By understanding the principles of AI, ML, and DL, it will be felicitating the more use with major advantages in our today practise. For the very successful implementation of AI in medical imaging, the component of the advanced technology along with the various facets will be useful for its impact on the imaging.

Since the beginning of radiology, this speciality is based more on the technological development. Today, radiologist needs to be updated and trained for the various principles of ML/DL systems and also know their limitations. Thus, radiologists have to work for and with AI in the coming years, ultimately leading to the best harmony as well for the best outcome for the patient care.

References

1. McBee MP, Awan OA, Colucci AT, et al. Deep learning in radiology. Acad Radiol. 2018;25(11):1472–80.
2. Langlotz C, Allen B, Erickson B, et al. A roadmap for foundational research on artificial intelligence in medical imaging: from the 2018 NIH/RSNA/ACR/The academy workshop. Radiology. 2019;291(3):781–91.
3. Liew C. The future of radiology augmented with artificial intelligence a strategy for success. Eur J Radiol. 2018;102:152–6.
4. Tajmir SH, Alkasab TK. Toward augmented radiologists: changes in radiology education in the era of machine learning and artificial intelligence. Acad Radiol. 2018;25(6):747–50.
5. Thrall JH, Li X, Li Q, et al. Artificial intelligence and machine learning in radiology: opportunities, challenges, pitfalls, and criteria for success. J Am Coll Radiol. 2018;15(3 Pt B):504–8.
6. Currie G. Intelligent imaging: radiomics and artificial neural networks in heart failure. J Med Imaging Radiat Sci. 2019. in press.
7. Tang A, Tam R, Cadrin-Chenevert A, et al. Canadian association of radiologists white paper on artifi-

cial intelligence in radiology. Can Assoc Radiol J. 2018;69(2):120–35.
8. Yamashita R, Nishio M, Do RKG, Togashi K. Convolutional neural networks: an overview and application in radiology. Insights Imaging. 2018;9(4):611–29.
9. Lundervold AS, Lundervold A. An overview of deep learning in medical imaging focusing on MRI. Z Med Phys. 2019;29:102–27.
10. Goodfellow I, Bengio Y, Courville A. Deep learning. MIT Press; 2016. Available at: http://www.deeplearningbook.org/. Accessed 6 June 2019.
11. Nielsen MA. Neural networks and deep learning. Determination Press; 2015. Available at: http://neuralnetworksanddeeplearning.com/index.html. Accessed 6 June 2018.
12. Currie G. Intelligent imaging: anatomy of machine learning and deep learning [e-pub ahead of print]. J Nucl Med Technol. 2019;47(4) https://doi.org/10.2967/jnmt.119.232470.
13. Maier A, Syben C, Lasser T, Riess C. A gentle introduction to deep learning in medical imaging processing. Z Med Phys. 2018;29:86–101.
14. Shen D, Wu G, Suk H. Deep learning in medical image analysis. Annu Rev Biomed Eng. 2017;19:221–48.
15. Lin M, Chen Q, Yan S. Network in network. CoRR. 2013. Available at http://arxiv.org/abs/1312.4400.
16. Currie G, Hewis J, Bushong S. Tomographic reconstruction; a non-mathematical overview. J Med Imaging Radiat Sci. 2015;46(4):403–12.
17. Lambin P, Rios-Velazquez E, Leijenaar R, et al. Radiomics: extracting more information from medical images using advanced feature analysis. Eur J Cancer. 2012;48:441–6.
18. Vial A, Stirling D, Field M, et al. The role of deep learning and radiomic feature extraction in cancer-specific predictive modelling: a review. Transl Cancer Res. 2018;7:803–16.
19. Clifton H, Vial A, Stirling D, et al. Using machine learning applied to radiomic image features for segmenting tumour structures. In: Asia-Pacific Signal and Information Processing Association annual summit and conference (APSIPA); 2019.
20. Currie G. Intelligent imaging: artificial intelligence augmented nuclear medicine. J Nucl Med Technol. 2019;47:217–22.
21. From $600 M to $6 billion, artificial intelligence systems poised for dramatic market expansion in healthcare. Frost & Sullivan website. http://ww2.frost.com/news/press-releases/600-m-6-billion-artificial-intelligence-systems-poised-dramatic-market-expansion-healthcare/. Accessed 2 Sept 2016.
22. Schoepf UJ, Costello P. CT angiography for diagnosis of pulmonary embolism: state of the art. Radiology. 2004;230(2):329–37.
23. Schoepf UJ, Schneider AC, Das M, Wood SA, Cheema JI, Costello P. Pulmonary embolism: computer-aided detection at multidetector row spiral computed tomography. J Thorac Imaging. 2007;22(4):319–23.
24. Dundar MM, Fung G, Krishnapuram B, Rao RB. Multiple instances learning algorithms for computer-aided detection. IEEE Trans Biomed Eng. 2008;55(3):1015–21.
25. Summers RM. Improving the accuracy of CTC interpretation: computer-aided detection. Gastrointest Endosc Clin N Am. 2010;20(2):245–57.
26. Yoshida H, Näppi J. CAD in CT colonography without and with oral contrast agents: progress and challenges. Comput Med Imaging Graph. 2007;31(4-5):267–84.
27. Chan HP, Lo SC, Sahiner B, Lam KL, Helvie MA. Computer aided detection of mammographic microcalcifications: pattern recognition with an artificial neural network. Med Phys. 1995;22(10):1555–67.
28. Bauer S, Wiest R, Nolte LP, Reyes M. A survey of MRI-based medical image analysis for brain tumor studies. Phys Med Biol. 2013;58(13):R97–R129.
29. Mitchell TM, Shinkareva SV, Carlson A, et al. Predicting human brain activity associated with the meanings of nouns. Science. 2008;320(5880):1191–5.
30. Davatzikos C, Fan Y, Wu X, Shen D, Resnick SM. Detection of prodromal Alzheimer's disease via pattern classification of magnetic resonance imaging. Neurobiol Aging. 2008;29(4):514–23.
31. Kim D, Burge J, Lane T, Pearlson GD, Kiehl KA, Calhoun VD. Hybrid ICA-Bayesian network approach reveals distinct effective connectivity differences in schizophrenia. Neuroimage. 2008;42(4):1560–8.
32. Nixon M, Nixon MS, Aguado AS. Feature extraction & image processing for computer vision. London, England: Academic; 2012.
33. Wang Y, Yuhang W. Spatial feature extraction algorithms. Master's thesis. Hanover, NH: Dartmouth College; 2005.
34. Way TW, Sahiner B, Hadjiiski LM, Chan HP. Effect of finite sample size on feature selection and classification: a simulation study. Med Phys. 2010;37(2):907–20.
35. Saeys Y, Inza I, Larrañaga P. A review of feature selection techniques in bioinformatics. Bioinformatics. 2007;23(19):2507–17.
36. Kuhn M, Johnson K. An introduction to feature selection. In: Applied predictive modelling. New York: Springer; 2013. p. 487–519.
37. Kohavi R, Ron K, John GH. Automatic parameter selection by minimizing estimated error. In: Proceedings of the twelfth international conference on machine learning, Tahoe City, Calif. New York: Elsevier; 1995. p. 304–12.
38. Arlot S, Celisse A. A survey of cross-validation procedures for model selection. Stat Surv. 2010;4:40–79.
39. Zhang T, Tong Z. A leave-one-out cross validation bound for kernel methods with applications in learning. Lect Notes Comput Sci. 2001;2111:427–43.

40. Szegedy C, Toshev A, Erhan D. Deep neural networks for object detection. In: Burges CJC, Bottou L, Welling M, Ghahramani Z, Weinberger KQ, editors. Advances in neural information processing systems. Red Hook, NY: Curran; 2013. p. 2553–61.
41. Brosch T. Efficient deep learning of 3D structural brain MRIs for manifold learning and lesion segmentation with application to multiple sclerosis. The University of British Columbia Library website. https://open.library.ubc.ca/collections/ubctheses/24/items/1.0305854. Published 2016. Accessed October 2016.
42. Abadi M, Agarwal A, Barham P, et al. TensorFlow: large-scale machine learning on heterogeneous distributed systems. Cornell University Library website. http://arxiv.org/abs/1603.04467. Published 2016. Accessed October 2016.
43. Srivastava N, Hinton GR, Krizhevsky A, Sutskever I, Salakhutdinov R. Dropout: a simple way to prevent neural networks from overfitting. J Mach Learn Res. 2014;15(7):1929–58.
44. Erickson BJ, Korfiatis P, Akkus Z, Kline TL. Machine learning for medical imaging. RadioGraphics. 2017;37:505–15. [PubMed: 28212054]
45. Yosinski J, Clune J, Bengio Y, Lipson H. How transferable are features in deep neural networks? In: Advances in neural information processing systems. 2014. p. 3320–8.
46. Sharif Razavian A, Azizpour H, Sullivan J, Carlsson S. CNN features off-the-shelf: an astounding baseline for recognition. In: Proceedings of the IEEE Computer Society conference on computer vision and pattern recognition. 2014. p. 806–13.
47. Ahmed KB, Hall LO, Goldgof DB, Liu R, Gatenby RA. Fine-tuning convolutional deep features for MRI based brain tumor classification. In: Proceedings of the medical imaging 2017: computer-aided diagnosis, Orlando, FL, USA. 2017. p. 101342E.
48. Esteva A, Kuprel B, Novoa R, Ko J, et al. Dermatologist-level classification of skin cancer with deep neural networks. Nature. 2017;542(7639):115–8. www.nature.com.
49. Paul R, et al. Deep feature transfer learning in combination with traditional features predicts survival among patients with lung adenocarcinoma. Tomography. 2016;2(4):388–95.
50. Wang X, Yang W, Weinreb J, et al. Searching for prostate cancer by fully automated magnetic resonance imaging classification: deep learning versus non-deep learning. Sci Rep. 2017;7:15415. [PubMed: 29133818]
51. Kumar A, Kim J, Lyndon D, Fulham M, Feng D. An ensemble of fine-tuned convolutional neural networks for medical image classification. IEEE J Biomed Heal Inform. 2017;21:31–40.
52. Zhu Z, Albadawy E, Saha A, Zhang J, Harowicz MR, Mazurowski MA. Deep learning for identifying radiogenomic associations in breast cancer. Comput Biol Med. 2019;109:85–90.
53. Ortiz A, Munilla J, Martínez-Murcia FJ, Górriz JM, Ramírez J. Learning longitudinal MRI patterns by SICE and deep learning: assessing the Alzheimer's disease progression. Commun Comput Inf Sci. 2017;723:413–24.
54. Yoo Y, Tang LYW, Brosch T, et al. Deep learning of joint myelin and T1w MRI features in normal-appearing brain tissue to distinguish between multiple sclerosis patients and healthy controls. NeuroImage Clin. 2018;17:169–78. [PubMed: 29071211]
55. Akkus Z, Ali I, Sedlář J, et al. Predicting deletion of chromosomal arms 1p/19q in low-grade gliomas from MR images using machine intelligence. J Digit Imaging. 2017;30:469–76. [PubMed: 28600641]
56. Li Z, Wang Y, Yu J, Guo Y, Cao W. Deep Learning based Radiomics (DLR) and its usage in noninvasive IDH1 prediction for low grade glioma. Sci Rep. 2017;7:5467. [PubMed: 28710497]
57. Havaei M, Davy A, Warde-Farley D, et al. Brain tumor segmentation with deep neural networks. Med Image Anal. 2017;35:18–31. [PubMed: 27310171]
58. Milletari F, Ahmadi S-A, Kroll C, et al. Hough-CNN: deep learning for segmentation of deep brain regions in MRI and ultrasound. Comput Vis Image Underst. 2017;164:92–102.
59. Hussain S, Anwar SM, Majid M. Brain tumor segmentation using cascaded deep convolutional neural network. In: 39th annual international conference of the IEEE Engineering in Medicine and Biology Society (EMBC). 2017:1998–2001. Mazurowski et al. Page 17 J Magn Reson Imaging. Author manuscript available in PMC 1 Apr 2020.
60. Valverde S, Cabezas M, Roura E, et al. Improving automated multiple sclerosis lesion segmentation with a cascaded 3D convolutional neural network approach. Neuroimage. 2017;155:159–68. [PubMed: 28435096]
61. Wachinger C, Reuter M, Klein T. DeepNAT: deep convolutional neural network for segmenting neuroanatomy. Neuroimage. 2017;170:434–45.
62. Trebeschi S, van Griethuysen JJM, Lambregts DMJ, et al. Deep learning for fully automated localization and segmentation of rectal cancer on multiparametric MR. Sci Rep. 2017;7:5301. [PubMed: 28706185]
63. Long J, Shelhamer E, Darrell T. Fully convolutional networks for semantic segmentation. In: Proceedings of the IEEE Computer Society conference on computer vision and pattern recognition. 2015. p. 3431–40.
64. Poudel RPK, Lamata P, Montana G. Recurrent fully convolutional neural networks for multi-slice MRI cardiac segmentation. In: International workshops on reconstruction and analysis of moving body organs. 2016. p. 83–94.
65. Cai J, Lu L, Xie Y, Xing F, Yang L. Improving deep pancreas segmentation in CT and MRI images via recurrent neural contextual learning and direct loss function. In: MICCAI. 2017.

66. Hochreiter S, Schmidhuber J. Long short-term memory. Neural Comput. 1997;9:1735–80. [PubMed: 9377276]
67. Jaccard P. The distribution of the flora in the alpine zone. New Phytol. 1912;11:37–50. Mazurowski et al. Page 18 J Magn Reson Imaging. Author manuscript; available in PMC 1 Apr 2020.
68. Avendi MR, Kheradvar A, Jafarkhani H. A combined deep-learning and deformable-model approach to fully automatic segmentation of the left ventricle in cardiac MRI. Med Image Anal. 2016;30:108–19. [PubMed: 26917105]
69. Rey D, Subsol G, Delingette H, Ayache N. Automatic detection and segmentation of evolving processes in 3D medical images: application to multiple sclerosis. Med Image Anal. 2002;6:163–79. [PubMed: 12045002]
70. Roth HR, Lu L, Seff A, et al. A new 2.5 D representation for lymph node detection using random sets of deep convolutional neural network observations. In: International conference on medical image computing and computer-assisted intervention. 2014. p. 520–7.
71. Dou Q, Chen H, Yu L, et al. Automatic detection of cerebral microbleeds from MR images via 3D convolutional neural networks. IEEE Trans Med Imaging. 2016;35:1182–95. [PubMed: 26886975]
72. Shin H-C, Roth HR, Gao M, et al. Deep convolutional neural networks for computer-aided detection: CNN architectures, dataset characteristics and transfer learning. IEEE Trans Med Imaging. 2016;35:1285–98. [PubMed: 26886976]
73. Tajbakhsh N, Shin JY, Gurudu SR, et al. Convolutional neural networks for medical image analysis: full training or fine tuning? IEEE Trans Med Imaging 2016;35:1299–312. [PubMed: 26978662]. Mazurowski et al. Page 16 J Magn Reson Imaging. Author manuscript; available in PMC 1 Apr 2020.
74. Sa R, Owens W, Wiegand R, et al. Intervertebral disc detection in X-ray images using faster RCNN. In: 2017 39th annual international conference of the IEEE Engineering in Medicine and Biology Society (EMBC). 2017. p. 564–7.
75. Liu J, Wang D, Lu L, et al. Detection and diagnosis of colitis on computed tomography using deep convolutional neural networks. Med Phys. 2017;44(9):4630–42.
76. Redmon J, Divvala S, Girshick R, Farhadi A. You only look once: unified, real-time object detection. In: Proceedings of the IEEE Computer Society conference on computer vision and pattern recognition. 2016. p. 779–88.
77. Cao Z, Duan L, Yang G, et al. Breast tumor detection in ultrasound images using deep learning. In: International workshop on patch-based techniques in medical imaging. 2017. p. 121–8.
78. de Vos BD, Wolterink JM, de Jong PA, Viergever MA, Isgum I. 2D image classification for 3D anatomy localization: employing deep convolutional neural networks. In: Medical imaging: image processing. 2016. p. 97841Y.
79. Prasoon A, Petersen K, Igel C, Lauze F, Dam E, Nielsen M. Deep feature learning for knee cartilage segmentation using a triplanar convolutional neural network. In: International conference on medical image computing and computer-assisted intervention. 2013. p. 246–53.
80. Roth HR, Lu L, Liu J, et al. Improving computer-aided detection using convolutional neural networks and random view aggregation. IEEE Trans Med Imaging. 2016;35:1170–81. [PubMed: 26441412]
81. Roth HR, Wang Y, Yao J, Lu L, Burns JE, Summers RM. Deep convolutional networks for automated detection of posterior element fractures on spine CT. In: Medical imaging 2016: computer-aided diagnosis—proceedings of SPIE. Bellingham, WA: SPIE; 2016.
82. Li N, Liu H, Qiu B, et al. Detection and attention: diagnosing pulmonary lung cancer from CT by imitating physicians. arXivPrepr arXiv171205114. 2017.
83. Simonovsky M, Gutiérrez-Becker B, Mateus D, Navab N, Komodakis N. A deep metric for multimodal registration. In: International conference on medical image computing and computer-assisted intervention. Springer; 2016. p. 10–8. Mazurowski et al. Page 19 J Magn Reson Imaging. Author manuscript; available in PMC 1 April 2020.
84. Maes F, Collignon A, Vandermeulen D, Marchal G, Suetens P. Multimodality image registration by maximization of mutual information. IEEE Trans Med Imaging. 1997;16
85. Bahrami K, Shi F, Zong X, Shin HW, An H, Shen D. Reconstruction of 7T-Like Images from 3T MRI. IEEE Trans Med Imaging. 2016;35:2085–97. [PubMed: 27046894]
86. Schlemper J, Caballero J, Hajnal JV, Price A, Rueckert D. A deep cascade of convolutional neural networks for dynamic MR image reconstruction. IEEE Trans Med Imaging. 2018;37(2):491–503.
87. Chen H, Zhang Y, Zhang W, et al. Low-dose CT via convolutional neural network. Biomed Opt Express. 2017;8:679–94. [PubMed: 28270976]
88. Kang E, Min J, Ye JC. A deep convolutional neural network using directional wavelets for low-dose X-ray CT reconstruction. Med Phys. 2017;44:e360–75. [PubMed: 29027238]
89. Nie D, Cao X, Gao Y, Wang L, Shen D. Estimating CT image from MRI data using 3D fully convolutional networks BT. In: Carneiro G, Mateus D, Peter L, et al., editors. Deep learning and data labeling for medical applications: first international workshop, LABELS 2016, and second international workshop, DLMIA 2016, held in conjunction with MICC. Cham: Springer; 2016. p. 170–8.
90. Han X. MR-based synthetic CT generation using a deep convolutional neural network method. Med Phys. 2017;44:1408–19. [PubMed: 28192624]

91. Li R, Zhang W, Suk H-I, et al. Deep learning based imaging data completion for improved brain disease diagnosis. Med Image Comput Comput Assist Interv. 2014;17(03):305–12. [PubMed: 25320813]
92. Jiang D, Dou W, Vosters L, Xu X, Sun Y, Tan T. Denoising of 3D magnetic resonance images with multi-channel residual learning of convolutional neural network. Jpn J Radiol. 2018;36(9):566–74.
93. Qayyum A, Anwar SM, Awais M, Majid M. Medical image retrieval using deep convolutional neural network. Neurocomputing. 2017;266:8–20.
94. Chow LS, Paramesran R. Review of medical image quality assessment. Biomed Signal Process Control. 2016;27:145–54.
95. Wu L, Cheng J-Z, Li S, Lei B, Wang T, Ni D. FUIQA: Fetal ultrasound image quality assessment with deep convolutional networks. IEEE Trans Cybern. 2017;45:1336–49.
96. Buda M, Maki A, Mazurowski MA. A systematic study of the class imbalance problem in convolutional neural networks. Neural Netw. 2018;106:249–59.
97. OECD. Computed tomography (CT) exams. 2018. https://doi.org/10.1787/3c994537-en.
98. OECD. Magnetic resonance imaging (MRI) exams. 2018. https://doi.org/10.1787/1d89353f-en.
99. Kamnitsas K, et al. Information processing in medical imaging. Cham: Springer; 2017. p. 597–609.
100. Gilad-Bachrach R, et al. CryptoNets: applying neural networks to encrypted data with high throughput and accuracy. In: Proceedings of the 33rd international conference on machine learning, New York, NY; 2016. p. 201–10.

Molecular Imaging and Radiomics 25

Key Points (Abstract)

Radiomics is a defined as the multidisciplinary field, which is the combination of technology, comprising of data acquisition, feature selection, model building, and analysis, thus having the capability to convert the routine clinical images into mineable data, a very high fidelity, and high throughput. With the significant research in this fields, it has become an important component especially in the imaging and also clinical oncology where more precise diagnosis, evaluation, and management plans can be tailor made with more perfection thus reducing the morbidity and mortality. Again, here it is the amalgamation of the various biomarkers, various genetic indices, as well as the multiple newly developed biochemical and also image-based signatures which are put together for the better diagnosis and prognosis of various human diseases.

Keywords

Radiomics · Radiogenomics · PET · MRI · Cancer · Radiotherapy · Biomarkers

25.1 Introduction

25.1.1 Definition

The term "radiomics" was first mentioned by Gillies et al. [1] in 2010 while formulating the process of extraction of various quantitative features from images. In 2012, Lambin et al. [2] gave the definition of "radiomics" for the first time as analysing medical image data quantitatively by extracting high-throughput quantitative features from medical images and further transforming these images into the very high-resolution and deep-going mineable automatic or semi-automatic software. Later, Kumar et al. [3] further expanded the definition of radiomics for the extraction and analysis of the quantitative medical images from various modalities like computed tomography (CT), positron emission tomography (PET), or MRI with high throughput.

25.2 Process of Radiomics

Radiomics is now a newer concept of the multidisciplinary technology, which involves the various aspects of the data acquisition, feature selection, model building, and analysis. These are capable of converting the basic images into mineable data, which is having very high fidelity and high throughput.

The important steps involved in the process of radiomics are as follows:

1. High-quality imaging data sets are acquired and reconstructed.
2. The image data sets need to have the region of interest (ROI) or the volume of interest (VOI)

S. Shaikh, *Advances in Imaging*, https://doi.org/10.1007/978-981-16-9535-3_25

segmentation which can be done manually or by planning with the computer.
3. Extraction and quantification is having very high throughput.
4. Various clinical models can be selected, and based on this, the various clinical models can be made.
5. After this is the proper validation of the shared databases [2–4].

Imaging is an important component for the diagnosis and staging of various pathologies, one of the main pillars of cancer care, and this can also be used for the various treatment planning evaluation and for the assessment of the therapeutic response. This extraction of the clinical images can be used as an important information for the evaluation of the tumor which will be more useful for the diagnosis and prognosis of the cancer. These data can be also linked to the genomic data, forming the basis of the radiogenomics. With this concept, it will be helpful for the more specific prediction of accuracy of various clinical outcomes.

Imaging is the main component of the clinical oncology, which is playing an important role for the diagnosis, staging, radiation treatment planning, therapeutic response evaluation, follow-up, and monitoring of the disease [5–8]. Our routine images are based on our visual assessment. The precision medicine concept has led to the various newer modalities which are playing an important role in characterization, treatment response assessment, and further the overall prognosis of the patient. Radiomics is now an established imaging modality which is based on the newer biomarkers and various features of the tumor heterogeneity [9–13]. All our routine imaging modalities CT, MRI, or PET can be applied for the radiomics for the diagnosis, evaluation of treatment response, and finally prediction of the prognosis of the disease. However, these modalities are having issues related with the reconstruction, resolution, and sometimes artefacts due to various reasons that lie on patient movement, etc. To prevent these, the development of radiomics is present which can be done using the various statistical or bioinformatics tools, to develop the various models which are very sensitive for the prediction and accuracy of clinical outcomes. Afterwards, the imaging findings in these modalities are being validated by the experts in the field of the imaging and then based on the regions of interest (ROIs). Then processing of these which are the quantitative parameters of the imaging after the extraction of the data matrix also and all clinical data which is integrated into a particular model for the patient with study. Then again, this needs to be validated for accuracy before applying and using on the patient. Radiogenomics uses the concept of the radiomic features at the tissue level with genomic, transcriptomic, or proteomic typing [14–21]; this will be more useful for the characterization of the biological basis phenotypes. Here the various concepts of the radiomic imaging will be using the signature for significant diagnostic, prognostic, or predictive advantage over the pre-existing imaging modalities in cancer.

Thus, radiomics is having the significant impact on the radiology and oncology [22–25]. Regions of interest (ROIs) are marked on the images having the heterogenicity and can give more precise information for the overall management of the cancers [9, 26, 27]. Here the radiomics uses various biomarkers, genetic, and biochemical parameters having the heterogeneity where the various signatures of images are developed for the better diagnosis and prognosis [28, 29]. Computed tomography (CT), positron emission tomography (PET), and magnetic resonance imaging (MRI) are the most used imaging modalities for the evaluation of the cancers. Manual or automatic segmentation of the images is developed in the regions of interest (ROIs). The various data matrix and various clinical indicators are used for more accurate outcome [30–32]. Radiomics will cause the acquisition of image information like the traditional CADs [4]. Severity of the tumour, progression of the tumour, or recurrence is easily quantified by radiomics [33–36]. Radiomics are very important for the prediction of lymphatic metastasis from colorectal cancer [37], nasopharyngeal carcinoma [38], lung cancer therapeutic response [39], and evaluation of gene expressions [40, 41].

25.3 Workflow and Functioning of the Radiomics

Radiomics involves the image acquisition, tumor segmentation, extraction of the information, predictive modelling, and final model validation. The routine imaging modalities CT, MRI, and FDG-PET are the well-established modalities for the analysis of the anatomical or physiological information in each patient [42]. The basis of the image formation and analysis is the contrast difference between normal and abnormal tissue. Image acquisition then tumor segmentation entire tumour or the region of the interest. Posttreatment analysis which includes post-radiotherapy changes as well as the evaluation of the residual tumour can be done for radiomics analysis. With the development of artificial intelligence, the newer deep learning-based tools are used for radiomics applications. The two radiomics tools used for the data acquisition of different tumour phenotypes are semantic and agnostic which are based on the American College of Radiology; thus, lexicon is used to describe tumours. Agnostic features will define the tumor shape and the intratumoral heterogeneity [11, 43].

25.4 Predictive Modelling

Artificial intelligence can define various biological/genomic traits which can have large number of the features and small sample number [44]. This will have more precise information and will show the minimal changes to tumor contour and variations. By these, different algorithms can be developed for a particular disease or group of disease [17, 18].

25.5 Model Validation

These various radiomic signatures have to be validated on various external cohorts, that is, independent and multiple, based on the characteristics. The concept of the prospective validation is used for the fast assessment of various models. These signatures have to be validated and tested based on the clinical data or available datasets [45]. These will have signatures from clinical and pathologic factors, and both can be combined for a multivariate model. By the use of these signatures, the patient management, quality score, and ultimate practical implementation of the radiomics can be done. The various acquisition protocols, image pre-processing, image extraction, and statistical modelling are important for the future (Diagram 25.1).

25.6 Current Status and Future Prospectives

Various studies are being used to validate the radiomics pattern

One of the studies by Aerts and colleagues showed the use of the radiomic signature for predicting survival rate in the patients who are having lung cancer and underwent radiotherapy [46]. They studied different 400 features of CT images to analyse the tumor intensity, shape, and texture. Radiomic signature is an important tool to define the various intra-tumour heterogeneity, and MRI in glioblastoma will define the response to the treatment [47]. Wu et al. used the radiomic features by use of the FDG-PET and CT for distant metastasis in early-stage non-small cell lung cancer (NSCLC) the role of the stereotactic ablative radiotherapy (SABR) [48]. Based on these structures, the tumor morphology and intratumoral metabolic activity will create the radiomic signature, which will be used for the significant increased prognostic value in comparison to the conventional imaging. El Naqa and colleagues also studied FDG-PET/CT radiomics with associated clinical information for the evaluation of the locoregional nodes, tumour recurrences, and distant metastases in head and neck cancer [49].

25.7 Emerging Paradigms of Radiomics for Precision Radiotherapy

The newer concept of habitat imaging is the acquisition of the heterogeneity more commonly seen at the local level [12, 50]. Cao and colleagues showed dynamic contrast-enhanced (DCE) MR

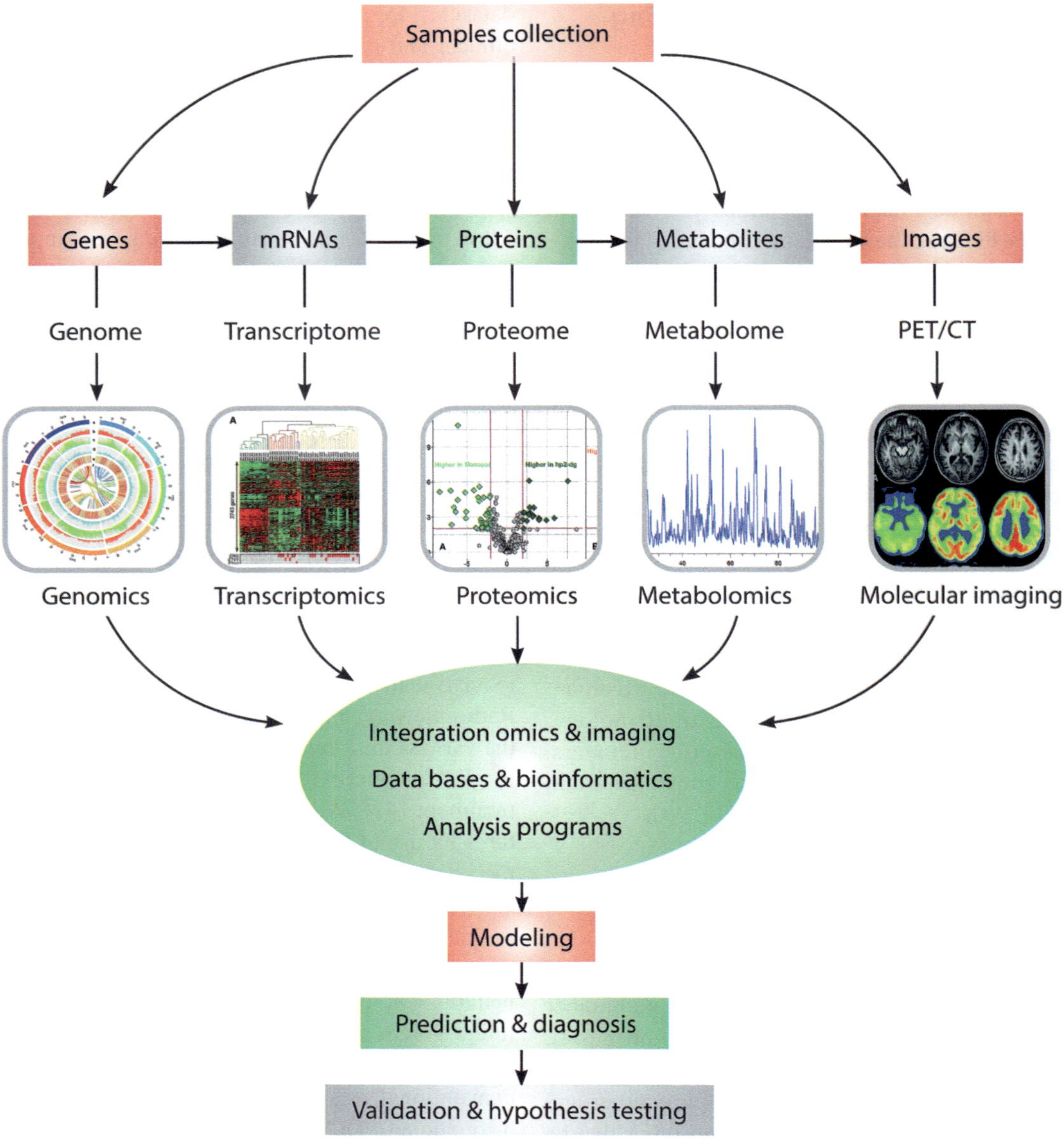

Diagram 25.1 Different models and algorithms for the radiomics

imaging more precise in the head and neck cancer [51]. The perfusion characteristics will be showing the response to the primary tumor at baseline and during the early course of chemoradiotherapy. This is based on the metabolically active heterogeneous lesions preferably the solid component of the tumor, which is always more variable. This will help in the evaluation of the distant metastasis and prognosticate the overall survival in patients with NSCLC. Hence, we have seen the significant growth in the radiomics which has significantly changed the way the diagnosis and staging of the various tumours, the tumor classification, treatment outcome, survival rates of the patients, and also the other clinical aspects of various diseases. Thus, radiomics will be the most important support for more precise results for every aspect of the disease.

25.8 Radio Genomics: Integrating Imaging with Genomics

Radiogenomics uses the imaging and genomic data for better biological interpretation for precision medicine [14–19, 52–56]. Two radiogenomic-related studies are present; CT semantic and radiomic image features are associated with the EGFR mutations in lung cancer [57, 58]; radiogenomics is also based on molecular features rather than different imaging phenotypes for different tumours. The best example is the higher maximum standardized uptake value from FDG-PET scan which is usually associated with the related pathological variants like epithelial–mesenchymal non-small cell lung cancer [59]. The role of radiogenomics is to classify tumours in various subtypes depending on the imaging phenotypes rather than molecular features. Wu et al. [18] evaluated and validated the three breast cancer imaging subtypes, based on the intratumoral enhancement pattern, more or less parenchymal enhancement.

Precision medicine is an important approach as it can acquire the imaging and molecular data simultaneously for better accuracy and outcome. Cottereau et al. [60] analysed the molecular profile and the associated metabolic tumor volume at FDG-PET imaging; this showed the significantly increased survival in diffuse large B-cell lymphoma. Studies of Grossmann et al. [61] show that the image-based biomarkers provide more valuable information for tumour assessment.

Genomics and medical imaging modalities and the various techniques are more specific [62]. Different tumours like brain, lung, or liver [62, 63] possess different features. Prostate carcinoma is known to be related to phosphatase and tensin homolog (PTEN), which has more aggressiveness and mortality.

25.9 Conclusion

Radiomics has become the very important tool especially in clinical oncology, which is used for the characterization, prognosis, treatment prediction, and assessment of the treatment response. However, a lot of the research in relation to the various developments in radiomics, the current practising trends, and future developments are not still validated due to the scarcity of the various aspects. Still, a lot of advancements have to be done to see the potential value of radiomics to be used for the best possible extent. This will further propagate the concept of the precision medicine further leading to the personalized medicine.

References

1. Gillies RJ, Anderson AR, Gatenby RA, Morse DL. The biology underlying molecular imaging in oncology: from genome to anatome and back again. Clin Radiol. 2010;65(7):517–21. https://doi.org/10.1016/j.crad.2010.04.005.
2. Lambin P, Rios-Velazquez E, Leijenaar R, Carvalho S, van Stiphout RG, Granton P, et al. Radiomics: extracting more information from medical images using advanced feature analysis. Eur J Cancer (Oxf Engl 1990). 2012;48(4):441–6. https://doi.org/10.1016/j.ejca.2011.11.036.
3. Kumar V, Gu Y, Basu S, Berglund A, Eschrich SA, Schabath MB, et al. Radiomics: the process and the challenges. Magn Reson Imaging. 2012;30(9):1234–48. https://doi.org/10.1016/j.mri.2012.06.010.
4. Gillies RJ, Kinahan PE, Hricak H. Radiomics: images are more than pictures, they are data. Radiology. 2016;278(2):563–77. https://doi.org/10.1148/radiol.2015151169.
5. O'Connor JP, Aboagye EO, Adams JE, et al. Imaging biomarker roadmap for cancer studies. Nat Rev Clin Oncol. 2017;14:169–86.
6. Yankeelov TE, Mankoff DA, Schwartz LH, et al. Quantitative imaging in cancer clinical trials. Clin Cancer Res. 2016;22:284–90.
7. Weissleder R, Schwaiger MC, Gambhir SS, et al. Imaging approaches to optimize molecular therapies. Sci Transl Med. 2016;8:355ps16.
8. O'Connor JPB. Cancer heterogeneity and imaging. Semin Cell Dev Biol. 2017;64:48–57.
9. Aerts HJ. The potential of radiomic-based phenotyping in precision medicine: a review. JAMA Oncol. 2016;2(12):1636–42.
10. Sala E, Mema E, Himoto Y, et al. Unravelling tumour heterogeneity using next-generation imaging: radiomics, radiogenomics, and habitat imaging. Clin Radiol. 2017;72:3–10. Radiomics and radiogenomics • i29 Downloaded from https://academic.oup.com/jrr/article/59/suppl_1/i25/4827067 by guest on 19 Mar 2021.

11. Lambin P, Leijenaar RT, Deist TM, et al. Radiomics: the bridge between medical imaging and personalized medicine. Nat Rev Clin Oncol. 2017;14:749–62.
12. Gillies RJ, Kinahan PE, Hricak H. Radiomics: images are more than pictures, they are data. Radiology. 2015;278:563–77.
13. Limkin E, Sun R, Dercle L, et al. Promises and challenges for the implementation of computational medical imaging (radiomics) in oncology. Ann Oncol. 2017;28:1191–206.
14. Diehn M, Nardini C, Wang DS, et al. Identification of noninvasive imaging surrogates for brain tumor gene-expression modules. Proc Natl Acad Sci U S A. 2008;105:5213–8.
15. Gevaert O, Xu JJ, Hoang CD, et al. Non-small cell lung cancer: identifying prognostic imaging biomarkers by leveraging public gene expression microarray data-methods and preliminary results. Radiology. 2012;264:387–96.
16. Segal E, Sirlin CB, Ooi C, et al. Decoding global gene expression programs in liver cancer by noninvasive imaging. Nat Biotechnol. 2007;25:675–80.
17. Itakura H, Achrol AS, Mitchell LA, et al. Magnetic resonance image features identify glioblastoma phenotypic subtypes with distinct molecular pathway activities. Sci Transl Med. 2015;7:303ra138.
18. Wu J, Cui Y, Sun X, et al. Unsupervised clustering of quantitative image phenotypes reveals breast cancer subtypes with distinct prognoses and molecular pathways. Clin Cancer Res. 2017;23:3334–42.
19. Wu J, Li B, Sun X, et al. Heterogeneous enhancement patterns of tumor-adjacent parenchyma at MR imaging are associated with dysregulated signaling pathways and poor survival in breast cancer. Radiology. 2017;285:401–13.
20. Colen R, Foster I, Gatenby R, et al. NCI workshop report: clinical and computational requirements for correlating imaging phenotypes with genomics signatures. Transl Oncol. 2014;7:556–69.
21. Fehr D, Veeraraghavan H, Wibmer A, et al. Automatic classification of prostate cancer Gleason scores from multiparametric magnetic resonance images. Proc Natl Acad Sci U S A. 2015;112:E6265–73.
22. Wang K, Lu X, Zhou H, Gao Y, Zheng J, Tong M, Wu C, Liu C, Huang L, Jiang T, Meng F, Lu Y, Ai H, Xie XY, Yin LP, Liang P, Tian J, Zheng R. Deep learning Radiomics of shear wave elastography significantly improved diagnostic performance for assessing liver fibrosis in chronic hepatitis B: a prospective multicentre study. Gut. 2019;68(4):729–41.
23. Liu Z, Zhang XY, Shi YJ, Wang L, Zhu HT, Tang Z, Wang S, Li XT, Tian J, Sun YS. Radiomics analysis for evaluation of pathological complete response to neoadjuvant chemoradiotherapy in locally advanced rectal cancer. Clin Cancer Res. 2017;23(23):7253–62.
24. Huang Y, Liu Z, He L, Chen X, Pan D, Ma Z, Liang C, Tian J, Liang C. Radiomics signature: a potential biomarker for the prediction of disease-free survival in early-stage (I or II) non-small cell lung cancer. Radiology. 2016;281(3):947–57.
25. Aerts HJ, Velazquez ER, Leijenaar RT, Parmar C, Grossmann P, Carvalho S, Bussink J, Monshouwer R, Haibe-Kains B, Rietveld D, Hoebers F, et al. Decoding tumour phenotype by noninvasive imaging using a quantitative radiomics approach. Nat Commun. 2014;5:4006.
26. Lambin P, Leijenaar RTH, Deist TM, Peerlings J, de Jong EEC, van Timmeren J, Sanduleanu S, Larue R, Even AJG, Jochems A, van Wijk Y, Woodruff H, van Soest J, Lustberg T, Roelofs E, van Elmpt W, Dekker A, Mottaghy FM, Wildberger JE, Walsh S. Radiomics: the bridge between medical imaging and personalized medicine. Nat Rev Clin Oncol. 2017;14(12):749–62.
27. Gerlinger M, Rowan AJ, Horswell S, Math M, Larkin J, Endesfelder D, Gronroos E, Martinez P, Matthews N, Stewart A, Tarpey P, Varela I, Phillimore B, Begum S, McDonald NQ, Butler A, Jones D, Raine K, Latimer C, Santos CR, Nohadani M, Eklund AC, Spencer-Dene B, Clark G, Pickering L, Stamp G, Gore M, Szallasi Z, Downward J, Futreal PA, Swanton C. Intratumor heterogeneity and branched evolution revealed by multiregional sequencing. N Engl J Med. 2012;366(10):883–92.
28. Itakura H, Achrol AS, Mitchell LA, Loya JJ, Liu T, Westbroek EM, Feroze AH, Rodriguez S, Echegaray S, Azad TD, Yeom KW, Napel S, Rubin DL, Chang SD, Harsh GRT, Gevaert O. Magnetic resonance image features identify glioblastoma phenotypic subtypes with distinct molecular pathway activities. Sci Transl Med. 2015;7(303):303ra138.
29. Gevaert O, Mitchell LA, Achrol AS, Xu J, Echegaray S, Steinberg GK, Cheshier SH, Napel S, Zaharchuk G, Plevritis SK. Glioblastoma multiforme: exploratory radiogenomic analysis by using quantitative image features. Radiology. 2014;273(1):168–74.
30. Aerts H. Data science in radiology: a path forward. Clin Cancer Res. 2018;24(3):532–4.
31. Lambin P, Rios-Velazquez E, Leijenaar R, Carvalho S, van Stiphout RG, Granton P, Zegers CM, Gillies R, Boellard R, Dekker A, Aerts HJ. Radiomics: extracting more information from medical images using advanced feature analysis. Eur J Cancer. 2012;48(4):441–6.
32. Kumar V, Gu Y, Basu S, Berglund A, Eschrich SA, Schabath MB, Forster K, Aerts HJ, Dekker A, Fenstermacher D, Goldgof DB, Hall LO, Lambin P, Balagurunathan Y, Gatenby RA, Gillies RJ. Radiomics: the process and the challenges. Magn Reson Imaging. 2012;30(9):1234–48.
33. Li Q, Kim J, Balagurunathan Y, Liu Y, Latifi K, Stringfield O, Garcia A, Moros EG, Dilling TJ, Schabath MB, Ye Z, Gillies RJ. Imaging features from pretreatment CT scans are associated with clinical outcomes in nonsmall-cell lung cancer patients treated with stereotactic body radiotherapy. Med Phys. 2017;44(8):4341–9.

34. Li H, Zhu Y, Burnside ES, Drukker K, Hoadley KA, Fan C, Conzen SD, Whitman GJ, Sutton EJ, Net JM, Ganott M, Huang E, Morris EA, Perou CM, Ji Y, Giger ML. MR imaging radiomics signatures for predicting the risk of breast cancer recurrence as given by research versions of MammaPrint, Oncotype DX, and PAM50 Gene Assays. Radiology. 2016;281(2):382–91.
35. Song J, Shi J, Dong D, Fang M, Zhong W, Wang K, Wu N, Huang Y, Liu Z, Cheng Y, Gan Y, Zhou Y, Zhou P, Chen B, Liang C, Liu Z, Li W, Tian J. A new approach to predict progression-free survival in stage IV EGFR-mutant NSCLC patients with EGFR-TKI therapy. Clin Cancer Res. 2018;24(15):3583–92.
36. van Griethuysen JJM, Fedorov A, Parmar C, Hosny A, Aucoin N, Narayan V, Beets-Tan RGH, Fillion-Robin JC, Pieper S, Aerts H. Computational radiomics system to decode the radiographic phenotype. Cancer Res. 2017;77(21):e104–7.
37. Huang YQ, Liang CH, He L, Tian J, Liang CS, Chen X, Ma ZL, Liu ZY. Development and validation of a radiomics nomogram for preoperative prediction of lymph node metastasis in colorectal cancer. J Clin Oncol. 2016;34(18):2157–64.
38. Zhang B, Tian J, Dong D, Gu D, Dong Y, Zhang L, Lian Z, Liu J, Luo X, Pei S, Mo X, Huang W, Ouyang F, Guo B, Liang L, Chen W, Liang C, Zhang S. Radiomics features of multiparametric MRI as novel prognostic factors in advanced nasopharyngeal carcinoma. Clin Cancer Res. 2017;23(15):4259–69.
39. Song J, Liu Z, Zhong W, Huang Y, Ma Z, Dong D, Liang C, Tian J. Non-small cell lung cancer: quantitative phenotypic analysis of CT images as a potential marker of prognosis. Sci Rep. 2016;6:38282.
40. Zhou M, Leung A, Echegaray S, Gentles A, Shrager JB, Jensen KC, Berry GJ, Plevritis SK, Rubin DL, Napel S, Gevaert O. Non-small cell lung cancer radio genomics map identifies relationships between molecular and imaging phenotypes with prognostic implications. Radiology. 2018;286(1):307–15.
41. Gevaert O, Xu J, Hoang CD, Leung AN, Xu Y, Quon A, Rubin DL, Napel S, Plevritis SK. Non-small cell lung cancer: identifying prognostic imaging biomarkers by leveraging public gene expression microarray data–methods and preliminary results. Radiology. 2012;264(2):387–96.
42. Timmerman R, Xing L. Image guided and adaptive radiation therapy. Baltimore: Lippincott Williams & Wilkins; 2009.
43. Larue RT, Defraene G, De Ruysscher D, et al. Quantitative radiomics studies for tissue characterization: a review of technology and methodological procedures. Br J Radiol. 2017;90:20160665.
44. Chandrashekar G, Sahin F. A survey on feature selection methods. Comput Electr Eng. 2014;40:16–28.
45. Subramanian J, Simon R. What should physicians look for in evaluating prognostic gene-expression signatures? Nat Rev Clin Oncol. 2010;7:327–34.
46. Aerts HJ, Velazquez ER, Leijenaar RT, et al. Decoding tumour phenotype by non-invasive imaging using a quantitative radiomics approach. Nat Commun. 2014;5:4006.
47. Grossmann P, Narayan V, Chang K, et al. Quantitative imaging biomarkers for risk stratification of patients with recurrent glioblastoma treated with bevacizumab. Neuro Oncol. 2017;19:1688–97.
48. Wu J, Aguilera T, Shultz D, et al. Early-stage non-small cell lung cancer: quantitative imaging characteristics of 18F fluorodeoxyglucose PET/CT allow prediction of distant metastasis. Radiology. 2016;281:270–8.
49. Vallieres M, Kay-Rivest E, Perrin LJ, et al. Radiomics strategies for risk assessment of tumour failure in head-and-neck cancer. Sci Rep. 2017;7:10117.
50. Gatenby RA, Grove O, Gillies RJ. Quantitative imaging in cancer evolution and ecology. Radiology. 2013;269:8–15.
51. Wang P, Popovtzer A, Eisbruch A, et al. An approach to identify, from DCE MRI, significant sub volumes of tumours related to outcomes in advanced head-and-neck cancer. Med Phys. 2012;39:5277–85.
52. Bakas S, Akbari H, Pisapia J, et al. In vivo detection of EGFRvIII in glioblastoma via perfusion magnetic resonance imaging signature consistent with deep peritumoral infiltration: the φ index. Clin Cancer Res. 2017;23:4724–34.
53. Smits M, van den Bent MJ. Imaging correlates of adult glioma genotypes. Radiology. 2017;284:316–31.
54. Vargas HA, Huang EP, Lakhman Y, et al. Radio genomics of high-grade serous ovarian cancer: multileader multi-institutional study from the Cancer Genome Atlas Ovarian Cancer Imaging Research Group. Radiology. 2017;285:482–92.
55. Lee J, Cui Y, Sun X, et al. Prognostic value and molecular correlates of a CT image-based quantitative pleural contact index in early-stage NSCLC. Eur Radiol. 2018;28:736–46.
56. Zhu Y, Li H, Guo W, et al. Deciphering genomic underpinnings of quantitative MRI-based radiomic phenotypes of invasive breast carcinoma. Sci Rep. 2015;5:17787.
57. Liu Y, Kim J, Balagurunathan Y, et al. Radiomic features are associated with EGFR mutation status in lung adenocarcinomas. Clin Lung Cancer. 2016;17:441–8.e6.
58. Rios Velazquez E, Parmar C, Liu Y, et al. Somatic mutations drive distinct imaging phenotypes in lung cancer. Cancer Res. 2017;77:3922–30.
59. Yamamoto S, Huang D, Du L, et al. Radio genomic analysis demonstrates associations between 18F-fluoro-2-deoxyglucose PET, prognosis, and epithelial-mesenchymal transition in nonsmall cell lung cancer. Radiology. 2016;280:261–70.
60. Cottereau AS, Lanic H, Mareschal S, et al. Molecular profile and FDG-PET/CT total metabolic tumor volume improve risk classification at diagnosis for

patients with diffuse large B-cell lymphoma. Clin Cancer Res. 2016;22:3801–9.
61. Grossmann P, Stringfield O, El-Hachem N, et al. Defining the biological basis of radiomic phenotypes in lung cancer. Elife. 2017;6:e23421.
62. Bodalal Z, Trebeschi S, Nguyen-Kim TDL, Schats W, BeetsTan R. Radio genomics: bridging imaging and genomics. Abdom Radiol (New York). 2019;44(6):1960–84. https://doi.org/10.1007/s00261-019-02028-w.
63. Pinker K, Shitano F, Sala E, Do RK, Young RJ, Wibmer AG, et al. Background, current role, and potential applications of radio genomics. J Magn Reson Imaging JMRI. 2018;47(3):604–20. https://doi.org/10.1002/jmri.25870.

Quantitative Imaging Biomarkers in Precision Medicine

26

Key Points (Abstract)

The first discovery of X-rays is 125 years ago now, and medical imaging is growing in the very fast mode in every aspect of the anatomical and molecular imaging (Kamel SI, Levin DC, Parker L, Rao VM. J Am Coll Radiol 14(3):337–342, 2017). The routine anatomical modalities are growing very fast together with this newer modality which is advanced structural and hybrid modalities which are capable of giving a more structural and functional detail (Herold CJ, Lewin JS, Wibmer AG, et al. Radiology 279(1):226–238, 2016). Thus, the newer methods along with the newer concepts of the acquisition of the image, processing of the image, archiving of the image, and also displaying the analysis are significantly changed. Many changes are happening in the various molecular levels for better, more precise, and systematic approach to the diagnosis and treatment of the diseases.

Keywords

Quantitative imaging · CT · MRI · Biomarkers · QIBA · RSNA · COPD · Alzheimer's disease

Significant pharmaceutical and medical device developments are happening rapidly. The newer quantitative imaging techniques and biomarkers will be having significant impact. These impacts will have more sensitivity, specificity, and all the statistical parameters related in both the diagnostic and therapeutic applications. Various imaging biomarkers are being used for identification, characterization, and validation of various applications resulting in the higher image quality along with processing and detailed analysis. These various quantitative imaging biomarkers will redefine the newer concepts for better image processing and also the analysis for newer clinical applications. This will be more helpful in biomarker research of various common diseases like osteoarthritis (OA), Alzheimer's disease (AD), and cancer which is being presented and further validated for clinical use in the future.

26.1 Introduction

The definition of quantitative imaging biomarker is derived from one or more in vivo images based on the ratio or interval scale which will be an indicator for the normal biologic along with the pathogenic processes and also for therapeutic intervention [1]. Quantitative Imaging Biomarkers Alliance (QIBA) was launched in 2007 by the Radiological Society of North America. There is collaboration of the researchers, healthcare professionals, and health industry for research of this quantitative imaging which will be useful for clinical practice [2]. The Quantitative Imaging Biomarkers Alliance

S. Shaikh, *Advances in Imaging*, https://doi.org/10.1007/978-981-16-9535-3_26

(QIBA), organized by the Radiological Society of North America (RSNA), defined a QI biomarker as "an objective characteristic features of taking the information from the in vivo image and quantified as the indicator of various normal biological processes, pathogenic processes, or a response to a therapeutic intervention". These concepts of the ratio or the interval variables is applied to the various tumor volumes or PET standardized uptake values (SUVs), as they are the quantitative markers. Breast Imaging Reporting and Data System (BIRADS) assessment is one of the systems. QI research is for the biomarkers which are being evaluated by the various robust parameters like frequency distributions, medians, means, standard deviations, and standard errors of the mean [1]. The QIBA's mission as stated is "to improve the value and practicality of quantitative imaging biomarkers by reducing variability across devices, sites, patients and time" [2]. QIBA is also based on the analysis of the clinical situation and accordingly proposing different biomarkers, along with the various protocol and profile developments and then the validation, promulgation, and maintenance of the allotted profile [2]. Different proposed protocols are present for documenting the various imaging acquisition and analysis protocols. Sullivan et al. [1] metrology standards proposed for quantitative imaging are mentioned.

26.2 Various Applications

26.2.1 Cardiothoracic Applications

The role of the CT chest is very important in precision medicine having the various quantitative imaging initiatives and correlation between the anatomical regions like ischemic heart disease, lung cancer, and chronic obstructive pulmonary disease (COPD) which are causes of mortality in the USA [3]. QIBA defines the more precise accurate, reproducible, and meaningful uses of volumetric data analysis for lung lesions in chest CT. The different changes in the parenchyma and airway in the COPD patients are important biomarkers for the study of the dual-energy analysis of the CT for the lung perfusion evaluation and research. The most important clinical applications in chest CT are for the analysis of the parenchymal nodule along with the various anatomic features, being converted into the reports. The film-based archiving of the images is being done [4]. By this technique, huge data can be analysed easily by the prospective or retrospective analysis. The different aspects of the images can be done for the subjective interpretation [5]. Here the quantitative imaging can also be programmed along with the machine learning [6], by which the radiology services can be altered to the highest standards.

26.2.2 Biomarkers and the Quantitative Imaging

Biomarkers Alliance Biologic markers are also known as biomarkers, and these are defined as the measurable objective used to assess the various normal biologic or pathogenic processes [7]. These biomarkers will be useful for the diagnosis and prognosis of the information.

A quantitative imaging biomarker is defined as a characteristic which can be derived from one or more in vivo images and can be objectively measured based on the ratio or interval for the biologic processes, pathogenic processes, or response to the various therapeutic interventions. Chest CT acquisition can be done for the non-cardiac applications without electrocardiographic (ECG) gating as compared to the ECG-gated CT examinations for the coronary artery evaluation. The lung nodule size is also one of the important predictive behaviours for the quantitative analysis. The end-inspiratory images of the low attenuation areas in correlation with the coronary artery calcification can be used to quantify the scores which are greater than 400 on non-ECG-gated chest CT images, and this is the important predictive factor for the future cardiovascular events. The coronary artery calcification which can be quantified on chest CT for coronary atherosclerosis in non-cardiac CT is also important [8]. The coronary calcium, epicardial, and thoracic fat can be used as the biomarkers for the quantification and progression of coronary disease and various future cardiovascular events [9]. The lung nodule which can be metastatic is also being considered as a major cause of the death in lung cancer [10]. Low-dose CT screening reduces lung cancer mortality by more than 20% when compared with chest radiographs [11]. Lung nodule characterisation in the chest CT is an important indicator for the identification of the associated risk factors based on its morphology and characteristics.

26.2.3 Cardiovascular Risk Screening

Due to the advancements in the technologies, there is significant reduction in the possible risk of the cardiovascular diseases and for the management options [12]. One of the important quantification factors is the coronary artery calcification for the evaluation of the atherosclerosis along with the various cardiovascular risk factors in both symptomatic and asymptomatic patients [13–15]. Thus, CT is an important modality for the evaluation of cardiovascular disease risk factors and for the various management options. The various noncardiac indications of the CT for the detection of coronary artery calcification from the ECG-gated scans [16] along with scoring of the low-dose CT is impacting the quality of patient care [17, 18]. The American College of Radiology guidelines for CT screening are defined for the [19] nodule which will be solid, semi-solid, and mixed entity. The Fleischer Society for the incidental lung nodules can be seen on the chest CT, which will be re upgraded [20]. The different features and the morphology of lung nodules, which will be based on the calcification and the this morphology is very difficult for the analysis in very small nodules [21, 22].

The various automated and semi-automated segmentations are used for the precise location and the reproduction of the lung [1]] nodule [23]. Hein et al [24] the automated segmentation for the various volumetric lung nodule analysis, in comparison to the various measurements, between two readers at different CT dose levels. The quantitative analysis of Agatston score of 2579 is always greater than the 95th percentile for the Multi-Ethnic Study of Atherosclerosis [25]. The QIBA profiling of the "Small Lung Nodule Volume Assessment and Monitoring in Low Dose CT Screening" [26], the exact analysis of the volumes and changes for the solid nodules which will be 6 and 10 mm in diameter. The QIBA CT-Volumetry Technical Committee [26] for the better quantification there should be more than 95% CIs of nodule volumes.

QIBA profile for the nodules and masses is present for quantification [27]. With this protocol, the changes in the tumor volume will have 95% confidence and if the volume changes are greater than 39%, 29%, and 24%, then the size of the lesions is between 10 and 34 mm, 35 and 49 mm, and 50 and 100 mm, respectively. Thus, the different characteristics of the nodules will be based on the content like semisolid will have different from the very high solid nodules [28]. The radiomics-based quantitative analysis will be helpful for future prognostication of patients with lung cancer [29–32]. The availability of the dual-energy CT along with the various radiomic features can play an important role for the characterization of lung nodule. Lung perfusion is also another parameter of characterization for differentiating the benign and malignant lung nodules [33, 34]. The contrast enhancement pattern is also a useful parameter for the characterization and distribution of the contrast in the pulmonary nodules [35], by which the different phases of the scans can be avoided. The iodine quantification in the diagnosed lung cancers will be having a positive correlation ($r = 0.51$) along with the metabolic activity in primary lesion and in metastatic lymph nodes [36]. The available biomarkers along with the iodine attenuation can differentiate between the metastatic and nonmetastatic mediastinal lymph nodes in non-small cell lung cancer. The COPD is related with emphysema, chronic bronchitis, and small airway obstruction in various conditions [37]. The diagnosing and staging of the COPD is done by spirometry. The severity of emphysematous changes can be classified into "trace" if the percentage of low-attenuation areas is less than 0.5%, "mild" if low-attenuation areas is between 0.5 and 5%, and "moderate" if the low-attenuation areas is more than 5%.

Tracheomalacia is a condition where the weakness of the cartilaginous rings of the tracheal wall collapses during expiration which is again due to the increased laxity of the membranous portion in the airway collapse [38]. The common clinical symptoms in the tracheomalacia are the dyspnoea, cough, and haemoptysis [39]. Dynamic collapse evaluation can be done with the expiratory CT for the diagnosis of tracheomalacia.

Interstitial lung disease is one of the common presentations in the COPD. Thus, the various imaging biomarkers are being studied and evaluated [40]. Bronchial asthma patients will be showing the structural changes more in the large and small airways due to the various degrees of the airflow obstruction [41].

Pulmonary thromboembolism iodine mapping in the dual-energy CT is evolving newer biomarker of pulmonary perfusion. Dual-energy CT perfusion and along with the pulmonary blood flow [42] different stages of the acute and chronic pulmonary embolism can be diagnosed and evaluated based on the various dual-energy CT biomarkers, for perfusion of the lung. Blood flow images with CT angiography fusion will be showing the significant increased sensitivity and specificity of 100 and 98%, for pulmonary embolism evaluation [43]. Dual-energy CT biomarkers for lung perfusion and the various clinical biomarkers can show high risk in patients for evaluation and post-thrombolysis also. CT biomarkers of the dual energy can have pulmonary hypertension correlation with the various pulmonary arterial pressures [44, 45]. Monitoring response to treatment can also be done for the chronic thromboembolic phenomenon with the pulmonary hypertension and after balloon angioplasty [46]. QIBA is also important for the evaluation of translating research for various clinical indications.

The QI concept is defined as a characteristic which is measured and evaluated in the various normal physiological process, pathological process, and also the therapeutic response to the various conditions by using the various biomarkers [7]. Biomarker is usually derived from the medical image and can be correlated anatomically and physiologically for various diseases, for the evaluation of the severity of the disease, and also for the molecular level quantification for the prediction of the course of the disease. The QIBA's definition also states that the tumor volume evaluation or standardized uptake values (SUVs) in the PET are also the QI biomarkers. These different criteria for the QI research for the various biomarkers are based on the various medians, means, standard deviations, and standard errors of the mean [47]. By using them, more diagnostic accuracy, different variables, and subjectivity will be there for image analysis; and the imaging findings will be more perfect along with the various biological and clinical applications and for the various phenotypic genomic profiles based on the various imaging patterns [48]. QI is also based on the evidence-based medicine on the quantitative data [49, 50]. The cancer trials are also based on the various quantitative measurements of tumor response; for example, the Response Evaluation Criteria in Solid Tumours (RECIST) [51] is being used in the various oncological settings [52, 53].

The Institute of Medicine (IOM) biomarker evaluation is divided into three parts: analytical validation, qualification, and utilization [54].

26.3 Analytical Validation

The analytical validation will be based on the exact accuracy, for more precision, and also on the feasibility of various biomarker measurements. The different validation studies are based on the standards for QI biomarkers reporting parameters [55]. The QI biomarker is an important indicator for the biological and pathologic process and also response to therapy evaluations [1, 56–60].

These biomarkers can be used in the various clinical and research applications, having the various regulations for the evaluation of the drugs and devices [55]. By using the various biomarker performances, the correlation of the various biomarker disease quantification along with the clinical outcome can be done. Different designs can be used for the evaluation of the patients for the various biomarker status. With the various prospective, randomized studies, and also retrospective analyses, this will give the more important aspect of biomarker qualification [61].

26.4 Utilization

Utilization is also used for the assessment of biomarker performance for the specific pathology. This shows the various aspects of the validation and qualification for the proper use of the biomarkers [54]. The different QI aspects can also be related to the various equipment upgrades, phantoms, software, image processing and interpretation, altered workflow, and ongoing quality assurance which are also based on the various recommendations by expert panels [62]. QIBA in May 2014 has reviewed different DCE-MRI, CT tumor volume, and FDG-PET/CT imaging biomarker profiles for measuring response to cancer therapy [63]. QI biomarker research can also be related for the evaluation of the various aspects of the basic imaging science and also the clinical research having the novel techniques which can be used in our daily routine practise.

Quantitative imaging biomarkers used are very sensitive, specific, accurate, and reproducible imaging which can be used for the various disease diagnosis, treatment planning, and medical product development. Digital image processing and analysis is playing an important role for identification, characterization, validation, and application of various quantitative imaging biomarkers. Semi-automated or automated segmentation and registration aspects are more efficient for the various quantitative imaging biomarkers. Here the [64] concepts of the various quantitative imaging biomarkers are studied [65]; various validations of various quantitative imaging biomarkers [66]; to see the advanced image processing and analysis for quantitative imaging biomarker characterization, in Osteoarthritis (OA), Alzheimer's disease (AD) and various cancers [67]; various challenges used in the quantitative imaging biomarker research and [68] for the image processing and analysis along with the development of quantitative imaging biomarkers. Thus, the biological biomarker will be able to differentiate the normal physiological and various pathologic processes and also for the therapeutic response evaluation [7]. The other end is having "a characteristic which will be reflecting on the patient related aspects" [7]. These end points are also seen in the various morbidity aspects of the various diseases like cancer.

The automated segmentation of the articular cartilage sometimes is used as the potential quantitative imaging biomarkers of OA [69–71].

Alzheimer's disease (AD) is a cortical, neurodegenerative dementia [72]. This condition will be accounting 70% of all cases of dementia in the elderly and about 30% of the adults affecting around five million people in the USA [72].

26.5 Cancer

Different criteria of the structural or functional image processing and analysis can be done for the various types of solid malignant neoplasms. Many processing and analysis of the images can be done for the different types of solid tumours. As per the FDA data, the commonest application of this is in cancer for various clinical and diagnostic applications [73]. Newer biomarkers are having the intratumoral arterial enhancement, and these are also used for tracking treatment response [74, 75]. Biomarker discovery, their characterization, validation for various applications, and application in various clinical situations are challenging. The validation criteria of a quantitative imaging biomarker ("Validation of Quantitative Imaging Biomarkers") are very precise. Here the biomarker for the preclinical or clinical evaluation should be consistent and accurate (Figs. 26.1 and 26.2).

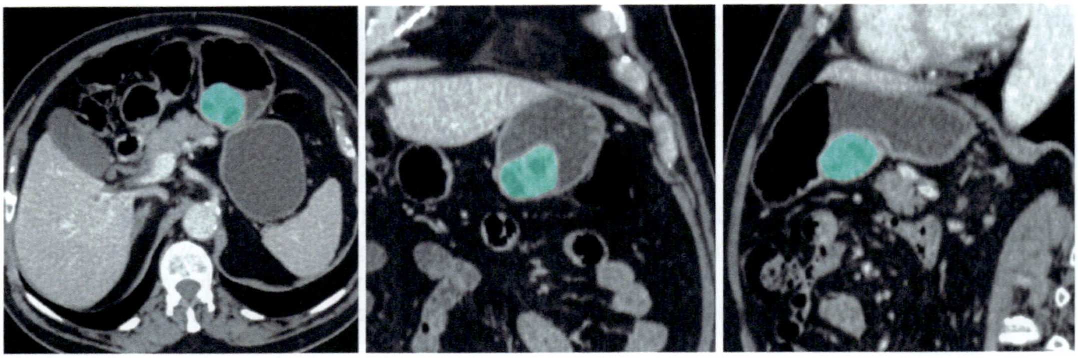

Fig. 26.1 The quantification of the gall bladder lesion which turned out to be malignant

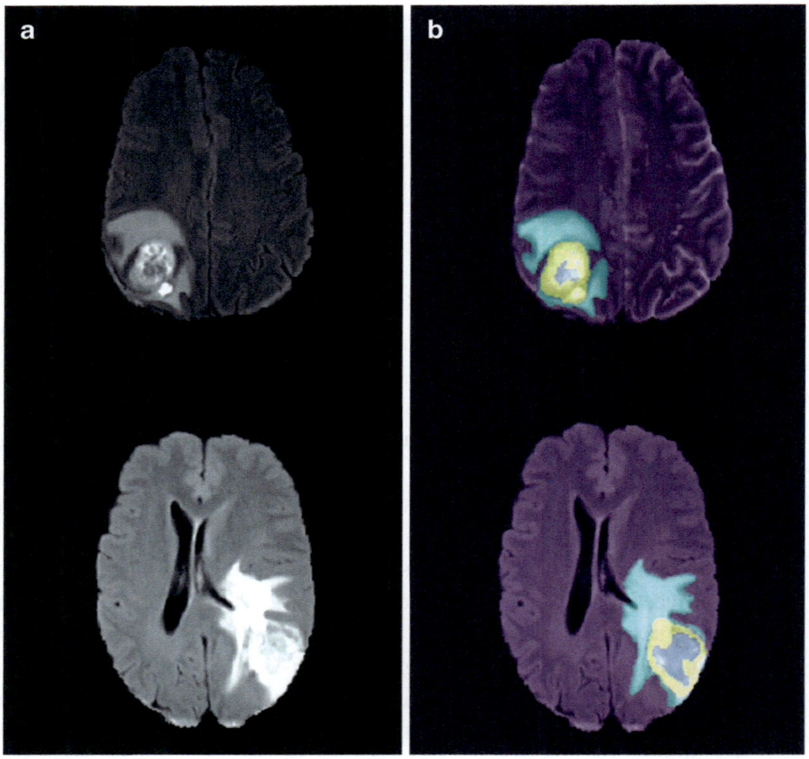

Fig. 26.2 Two different lesions with two different quantification parameters **a** and **b** which show the difference in the earlier and better evaluation

26.6 Quantification Parameters

The reporting parameters are also in relation for quantifying the atrophy for the brain volume loss, for example, 24% which will depend on the age of the patient and commonly seen in the middle temporal lobe. Tumour characteristics is also based on the various aspects of tumour characteristics: malignant, metastatic, and response to treatment. Quantification can be done on the various different algorithms, for example, the bone abnormalities in the MR do not correlate with the amount of the trabecular bone loss and the amount of osteoporosis and risk of fracture. Thus, imaging biomarkers are crucial in the evaluation of various algorithms which are based on the use of the modality and pathology to be evaluated. These imaging biomarkers have variable quanti-

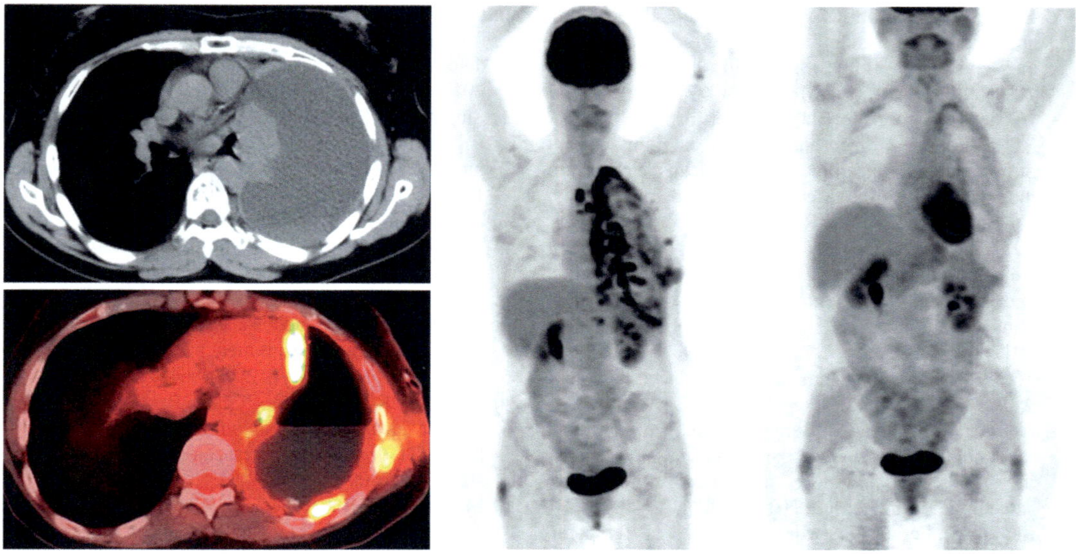

Fig. 26.3 Whole body PET-CT with carcinoma lung involving the mediastinal pleura and infiltrating into the both costal and mediastinal pleura on the left side

tative parameters based on the different parameters, which are needed for the spatial distribution of the biomarker. The common imaging modalities are radiography, ultrasound, CT, MRI, Single Photon Emission Computed Tomography (SPECT), or Positron Emission Tomography (PET). Image quality can be evaluated based on the signal-to-noise ratio (SNR) and contrast-to-noise ratio (CNR). Functional and dynamic studies will need very good spatial and temporal resolution. SNR and CNR can have different phantoms based on different frequency tuning, different spatial resolution, and degree of changes for different variables in the region of the interest (Fig. 26.3).

26.7 Conclusion

Imaging biomarkers is defining the various objectives which can be extracted from medical images which are related to the various normal biological processes, diseases, or the response to treatment. Developing the imaging biomarker needs to have the different steps for the validation and needs to be checked for the clinical and technical validity. This will involve various concepts and mechanisms along with obtaining standardized and optimized anatomic, functional, and molecular images, analysing various data sets with computer models, displaying data appropriately, obtaining the appropriate statistic measures, and conducting tests on the principle, efficacy, and effectiveness.

References

1. Sullivan DC, Obuchowski NA, Kessler LG, et al. Metrology standards for quantitative imaging biomarkers. Radiology. 2015;277(3):813–25.
2. Quantitative Imaging Biomarkers Alliance. Radiological Society of North America website. https://www.rsna.org/QIBA/. Published 2018. Accessed 6 Apr 2019.
3. Mokdad AH, Ballestros K, Echko M, et al. US Burden of Disease Collaborators. The state of US health, 1990-2016: burden of diseases, injuries, and risk factors among US states. JAMA. 2018;319(14): 1444–72.
4. Cox GG, Templeton AW, Dwyer SJ 3rd. Digital image management: networking, display, and archiving. Radiol Clin North Am. 1986;24(1):37–54.
5. Sullivan DC. Imaging as a quantitative science. Radiology. 2008;248(2):328–32.
6. Erickson BJ, Korfiatis P, Akkus Z, Kline TL. Machine learning for medical imaging. Radiographics. 2017;37(2):505–15.

7. Biomarkers Definitions Working Group. Biomarkers and surrogate endpoints: preferred definitions and conceptual framework. Clin Pharmacol Ther. 2001;69(3):89–95. [PubMed: 11240971]
8. Hecht HS, Cronin P, Blaha MJ, et al. 2016 SCCT/STR guidelines for coronary artery calcium scoring of noncontrast noncardiac chest CT scans: a report of the Society of Cardiovascular Computed Tomography and Society of Thoracic Radiology. J Thorac Imaging. 2017;32(5):W54–66.
9. Dey D, Nakazato R, Li D, Berman DS. Epicardial and thoracic fat: noninvasive measurement and clinical implications. Cardiovasc Diagn Ther. 2012;2(2):85–93.
10. Torre LA, Siegel RL, Jemal A. Lung cancer statistics. Adv Exp Med Biol. 2016;893:1–19.
11. Aberle DR, Adams AM, Berg CD, et al. National Lung Screening Trial Research Team. Reduced lung-cancer mortality with low-dose computed tomographic screening. N Engl J Med. 2011;365(5):395–409.
12. Moran AE, Forouzanfar MH, Roth GA, et al. Temporal trends in ischemic heart disease mortality in 21 world regions, 1980 to 2010: the Global Burden of Disease 2010 study. Circulation. 2014;129(14):1483–92.
13. Budoff MJ, Achenbach S, Blumenthal RS, et al. Assessment of coronary artery disease by cardiac computed tomography: a scientific statement from the American Heart Association Committee on Cardiovascular Imaging and Intervention, Council on Cardiovascular Radiology and Intervention, and Committee on Cardiac Imaging, Council on Clinical Cardiology. Circulation. 2006;114(16):1761–91.
14. Hou ZH, Lu B, Gao Y, et al. Prognostic value of coronary CT angiography and calcium score for major adverse cardiac events in outpatients. JACC Cardiovasc Imaging. 2012;5(10):990–9.
15. Budoff MJ, Mayrhofer T, Ferencik M, et al. Prognostic value of coronary artery calcium in the PROMISE study (prospective multicenter imaging study for evaluation of chest pain). Circulation. 2017;136(21):1993–2005.
16. Hughes-Austin JM, Dominguez A 3rd, Allison MA, et al. Relationship of coronary calcium on standard chest CT scans with mortality. JACC Cardiovasc Imaging. 2016;9(2):152–9.
17. Yip R, Henschke CI, Yankelevitz DF, Smith JP. CT screening for lung cancer: alternative definitions of positive test result based on the National Lung Screening Trial and International Early Lung Cancer Action Program databases. Radiology. 2014;273(2):591–6.
18. Pinsky PF, Gierada DS, Black W, et al. Performance of LungRADS in the National Lung Screening Trial: a retrospective assessment. Ann Intern Med. 2015;162(7):485–91.
19. American College of Radiology. Lung CT Screening Reporting & Data System. https://www.acr.org/Clinical-Resources/Reporting-and-Data-Systems/Lung-Rads. Published 2018. Accessed 6 Apr 2019.
20. MacMahon H, Naidich DP, Goo JM, et al. Guidelines for management of incidental pulmonary nodules detected on CT images: from the Fleischner Society 2017. Radiology. 2017;284(1):228–43.
21. Siegelman SS, Khouri NF, Leo FP, Fishman EK, Braverman RM, Zerhouni EA. Solitary pulmonary nodules: CT assessment. Radiology. 1986;160(2):307–12.
22. Zwirewich CV, Vedal S, Miller RR, Müller NL. Solitary pulmonary nodule: high-resolution CT and radiologic-pathologic correlation. Radiology. 1991;179(2):469–76.
23. Ko JP, Rusinek H, Jacobs EL, et al. Small pulmonary nodules: volume measurement at chest CT—phantom study. Radiology. 2003;228(3):864–70.
24. Hein PA, Romano VC, Rogalla P, et al. Linear and volume measurements of pulmonary nodules at different CT dose levels: intrascan and interscan analysis. Rofo. 2009;181(1):24–31.
25. McClelland RL, Jorgensen NW, Budoff M, et al. 10-Year coronary heart disease risk prediction using coronary artery calcium and traditional risk factors: derivation in the MESA (Multi-Ethnic Study of Atherosclerosis) with validation in the HNR (Heinz Nixdorf Recall) Study and the DHS (Dallas Heart Study). J Am Coll Cardiol. 2015;66(15):1643–53.
26. QIBA CT Volumetry Technical Committee. QIBA profile: small lung nodule volume assessment and monitoring in low dose CT screening—publicly reviewed draft. Radiological Society of North America website. http://qibawiki.rsna.org/index.php/Profiles. Updated 15 June 2018. Accessed 6 Apr 2019.
27. QIBA CT Volumetry Technical Committee. QIBA profile: CT tumor volume change for advanced disease (CTV-AD)—technically confirmed profile. Radiological Society of North America website. http://qibawiki.rsna.org/index.php/Profiles. Updated 22 June 2018. Accessed 6 Apr 2019.
28. Tirkes T, Hollar MA, Tann M, Kohli MD, Akisik F, Sandrasegaran K. Response criteria in oncologic imaging: review of traditional and new criteria. RadioGraphics. 2013;33(5):1323–41.
29. Grove O, Berglund AE, Schabath MB, et al. Quantitative computed tomographic descriptors associate tumor shape complexity and intratumor heterogeneity with prognosis in lung adenocarcinoma. PLoS One. 2015;10(3):e0118261. https://journals.plos.org/plosone/article?id=10.1371/journal.pone.0118261. Published 4 Mar 2015.
30. Huang Y, Liu Z, He L, et al. Radiomics signature: a potential biomarker for the prediction of disease-free survival in early-stage (I or II) non-small cell lung cancer. Radiology. 2016;281(3):947–57.
31. Li B, Cui Y, Diehn M, Li R. Development and validation of an individualized immune prognostic signature in early stage non squamous non–small cell lung cancer. JAMA Oncol. 2017;3(11):1529–37.
32. Coroller TP, Agrawal V, Huynh E, et al. Radiomic based pathological response prediction from primary

tumours and lymph nodes in NSCLC. J Thorac Oncol. 2017;12(3):467–76.
33. Ohno Y, Koyama H, Matsumoto K, et al. Differentiation of malignant and benign pulmonary nodules with quantitative first-pass 320–detector row perfusion CT versus FDG PET/ CT. Radiology. 2011;258(2):599–609.
34. Yuan X, Zhang J, Quan C, et al. Differentiation of malignant and benign pulmonary nodules with first-pass dual-input perfusion CT. Eur Radiol. 2013;23(9):2469–74.
35. Thieme SF, Johnson TR, Lee C, et al. Dual-energy CT for the assessment of contrast material distribution in the pulmonary parenchyma. AJR Am J Roentgenol. 2009;193(1):144–9.
36. Schmid-Bindert G, Henzler T, Chu TQ, et al. Functional imaging of lung cancer using dual energy CT: how does iodine related attenuation correlate with standardized uptake value of 18FDG-PET-CT? Eur Radiol. 2012;22(1):93–103.
37. Petty TL, Weinmann GG. Building a national strategy for the prevention and management of and research in chronic obstructive pulmonary disease. National Heart, Lung, and Blood Institute Workshop summary. JAMA. 1997;277(3):246–53.
38. Murgu SD, Colt HG. Tracheobronchomalacia and excessive dynamic airway collapse. Respirology. 2006;11(4):388–406.
39. Carden KA, Boiselle PM, Waltz DA, Ernst A. Tracheomalacia and Tracheobronchomalacia in children and adults: an in-depth review. Chest. 2005;127(3):984–1005.
40. Ohkubo H, Nakagawa H, Niimi A. Computer-based quantitative computed tomography image analysis in idiopathic pulmonary fibrosis: a mini review. Respir Investig. 2018;56(1):5–13. 976, July-August 2019. https://radiographics.rsna.org
41. Gono H, Fujimoto K, Kawakami S, Kubo K. Evaluation of airway wall thickness and air trapping by HRCT in asymptomatic asthma. Eur Respir J. 2003;22(6):965–71.
42. Fuld MK, Halaweish AF, Haynes SE, Divekar AA, Guo J, Hoffman EA. Pulmonary perfused blood volume with dual-energy CT as surrogate for pulmonary perfusion assessed with dynamic multidetector CT. Radiology. 2013;267(3):747–56.
43. Zhang LJ, Chai X, Wu SY, et al. Detection of pulmonary embolism by dual energy CT: correlation with perfusion scintigraphy and histopathological findings in rabbits. Eur Radiol. 2009;19(12):2844–54.
44. Meinel FG, Graef A, Thierfelder KM, et al. Automated quantification of pulmonary perfused blood volume by dual-energy CTPA in chronic thromboembolic pulmonary hypertension. Rofo. 2014;186(2):151–6.
45. Takagi H, Ota H, Sugimura K, et al. Dual-energy CT to estimate clinical severity of chronic thromboembolic pulmonary hypertension: comparison with invasive right heart catheterization. Eur J Radiol. 2016;85(9):1574–80.
46. Koike H, Sueyoshi E, Sakamoto I, Uetani M, Nakata T, Maemura K. Quantification of lung perfusion blood volume (lung PBV) by dual-energy CT in patients with chronic thromboembolic pulmonary hypertension (CTEPH) before and after balloon pulmonary angioplasty (BPA): preliminary results. Eur J Radiol. 2016;85(9):1607–12.
47. Kessler LG, Barnhart HX, Buckler AJ, et al. The emerging science of quantitative imaging biomarkers terminology and definitions for scientific studies and regulatory submissions. Stat Methods Med Res. 2015;24(1):9–26.
48. Sullivan DC. Imaging as a quantitative science. Radiology. 2008;248(2):328–32 [PubMed: 18641239] Abramson et al. Page 9 Acad Radiol. Author manuscript; available in PMC 1 Jan 2016. NIH-PA Author Manuscript.
49. Boone JM. Radiological interpretation 2020: toward quantitative image assessment. Med Phys. 2007;34(11):4173–9. [PubMed: 18072481]
50. Choong MK, Tsafnat G. The implications of biomarker evidence for systematic reviews. BMC Med Res Methodol. 2012;12:176. [PubMed: 23173809]
51. Eisenhauer EA, Therasse P, Bogaerts J, et al. New response evaluation criteria in solid tumours: revised RECIST guideline (version 1.1). Eur J Cancer. 2009;45(2):228–47. [PubMed: 19097774]
52. Vidaurre T, Wilkerson J, Simon R, Bates SE, Fojo T. Stable disease is not preferentially observed with targeted therapies and as currently defined has limited value in drug development. Cancer J. 2009;15(5):366–73. [PubMed: 19826355]
53. Buyse M, Thirion P, Carlson RW, Burzykowski T, Molenberghs G, Piedbois P. Relation between tumour response to first-line chemotherapy and survival in advanced colorectal cancer: a meta-analysis. Meta-Analysis Group in Cancer. Lancet. 2000;356(9227):373–8. [PubMed: 10972369]
54. Institute of Medicine. Evaluation of biomarkers and surrogate endpoints in chronic disease. Washington, DC: National Academies Press; 2010.
55. Katz R. Biomarkers and surrogate markers: an FDA perspective. NeuroRx. 2004;1(2):189–95. [PubMed: 15717019]
56. Wintermark M, Albers GW, Alexandrov AV, et al. Acute stroke imaging research roadmap. AJNR Am J Neuroradiol. 2008;29(5):e23–30. [PubMed: 18477656]
57. Bruns A, Kunnecke B, Risterucci C, Moreau JL, von Kienlin M. Validation of cerebral blood perfusion imaging as a modality for quantitative pharmacological MRI in rats. Magn Reson Med. 2009;61(6):1451–8.
58. Yoo AJ, Sheth KN, Kimberly WT, et al. Validating imaging biomarkers of cerebral edema in patients with severe ischemic stroke. J Stroke Cerebrovasc Dis. 2013;22(6):742–9.
59. Wintermark M, Albers GW, Broderick JP, et al. Acute stroke imaging research roadmap II. Stroke. 2013;44(9):2628–39.

60. Huynh TJ, Flaherty ML, Gladstone DJ, et al. Multicentre accuracy and interobserver agreement of spot sign identification in acute intracerebral haemorrhage. Stroke. 2014;45(1):107–12.
61. Green E, Yothers G, Sargent DJ. Surrogate endpoint validation: statistical elegance versus clinical relevance. Stat Methods Med Res. 2008;17(5):477–86. [PubMed: 18285438]
62. Institute of Medicine. Developing biomarker-based tools for cancer screening, diagnosis and treatment: workshop summary. Washington, DC: National Academies Press; 2007.
63. Radiological Society of North America. QIBA protocols and profiles. Available at: https://www.rsna.org/QIBA_Protocols_and_Profiles.aspx. Accessed 20 May 2014.
64. US Food and Drug Administration: Innovation or stagnation: challenge and opportunity on the critical path to new medical products. 2004.
65. Administration USFaD: FDA New Molecular Entities. 2011.
66. US Food and Drug Administration: Innovation or stagnation: critical path opportunities report. 2006.
67. Obuchowski NA, Reeves AP, Huang EP, et al. Quantitative imaging biomarkers: a review of statistical methods for computer algorithm comparisons. Stat Methods Med Res. 2015;24(1):68–106.
68. US Food and Drug Administration: The Sentinel Initiative: national strategy for monitoring medical product safety. 2008.
69. Fripp J, Crozier S, Warfield SK, Ourselin S. Automatic segmentation and quantitative analysis of the articular cartilages from magnetic resonance images of the knee. IEEE Trans Med Imaging. 2010;29:55–64.
70. Dodin P, Pelletier J, Martel-Pelletier J, Abram F. Automatic human knee cartilage segmentation from 3-D magnetic resonance images. IEEE Trans Biomed Eng. 2010;57:2699–711.
71. Yin Y, Zhang X, Williams R, Wu X, Anderson DD, Sonka M. LOGISMOS—layered optimal graph image segmentation of multiple objects and surfaces: cartilage segmentation in the knee joint. IEEE Trans Med Imaging. 2010;29:2023–37.
72. Andreoli TE, Carpenter CCJ, Griggs RC, Benjamin IJ. Andreoli and Carpenter's Cecil essentials of medicine. Philadelphia: Saunders Elsevier; 2007.
73. Hampel H, et al. Biomarkers for Alzheimer's disease: academic, industry and regulatory perspectives. Nat Rev Drug Discov. 2010;9:560–74.
74. Sullivan DC, Gatsonis C. Response to treatment series: part 1 and introduction, measuring tumor response—challenges in the era of molecular medicine. Am J Roentgenol. 2011;197:15–7.
75. Yaghmai V, Miller FH, Rezai P, Benson AB III, Salem R. Response to treatment series: part 2, tumor response assessment— using new and conventional criteria. Am J Roentgenol. 2011;197:18–27.

GPSR Compliance

The European Union's (EU) General Product Safety Regulation (GPSR) is a set of rules that requires consumer products to be safe and our obligations to ensure this.

If you have any concerns about our products, you can contact us on ProductSafety@springernature.com

In case Publisher is established outside the EU, the EU authorized representative is:

Springer Nature Customer Service Center GmbH
Europaplatz 3
69115 Heidelberg, Germany

Batch number: 10732809

Printed by Printforce, the Netherlands